Manual of
Surgical
Pathology

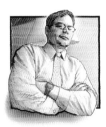

Illustrator:
Christopher A French MD

Assistant Professor of Pathology
Harvard Medical School
Brigham and Women's Hospital
Boston, Massachusetts
USA

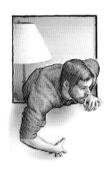

Illustrator:
Glenn Curtis BA

Boston, Massachusetts
USA

Manual of
Surgical
Pathology

Second Edition

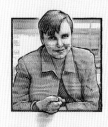

Susan C Lester MD PhD

Assistant Professor of Pathology
Harvard Medical School
Director, Breast Pathology Services
Brigham and Women's Hospital
Boston, Massachusetts
USA

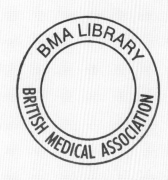
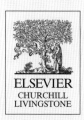
ELSEVIER
CHURCHILL
LIVINGSTONE

ELSEVIER
CHURCHILL
LIVINGSTONE

An imprint of Elsevier Inc

First edition 2000
Second edition 2006

ISBN 0 4430 6645 0

British Library Cataloguing in Publication Data
A catalogue record for this book is available from the British Library

Library of Congress Cataloging in Publication Data
A catalog record for this book is available from the Library of Congress

Notice
Medical knowledge is constantly changing. Standard safety precautions must be followed, but as new research and clinical experience broaden our knowledge, changes in treatment and drug therapy may become necessary or appropriate. Readers are advised to check the most current product information provided by the manufacturer of each drug to be administered to verify the recommended dose, the method and duration of administration, and contraindications. It is the responsibility of the practitioner, relying on experience and knowledge of the patient, to determine dosages and the best treatment for each individual patient. Neither the Publisher nor the author assume any liability for any injury and/or damage to persons or property arising from this publication.

The Publisher

Printed in China
Last digit is the print number : 9 8 7 6 5 4 3 2 1

For Elsevier:
Commissioning Editor: Michael J Houston
Project Development Manager: Cecilia Murphy, Louise Cook
Project Manager: Cheryl Brant
Designer: Sarah Russell
Illustrations Manager: Mick Ruddy
Illustrators: Christopher French, Glenn Curtis
Marketing Managers: Gaynor Jones (UK), Ethel Cathers (US)

Contents

Foreword

Almost 40 years ago, a young pathology resident friend at one of the main Harvard teaching hospitals asked in the greatest degree of respect and admiration how any mere mortal could attain such comprehensive knowledge of all areas of surgical pathology as his senior professor. The question was asked in particular reference to renal pathology, which was at that time beginning its development into the major subspecialty it has become today. The reply was suprisingly straightforward, since glomerular disease in his estimation was really only three entities, better known then as acute glomerulonephritis, subacute glomerulonephritis and chronic glomerulonephritis. Yes, life was simpler then. Through the 1970s, many of the tools that we take for granted today, such as immunohistochemistry, did not exist. Thus, many of us have watched during our careers the birth of the subspecialty called surgical pathology, and its further refinement into areas where some experts specialize in but a single disease or organ. The superb textbook entitled "Systemic Pathology" by Wright and Symmers best reflects the growth of our specialty. Edition one published in 1966 compressed all of surgical pathology into two volumes. Edition two, published in 1978, required six volumes. The third and final edition, printed largely during the 1990s, exploded to over 30 volumes.

Simultaneously with this ever expanding wealth of knowledge, techniques and expectations in pathology, we have all experienced similar changes in what medical students are now expected to know. Medical education currently stresses the clinical years, so that students now have greatly expanded experiences in clinical medicine, and not surprisingly, far more emphasis on sociological and humanistic facets, never forgetting the ever looming medical jurisprudence. As a consequence, the time allocated to the basic sciences, including pathology, has dwindled from an intensive full-year program to a partial year in some institutions, and in some to isolated lectures within core blocks devoted to some broad aspect of medicine.

With this in mind, the ability for any single person to master the entire field of surgical pathology is a tutorial in impracticability. It is daunting at best for the experienced pathologist and absolutely unattainable for the neophyte. To help fill this void, virtually every department of pathology in the United States has developed some form of a laboratory manual for its incoming students. The goal has been straightforward. The manual is to provide a framework for helping the student achieve a foothold to begin his experience in pathology. Several of these manuals have developed into full-fledged books. One of the earliest (1983) and most successful was Dr. Waldemar Schmidt's "Principles and Techniques of Surgical Pathology". Multiple copies dotted the surgical pathology bench and was the benchmark of the smart laboratory. It is certainly worthwhile to compare that book with today's endeavors. Many of the techniques about how to examine a specimen are similar and were well developed at that time. But as the field has become more complicated, additional books have appeared. Beginning in 1991, Dr. Susan Lester, at the instigation of and collaboration with Dr. Joseph "Mac" Corson and Dr. Geraldine Pinkus, began issuing yearly an ever expanding in-house laboratory manual at the Brigham and Women's Hospital in Boston, which in its initial publication by Churchill Livingstone (now Elsevier) was 327 pages long. The manual was enormously impressive. Part of my review in 2001 for the International Journal of Gynecologic Pathology is excerpted below:

> "Part I of the book, nearly 100 pages long, consists of nine chapters that examine various aspects of cutup. It begins with the clinician's request for consultation, general rules for processing from gross specimen to tissue cassettes, photography and synoptic reporting. There are a great many tables and discussions I found valuable. A particularly useful table on antibodies for histochemistry lists virtually all of the commonly used and some of the newer and more important immunocytochemical tests. Multiple columns detail each antigen being identified, its location with the cell,

the types of normal cells and tissues that are identified, the particular tumors commonly identified, the general uses for the marker, and finally comments. This is the only place where I have seen such a table in print. A complementary table lists histochemical stains, the components of tissues stained and possible uses, as well as comments about the stain. Multiple tables list differential diagnoses. Examples include mesothelioma vs adenocarcinoma; differential diagnosis of spindle cell lesions; tumors with characteristic findings by electron microscopy; solid neoplasms with diagnostically useful cytogenetic changes and the histologic appearances of infectious agents in surgical tissues. This book, especially with its quite inexpensive price, is a must for every surgical lab. And beyond that, simply, it is an excellent reference book chuck full of information that is otherwise hard to find, but which every pathologist often wishes he had at his fingertips at certain critical moments."

The second edition of Dr. Lester's book is 627 pages long and virtually rewritten from beginning to end. This virtuoso is a truly major contribution to the field of Surgical Pathology and chock full of helpful information for every person involved in pathology, be it the novice resident or pathology assistant, the experienced resident or the highly accomplished practitioner. The table on immunocytochemistry, done so well in the first edition, is now double in size, or 38 pages long. I suspect that these pages will soon be conveniently available at the surgical path bench or at the digital fingertips of most pathologists worldwide. The new edition also greatly expands upon common differential diagnoses, and the use of immunocytochemistry to help resolve the differences. The areas covered in the earlier edition are all expanded and include proper identification, sectioning, processing, pathologic assessment of tissue specimens, and what is optimal and sub optimal handling. Sections relevant to the daily practice of pathology include issues of health and safety in pathology, regulatory policy and medical legal and ethical matters, which respond to the rapidly growing literature together and the invigorated regulatory climate hoping to reduce medical errors. These sections complement the growing widespread adoption of synoptic reporting by pathologists as well as use of the College of American Pathologists (CAP) checklists for standardized reporting of cancer findings. Since January 2004, the American College of Surgeons has required for certification of cancer registries that all surgical pathology reports of cancer include the CAP's prescribed cancer data elements. Lester and her co-authors masterfully show how pathology specimens can be examined to reliably capture these critical items.

This book will be an invaluable aid to every person involved in surgical pathology. Bravo to Dr. Lester and her colleagues.

Stanley J. Robboy, MD
Professor of Pathology
Professor of Obstetrics & Gynecology
Vice Chairman for Diagnostic Services
Department of Pathology
Duke University Medical Center
Durham, North Carolina

Preface to
the first edition

I was first asked to edit the procedure manual for the Brigham and Women's Hospital Pathology Department in 1991. Over the years, the manual has been a collaborative effort, involving staff pathologists, residents, clinicians, pathology assistants, secretaries, and histotechnologists. This is the manual's greatest strength. It reflects the combined knowledge, experience, and opinions of a multitude of people who produce and use pathologic information. It has been refined by almost a decade of use by staff, residents, and pathology assistants on the front lines of pathology.

This manual has grown over the years from instructors for the gross examination of specimens to a comprehensive guide for the making of a pathologic diagnosis – from the submission of pathology specimens to the preparation of the final surgical pathology report. Tables describing histochemical stains, immunoperoxidase studies, and electron microscopy findings can facilitate the interpretation of special studies. Checklists for diagnostic and prognostic information to be included for major tumor resections are provided, as well as information for standard tumor classification and staging. It is hoped that simplifying the access to this information, currently only available from numerous diverse sources, will enhance the provision of important pathologic information in pathology reports. Complementary recommendations have been published by the Association of Directors of Anatomic and Surgical Pathology, the College of American Pathologists, and individual institutions, and information from theses sources has been incorporated when appropriate.

The *Manual of Surgical Pathology* is not intended to be, and should not be misconstrued to be, a "standard of care". The "correct" method to process or report a specimen can vary, depending on the specifics of a case, institutional policies, and the personal preferences of clinicians and pathologists, and will change over time. In addition, since unlimited budgets for specimen processing is an unobtainable goal, the cost of examining a specimen must be balanced against the clinical significance of the information obtained.

From the surgical cutting room to the senior sign out area, we keep this manual close at hand as a helpful reference. It is our sincere hope that others will find it equally as useful in their practice.

Susan C. Lester MD PhD

Preface to the second edition

A major advantage of pathology as a medical specialty is that the *biology* of disease remains constant for the most part, resulting in a large body of knowledge that will never change. On the other hand, our *understanding* of disease is expanding rapidly. Pathologists are being asked to use new information to re-classify disease, provide better prognostic information, and to predict response to therapy. The growing amount of relevant data and the expanding role of pathologists has created the need for an updated version of this manual. In particular, every table in the manual has been revised and updated and many new tables added.

New antibodies with value for clinical diagnosis are introduced almost monthly. Since the last edition, the number of antibodies used for diagnostic purposes has almost doubled and is now approaching 200. To facilitate the use of these markers, all of the immunohistochemistry tables have been updated with many new tables for differential diagnosis added.

Pathologists are also playing a larger role in determining tumor response to therapy. HER2/neu and breast cancer, CD117 (c-kit) and GIST, along with EGFR and colon carcinoma, herald a new era of targeted therapy. Information is provided about when these tests are appropriate, and the reporting of results.

Cytogenetic studies are increasingly important in tumor classification and prognosis. The recent discovery of a group of lung adenocarcinomas that are particularly susceptible to treatment due to specific mutations in EFGR is only one example. Expanded tables that list cytogenetic changes in solid tumors and hematological malignances provide many more examples of how this information is being used for diagnosis, prognosis, and treatment. Pathologists can also play an important role in suggesting which patients may carry germline mutations that cause susceptibility to cancer. New tables provide the tumors and clinical settings in which a germline mutation is highly probable, and syndromes associated with pathologic findings.

The gross examination of specimens and histologic features of carcinomas continue to be the most important factors for predicting a patient's course. This information has been critically evaluated and the College of American Pathologists has issued new guidelines for the reporting of tumors. Information now considered to be required has been highlighted in the "Pathologic Prognostic and Diagnostic Features Sign-out Checklists". In addition, specific criteria have been provided for the grading or assessment of other relevant pathologic features.

Concern about disease as a weapon of mass destruction is, unfortunately, also a new development since publication of the first edition. Pathologists may have the opportunity to be the first to recognize an agent of bioterrorism, but these are not typically encountered in ordinary practice and may present a diagnostic challenge. A new table gives information on the most likely agents, their pathologic features, and contact information for the CDC if such an agent is suspected.

The illustrations by Dr. Christopher French and Mr. Glenn Curtis are another very important addition to the second edition. Although some of the figures from the first edition have been maintained, all new illustrations are theirs. As an experienced pathologist and an accomplished artist, Dr. French has been able to capture the essential morphological differences among tumors that allow for gross diagnosis. Excellent examples include his illustrations of adrenal, kidney, liver, and pancreatic tumors.

Finally, the manual has been refined through another four years of exacting criticism by the residents of BWH. Their constant vigilance keeps me on my toes and the manual on the path to perfection.

Susan C. Lester MD PhD

List of Consultants

Jon Christopher Aster MD PhD
Associate Professor of Pathology, Harvard Medical School; Associate Pathologist, Brigham and Women's Hospital, Boston, Massachusetts
Lymph Nodes, Spleen, and Bone Marrow; Special Studies

Thomas Brenn MD PhD
Instructor in Pathology, Harvard Medical School; Associate Pathologist, Brigham and Women's Hospital, Boston, Massachusetts
Dermatopathology Specimens

Gilbert Brodsky MD
Assistant Professor of Pathology, Harvard Medical School; Associate Director, Surgical Pathology, Department of Pathology and Laboratory Medicine, Harvard Vanguard Medical Associates; Consultant Pathologist, Brigham and Women's Hospital, Boston, Massachusetts
Specimen Processing; Genitourinary Specimens; Head and Neck Specimens

Edmund S. Cibas MD
Associate Professor of Pathology, Harvard Medical School; Director, Cytology Division, Brigham and Women's Hospital, Boston, Massachusetts
Cytology Specimens

Joseph M. Corson MD
Professor of Pathology, Harvard Medical School; Director, Senior Pathologist, Brigham and Women's Hospital, Boston, Massachusetts
Lung and Pleura Specimens; Bone and Joint Specimens; Special Studies

James M. Crawford MD PhD
Professor of Pathology, Chairman, Department of Pathology, Immunology, and Laboratory Medicine, University of Florida, Gainesville, Florida
Gastrointestinal Specimens

Christopher P. Crum MD
Professor of Pathology, Harvard Medical School; Director, Women's and Perinatal Pathology Division, Brigham and Women's Hospital, Boston, Massachusetts
Gynecologic and Perinatal Specimens

Paola Dal Cin PhD
Associate Professor of Pathology, Harvard Medical School; Associate Cytogeneticist, Brigham and Women's Hospital, Boston, Massachusetts
Cytogenetics

Umberto De Girolami MD
Professor of Pathology, Harvard Medical School; Director of Neuropathology, Brigham and Women's Hospital and Children's Hospital, Boston, Massachusetts
Neuropathology Specimens

David M. Dorfman MD PhD
Associate Professor of Pathology, Harvard Medical School; Medical Director, Hematology Laboratory, Brigham and Women's Hospital, Boston, Massachusetts
Thymus Specimens; Bone and Joint Specimens; Analytical Cytology (Flow Cytometry)

Christopher D. M. Fletcher MD FRCPATH
Professor of Pathology, Harvard Medical School; Director, Surgical Pathology Division, Brigham and Women's Hospital; Chief of Onco-Pathology, Dana Farber Cancer Institute, Boston, Massachusetts
The Surgical Pathology Report, Consultation Reports, Soft Tissue Tumor (Sarcoma) Specimens; Special Studies

Jonathan A. Fletcher MD
Associate Professor of Pathology and Pediatrics, Harvard Medical School; Cytogeneticist, Brigham and Women's Hospital, Boston, Massachusetts
Cytogenetics

Christopher A. French MD
Assistant Professor, Harvard Medical School; Associate Pathologist, Brigham and Women's Hospital, Boston, Massachusetts
Artist

Rebecca D. Folkerth MD
Associate Professor of Pathology, Harvard Medical School; Associate Pathologist, Brigham and Women's Hospital; Consultant in Neuropathology, Children's Hospital, Boston, Massachusetts
Neuropathology Specimens

David R. Genest MD
Associate Professor of Pathology, Harvard Medical School; Associate Pathologist, Brigham and Women's Hospital, Boston, Massachusetts
Gynecologic and Perinatal Specimens

Jonathan N. Glickman MD PhD
Assistant Professor of Pathology, Harvard Medical School; Associate Pathologist, Brigham and Women's Hospital, Boston, Massachusetts
Gastrointestinal Specimens

John J. Godleski MD
Associate Professor of Pathology, Harvard Medical School; Chief, Pulmonary Pathology Division, Brigham and Women's Hospital, Boston, Massachusetts
Lung and Pleura Specimens

Scott R. Granter MD
Associate Professor of Pathology, Harvard Medical School; Associate Pathologist, Brigham and Women's Hospital, Boston, Massachusetts
Dermatopathology Specimens, Special Studies

Michelle S. Hirsch MD PhD
Instructor in Pathology, Harvard Medical School; Associate Pathologist, Brigham and Women's Hospital, Boston, Massachusetts
Genitourinary Specimens, Special Studies

Jason L. Hornick MD PhD
Instructor in Pathology, Harvard Medical School; Associate Pathologist, Brigham and Women's Hospital, Boston, Massachusetts
Gastrointestinal Specimens, Lymph Nodes, Spleen, and Bone Marrow Specimens, Soft Tissue (Sarcoma) Specimens, Special Studies

Lester Kobzik MD
Associate Professor of Pathology, Harvard Medical School; Associate Pathologist, Brigham and Women's Hospital, Boston, Massachusetts
Lung and Pleura Specimens

Jeffrey F. Krane MD PhD
Assistant Professor of Pathology, Harvard Medical School; Chief, Head and Neck Pathology, Brigham and Women's Hospital, Boston, Massachusetts
Head and Neck Specimens, Thyroid and Parathyroid Specimens

Frank C. Kuo MD PhD
Assistant Professor of Pathology, Harvard Medical School; Associate Pathologist, Brigham and Women's Hospital, Boston, Massachusetts
The Surgical Pathology Report, Lymph Nodes, Spleen, and Bone Marrow Specimens

Jeffery L. Kutok MD PhD
Assistant Professor of Pathology, Harvard Medical School; Associate Pathologist, Brigham and Women's Hospital, Boston, Massachusetts
Lymph Nodes, Spleen, and Bone Marrow Specimens, Special Studies

Keith L. Ligon MD PhD
Instructor in Pathology, Harvard Medical School, Associate Pathologist, Brigham and Women's Hospital, Boston, Massachusetts
Neuropathology Specimes

Massimo F. Loda MD
Associate Professor of Pathology, Harvard Medical School; Associate Pathologist, Brigham and Women's Hospital, Boston, Massachusetts
Genitourinary Specimens

Janina A. Longtine MD
Associate Professor of Pathology, Harvard Medical School; Chief, Molecular Diagnostics, Brigham and Women's Hospital, Boston, Massachusetts
Molecular Genetic Pathology, Lymph Nodes, Spleen, and Bone Marrow Specimens, Special Studies

Richard N. Mitchell MD PhD
Associate Professor of Pathology, Harvard Medical School; Associate Pathologist, Brigham and Women's Hospital, Boston, Massachusetts
Cardiovascular Specimens

Vânia Nosé MD PhD
Associate Professor of Pathology, Harvard Medical School; Associate Director of Surgical Pathology, Brigham and Women's Hospital, Boston, Massachusetts
Adrenal Specimens, Thyroid and Parathyroid Specimens, Special Studies

Marisa R. Nucci MD PhD
Assistant Professor of Pathology, Harvard Medical School; Associate Pathologist, Brigham and Women's Hospital, Boston, Massachusetts
Gynecologic and Perinatal Specimens, Special Studies

Robert D. Odze MD
Associate Professor of Pathology, Harvard Medical School; Chief, Gastrointestinal Pathology, Brigham and Women's Hospital, Boston, Massachusetts
Gastrointestinal Specimens

Geraldine S. Pinkus MD
Professor of Pathology, Harvard Medical School; Director of Hematopathology, Brigham and Women's Hospital, Boston, Massachusetts
Lymph Nodes, Spleen, and Bone Marrow Specimens, Special Studies

Bradley J. Quade MD PhD
Associate Professor of Pathology, Harvard Medical
School; Associate Pathologist, Brigham and Women's
Hospital, Boston, Massachusetts
Gynecologic and Perinatal Specimens

Mark S. Redston MD
Assistant Professor of Pathology, Harvard Medical
School; Associate Pathologist, Brigham and Women's
Hospital, Boston, Massachusetts
Gastrointestinal Specimens

Helmut G. Rennke MD
Professor of Pathology, Harvard Medical School; Chief,
Kidney Pathology Service, Brigham and Women's
Hospital, Boston, Massachusetts
Kidney Specimens, Special Studies

Andrea L. Richardson MD PhD
Instructor in Pathology, Harvard Medical School;
Associate Pathologist, Brigham and Women's Hospital,
Boston, Massachusetts
Breast Specimens

Drucilla J. Roberts MD
Assistant Professor of Pathology, Harvard Medical
School; Associate Pathologist, Massachusetts General
Hospital, Boston, Massachusetts
Perinatal Specimens

Mark A. Rubin MD
Associate Professor of Pathology, Harvard Medical
School; Chief, Genitourinary Pathology, Brigham and
Women's Hospital, Boston, Massachusetts
Genitourinary Specimens, Special Studies

Frederick J. Schoen MD PhD
Professor of Pathology and Health Sciences and
Technology (HST), Harvard Medical School; Executive
Vice-Chairman, Chief, Cardiac Pathology, Brigham and
Women's Hospital, Boston, Massachusetts
Cardiovascular Specimens

Sara O. Vargas MD
Assistant Professor of Pathology, Harvard Medical
School; Associate Pathologist, Brigham and Women's
Hospital, Children's Hospital, Boston, Massachusetts
Lung and Pleura Specimens

William R. Welch MD
Associate Professor of Pathology, Harvard Medical
School; Associate Pathologist, Brigham and Women's
Hospital; Boston, Massachusetts
*Women's and Perinatal Specimens, Genitourinary
Specimens*

Tad J. Wieczorek MD
Instructor in Pathology, Harvard Medical School;
Consultant in Cytopathology, Brigham and Women's
Hospital; Staff Pathologist, Faulkner Hospital, Boston,
Massachusetts
Cytology Specimens

Gayle L. Winters MD
Associate Professor of Pathology, Harvard Medical
School; Director, Pathology Residency and Training
Program, Brigham and Women's Hospital, Boston,
Massachusetts
Cardiovascular Specimens

Acknowledgments

The requirement for a comprehensive, detailed procedure manual grew out of the needs of a large pathology department handling numerous specimens using state-of-the-art techniques. The Brigham and Women's Hospital Pathology Department will always be indebted to Dr. Ramzi Cotran, as the department flourished under his outstanding leadership and I am truly fortunate to have been both his trainee and, later, a member of his staff. Our current Chairman, Dr. Michael Gimbrone, has continued his legacy of excellence in pathology service, teaching, and research.

I must also credit Dr. Stan Robbins, whose glimpses of gentle humor in "The Pathologic Basis of Disease" were treasures for a medical student to find while studying late at night. He proved that a serious textbook need not be devoid of humanity.

This manual grew out of the original Brigham and Women's departmental manual that was edited by Dr. Joseph Corson and Dr. Geraldine Pinkus for many years. Dr. Corson continued to co-edit the current manual during his tenure as the Director of Surgical Pathology. His meticulous attention to detail, as well as his enthusiastic love for pathology, are just two of the many important things he taught me. As Dr. Corson's successor, Dr. Christopher Fletcher has continued to set the highest standards for the department.

The consulting authors have provided their expertise in all facets of pathology and I am grateful for their willingness to lend their names and talents to the preparation of the published manual. All credit should be given to them. Any deficiencies or errors are mine alone.

Many other individuals have contributed over the years and their help is also gratefully acknowledged: Dr. Douglas Anthony, Dr. Kamran Badizadegan, Dr. Raymond Barnhill, Dr. Michael Bennett, Dr. Frederick Bieber, Dr. Ramon Blanco, Ms. Holly Bodman, Dr. Marcus Bosenberg, Mr. David Bowman, Mr. Lynroy Brade, Dr. Felix Brown, Dr. Elizabeth Bundock, Dr. Joseph Carlson, Dr. Diego Castrillon, Dr. Young Chang, Ms. Ghizlane Charki, Dr. Gerald Chu, Ms. Margaret Cialdea, Dr. James Connolly, Dr. Christopher Corless, Dr. Milton Data, Dr. Deborah Dillon, Ms. Marilyn Donovan, Mr. Thomas Dunphy, Mr. Dan Faasse, Mr. John Fahey, Dr. Carol Farver, Dr. Mark Fleming, Dr. Matthew Frosch, Dr. Eleanora Galvanek, Ms. Kristi Gill, Dr. Meryl Goldstein, Dr. James Gulizia, Dr. Julie Gulizia, Dr. Susan Hasegawa, Dr. Robert Hasserjian, Dr. Jonathan Hecht, Dr. Jay Hess, Mr. Mark Knowlton, Dr. Madeleine Kraus, Dr. Todd Kroll, Dr. Frank Lee, Dr. Kenneth Lee, Dr. Michelle Mantel, Dr. James McGuire, Dr. Phillip McKee, Dr. Mairin McMenamin, Mr. Steve Mello, Ms. Kathleen Mitchell, Dr. George Mutter, Dr. Kirstine Oh, Ms. Lori Patruno, Dr. German Pihan, Mrs. Cathy Quade, Ms. Catherine Quigley, Dr. Andrew Rosenberg, Dr. Andrew Renshaw, Ms. Chris Ridolphi, Dr. Brian Rubin, Mr. Richard Sartorelli, Dr. Birgitta Schmidt, Dr. Stuart Schnitt, Dr. Joseph Semple, Mr. Aliakbar Shahsafaer, Ms. Kathleen Sirois, Dr. Jeffrey Sklar, Ms. Alyson Smeedy, Dr. Lincoln Stein, Dr. Howard Stern, Dr. James Stone, Dr. Jerrold Turner, Dr. Franz von Lichtenberg, Dr. Peter Wang, Dr. David Weinberg, Dr. Michael Weinstein, Dr. William Welch, Dr. Frances White, Dr. Greg Wolgamot, and Mr. Keith Yarid.

Our publisher, Elsevier (under the imprint of Churchill Livingstone), must be acknowledged and especially Michael Houston, Ruth Swan and Nora Naughton, whose patience and support made this project possible. I am sure there are other individuals who deserve my sincere thanks and I apologize for not naming each person individually.

My parents, Dr. Richard Lester and Mrs. Mary Lester, introduced me to laboratories, microscopes, and the treat of drinking soda out of lab beakers, which is now, unfortunately, in violation of current regulations. However, I survived, and developed an appreciation of science and writing, for which I will always be grateful to them.

Finally, without support at home such a project would never be possible. My husband, Dr. Lloyd Klickstein has been a steadfast supporter, computer crisis consultant, and best friend. My three children, Isaac, Jacob, and Naomi have, hopefully, enjoyed their trips to the pathology department, peering down microscopes, and drinking sodas (but not out of beakers) as much as I have enjoyed showing them what I do. Tanya Badder, Heather McCartney, Fritzi Rother, Sarah Schneemann, or Steffi Bauer were always home when Lloyd or I couldn't be there. The last person in my family to write or edit a book was my great-great-grandfather John Reagan, who traveled to America from Scotland and published "Backwoods and Prairies" in 1850 to encourage other people to emigrate to the United States. I hope my children have inherited his spirit of adventure, love of writing and of the United States, and that it won't be another 151 years before another book is written.

Susan C. Lester MD PhD

In loving memory of my mother, Mary Innocent Cullings Lester

Part 1

Requests for pathologic evaluation

1

The pathologist has an essential role in patient care as diagnostician, patient advocate, and clinical teacher. The surgical pathologist examines all tissues and foreign objects removed from patients to identify disease processes, document surgical procedures, and release tissue for research. Specimens submitted for examination include:

- Fluids, cells, and tissues. Hair, fingernails, and toenails removed for cosmetic reasons are not included, unless there are specific indications for examination.
- Products of conception.
- Medical devices that have been implanted in the body. Temporary devices (such as intravenous [IV] catheters, endotracheal tubes, etc.) usually are not examined.
- Foreign objects removed from the body, including objects introduced by trauma such as bullets.

A decision to not submit specific types of specimens for pathologic examination should be made jointly by the department of pathology, other involved departments, and the institution's legal department to ensure that the best interests of the patient, physicians, and hospital are being served. Such decisions should be documented as written hospital policy according to the Joint Commission on Accreditation of Healthcare Organizations (JCAHO) guidelines. Guidelines for submitting certain specimens for pathologic examination are discussed further in Chapter 21.

■ SUBMITTING PATHOLOGY SPECIMENS

It is the responsibility of all hospital personnel involved to ensure that each patient's specimen is appropriately and safely handled and processed for the maximum benefit to the patient and the physicians caring for him or her.[1] JCAHO standards require that requests for pathologic examination be made in writing or electronically and that the request be kept on file for 2 years. When a pathologic examination is requested, the following information must be provided:

- Patient identification
- Identification of the individual(s) requesting the examination
- Procedure date; the time also should be included, if relevant
- Adequate clinical history
- Specimen identification, including tests requested and any special handling required
- Timely and appropriate transport to the laboratory
- Instructions for the disposition of gross specimens, if not routine disposal (e.g., specimens to be returned to the patient, products of conception, medical devices to be returned to the manufacturer).

Patient identification

Misidentification of specimens can lead to serious errors in diagnosis or failure to diagnose. The identification of specimens must include, as a minimum, the patient's full name and date of birth. A hospital or clinic identification number should also be provided. This information *must* be attached firmly to the specimen container. Unattached paperwork is easily separated from an unlabeled container and is **not acceptable** for definitive identification.

Inappropriately identified specimens must be brought to the attention of the submitting clinician immediately. If there is any uncertainty in determining the identity of the patient, the clinician should come to the pathology department to identify the specimen. If the nature of the specimen is such that gross identification is not possible (e.g., a small biopsy), and identification is uncertain, a repeat specimen should be obtained if possible. There are tissue typing methods that can match tissues from patients and specimens, but such techniques are time consuming and costly and are best avoided by ensuring appropriate identification at the time the biopsy is performed (see Chapter 3, "Identification of Tissue").

Identification of the individual(s) requesting the examination

The names of all clinicians caring for the patient should be provided in order for them to receive a copy of the completed report. This includes not only the physician sending the specimen (e.g., a surgeon or gastro enterologist) but also the primary care physician and any specialists involved (e.g., an oncologist caring for a cancer patient).

If a rush reading is requested, the name or names of physicians to be contacted as well as a means to reach them (e.g., a beeper number or extension) must be provided.

The name of the submitting individual may also be needed if additional clinical history or other information is required before processing.

Procedure date

The date of the procedure (day, month, and year) must be documented to:

1. Correlate the biopsy findings with other clinical tests (e.g., radiologic examinations or serum chemistries)
2. Determine if there is a delay during transport to the pathology department
3. Monitor turnaround time for pathology specimens.

If the specimen is placed in a fixative for which the time of fixation is important (e.g., bone marrow biopsies in Zenker's fixative), the time of placing the specimen in the fixative should also be recorded.

Adequate clinical history

As for any medical consultation, the consultant can provide the most helpful additional information when an adequate history is provided. The clinical history helps define the need for, and nature of, special studies that can be performed. It has been shown that pathologists cannot accurately predict clinical information from the glass slides alone.[2] An adequate clinical history includes:

Purpose for removal of the specimen and type of specimen

- Diagnostic biopsy
- Resection of tumor or reexcision of tumor site
- Surgery for therapeutic purposes (e.g., colostomy takedown or joint replacement).

Note: The purpose of the surgery often determines the type of pathologic examination required (e.g., inking of margins, tissue allocation for special studies). Inaccurate or insufficient labeling may lead to a suboptimal pathologic examination. The type of specimen is also important for accurate billing.

Gross appearance and location of any lesions present

Note: Some lesions that are grossly evident in vivo may become less evident after excision (e.g., vascular lesions, cystic lesions if incised). Radiologic lesions (e.g., breast calcifications or areas of octreotide uptake) may require radiologic specimen imaging for identification. Cancers after treatment may no longer be grossly identifiable.

Prior diagnoses

- History of prior known tumors (including type, site, date of removal, and stage of disease).
- Immune system status. It is important to know if the patient has a reason for being immunocompromised, such as being human immunodeficiency virus (HIV) positive, on assisted ventilation or chronic ambulatory peritoneal dialysis, or having an indwelling catheter or monitoring device, having received an organ transplant or suffering from extensive burns, chronic sinusitis, or diabetes. This information is important to help guide special studies (i.e., characteristic histologic responses to infectious disease organisms may be absent), to interpret histologic findings, and to aid in ensuring the safety of pathology personnel handling specimens with infectious organisms.
- Current or recent pregnancy—pregnancy-related changes can mimic malignancies.

Prior or current treatment

- Radiation or chemotherapy. Treatment-related changes in the histologic appearance of tissues can be mistaken for malignancy if this history is not provided. Carcinomas can be difficult to find grossly after treatment, although extensive disease may be present microscopically.
- Drug use that can alter the histologic appearance of tissues (especially important for the evaluation of liver and endometrial biopsies).
- Drug use that could make the patient susceptible to unusual infections (corticosteroid therapy, chemotherapy, prophylactic antibacterial or antifungal therapy).

Specific purpose of consultation

- The requisition should state if special studies are needed clinically, especially those studies requiring special handling of the tissue (e.g., suspected lymphoma possibly requiring marker studies, microbiologic culture of suspected infection, examination of crystals in joint tissues).

Rush diagnoses

- Specimens from critically ill patients can be given priority over other specimens if this would lead to better clinical management. If a specimen requires a rapid diagnosis, a means to reach the appropriate clinician (e.g., a beeper number) must be supplied.

For the great majority of specimens, a history adequate for the pathologic examination can be given in one or two sentences. For example:

History of diverticulitis. Colostomy takedown.
History of colon carcinoma with multiple positive nodes one year ago. Now with ulcerated mass at colostomy site, biopsy shown to be carcinoma.

Woman s/p invasive breast cancer (ER and PR positive) resected here in 1989 with 3 lymph nodes positive, s/p radiation and chemotherapy, now with subcutaneous nodule in old skin scar. Please do receptor studies if tumor.

52-year-old male s/p bone marrow transplant for large cell lymphoma, now with bilateral pulmonary infiltrates, suspect opportunistic infection. Open lung biopsy for culture and histologic examination. R/o recurrent lymphoma.

Specimens requiring special processing
(Table 1-1)

The type of specimen will determine how it is processed. Specimens requiring special studies must be clearly identified. Most such specimens can be transported moist on saline.

Timely and appropriate transport to the laboratory

Autolysis begins immediately after the surgical removal of tissues. Although it can be reduced by refrigeration, extended delays before fixation adversely affect the diagnostic quality of tissues. Immunoreactivity is diminished for some markers (e.g., receptors in breast cancers).

In some cases, it is appropriate for clinicians to place specimens directly into fixative at 15 to 20× the volume of the tissue. The type of fixative must be identified on the container, with a warning label identifying the fixative. The time of placing the specimen in the fixative should be included when appropriate (e.g., for fixatives containing mercury such as Zenker's, or if rush processing is requested).

All tissues and objects removed from patients may be hazardous and must be transported in a safe fashion. The container must be leak proof. Either plastic rigid containers (preferably with a screw cap lid) or bags (but not if there is liquid with the specimen) may be used.

Clinicians submitting specimens in containers that are inappropriate, unlabeled, or with the outside surface grossly contaminated must be contacted and advised of the hazards such actions pose to patients and hospital personnel.

Instructions for the disposition of gross specimens

If a patient wants to keep a specimen (e.g., a limb, products of conception for burial, a breast implant for legal purposes, or hardware from a joint prosthesis) this request should be stated on the requisition form to avoid routine disposal of specimen after the final report is issued. To avoid later misunderstandings, patients should be informed that their specimens will be discarded.

The following are JCAHO recommendations for retention times:

Pathology report	10 years
Slides	10 years
Gross specimens	7 days after report issued
Paraffin blocks	At least 2 years

Institutional practices vary and in some cases materials may be kept for longer periods of time.

The disposal of human tissues may be subject to state law (usually requiring incineration and/or internment); however, the wishes of patients should always be respected. A legal opinion may be required if a patient request would interfere with optimal patient care or could endanger him or her. There may be specific legal requirements to inform parents of their rights and for appropriate disposition of products of conception (including stillborn fetuses and fetal deaths).

■ ORIENTATING PATHOLOGY SPECIMENS

The orientation of some specimens is evident from anatomic landmarks (e.g., a right colectomy). However, many specimens are either difficult or impossible to orient once they have been removed from the patient.

If orientation is important for the evaluation of a specimen (e.g., excisions of malignant tumors), and orientation has not been provided or is unclear, the pathologist should contact the surgeon before processing the specimen. It is always preferable for the surgeon to discuss complicated specimens personally with the pathologist.

For most specimens, external markers must be used to provide information about orientation for the pathologist. The pathologist can then identify the site of the sections taken and relate them to the anatomic location in the patient. Possible techniques include:

1. **Sutures.** Sutures of variable composition, length, or number can be used to mark anatomic sites (e.g., "deep margin") or areas of greatest concern (e.g., "closest margin"). Two sutures at right angles are necessary to

Table 1-1 Specimens requiring special processing

TYPE OF SPECIMEN OR REQUESTED STUDY	CONDITION OF SPECIMEN	COMMENTS
Bone marrow biopsy	Zenker's fixative	Provides optimal cytologic detail and decalcifies the bone
Bullets or other specimens of potential medicolegal importance	Direct transfer	A direct chain of custody must be maintained
Cytogenetics (e.g., some products of conception, some unusual tumors)	Unfixed, viable	Cytogenetic studies require viable cells. Some specific studies can be performed on fixed tissue (e.g., FISH)
Flow cytometric analysis	Unfixed	Flow cytometry is optimally performed on fresh tissue, either for marker analysis (e.g., lymphomas) or for ploidy and S-phase fraction (e.g., carcinomas). Although flow cytometry can be performed on fixed tissue, S-phase determination is less accurate due to fragmentation of nuclei
Frozen section for rapid diagnosis	Unfixed	Fixed tissues do not adhere well to slides
Gout	Unfixed	Uric acid crystals dissolve in formalin. Tissue should be fixed in 100% ethanol for anaqueous processing
Infections	Unfixed	Tissue should be taken for culture. In some cases (e.g., tuberculosis and Creutzfeldt–Jakob disease), special procedures may be required to protect pathology personnel and to decontaminate equipment
Kidney biopsy	Unfixed	Tissue should be fixed for immunofluorescence and electron microscopy (EM)
Liver: acute fatty liver	Unfixed	Lipids are dissolved during routine processing. Demonstration of microvesicular fat requires frozen section and special stains
Liver: copper	Special	The specimen must not be touched with metal tools to avoid trace contamination
Lymphomas	Unfixed	Special studies—including flow cytometry, DNA analysis, and some marker studies—are optimally performed on fresh or frozen tissue
Muscle biopsy	Unfixed	The specimen should be well orientated and frozen for enzyme studies and fixed for EM
Skin biopsies for bullous disease or systemic lupus erythematosus	Unfixed or in IF transport media	Tissue needs to be fixed for immunofluorescence
Unusual tumors: sarcomas, small round blue cell tumors, mesotheliomas, metastatic tumor of unknown primary	Unfixed	Special studies may be helpful for classification and may require fresh tissue (cytogenetics) or special fixatives (EM)

identify the remaining four margins. Whip stitches can also be used to mark a region of a specimen. Sutures of different colors may be problematic as the color may be obscured after inking margins. A common, and easily remembered, system is to use a Long suture for the Lateral margin and a Short suture for the Superior margin.

2. **Subdividing a specimen.** Different areas are submitted as separate specimens (e.g., separating the levels of an axillary dissection for breast carcinoma or compartments of a radical neck dissection).

3. **Suturing a specimen to a surgical drape.** The surrounding cloth can be used to label areas or to draw the anatomic location.

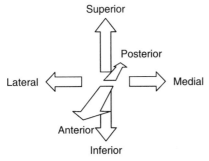

Most specimens can be visualized
as a box with six sides

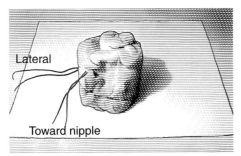

Cannot determine superior/inferior

Two orientating sutures must be at
right angles, in the center of the
"side" of the box, in order to identify
the remaining four margins

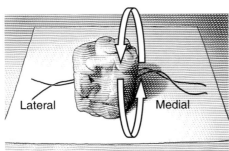

Too complex

If the sutures are at the junction of
two margins, it is difficult to identify
the boundaries of the other margins

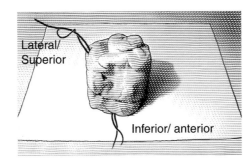

Cannot determine superior/inferior
(e.g. is nipple inferior or superior?)

If the sutures are not given standard
designations, the other margins
cannot be identified with respect
to the patient

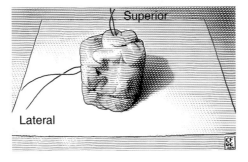

Preferred
(Short = Superior; Long = Lateral)

A simple method uses two sutures:
Short suture = Superior margin;
Long suture = Lateral margin.

Figure 1-1 Orientation of specimens.

A

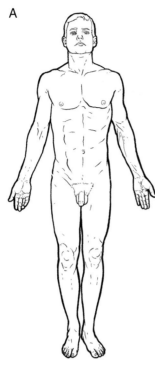

B

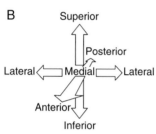

C

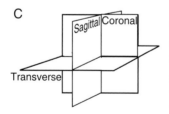

The (almost) anatomic position

Person erect with head, eyes, and toes directed foward

Arms to the side with palms forward

Legs straight and feet together

Penis erect

All designations refer to the patient in the **anatomic position**. The actual position of the patient at the time of removing the specimen is irrelevant (e.g. supine, prone, sitting). Thus, superior is always cephalad, inferior caudad, etc.

Terms for orientation

Anterior (ventral): towards the front of the body

Posterior (dorsal): towards the back of the body. The upper surface of the foot is termed the dorsal surface because this is the position of the foot during embryonic development. The upper surface of the penis is the dorsal surface because whoever made up this system thought the penis should be erect

Superior (cephalic, cephalad): towards the head

Inferior (caudal, caudad): towards the feet. The inferior surface of the foot is termed the plantar surface

Medial: median (midline) plane of the body

Lateral: away from the median plane of the body

Proximal: nearest the trunk or point of origin

Distal: farthest from the trunk or point of origin

Superficial: nearest to the skin surface

Deep: furthest from the skin surface

Transverse section: a horizontal plane at right angles to the longitudinal axis of the body or a body part with division into superior and inferior parts

Coronal section: a vertical plane that divides the body or body structure into anterior and posterior parts

Sagittal section: a vertical plane parallel to the median plane that divides the body or body structure into medial and lateral parts

Figure 1-2 The (almost) anatomic position.

4. **Drawing a diagram.** Anatomic landmarks from the specimen or markers attached to the specimen (e.g., sutures) can be used to correlate the diagram to the specimen.
5. **Small specimens.** Orientation can be provided by placing the base of the biopsy on a plastic mesh (e.g., small bowel biopsies).
6. **Colored inks.** Specific areas of the specimen (e.g., margin locations) can be identified by using colored inks.

REFERENCES

1. Nakhleh RE, Zarbo RJ. Surgical pathology specimen identification and accessioning—A College of American Pathologists Q-Probes study of 1,004,115 cases from 417 institutions. Arch Pathol Lab Med 120:227-233, 1996.
2. Bull AD, Cross SS, James DS, Silcocks PB. Do pathologists have extrasensory perception? BMJ 303:1604-1605, 1991.

Specimen processing: from gross specimens to tissue cassettes

2

Surgical pathologists should deal with each specimen as if they were the clinician—or, better yet, the patient—awaiting the surgical pathology report. Questions such as whether to photograph a gross specimen, how many sections to submit of a particular lesion, how carefully to search for lymph nodes in a radical procedure, whether to order recuts or special stains, whether to write or dictate a microscopic description, and so forth all become answerable in terms of the single basic question, "Were I either the clinician or the patient in this case, what information would I need about this specimen, and how can that information best be supplied?"

STEVEN SILVERBERG, PRINCIPLES AND PRACTICE OF SURGICAL PATHOLOGY AND CYTOPATHOLOGY, 1997

The gross evaluation and processing of specimens is the cornerstone upon which all other pathologic diagnoses rest.

■ GENERAL PRINCIPLES OF PROCESSING SPECIMENS

The following discussion highlights principles common to all specimens. Each type of specimen is described in detail, along with any special procedures that apply, in the specific sections of Part 2 (Chapters 11 to 34).

Specimen identification

Most pathology departments assign each case a unique identification number that includes the year (e.g., S05-4382). This number is used to identify all specimen containers, additional materials (e.g., specimen radiographs), and paperwork. Each "case" is usually defined as all specimens derived from the same surgical procedure. For example, five skin biopsies from the same patient, performed on the same day, would be given the same pathology number.

The first step in specimen processing is identification of all components of a specimen. The specimen container label must include the patient's name and date of birth or the patient's assigned hospital or clinic number. The name or number is matched with any accompanying paperwork. The number and types of specimens received are checked against the list given on a requisition form. Additional parts of the specimen generated by the pathology department (e.g., frozen-section remnants or tissue taken for special studies) are identified.

Any inconsistencies in labeling or missing specimens should be resolved the same day while memories are fresh and when it may be possible to recover a misplaced specimen or acquire a new specimen. The clinician submitting the specimen is called as soon as a problem is found. If the clinician cannot be reached, the call and the time it was made should be documented.

Gross examination and dissection

Each specimen is approached with clear goals in mind based on the type of specimen and the reason for the surgical procedure. If it is unclear why a procedure was performed, it is always preferable to contact the clinician before proceeding. If it is a photogenic specimen or photography is recommended, as in medicolegal cases, consider the best method to illustrate the pathology before inking or dissecting (see Chapter 9).

Identify all anatomic structures present. This might include determining the parts of the bowel present, the lobe of lung, or muscle, bone, and nerve present in an amputation for tumor. Figures in Part 2 illustrate the anatomic components of large resections.

Orientation markers. Anatomic landmarks (e.g., an axillary tail on a mastectomy) or surgically designated orientation marks (e.g., sutures) must be identified. These landmarks should not be obscured or removed during dissection if they are necessary for orientation. If a landmark must be removed, its location should be identified by colored inks, sutures added by the pathologist, or nicks in the attached skin.

Sometimes, radiologic studies, operative notes, or additional information from the surgeon can aid in understanding the orientation. If orientation is unclear from gross examination and the information available (e.g., an unoriented simple mastectomy), the surgeon should be called to provide additional information.

Measurements. Dimensions (in metric units) and, for some specimens, weights should be taken on intact specimens prior to dissection and fixation.

Inking margins. Small biopsies taken for non-neoplastic disease (e.g., colon biopsies), incisional biopsies of tumors, or large specimens for non-neoplastic disease (e.g., diverticulitis) are usually not inked. In some cases, inking small specimens such as skin may help to ensure that the entire face of a specimen fragment is present on the glass slide.

Small simple specimens with known or potential neoplasias are often best inked in their entirety before proceeding (e.g., primary breast biopsies or the soft tissue of skin excised for pigmented lesions). All large resections with margins with areas of gross tumor involvement are inked. However, for large complicated resections with grossly negative margins, it may be better to delay inking until the area of the tumor closest to the margin is identified after sectioning. Global inking of large complicated specimens may obscure anatomic landmarks and can increase the likelihood of artifactually introducing ink into non-marginal tissue.

Care must be taken to either blot specimens dry after inking or allow the specimen to air dry before cutting to avoid such artifacts. If ink is present on non-marginal tissue, tissue sections should be taken and described adequately to avoid interpretation of this ink as indicating margin involvement.

Dissection. No specimen is adequately examined until it has been completely dissected and serially sectioned. Although there are advantages to keeping specimens relatively intact, this is not an excuse for a limited and inadequate examination. With experience, specimens can be thoroughly sectioned without rendering them unrecognizable.

The initial examination is simplified by opening all hollow structures (e.g., bowel resections for tumors and uteri) except in cases in which inflation provides better preservation (e.g., bladders and colon resections for diverticular disease). For tumor specimens, the examination is directed towards determining the site and size of the tumor, location and identity of structures invaded by tumor, vascular invasion, distance from resection margins, and the presence of lymph nodes in the specimen. For other specimens, identification of the suspected disease process (e.g., chronic cholecystitis and cholelithiasis), any incidental findings (e.g., serosal tumor implants on a cholecystectomy specimen), and the identification of abnormal lymph nodes are important.

Identification of pathologic processes. All pathologic lesions have characteristic gross appearances. Part 2 provides brief gross differential diagnoses of common lesions. If a lesion reported to be present, or previously diagnosed by biopsy, cannot be found (e.g., a fistula tract or avascular necrosis of the femoral head), or if the lesion is unusual in appearance, it is advisable to consult the surgeon and the attending pathologist before further processing of the specimen. It is important to document the absence of a lesion if the surgical intent was to remove one (e.g., the absence of a biopsy cavity in a breast re-excision specimen or the absence of a large polyp in a bowel resection).

Histologic sections. Sections that best demonstrate the features seen on gross examination should be taken, not simply random sections. For example, the best section to demonstrate penetration of the bowel wall by a colon carcinoma is the one showing the deepest extent of tumor. To find this area, the entire carcinoma must be carefully sectioned. Similarly, margins must be taken at the sites most likely to show tumor at the margin.

Residents or pathology assistants should show gross specimens to more senior pathologists in the following circumstances:

- Complex specimens
- Specimens with difficult or ambiguous orientation
- Specimens with an unusual gross appearance
- Specimens that will be difficult to interpret or reconstruct once sectioned
- Specimens in which there is uncertainty about why the surgery was performed or the purpose of the pathologic examination

This will enhance the learning experience, as well as facilitate the optimal evaluation and sign-out of the case.

It is extremely difficult for a senior pathologist to sign out a case that has been randomly sectioned by a prosector who is unaware of the reason for the pathologic examination. If a picture is worth a thousand words, a good gross examination is better than a thousand slides!

Special issues in specimen processing

Lymph nodes

Lymph nodes are the most important component of all tumor resections. Gross primary tumors tend to distract the prosector because the tumor is more interesting than lymph nodes, which may be small and difficult to find. However, in terms of a patient's prognosis, and thus the planning of therapeutic options, the status of the lymph nodes is almost always more important than documenting a known primary tumor. Lymph nodes free of tumor may indicate a surgical cure, whereas tumor metastatic to lymph nodes signifies a worse prognosis and is often an indication for systemic chemotherapy or hormonal therapy. Fixing fatty tissue in Bouin's solution facilitates finding small nodes (see Chapter 27), but small nodes can also be found with careful sectioning and palpation.

Enlarged lymph nodes should be searched for diligently in any resection. Occasionally, an occult primary or as yet unsuspected lymphoma comes to light because an involved lymph node is present in a resection for benign disease.

If a resection is performed in order to remove lymph nodes for staging, and fewer than expected lymph nodes are found, the differential diagnosis includes the following:

- The patient is unusual and has few lymph nodes (this is the least likely possibility).
- The patient has undergone treatment that can diminish the size and number of lymph nodes (e.g., radiation therapy or chemotherapy).
- The surgeon failed to remove the tissue that contained lymph nodes.
- The pathologist failed to find the lymph nodes in the specimen.

Studies have shown that the documentation of only a few negative lymph nodes is a poor prognostic factor for patients with colon carcinoma, when compared to patients with large numbers of negative nodes. In part, this may be due to patient and surgical factors, but at least some of these cases may be due to pathologists missing positive lymph nodes. Pathologists should diligently work to eliminate this possibility. If only a few lymph nodes are found, it is usually of value to re-examine the specimen and to submit any tissue that may contain nodes. Nodes with extensive fatty replacement may be difficult to see grossly. It is helpful to document this diligent search in the report (e.g., "The axillary tail is thinly sectioned and palpated and all firm tissue is submitted for histologic examination.").

Margins

Margins are taken on all resections to document the presence or absence of tumor and the viability of the resection margin. India ink (or other colored inks) may be used to cover an entire specimen after the outside has been carefully examined grossly, or used selectively on large and complicated specimens. Several colors of ink may be used when multiple margins need to be evaluated and histologic sections may include more than one margin (e.g., excisional breast biopsies). *Gross and microscopic correlation is very important for margin evaluation because ink very frequently runs onto tissue not at the margin and can be interpreted erroneously as margin involvement.*

All margins are taken in the area most likely to show involvement by tumor, that is, at the closest approach of the tumor.

There are two types of margins: en face and perpendicular to the plane of resection. The type of margin must be specified in the dictation, as this will determine whether or not a margin should be considered positive.

For some specimens, such as skin excisions, a combination of en face and perpendicular margins may be useful.[1]

En face margins (shave, parallel, orange peel; Fig. 2-1). The margin is taken parallel to the plane of resection. This has been likened to taking off an orange peel.

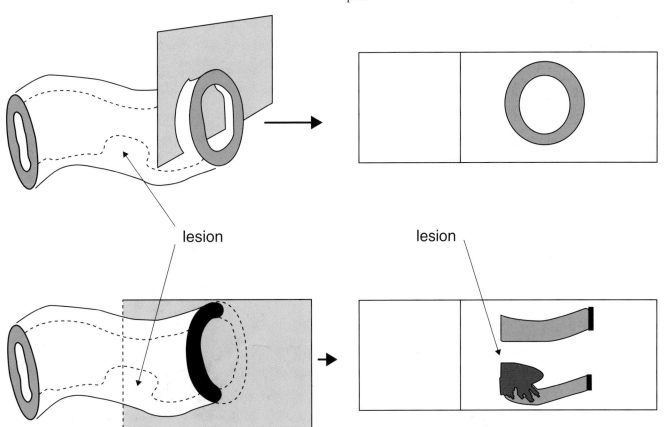

Figure 2-1 En-face margin (above) and perpendicular margin (below).

Advantages

- A surface area 10- to 100-fold greater can be examined than when sections are taken in a perpendicular plane.
- An entire anatomic structure can be evaluated (e.g., a bronchus or ureter).

Disadvantages

- The exact distance of the tumor from the margin cannot be measured. Tumor can be reported to be within the width of the section to the margin (usually within 0.2 to 0.3 cm).
- This type of margin must be specified in the dictation as, unlike perpendicular margins, any tumor in the section is considered to be "at the margin" and ink will not be present.
- Most pathologists are accustomed to evaluating perpendicular margins.
- Cautery artifact is often present and can make interpretation difficult.

The orientation of an en face margin as it is embedded for histologic sections, either for frozen sections or in a paraffin block for permanent sections, is important for tumors for which a narrow rim of normal tissue would be considered to be a negative margin. The tissue may be embedded so that the first cut section is the true margin. If the opposite face is cut first, and tumor is present, then deeper sections may be obtained, or the tissue re-embedded in the opposite orientation, to evaluate the "true" margin.

Perpendicular margins (Fig. 2-1). The margin is taken perpendicular to the plane of resection.

Advantages

- The exact distance of the tumor from the margin can be determined. Perpendicular margins are recommended when a small rim (e.g., less than 0.2 cm) of uninvolved tissue would be considered a negative margin.
- Most pathologists are familiar with interpreting this type of margin.

Disadvantages

- Very little tissue at the margin is actually sampled in large resections.

Method of inking margins

The outer surface of the specimen should be relatively clean and dry. Ink may be applied with a gauze pad or a cotton swab, or by immersing the entire specimen in a container of ink. After the ink has been applied, Bouin's solution or methanol is applied: this acts as a mordant and helps to fix the ink to the tissue and to prevent it from dissolving in formalin. Bouin's solution should not be used prior to frozen section because it may prevent good adherence of tissue to the slide. The inked surfaces are blotted dry before cutting the specimen so as to prevent ink

artifactually marking interior surfaces. Multicolored inks are available for the orientation of complicated specimens.

Stapled margins

The staples cannot be removed without shredding the tissue. The staple line can be carefully cut away as close to the staples as possible and the next closest tissue taken as the margin. Sections that contain staples should never be submitted for histologic processing as the staples will damage or destroy microtome blades and the tissue adjacent to the staple cannot be examined.

Multiple lesions

Occasionally, multiple gross neoplastic lesions are found in a specimen. It is important for both diagnosis and prognosis to determine if these lesions represent: (1) the same lesion, there being a microscopic interconnection between the two gross lesions; (2) a primary tumor and a metastasis; or (3) two independent neoplasms. Each lesion is sampled separately and special studies taken as indicated. *Always* submit a section of tissue between two (or more) lesions for evaluation of whether they are truly separate or are interconnected.

Missing specimens

Possible scenarios with regard to specimens that cannot be found and were never documented as having arrived in the department include:

- The specimen may have been misidentified as a similar specimen received on the same day from a different patient.
- The patient's name may be incorrect (e.g., the first name may have been used as the last name).
- The specimen may be in another part of the hospital (e.g., clinic, transport).
- The specimen may be included with another specimen from the same patient, possibly from a different day or different procedure.
- The entire specimen may have been taken by mistake by a research laboratory.

Specimen containers occasionally arrive empty. The container, including the lid, must be carefully examined as small specimens may stick to the sides or top of the container. Check other containers associated with the case to identify any that may potentially contain the missing specimen. If the specimen is not present, the clinician who submitted it should be contacted the same day. The container should be retained until the issue is resolved. It may be possible to recover a specimen mislaid in the clinician's office, or the clinician may decide to submit additional tissue. Document in the dictation the person who was notified, and at what time.

Specimens are rarely lost after their arrival has been documented in a pathology department. Possible reasons for a specimen not being in the usual location are the following:

- The case was set aside because of precautions concerning infection.
- It is in a waste container. It may be useful to save the waste containers from the gross processing room for an extra day to allow for recovery of lost specimens (or cassettes) if necessary.

Specimens in cassettes also are rarely lost. The most common problem is that the cassette failed to go into the container for processing and was inadvertently placed somewhere else. The container for sharps, the original container (if not all the tissue was submitted), sinks, and waste containers are the most likely locations.

Occasionally, the cassette is present but there is no tissue. Usually either the cassette was not properly closed and it opened during processing or the fragment was small enough to slip through the holes. The latter can be avoided by always wrapping small specimens in lens paper.

■ GENERAL PRINCIPLES OF GROSS DESCRIPTIONS

The ability to accurately examine, describe, and process gross specimens is one of the most important skills of the pathologist. Based on keen observation and detailed dissection, the microscopic sections are taken that best yield important diagnostic and prognostic information for patients. Without these skills, many diagnoses will be left in the formalin jar, and even the most skilled microscopic examination cannot overcome an inept gross one.

A study of the gross examination of breast specimens revealed that reexamination of mastectomies showed discrepancies in 18% of the specimens.[2] Approximately half of the discrepancies were considered major: new diagnosis of cancer, different TNM stage, or new information leading to additional diagnostic or therapeutic procedures. In contrast, review of the glass slides revealed major diagnostic discrepancies in only 1% of cases. Many of the errors occurred during the pathologists' first few months of residency training.

The description of a surgical specimen provides a permanent record of all pertinent information regarding a specimen, including the information provided by the submitting clinician, procedures taking place during operating room consultations, the description of the specimen as it was received and observations after dissection, disposition of all tissues submitted for special studies or for research, and a description of the microscopic sections taken.

In some cases, for routine specimens, standard descriptive text can be used and specific descriptors added as appropriate. However, the use of such forms should never take the place of a careful gross examination.

Accurate and complete descriptions are very important for the following reasons:

Diagnosis. Gross descriptions provide important diagnostic information that is used for staging and prognosis. Microscopic sections alone cannot always provide information about the size of tumors, multiple tumors, distance from margins, or number of lymph nodes examined.

Correlation. Good gross descriptions allow the pathologist to correlate the microscopic findings with the gross findings. Artifacts (e.g., ink present on tissue not at a margin) or errors (e.g., cassettes labeled with the wrong number) can be detected if there are discrepancies between the gross description and what is present on the glass slide.

Documentation. Each specimen and the condition in which it arrived must be carefully documented for medical and legal purposes. The gross description is the only record of the specimen as it was received in the department.

Training. Accurate gross descriptions reveal the strengths and limitations of the gross examination as compared to microscopic examination. For some specimens, such as colon carcinoma, almost the entire diagnosis can be made grossly. This skill is especially important for operating room consultations in which the pathologist must be able to rapidly select the tissue most likely to reveal important diagnostic information. In some cases a good gross examination can yield more information than a frozen-section diagnosis.

Gross descriptions

A good gross description has the following qualities:

Succinct and precise expression. The important information can usually be captured in a few sentences. Long rambling descriptions are often poor because important information is buried in, or replaced by, irrelevant details.

Good organization. Information is easily overlooked if it is not readily accessible and in the right location.

Adequate dissection. A specimen cannot be described accurately until it has been completely dissected and examined. Initial impressions often change after a thorough examination. Important findings and measurements can be recorded in a notebook to aid in dictation after the specimen has been completely examined. This also provides a back-up gross description for transcriptions.

Standardization. Most specimens can be dictated in a standard style. Standardization minimizes the risk of omitting important information. Creative dictations should be reserved for the very unusual or complicated specimen. Sample dictations for all large specimens are included in Part 2.

Diagrams. It can be helpful to make diagrams of complicated specimens, indicating the site of sections taken. Some departments make use of photocopied images of gross specimens for this purpose.[3]

Formatting the gross description

Even the most complex resections (e.g., extrapleural pneumonectomies, complex hemipelvectomies with multiple organs, Whipple pancreaticoduodenectomies) can be clearly described and sampled if the specimen is approached systematically.

There are six components to a gross description:

1. The first part documents the patient's name, the specimen label, whether it was received fresh or in a type of fixative, and anatomic structures present in the specimen (with dimensions and weight as appropriate).
2. The second part begins the description of the main pathologic findings that caused the specimen to be resected (type of lesion, size, relationship to normal structures and margins, etc.).
3. The third part describes any secondary pathology not described in the second part (incidental polyps, a second smaller lesion, diverticula, etc.).
4. The fourth part describes any other normal structures that do not conveniently fit into the first sentence (e.g., length and diameter of ureters from a bladder resection).
5. The fifth part lists frozen sections, photographs, radiographs, and any other special studies that were done. Note if the margins were inked and whether they are en face or perpendicular.
6. The sixth part is a list of all the microscopic sections that were taken.

The first part: Label, fixative, structures present

The gross description starts by documenting how the specimen was labeled and whether it was fresh or in fixative. Specimens first seen as an operating room consultation are dictated as they were received there. For example:

Received fresh labeled with the patient's name and unit number and "Ascending colon" is...

or

Received in formalin labeled with the patient's name and "PNBX" is...

Special note should be taken of specimens that are identified in unusual ways:

Received fresh in an unlabeled container hand-carried by Dr. G. Smith and identified as belonging to the patient, is...

The remainder of the first sentence documents all of the components of the specimen. In order to keep the dictation clear, measurements can be placed in parentheses. For example:

Received fresh, labeled with the patient's name and unit number and "MRM," is a 563-g left modified radical mastectomy specimen (15 × 12 × 4.5 cm) with a white/tan skin ellipse (14 × 12 cm) and with attached axillary tail (6 × 5 × 4 cm).

or

Received fresh, labeled with the patient's name and unit number and "Colon," is a right colectomy specimen consisting of terminal ileum (5 cm in length × 3 cm in circumference), cecum and ascending colon (30 cm in length × 6 cm in circumference), and appendix (7 cm in length × 0.8 cm in diameter).

The second part: Principal pathologic finding

The second sentence starts the description of the main pathologic findings. For example:

There is an ulcerated tan/pink lesion (5 × 4 × 3 cm in depth) with raised serpiginous borders 7 cm from the proximal margin and 22 cm from the distal margin. The lesion grossly extends through the muscularis propria and into pericolonic soft tissue and is present at the serosal surface.

or

There is a 4 cm well-healed surgical scar in the outer upper quadrant, 5 cm from the unremarkable nipple (1.0 × 0.9 cm). Two cm deep to the scar there is a biopsy cavity (4 × 3 × 2 cm) filled with red/brown organizing thrombus. The cavity is surrounded by firm white tissue, 0.2 to 1.0 cm in thickness, but no residual tumor is identified grossly. The cavity is 1 cm from the deep margin, which is a smooth fascial plane.

Dictate gross observations, not what was done with the specimen.

Verbose:

Upon opening the colon longitudinally with a pair of scissors, it can be seen there is a 4-cm lesion. On careful serial sectioning it can be seen to extend through the muscularis propria into pericolonic fat.

Precise:

There is a 4-cm lesion that extends through the muscularis propria into pericolonic fat...

A pathology report should not read like an operative note. In the words of Jack Webb, "the facts, ma'am, just the facts." It can be assumed that the colon was opened, a lesion was observed, and it was carefully sectioned.

However, there are specimens for which it will be necessary to stress an important negative finding in spite of meticulous dissection:

No lymph nodes are found in the area designated by the surgeon as the axillary tail after overnight Bouin's fixation, 1 mm sectioning, and careful palpation.

The third part: Secondary pathologic findings

After the main lesion has been dictated, all secondary lesions are dictated. This description always includes the relationship of multiple lesions to each other.

Three cm proximal to the ulcerated lesion is a tan/pink, soft, villous polyp (3.0 × 2.0 × 2.0 cm) with a stalk (1.0 cm in length × 0.4 cm in diameter).

The fourth part: Lymph nodes, incidental findings, and normal structures

Normal structures need not be dictated in detail. A pathologist or pathology assistant must be able to recognize what is normal and need not elaborate on these findings in the gross description. Summary statements are made such as *The remainder of the colonic mucosa is unremarkable* or *No other lesions are present.* On the other hand, when there is an abnormality, this finding is described: *The colonic mucosa is dusky red* or *The remainder of the breast parenchyma consists of firm white fibrous tissue with numerous blue dome cysts.* This section may also include additional measurements or documentary facts that do not comfortably fit into the first sentence:

Also received is a separate fragment of yellow/white adipose tissue (4.0 × 3.5 × 2.0 cm) without gross lesions.

The fifth part: Special methods

Routine procedures (fixing the specimen overnight in formalin or serially sectioning the breast) do not need to be specified. However, all procedures that are included in billing, in particular decalcification, must be specified. All non-routine procedures and special fixatives used must also be stated. This will be the only record of what was done with the tissue and what is available for special studies. For example:

A frozen section was performed on the tumor and the bronchial resection margin.

The bone is fixed in formalin and then decalcified.

Photographs and radiographs are taken. Portions of the tumor are fixed in Zenker's, B5, and Bouin's solutions and are snap-frozen. Samples are taken for cytogenetics,

and electron microscopy. Tumor (1 × 1 × 1 cm) and normal fat (1 × 1 × 1 cm) are given to Dr. Strangelove for special studies.

It is also helpful to state for some specimens, especially diagnostic breast biopsies, whether or not all of the tissue has been submitted. For example:

All of the tissue is submitted for histologic examination.

Seventy percent of the tissue is submitted for histologic examination, including all fibrous tissue.

The entire lesion and representative normal tissue are submitted for histologic examination.

The sixth part: Microscopic sections

The final section of the pathology report is a list of the microscopic sections submitted. The total number of submitted sections should be recorded by using consecutive numbers or letters.

The end of the gross description includes a list of each cassette and the tissue in the cassette, if cassettes contain different types of tissue. No new information should be included here that is not in the gross description; for example, cassette number 23 should not be *nodule found upon further sectioning* unless it has been described previously. Also included is the number of fragments in the cassette (helpful for the person embedding the tissue and sometimes in identifying possibly misidentified cassettes), the type of fixative (if not formalin), and whether all or only a portion of the tissue has been submitted. This can be denoted by:

RSS: representative sections submitted. Additional tissue could be submitted.
ESS: entire specimen (or designated portion of specimen) submitted. This indicates that no more tissue of this type can be submitted.

Groups of cassettes can be dictated together if they all contain the same category of tissue. For example:

Cassettes #21–23, 1 lymph node per cassette, 6 frags, ESS.

The following are examples of how cassettes from several specimens might be dictated:

Punch biopsy of skin:

Cassette: 1 fragment, ESS.

Basal cell carcinoma, small skin ellipse:

Cassette #1: cross-sections of lesion, 2 fragments, ESS.
Cassette #2: ellipse tips, 2 fragments, ESS.

Prostate, TURP:

Cassettes #1–6: multiple fragments, ESS.

Esophageal carcinoma resection:

Cassettes #1–3: Tumor including deepest extension and deep margin, 3 fragments, RSS.

Cassette #4: Proximal margin, perpendicular, 1 fragment, RSS.

Cassette #5: Distal margin, perpendicular, 2 fragments, RSS.

Cassette #6: Proximal granular pink mucosa, 2 fragments, RSS.

Cassettes #7–11: Ten lymph nodes, two per cassette, 10 frags, ESS.

If focal lesions are present, the cassettes containing the lesion must be specified as the gross lesion may not be apparent on microscopic examination or may not be present on the initial slides prepared.

Thyroid resection:

Cassettes 1–4: well-circumscribed nodule, 8 frags, ESS.

Cassettes 5 and 6: representative sections of normal-appearing thyroid, 2 frags, RSS.

An example of a gross description

The first part:

Received fresh, labeled with the patient's name and unit number and "Colon," is a segment of colon (30 cm in length × 8 cm proximal circumference and 5 cm distal circumference) with attached mesentery (30 cm × 5 cm) with a suture indicating the proximal margin.

The second part:

A centrally ulcerated firm tan/pink tumor (4.0 × 3.5 × 2.0 cm) with raised serpentine borders occupies approximately 90% of the colon circumference. The residual lumen is approximately 0.5 cm in diameter and the proximal bowel is markedly dilated. The tumor grossly extends through the muscularis propria into pericolonic fat and is 0.5 cm from the serosal surface, which is inked. The tumor is 5 cm from the distal margin and 19 cm from the proximal margin.

The third part:

A sessile firm tan/pink smoothly lobulated polyp (1 × 1 × 0.8 cm), is located 2 cm distal to the tumor and 1 cm from the distal margin. The intervening mucosa is normal in appearance.

The fourth part:

Approximately 30 diverticula are noted in the remainder of the colon, which is otherwise unremarkable. There are 14 fleshy tan lymph nodes in the pericolonic fat, the largest measuring 0.6 cm in greatest dimension.

The fifth part:

The specimen is photographed. Tumor (1.0 × 1.0 × 1.0 cm) is given to Dr. Brown for special studies.

The sixth part:

Cassettes #1 and 2: Tumor and serosal surface, 2 frags, RSS.

Cassettes #3 and 4: Tumor and normal colon, 3 frags, RSS.
Cassette #5: Polyp, 2 frags, ESS.
Cassette #6: Distal margin, perpendicular, 1 frag, RSS.
Cassette #7: Diverticula, 2 frags, RSS.
Cassette #8–14: Lymph nodes, 2 per cassette, 14 frags, ESS.

Components of the gross description

Specimens have dimensions of size and weight and features such as color, shape, smell, texture, and consistency. All of these are used to paint a picture for readers of the pathology report and to capture important gross features of pathologic processes.

Measurements

Measurements are in centimeters and fractions of centimeters and expressed as numbers (e.g., 3.5 cm not "three and a half cm"). They should be as accurate as they need to be. Tumor sizes are measured to the nearest millimeter (not rounded off), as these sizes will be used for staging and prognosis. On the other hand, lengths of colon segments cannot be measured accurately to the nearest millimeter and measuring to the nearest 0.5 centimeter is adequate. Include the dimension being measured when appropriate:

> **Imprecise:**
> *The colon measures 5 cm × 2 cm.*

> **Better:**
> *The colon measures 5 cm in circumference × 2 cm in length.*

> or

> **Imprecise:**
> *Received is a skin ellipse measuring 2.5 × 3.0 × 1.0 cm.*

> **Better:**
> *Received is a skin ellipse measuring 2.5 × 3.0 × 1.0 cm (depth).*

Fragmented specimens can be measured in aggregate. In selected cases such as fragmented tumors it is appropriate to indicate the size of the largest fragment or a range of sizes.

Do not over-measure normal structures (e.g., give seven dimensions of a normal cervix) or under-measure important ones (e.g., describe multiple tumors as "several" or "large").

Do not use analogies for size (e.g., "grapefruit size,"

"the size of a child's fist," "the size of a baseball"). While picturesque, these are imprecise and cannot be used for tumor staging.

Measurements can also change over time. Colon segments contract and need to be measured as soon as possible after surgical removal.[4] Lungs deflate. Tissues also shrink after fixation and should be measured when unfixed.

Numbers

Be specific about numbers by giving an accurate count or at least an estimate.

Imprecise:
There are several gallstones.

Better:
There are three gallstones

or

There are approximately 30 gallstones.

Weight

Weight is expressed in grams. All solid organs (lungs, spleens, hearts, kidneys, adrenals, thyroids, prostates, transurethral resections of the prostate [TURP]), mastectomies, and reduction mammoplasties are weighed before fixation. Parathyroid adenomas, adrenal tumors, and some sarcomas are weighed, as this information may be useful for either diagnosis or prognosis.

Colors

Color can be helpful in describing a specimen, especially if the normal color of the tissue or organ has been altered.[5] Few specimens have pure colors. However, instead of using "ish" words (e.g. "reddish," "brownish"), combinations of colors can be used to express the fact that the specimen varies slightly in color (e.g.. red/brown, white/tan). Don't get carried away. Almost all specimens are "grey/white to pink/tan to yellow/orange to red/brown with focal lighter and darker areas."

Colors are very important when describing small biopsies. Blood is usually red/brown and tissues are usually white/tan. If one of three fragments grossly looks like blood clot this correlates with there being only two tissue fragments along with disaggregated blood cells on the slide. Colors caused by increased blood flow or congestion (e.g., in vascular lesions or inflammatory carcinoma of the breast) are often lost once the blood supply is terminated during excision.

Some tumors, tissues, and pathologic processes have characteristic colors:

Renal cell carcinoma (clear cell type)	Golden yellow and hemorrhagic
Normal adrenal or adrenal cortical lesions	Orange yellow
Pheochromocytoma (*phaios* = dusky + *chromo* = color in Greek)	White to tan; chromaffin reaction changes color to mahogany brown to black or purple
Melanoma (if pigmented) (*melas* = black in Greek)	Black
Melanosis coli	Black mucosa
Xanthogranulomatous inflammation (*xanthos* = yellow in Greek)	Yellow
Steroid-producing tumors	Often pale or bright yellow
Chloroma or any purulent exudate (*chloros* = green in Greek)	Green
Prior hemorrhage with oxidation of blood	Green (e.g., in synovial tissue in hemochromatosis or pigmented villonodular synovitis)
Anthracotic pigment (*anthrax* = coal in Greek)	Black
Endometriotic (chocolate) cyst	Brown
Cirrhosis (*kirrhos* = orange yellow in Greek)	Yellow
Ochronosis (*ochros* = pale yellow in Greek)	Black or brown
Gout or chondrocalcinosis	Chalky white
Blue dome cysts of the breast	Dark blue or black

Consistency

Consistency can be a helpful descriptor in communicating whether a malignant lesion is present. Fortunately for pathologists, most tumors incite a desmoplastic response and are harder than the surrounding tissue. In contrast, tissues that are soft or rubbery are less likely to contain malignant tumors. However, tumors that occur in tissue that is normally firm, such as prostate, can be very difficult to detect grossly. Other tumors, such as some lobular carcinomas of the breast, can be associated with a minimal desmoplastic response and may not form a palpable mass.

Tumors often become softer after treatment and more difficult to define grossly. It is often necessary to determine the site of the tumor prior to treatment to guide tissue sampling.

Necrotic areas are usually soft and friable. Papillary tumors are also often soft and can be mistaken for necrosis.

Shape and texture

Malignant processes (but also many inflammatory processes) usually have infiltrative borders and shapes that are irregular or difficult to define. Lesions with well-defined shapes and borders are less likely to be malignant. Tumors usually efface the underlying tissue planes and

Well-circumscribed or pushing borders (e.g., a fibroadenoma)

Stellate or spiculated borders (= irregular)

Irregular, jagged, or notched borders (e.g., a cutaneous malignant melanoma)

Serpiginous (snake-like; e.g., the edges of colon carcinomas)

Smoothly lobulated (e.g., lipomas)

Bosselated (rounded protuberances)

Verrucous (resembling a wart)

Papillary (e.g., bladder tumors)

Villous (e.g., villous adenomas of the colon)

Eburnated ("like ivory"; used for exposed bone surface after loss of cartilage in degenerative joint disease; do not mistake eburnated bone for cartilage or vice versa)

Velvety (e.g., normal gallbladder mucosa)

Pedunculated (with a stalk) or sessile (broad-based)

Macule (flat lesion) or papule (raised lesion)

Friable (soft and falling apart or crumbly)

Excrescence (an irregular outgrowth)

Fimbriated (fringe-like; e.g., the end of the fallopian tube)

Exophytic (projecting out from a surface)

Endophytic (projecting into a space)

Scabrous (covered with small projections and rough to the touch)

Papyraceous (like parchment or paper; e.g., a fetus found within the membranes of a term pregnancy of a twin)

textures. Useful terms for describing shape and texture include:

Pathologists have traditionally used food analogies to describe specimens.[6] Gross descriptions can be spiced with the following:

Currant jelly	Postmortem blood clot
Chicken fat	Postmortem blood clot
Sugar-coated spleen	Perisplenitis
Chocolate cyst	Endometriotic cyst
Unripe pear	Gritty consistency of breast cancer
Grape vesicle	The villi of a hydatidiform mole
Sago spleen	Miliary nodules of amyloidosis (sago is a pearly starch such as tapioca made from the sago palm)
Strawberry gallbladder	Cholesterolosis
Nutmeg liver	Chronic congestion
Apple-core lesion	An obstructing colonic adenocarcinoma (as seen on x-ray)
Rice bodies	Loose bodies in a joint
Lardaceous spleen	Amyloidosis
Fish-mouth stenosis	Rheumatic heart valve
Vegetation	Thrombus on a heart valve
Caseous necrosis	Cheese-like material (especially in tuberculous granulomas)

However, "serially sectioned" is preferred to "bread-loafed."

Fluids can be described using the following terms:

Viscous	Thick
Serosanguinous	Serum tinged with blood
Serous	Like serum—watery
Mucinous	Thick and sticky or gelatinous
Tacky	Sticky, like silicone gel
Suppurative	Thick green exudate

Smell

Fortunately, few surgical specimens have a prominent odor. However, this is an important aspect to report because it usually indicates decomposition of the tissue. Sending tissue for cultures should be considered unless infection has already been documented. A foul smell may indicate decomposition within the patient (e.g., a necrotic bowel) or inappropriate delayed handling of a specimen (e.g., a fresh specimen left overnight without refrigeration).

Be brief, but be precise!

Descriptions should be simple and direct and use as few words as are necessary to convey a clear idea of the specimen.

Grossly recognizable. If a structure can be identified (e.g., appendix, gallbladder, lung), dictate it as such.

Verbose:
Received is a grossly recognizable gallbladder…

Precise:
Received is a gallbladder….

On the other hand, if the specimen is a portion of a structure that cannot be unequivocally identified, use *grossly consistent with*. For example:

Received labeled "gallbladder" is a 3 × 1 × 0.2 cm (wall thickness) portion of velvety pink mucosa grossly consistent with the wall of a gallbladder…

Seen, felt, palpated, found. State only the facts, not how they were observed.

Verbose:
After sectioning the axillary fat, five lymph nodes are found which are firm upon palpation…

Precise:
There are five firm lymph nodes in the axillary fat…

Avoid chains of single fact sentences when they can be condensed into a single sentence.

Verbose:
The specimen is received labeled with the patient's name. It is also labeled with the unit number. It is

received fresh. It is a right modified radical mastectomy. It measures 15 × 14 × 6 cm. There is an attached axillary tail. The axillary tail measures 6 × 4 × 2 cm. The entire specimen weighs 182 g. The white/tan skin ellipse is 13 × 11 cm. The nipple is located in the center of the ellipse. There is a 3-cm well-healed surgical scar. It is in the upper outer quadrant. It is 3 cm from the nipple. There is a fibrotic biopsy cavity measuring 3 × 3 × 2.5 cm. It is filled with red/brown friable material. The biopsy cavity is 1 cm from the skin. The biopsy cavity is 2 cm from the deep margin. The deep margin is a smooth fascial plane.

Precise:

Received fresh, labeled with the patient's name and unit number, is a 182-g right modified radical mastectomy specimen (15 × 14 × 6 cm) with a white/tan skin ellipse (13 × 11 cm) and attached axillary tail (6 × 4 × 2 cm). There is a 3-cm well-healed surgical scar in the upper outer quadrant, 3 cm from the unremarkable nipple (0.7 × 0.6 cm). One cm deep to the scar is a fibrotic biopsy cavity filled with red/brown friable material. The cavity is 2 cm from the deep margin, which is a smooth fascial plane.

Avoid making uncertain diagnoses. Describe what is seen and do not make uncertain assumptions based on possible diagnoses. Some gross diagnoses will later prove to be incorrect, although with experience this happens less often. For example, it may turn out that an enlarged firm lymph node was not "grossly involved by tumor" but actually was fibrotic or fatty. Recognize the difference between terms that are diagnostic and terms that are descriptive:

Diagnostic/interpretive terms	Descriptive terms
Carcinoma	Mass
Hemorrhagic	Red, brown
Necrotic	Soft, friable
Purulent	Green, foul-smelling
Malignant	Irregular border, hard
Mucinous	Sticky, viscous
Invasive	Irregular

In the completed pathology report, the gross description and the microscopic diagnosis should be in agreement. People who are not pathologists often do not realize that the gross description is not based on microscopic findings. If clinicians read in the gross description that there is an involved lymph node, but there is no mention of it in the final diagnosis, it will raise doubts about whether that node was forgotten in the final report. These inconsistencies should be corrected in the gross description or avoided initially. For example, it is just as accurate to describe a "2 cm firm white lymph node" and leave the diagnosis of tumor to the microscopic slides. Similarly, the final number of lymph nodes reported should ultimately correspond to the number of lymph nodes described grossly.

■ SELECTION OF TISSUE FOR MICROSCOPIC EXAMINATION

Tissue is selected for microscopic examination to document:

- All lesions. If multiple similar lesions are present, tissue between the lesions is submitted to determine whether the lesions are separate or interconnected.
- Lesional tissue placed in special fixatives (e.g., B5) for histologic examination.
- Representative sections of all normal structures not included in other sections.
- Lymph nodes.
- All margins when appropriate.
- Frozen-section remnants.

Most specimens (including large, complicated ones) can be adequately sampled in no more than 20 cassettes.

The section that best demonstrates pathologic features should be taken, after complete dissection and examination of the specimen. If a section is to document a normal structure, the best representative tissue should be taken. Random sections (equivalent to selecting tissue blindly) should not be taken.

The ideal number of tissue sections avoids both over- and undersampling:

Oversampling: Wasteful of resources and unnecessarily increases costs.

Undersampling: Important diagnostic or prognostic information may be lost, leading to suboptimal pathologic evaluation.

For some specimens, such as those from a TURP (see Chapter 20), studies have attempted to define the appropriate amount of sampling. Decisions to limit or eliminate tissue sections should be made in the context of such studies. The cost of examining a few more slides may be significant for a pathology department but it is trivial in the overall cost of caring for a patient (with surgical costs running into the thousands of dollars) as well as in the personal cost in morbidity and mortality for individual patients with a suboptimal diagnosis.

Clinical colleagues should be kept informed if significant changes in sampling protocols occur. For example, taking several sections of a biopsy cavity in a mastectomy specimen is much more likely to reveal residual disease than taking one section. If such sampling were reduced because it was unlikely to yield additional important information in women with relatively large previously excised invasive carcinomas, one would expect that the number of mastectomies with residual disease would decline. If surgeons are not aware of the reason for this decline, it erroneously could be perceived that mastectomies are being over-utilized or that pathologists are overcalling positive margins on the original excisions.

FIXATION

After the dissection and description of the gross specimen, tissues must be placed in a fixative. Ideally, fixation serves to:

Preserve tissue by preventing autolysis by cellular enzymes and prevent decomposition by the actions of bacteria and molds.

Harden tissue to allow thin sectioning.

Devitalize or inactivate infectious agents. However, Creutzfeldt–Jakob cases will remain infectious even in tissue on glass slides unless previously treated with formic acid.

Stabilize tissue components.

Enhance avidity for dyes.

However, fixation also has undesirable effects on tissues:

Alteration of protein structure: Proteins may be cross-linked, charges changed, and changes in tertiary structure may occur. This may result in loss of antigenicity that, to some extent, can be reversed by antigen retrieval methods. However, results based on tissue fixed by one method cannot be extrapolated to tissue fixed by another method.

Solubility of tissue components: Lipids and carbohydrates (e.g., glycogen) are often lost during processing unless special techniques are used.

Shrinkage of tissue: Most fixatives cause shrinkage of the tissue. If exact measurements are important (e.g., tumor size in breast carcinomas and sarcomas, distance to the distal margin in rectal resections), they should be taken prior to fixation.

DNA and RNA degradation: Some fixatives, especially those containing picric acid, degrade nucleic acids and must be avoided if studies of nucleic acids are anticipated.

Most fixatives in use are combinations designed to maximize the desirable properties of the fixatives and to minimize the undesirable properties.

Adequate fixation depends upon:

Sufficient volume. An adequate amount of fixative is usually considered to be 15 to 20 times the volume of the tissue. If a specimen is received in saline, this should be discarded prior to adding fixative. Fixative contaminated with blood or other fluids will be diluted and will not fix tissues well.

Access of fixative to tissue. Fixatives penetrate slowly, at approximately 1 mm per hour. Anatomic barriers such as fascia and capsules are barriers to fixative penetration and must be incised to allow optimal fixation. Large specimens must be thinly sectioned. Gauze pads can be used to wick fixative around each portion of the specimen and between the specimen and the container. Large, flat specimens (e.g., colon segments, stomachs, large skin excisions) can be pinned out on a paraffin block and floated upside down in a container containing fixative. A piece of gauze may be placed between the specimen and the paraffin to wick fixative around the tissue.

If adequate fixation of an entire specimen is difficult or may be delayed, small, thin sections of tumor should be taken and fixed separately ("quick fix formalin"). These sections should be cut small enough to fit easily into a cassette to optimize fixation.

Time. Usually, 6 to 8 hours is required for adequate fixation in formalin. Other fixatives may penetrate more rapidly or more slowly. Over-fixation may result in hard, brittle tissue in some fixatives or in increased loss of antigenicity.

Temperature. Increasing the temperature increases the rate of fixation but also increases the rate of autolysis and must be carefully monitored. Most laboratories fix specimens at room temperature.

Types of fixative

The choice of fixative may limit the opportunities for other special studies. Before fixing tissue, consideration should be given to cytogenetic (cell culture) studies and frozen-tissue (RNA and DNA) analysis, which require, or are best performed on, unfixed tissue. Flow cytometry is optimally performed using fresh tissue but can be performed on fixed tissue.

Special gloves (e.g., nitrile gloves) should be worn when handling fixatives or fixed tissues. Latex gloves offer protection from biohazards when handling fresh tissues but do not protect against absorption of chemicals.

Formalin (clear)

Composition. 10% phosphate-buffered formalin (formalin is 40% formaldehyde in water, therefore 10% formalin is 4% formaldehyde).

Indications. Formalin can be used for the routine fixation of all specimens.

Advantages. Formalin is the standard fixative for most pathology departments and has been used in many studies of special stains and immunohistochemistry. It fixes most tissues well and is compatible with most histologic stains. Tissue can be preserved in formalin for many months. Formalin is necessary to see the lacunar cells of the nodular sclerosing variant of Hodgkin's disease and may be used for a portion of the tissue if this diagnosis is suspected.

Disadvantages. Fixation occurs through cross-linking of proteins, and antigenicity decreases over time. This is reversed to some extent by antigen retrieval methods. Modifications adding zinc may also preserve antigenicity. Because of the slower fixation time in comparison to other fixatives, fine bubbling of nuclei may occur due to chromatin coalescence. Formalin penetrates tissue at a rate of approximately 4 mm/24 hours. Formalin dissolves uric acid crystals and specimens containing these should be fixed in absolute alcohol. Calcifications in the breast can also dissolve if fixed for more than 24 hours.

The major toxic effects of acute exposure are eye, upper respiratory tract, and dermal irritation. Very high levels can cause pulmonary edema, hemorrhage, and death in laboratory animals.

Most people can smell formaldehyde at levels of 0.1 to 1.0 ppm. These are levels at which irritant effects occur and indicate that exposure should be reduced.[7] However, the sense of smell adapts quickly and is not a reliable method of determining whether formaldehyde vapors are present.

Exposure to formaldehyde must be kept within federal and state limits (see www.osha.gov/ for federal regulations). Exposure can be monitored using individual badges and may be appropriate for individuals who might be exposed to high formaldehyde levels.

Although legal regulations only apply to workplaces, it is inadvisable to release specimens fixed in formalin to patients (see "Returning Specimens to Patients").

Non-formalin fixatives

Composition. Variable: many are alcohol based. The ingredients of proprietary solutions may not be available.

Indications. May be used to avoid formaldehyde or to fix tissues for molecular protocols (see cgap-mf.nih.gov/ for the use of 70% ethanol fixation for molecular studies).

Advantages. Most are not hazardous, do not require monitoring, and can be disposed of in the general sewer system. Although the purchase cost may be higher than formalin, this expense may be offset by cheaper disposal. Some types may be superior for immunoperoxidase studies because proteins are not cross-linked.

Disadvantages. Time of fixation may be critical, with under- and over-fixation leading to suboptimal results. Penetration into large or fatty specimens may be slow. Nuclear and cytologic detail may not be as good as with formalin and other traditional fixatives. Some of these fixatives may not be optimal for estrogen and progesterone immunoperoxidase studies.

Bouin's solution (yellow)

Composition. Picric acid, formaldehyde, and acetic acid.

Indications. Any tissue (but especially small biopsies).

Advantages. Fixation in Bouin's results in sharp H&E staining and is preferred by some pathologists. Bouin's fixation can facilitate finding small lymph nodes as the nodes remain white and the fat is stained yellow. Prolonged fixation can be used to decalcify tissue.

Disadvantages. Tissues become quite brittle and should not be fixed for more than 18 hours. Tissues can then be transferred to ethanol. Large specimens should not be fixed in Bouin's as it colors the entire specimen yellow, making it difficult to see details grossly. Red cells are lysed and iron and small calcium deposits dissolved. Immunoperoxidase studies performed on tissues fixed in Bouin's may be less sensitive. Picric acid can cause degradation of DNA and may interfere with the use of tissues for special studies requiring intact DNA, such as the polymerase chain reaction (PCR).

Caution: Picric acid is an explosive when dry and must be kept moist!

Hollande's solution (green)

Composition. Picric acid, formaldehyde, acetic acid, copper acetate.

Indications. Small biopsies, especially those of the gastrointestinal tract.

Advantages. This is a modification of Bouin's solution. The cupric acetate stabilizes red blood cell membranes and the granules of eosinophils and endocrine cells, resulting in less lysis than Bouin's solution.

Disadvantages. These are similar to those of Bouin's solution. Tissues must be washed before processing to remove salts that will precipitate.

Caution: Picric acid is an explosive when dry and must be kept moist!

B5 (clear)

Composition. Mercuric chloride, sodium acetate, and formalin.

Indications. B5 is often used for the routine fixation of lymph nodes, spleens, and other tissues if a lymphoproliferative disorder is suspected.

Advantages. B5 gives rapid fixation with excellent cytologic detail. Antigen preservation for lymphoid markers is excellent.

Disadvantages. The fixative is unstable as the salt is reduced to elemental mercury when formalin is added. Mercuric chloride and sodium acetate must be mixed with an equal volume of formalin immediately before use. Over-fixation causes the tissue to become brittle. Tissue is fixed in B5 for 2 to 4 hours and then transferred to formalin. Preservation of some antigens may be poor (e.g., keratin immunoreactivity may be weak or absent), and some histochemical stains (e.g., Ziehl–Neelsen) may be suboptimal. Tissue that has been fixed in formalin can be postfixed in B5. This method is not optimal but gives better results than formalin alone. Special procedures for disposal are required due to the presence of mercury. Mercury-containing fixative corrodes metal.

Caution: Do not allow contact with skin—contains

mercury!

Zenker's acetic fixative (orange)

Composition. Potassium dichromate, mercuric chloride, and acetic acid.

Indications. Zenker's fixative may be used for bone marrow biopsies: between 8 and 12 hours are required for decalcification and optimal cytologic preservation. Soft-tissue tumors suspected of having muscle differentiation (cross-striations are especially well preserved) may be fixed for 4 hours.

Advantages. Tissues are rapidly fixed with excellent histologic detail. Zenker's slowly decalcifies tissues. It can be used to demonstrate a chromaffin reaction in pheochromocytomas because of the potassium dichromate but may be less sensitive than solutions that do not contain acetic acid (see Chapter 11). Zenker's is sometimes preferred for bloody specimens, as red blood cells are lysed.

Disadvantages. Zenker's penetrates poorly. Fixation for longer than 24 hours may cause the tissue to become brittle. The tissue can be transferred to formalin to avoid this. Erythrocytes are lysed and iron may be dissolved. Tissues are rinsed in a water bath and then washed for several hours in tap water (bone marrow ≥1 hour; soft-tissue tumors ≥4 hours) after fixation to remove mercury precipitates before processing. Tissues cannot be over-washed. There is poor antigen preservation for immunohistochemistry, and Zenker's interferes with chloroacetate esterase activity. Special procedures for disposal are required because of the presence of mercury. Mercury-containing fixative corrodes metal.
Caution: Do not allow contact with skin—contains mercury!

Helly's solution (Zenker's formal solution)

Composition. Potassium dichromate, mercuric chloride, formaldehyde.

Indications. The indications for use of Helly's solution are similar to those for Zenker's.

Advantages. This fixative is similar to Zenker's but contains formaldehyde instead of acetic acid. Erythrocytes are preserved.

Disadvantages. The solution is unstable and the formaldehyde must be added immediately before use. Other disadvantages are similar to Zenker's.
Caution: Do not allow contact with skin—contains mercury!

Glutaraldehyde (clear)

Composition. Glutaraldehyde, cacodylate buffer.

Indications. Tissues to be preserved for electron microscopy.

Advantages. Excellent preservation of ultrastructural cellular detail.

Disadvantages. Glutaraldehyde penetrates slowly and poorly. Tissues must be minced into small cubes and fixed rapidly. Refrigeration is required for storage. Glutaraldehyde can result in false positive PAS stains.

Alcohol (clear)

Composition. Ethanol and methanol rapidly displace water and denature protein.

Indications. Alcohol is used for synovial specimens if gout is suspected since urate crystals will be dissolved by water-containing fixatives (e.g., formalin). The tissue is fixed in 100% alcohol for nonaqueous processing and H&E and Wright stains. Smears, touch preps, and frozen sections are fixed in methanol before staining.

Advantages. Many antigens are well preserved. Most alcohol fixatives do not require special disposal methods.

Disadvantages. Alcohol dissolves lipids and penetrates poorly. Fixation times must be carefully monitored (for both under and over-fixation). Ethanol and methanol will shrink and harden tissue left in these fixatives over time. This is not a problem with alcohol-based fixatives such as methacarn.

Carnoy's (clear)

Composition. Glacial acetic acid, absolute ethanol, chloroform.

Indications. Carnoy's can be used for any tissue.

Advantages. Carnoy's rapidly penetrates tissue and achieves good nuclear preservation. It can potentially be used for same-day tissue processing because the fixative does not contain water, and dehydration steps are not required.[8] Glycogen is preserved.

Disadvantages. Chloroform may be hazardous to handle. Collagen is not well preserved. Red blood cells are lysed. Acid-fast bacilli are not stained. Acid-soluble cell granules and pigments may be lost. Tissues should not be fixed more than 4 hours to avoid shrinking and hardening.

Methacarn (clear)

Composition. Chloroform, glacial acetic acid, and methanol.

Indications. Methacarn is sometimes used for soft-tissue tumors and mesotheliomas.

Advantages. Methacarn is similar to Carnoy's but results in less hardening and shrinking. Tissue may be left in this fixative for several days. It preserves intermediate filaments well in addition to other antigens for immunoperoxidase studies. Tissues that have been fixed in methacarn should not be placed in formalin.

Disadvantages. Chloroform may be hazardous to handle. Methacarn dissolves some inks.

Decalcification

Bone and other calcified tissues (blood vessels with calcified plaques, some teratomas, intervertebral discs, some meningiomas, some ovarian tumors, calcified infarcted epiploic appendages, etc.) must have the calcium removed in order to allow the specimen to be sectioned. Some fixatives (e.g., Bouin's and Zenker's solutions) will both fix and decalcify tissues. Other decalcifying agents are not fixatives, and tissues must be fixed first before using such agents. Small specimens require only 1 to 2 hours whereas femoral heads may require 1 to 2 days. Large calcified structures should be sectioned with a bone saw prior to fixation and decalcification.

Prolonged decalcification adversely affects histologic detail and the preservation of some nuclear antigens, especially ER, PR, p53, and Ki-67.[9] Other antigens are relatively unaffected. Specimens of diagnostic importance such as tumors should be decalcified for the least amount of time necessary, checking the tissue every few hours.

Undecalcified sections are sometimes examined in the study for metabolic bone disease (see Part 2, "Biopsy, Metabolic Bone Disease p. 227"). Special processing is required and sections must be embedded in plastic. Such studies are usually performed only by specialized laboratories.

■ DISPOSAL OF FIXATIVES AND TISSUES

Tissue not submitted for histologic sections is generally retained for a period of time after the final sign-out of the case. College of American Pathologists (CAP) guidelines are 14 days; JCAHO guidelines are 7 days. This allows enough time for the clinician to receive the report and ensures that additional tissue can be submitted if any issues arise. Most departments do not have facilities for long-term storage of unprocessed tissue. In certain cases, such as specimens of possible medicolegal importance, it may be important for the clinician to inform the patient prior to the operation to avoid the patient assuming that his or her specimens will be available indefinitely.

Chemicals used in pathology can pose toxic, fire, explosive, and corrosive hazards. Tissues are potentially infectious. Care must be taken in how these materials are handled and disposed of for the safety of human beings (both inside and outside the hospital) and to meet current hospital and state standards for waste disposal. Laboratories must conform to federal standards regulated by the Occupational Safety and Health Administration (OSHA; see www.osha.gov/).

Fixatives and chemicals cannot be disposed of into the general waste water system (i.e., down sink drains). All fixatives must be placed in special designated containers for disposal. Although adequate amounts of fixative should always be used, the use of unnecessary amounts of fixative must be avoided and fixative should be reused for the same specimen when being transferred into a new container. To remove excess formalin from fixed specimens before handling, tissues may be rinsed in a water bath and the water disposed of with the formalin waste.

Mercury-containing fixatives (e.g., B5 and Zenker's) must be disposed of according to institutional and legal standards.

Xylene and methanol must be disposed of into special waste containers. Xylene is a neurotoxin and short-term exposure can cause headaches, dizziness, lack of coordination, confusion, and fatigue.

Clean ethanol can be disposed of into sink drains. However, ethanol that has been contaminated with any other substance (e.g., xylene during staining) must be placed in special waste containers.

If specimen containers that contain fixative are discarded, the cap should be tightly screwed on. Otherwise the liquid fixative mixed with other garbage constitutes a hazard and increases the amount of formalin in the air. Formalin containers for holding cassettes should have a lid.

Tissues and explanted synthetic materials are discarded in biohazard bags in specifically marked boxes that are incinerated.

■ DISPOSAL OF SHARPS

All tools used to process specimens (forceps, scissors, scalpel handles, probes) must be rinsed and examined carefully between cases to prevent tissue being carried over to another case. A small piece of malignant tissue, barely visible to the eye, when transferred to the wrong cassette could result in a diagnostic error or require expensive tests (typically costing thousands of dollars) for tissue typing.

Scalpel blades must be changed between cases to prevent carrying over tissue from another case and to reduce the infection risk should an injury occur.

Scalpel blades, glass slides, and needles must be discarded in specific sharps containers. The person using the sharp is responsible for its proper disposal. It is preferable to discard a sharp immediately after use, rather than to set it down on the working area. Before leaving a work area, always check for scalpels, blades, or syringe needles. Serious injuries have resulted from sharp blades and needles concealed in surgical drapes or paper towels.

■ RETURNING SPECIMENS TO PATIENTS

Most pathology departments do not have a formal policy for returning specimens to patients.

Issues that need to be addressed are:

The rights of the patient. The legal ownership of tissues and materials removed from patients is not clear. In part, "ownership" of a specimen may be affected by the precise wording in a consent form for surgery or admission to a hospital. Some specimens may be classified legally as "medical waste" and may fall under state regulations for disposal of hazardous waste. In general, when release of a specimen does not involve the issues discussed below, the patient's wishes should be accommodated. However, in difficult cases a legal opinion may be necessary.

Diagnostic issues. It is rare that a patient asks for possession of a specimen prior to a diagnostic procedure being performed. However, should this happen, the rights of the patient need to be balanced against the duty of the hospital and physician to do what is in the best interest of the patient and to make sure that the patient is well informed of the possible consequences of this action.

Safety of the patient and public. Specimens that are clearly a hazard, in particular any tissue from a patient with Creutzfeldt–Jakob disease, should definitely not be released. In general, clean foreign objects (e.g., hardware, prostheses, teeth) pose little if any hazard. Tissue specimens may carry a risk of infection if not fixed, and fixatives are potentially hazardous. Such risks can be minimized, but the patient should be informed of potential hazards.

In general, fixatives should be removed and specimens washed clean. It is preferable to place the specimen in a heat-sealed plastic bag that allows viewing of the specimen without opening the container. An informational release form may also be included (see Fig. 2-2).

Medicolegal issues. Some specimens may become evidence in lawsuits. In such cases it is useful to photograph the specimen to retain a permanent visual record. For non-tissue specimens (e.g., breast implants or bullets), it is preferable to not alter the specimen (e.g., by sterilization or cleaning) and to release it in the same condition as it was received.

Recipient of specimen. In all cases (except bullets) it is preferable to release the specimen directly to the patient.

The patient may request that the specimen be released to a legal representative or other party. In such cases, a signed release form from the patient must be obtained and medical confidentiality must be maintained. Bullets, or other specimens serving as evidence of a crime, should only be released to a police officer, and appropriate chain of custody documentation must be maintained.

Specimens requested for burial (usually limbs or products of conception) are generally released directly to a funeral home.

Specimens that are commonly requested for return include:

- Orthopedic hardware
- Foreign bodies
- Gallstones
- Teeth

These specimens pose little threat to health if clean and placed in a clean container, and return of such specimens is unlikely to cause harm. It has been questioned whether gallstones placed in formalin are hazardous, as formalin is still detectable even after rinsing in water for 30 minutes. Although patients and their families are not included under government regulations concerning formalin exposure, it would be inappropriate for a physician to give a patient something that constitutes a health hazard as specimens can fall into the wrong hands. There is a report of two children ingesting gallstones fixed in formalin.[10] Although the children did not develop symptoms, the episode did prompt a visit to an emergency room, x-rays, and treatment with activated charcoal.

Given that the possibility of harm is low but that it does exist, the following procedures are suggested:

- If it is known that the patient wants the gallstones returned, the stones can be washed clean, dried, and placed in a sealed container.
- If the gallstones have been placed in formalin, they may be rinsed in water and then dried. The stones can be placed in a sealed container with a label indicating that the stones had been fixed in formalin.

In either case, the patient should be informed that the gallstones are best left within the sealed container.

Sample specimen release form

Figure 2-2 is an example of a form that could be used to inform patients of the potential risks, appropriate procedures for handling a specimen, and appropriate disposal, as well as to document the release of a specimen.

DEPARTMENT OF PATHOLOGY
REQUEST FOR RELEASE OF PATHOLOGY SPECIMENS

Patient name:_____   Date:_____

Surgical Pathology Number:_____

Name of person requesting specimen:_____

Name of person authorizing the release of the specimen:_____

Type of specimen:_____

Specimens received by the pathology department are examined and sampled for diagnostic purposes. Specimens are normally held for two weeks and then disposed by incineration. Requests for return of specimens must be made at the time of surgery or within two weeks.

Risks involved in handling pathology specimens

Pathology specimens consist of human tissues and/or prosthetic materials that have been in contact with human tissues. Although the specimen has been placed in an impermeable container, these tissues and materials may constitute a health hazard and must be handled and disposed of properly as described below. If you wish to discard a specimen, you may return it to the department for disposal.

Unfixed tissue (e.g., amputations, placentas): Unfixed human tissue potentially harbors infectious agents such as hepatitis B virus and the human immunodeficiency virus (HIV). Tissue must always be handled with protective gloves and must not be allowed to contaminate surfaces. It is strongly recommended that such specimens be handled directly and exclusively by a designated funeral home. Appropriate disposal is by burial or incineration only.

Fixed tissues (e.g., appendix, gallstones): Formalin is a fixative that will inactivate most infectious agents but will not destroy the agent responsible for Creutzfeldt–Jakob disease. Tissue must always be handled using protective gloves and must not be allowed to contaminate other surfaces. Tissues must be disposed of by incineration.

Formalin is a toxic respiratory irritant and potential carcinogen. It should never be inhaled, ingested, or allowed to come into contact with skin or mucosal surfaces. The container must be kept away from children and pets. Containers must only be opened in well-ventilated sites. The fixed specimen may have been washed, but small amounts of formalin may remain in or on the specimen.

Synthetic materials (e.g., orthopedic hardware, breast implants): This material may have been cleaned of all gross blood and tissue fragments but must be handled with caution. It is recommended that these materials be kept in a protective container and only handled using gloves. These materials should be disposed of by incineration.

I have read and understand the information provided above and accept responsibility for handling and disposing of the requested specimen appropriately.

Signature_____   **Date** _____

Relationship to patient: _____

Figure 2-2 Informational request form for release of specimens.

REFERENCES

1. Rapini RP. Comparison of methods for checking surgical margins. J Am Acad Dermatol 23:288-294, 1990.
2. Wiley EL, Keh P. Diagnostic discrepancies in breast specimens subjected to gross reexamination, Am J Surg Pathol 23:876-879, 1999.
3. Olson DR. Specimen photocopying for surgical pathology reports. Am J Clin Pathol 70:94-95, 1978.
4. Goldstein NS, Soman A, Sacksner J. Disparate surgical margin lengths of colorectal resection specimens between in vivo and in vitro measurements. The effects of surgical resection and formalin fixation on organ shrinkage. Am J Clin Pathol 111:349-351, 1999.
5. Dirckx JH. Chromatic fantasies. Color words in medicine. Am J Dermatopathol 7:157-161, 1985.
6. Bewtra C. Food in pathology. Am J Dermatopathol 18:555, 1996.
7. Loomis TA. Formalin toxicity. Arch Pathol Lab Med 103:321-324, 1979.
8. Dawson PJ, Deckys MC. Rapid (same day) processing of biopsies using Carnoy's fixative. Am J Surg Pathol 11:82, 1987.
9. Arber JM, Arber DA, Jenkins KA, Battifora H. Effect of decalcification and fixation in paraffin-section immunohistochemistry. Appl Immunohistochem 4:241-248, 1996.
10. Dunn E, Nolte T. The potential toxicity of preserved gallstones [letter]. Vet Hum Toxicol 36:478, 1994.

The histology laboratory—what the pathologist needs to know, from tissue cassettes to glass slides

3

The histotechnologist and the histology laboratory are essential for the accurate diagnosis of pathologic specimens. However, the process by which tissue in cassettes is converted into glass slides remains an enigma for many pathologists. A basic knowledge of the histology laboratory is necessary to facilitate communication between pathologists and histotechnologists. Poor communication can lead to suboptimal evaluation and possibly errors in diagnosis.

■ HISTOLOGIC PROCESSING

Standard tissue cassettes measure $3 \times 2.5 \times 0.4$ cm. Tissue must be cut to fit easily into the cassette and must be 0.3 cm or less in thickness. Thin sections taken from such tissue will fit onto standard microscope slides measuring 7.5×2.5 cm. Larger tissue sections can be processed using larger cassettes and glass slides, but require special equipment and training to produce.

Tissue processing (Fig. 3-1)

The tissue undergoes automated processing (usually requiring several hours) consisting of three steps:

Dehydration. The water in the tissue is replaced by alcohol. Nonaqueous embedding media (such as paraffin) cannot penetrate tissues containing water.

Clearing. The alcohol is replaced by a clearing agent that makes the tissue receptive to infiltration by the embedding medium. The clearing agent must be miscible with both alcohol and the embedding medium. Because xylene (a common clearing agent) has a high refractive index, the tissue also becomes transparent ("cleared").

Infiltration. The xylene is replaced by paraffin or another embedding medium. The paraffin stiffens the tissue, allowing very thin sections (only a few μm in thickness) to be cut with a microtome.

Problems with submitted tissue

Fatty tissue. Fixatives, and especially dehydrants, penetrate fatty tissues slowly. Fatty tissues must be cut very thin to fix and dehydrate them well.

Tissue too thick or too large for the cassette. It is often tempting for pathologists to stuff cassettes with tissue, either because it is easier than cutting thin sections, or in a futile attempt to have a larger area of tissue present on the slide. Fixatives and processing solutions cannot gain access to the tissue. The tissue will not process well and may remain soft; it is often impossible to section such tissue. This outcome can have a significant adverse affect on patient care if the tissue (e.g., lymph nodes on a tumor resection) can never be examined. Tissue sections should be no thicker than 0.2 to 0.3 cm.

Calcified substances. As a general rule of thumb, any tissue submitted for processing should be easy to section with a scalpel blade. Thick bone or calcified tissues cannot be cut by a microtome and must be decalcified prior to processing.

Hair. Hair can dull microtome blades and should be carefully shaved off if abundant on a skin specimen.

Hard foreign material. Staples and clips must be removed from tissue. Metallic objects can be located by radiographing tissue, if necessary.

Multiple small tissue fragments. Fragments of tissue small enough to be lost through the holes in the cassette (0.1 to 0.2 cm) must be placed in a specimen bag or wrapped in lens paper. This also aids in identifying all tissue fragments for embedding.

Tissue embedding

At the end of the processing step, the cassettes containing tissue are immersed in paraffin. The tissue is removed from the cassette and placed in a metallic mold. The tissue is oriented in an optimal fashion for sectioning in liquid paraffin. The paraffin is then solidified by cooling, and the block of paraffin and tissue is attached to the bottom of the corresponding cassette for identification.

Special instructions for embedding may be required for the following:

Cross-sections of tissues (e.g., colon, skin). Sections oriented to show the complete cross-section perpendicular to the surface of the tissue are optimal. This orientation may be obvious in large, flat sections. Sponges placed in a cassette are sometimes helpful in holding tissue flat.

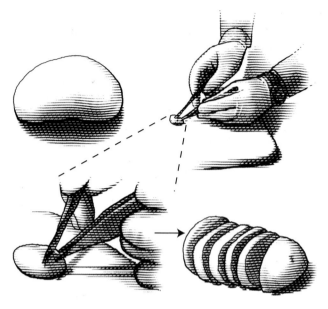

A. Tissue is grossly serially sectioned (0.2 to several mm) to look for small lesions.

B. **Cassette:** Tissue sections taken for histologic processing should be no thicker than 0.3 cm and should fit loosely in the cassette used to hold the tissue during processing.

A specimen is cut into thin sections

A

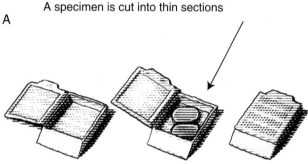

In general, tissue processing requires several hours and is usually performed overnight.

C. **Block:** Each block consists of the tissue in the cassette embedded in paraffin and attached to the bottom of the same cassette for identification.

Sections are placed into cassettes, fixed, and submitted for paraffin embedding

B

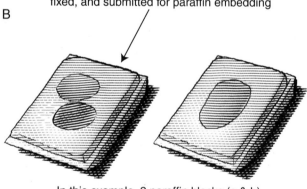

D. **Slide:** A microtome is used to generate a thin slice less than the thickness of a cell (typically 4 μm) from each block for mounting on a glass slide for microscopic examination.

Levels: If 4-μm slices are cut, a 0.3-cm thick tissue section can yield up to 750 glass slides (levels). For special stains, "no waste" slices (i.e., consecutive slices) can be used. To better evaluate small lesions, levels are typically from slices deeper in the block, 20 μm apart. In order to evaluate all the tissue in a block (e.g. sentinel lymph nodes for breast cancer) levers may need to be taken from slices several hundred μm apart.

In this example, 2 paraffin blocks (a & b) are produced

C

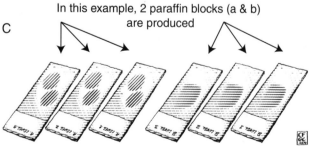

Glass slides (three levels in this example) are produced for each block

D

Figure 3-1 From specimen to slide: tissue processing.

Skin shave biopsies. These specimens often curl and are hard to orient. They may be submitted intact and sectioned and oriented perpendicularly at the time of embedding.

Small (<0.4 cm) punch biopsies. Small punch biopsies, especially those with vesicular lesions, may be submitted intact and bisected and oriented at the time of embedding.

Small lesions in large fragments of tissue (e.g., a hyperplastic polyp in the colon). Very small lesions may be seen only on one face of a tissue section. In such cases, one side of the tissue can be inked and specific instructions provided (e.g., "Embed with inked tissue surface up"). Avoid red ink—it may be difficult to see. Black ink is preferred.

Tubular structures (e.g., temporal arteries, vas deferens, fallopian tubes). It is preferable to submit the entire tubular structure in the cassette with instructions to cut into cross-sections before embedding. It may be difficult, or impossible, to orient multiple small fragments after processing.

Multiple fragments. The fragments should be embedded at the same level in the block in order to obtain a representative section of each piece on the glass slide. It is preferable to limit the number of fragments per cassette if it is expected that only some of the fragments may be diagnostic. In some cases, it may be helpful to separate fragments more likely to be diagnostic and to submit them in a separate cassette: for example, breast cancer cores with radiologic calcifications may be separated from those that do not have calcifications.

Small intestine biopsies. These biopsies may be placed on mesh by the endoscopist to aid in orientation. The entire mesh and tissue can be wrapped in paper and submitted. Each specimen should be placed in a separate cassette. The specimen can then be oriented for embedding.

Making glass slides

The "block" (the tissue embedded in paraffin attached to the bottom of the cassette) is mounted on a microtome and a 4-μm section is cut from the surface of the block. The cut tissue is floated in a water bath. In some cases thinner or thicker sections are appropriate. The tissue section is then placed on a glass slide. Plain glass slides are appropriate for most types of stains. Slides to be used for immunohisto-chemistry require a special adhesive surface on the glass to keep the tissue attached during the procedure. The slides are dried in an oven for variable periods of time to remove any water present. The tissue can then be stained and a coverslip added. When properly prepared, such slides will remain of good quality for many decades.

Problems with tissue sections on glass slides (e.g., holes, microscopic chatter, scratches) are often caused by

problems with tissue selection and fixation prior to arrival in the histology laboratory and can be minimized by careful gross processing by the pathologist.

Information for the histology laboratory

The histotechnologist often requires information about a specimen to optimize the embedding and staining procedures. This is most easily accomplished by keeping a list of cassettes submitted on each case with room for notation of the following information. This list can also be used to ensure that all cassettes submitted are received by the histology laboratory.

Type of tissue

The type of tissue can be important in deciding how a specimen should be embedded. For example, needle biopsies are ideally arranged in parallel rows perpendicular to the long axis of the slide. It is also helpful to indicate specimens in which problems may be encountered (e.g., possible small bone chips or metallic fragments).

Type of fixative

The type of fixative should be specified if it is not the usual fixative used by the laboratory. Some fixatives, such as those containing mercury, require special techniques for processing to remove precipitates and pigments. Nonaqueous processing (e.g., to demonstrate uric acid crystals) is often accomplished by hand and not in tissue processors.

Number of fragments

Documentation of the number of tissue fragments present is important to ensure that all tissue submitted is processed. It can also sometimes be helpful in detecting mislabeled cassettes.

Orientation

After processing, the tissue is removed from the cassette and re-embedded in a paraffin block. For most specimens, the orientation within the block is not important. Special instructions for the orientation of certain specimens for embedding should be provided. For example, some small specimens that are better processed intact and sectioned by the histotechnologist immediately before embedding include:

- Temporal arteries
- Vas deferens
- Small skin punch biopsies (<4 mm)
- Skin punch biopsies with vesicular lesions
- Skin shave biopsies.

Larger specimens that should be embedded face up or face down may be inked on one side and instructions provided: for example, "Please embed with the inked side face up." Such specimens might include:

- Small lesions within a larger piece of tissue
- En face margins for which specific orientation is important.

Small intestine biopsies submitted on mesh can be processed attached to the mesh. The histotechnologist can use the mesh as a guide to orientation.

Number of levels per paraffin block

The tissue in a paraffin block is 0.1 to 0.3 cm in thickness. Tens to hundreds of glass slides can potentially be prepared from this tissue. The first slide made is a representative section of the tissue. A "ribbon" of tissue may be made from small specimens and placed on the slide. This ribbon includes consecutive tissue sections and rarely reveals new information unless the pathologic finding is very small (e.g., viral inclusions). For large lesions, one slide representative of the tissue present is usually adequate.

Levels refer to sections taken at different depths through the block, typically 0.02 mm (20 μm) to 0.2 mm apart. Multiple levels can be helpful in the following circumstances:

Small lesions (less than the thickness of the block, typically 1 to 2 mm) may be present on some levels but not on others or better seen on some levels. Examples include small foci of prostatic carcinoma or breast ductal proliferations associated with calcifications.

Demonstrating the relationship of a lesion to a margin over a small area (e.g., a close margin on a prostatectomy).

Additional histochemical or immunoperoxidase studies: If it is anticipated that lesions will be small (e.g., prostate lesions and micrometastatic melanoma), intervening unstained levels may be cut up front. In most cases, enough tissue is left in the block in order to be able to order such studies, if necessary.

Evaluation of multiple fragments of tissue: Levels can ensure that all fragments are well represented. Many pathologists have experienced the "Atlantis phenomenon," when an entirely unexpected fragment of tissue appears on a deeper level. Although it is optimal to have all fragments embedded in the same plane, in practice this is difficult to achieve.

The number of routinely examined levels varies for different organ sites and among pathology departments. A reasonable approach is to obtain two to three levels (the first superficial and the last approximately halfway through the tissue) as standard processing for small biopsies. Good communication between the clinician taking the biopsy and the pathologist is very helpful to guide the need for additional levels if the initial slides do not correlate with the lesion biopsied.

The optimal number of levels has been critically examined for certain specimens:

Prostate needle biopsies. At least three levels were required for prostate needle biopsies.[1,2] An additional level was found to be helpful only in cases that revealed focal glandular atypia in the initial three slides.[3]

Endomyocardial biopsies for myocarditis. The majority of diagnoses could be made on a relatively superficial level (approximately 15% of the distance through the tissue) but some required sectioning at least halfway through the block, and 1 of 20 biopsies was only diagnostic when 70% of the tissue had been sectioned.[4]

Endoscopic colon biopsies. If additional levels are obtained on colon biopsies that are initially nondiagnostic (either by taking levels deeper into the block or by re-embedding the tissue and taking levels from the opposite side), 10% to 31% of cases reveal diagnostic features of either adenomatous or hyperplastic polyps.[5-7]

Breast core needle biopsies. Examination of the fifth (of eight) levels was required to accurately classify atypical ductal hyperplasia and atypical small acinar proliferations in breast core needle biopsies.[8] However, since the fifth level was essentially halfway through the tissue, the depth of leveling may be more important than the number of levels.

Sentinel lymph nodes. Numerous studies have shown that additional levels detect additional small tumor deposits in lymph nodes. It is universally agreed that metastases >0.2 cm in size are of prognostic significance and sampling techniques should be designed to detect all such macrometastases (see p. 525, "Sentinel lymph nodes"). The value of serendipitously finding micrometastases by examining multiple levels has not been established.

Special stains

For some types of small biopsies, special stains are almost always helpful and may be ordered on every case (liver, transbronchial, kidney, transplant kidney, bone marrow, testicular, and temporal artery biopsies; Table 3-1). The types of stains ordered vary among institutions. For large specimens it is preferable to view the H&E sections first to decide whether special stains are needed and, if so, to choose the optimal blocks for the performance of the studies.

Identification of tissue

Extreme care must be taken to ensure that tissues always correspond to the correct patient. The cassette number must always be checked against the number of the case on the specimen requisition form and the number on the specimen container before tissue is placed in the cassette. It is useful to keep a log-in sheet that records the specimen number, the number of cassettes, and the number of tissue fragments in each cassette. Special care must be taken when two similar specimens (e.g., two liver biopsies or two transbronchial biopsies) are received at the same time. Consecutive numbers should be avoided for such specimens, if possible.

If specimens are placed into the incorrect cassette, it may be impossible to correctly identify the case

Table 3-1 Routine stains and levels and instructions for biopsies

Bladder	2 H&E	
Bone marrow	1 H&E (3L), 2 Giemsa (1L & 4L)	
Breast, needle biopsy	3 H&E	Indicate cassettes containing calcifications
Cell block	2 H&E	Special stains are ordered if needed
Endobronchial	3 H&E	Special stains are ordered if needed
Heart	3 H&E, 1 unstained	Unstained used for special stains if needed
Kidney	3 H&E (1L, 3L, 5L), 2 PAS (2L, 6L), 1 AFOG (4L)	
Large bowel biopsy	2 H&E	
Polyps	2 H&E	Bisect along stalk, if too wide to fit into a cassette; trim the edges and submit in a separate cassette
Larynx/oropharynx	3 H&E	
Liver (needle)*	2 H&E (1L, 5L), 1 TRI (2L), 1 IRON (3L), 1 RETIC (4L)	Non-neoplastic disease.
	3 H&E	Tumors
Prostate (needle)	3 H&E (levels 1, 3, 5), 2 unstained (levels 2, 4)	
Prostate TURP	1 H&E	Submit 12 cassettes (if 1 to 2, order 2 L)
Sentinel lymph nodes	3 H&E	3 equally spaced levels (melanoma and breast)
Skin		
Punch >0.3 cm	3 H&E	Bisect or trisect
Punch <0.3 cm	3 H&E	Submit entire. Laboratory will bisect.
Punch with vesicle	3 H&E	Submit entire. Laboratory will bisect.
Shave	2 H&E	The specimen is bisected by the laboratory and embedded on edge
Ellipse	2 H&E if < 2 cm	
	1 H&E if > 2 cm	
Small bowel		Wrap each mesh with biopsy in lens paper, submit in separate
Hollandes:	3 H&E	cassettes, wash in tap water
Formalin:	3 H&E	
Stomach	2 H&E	Alcian yellow added if bx is for gastritis from the antrum
Testicle	2 H&E (1L, 5L), 1 PAS (2L), 1 ET (3L), 1 TRI (4L)	
Temporal artery	3 H&E (1L, 3L, 5L) 2 ET (2L, 4L)	Submit uncut. Laboratory will cut into sections and embed on end.
Transbronchial*	3 H&E, 1 MSS	If granulomatous disease is probable, order AFB and Gram
	3 L if probable tumor	Submit uncut. Laboratory will cut into sections and embed
Vas deferens	1 L	on end

* Special stains should not be ordered on liver or transbronchial biopsies for suspected tumor.
See Table 7.1; Histochemical stains, p 71 for a description of special stains

histologically if the types of tissue confused are similar (e.g., two skin punch biopsies). The gross description of the number and size of fragments may sometimes help in identifying the correct case number.

In some cases it may be necessary to use special techniques to correctly identify specimens. However, these methods are costly and time consuming and should be avoided if possible.

Methods used to identify specimens have included the following:

Immunoperoxidase studies for ABH blood group antigens can be performed but they require a relatively large piece of tissue in order to have enough blood vessels (endothelial cells and red blood cells) to evaluate. This method is most useful to identify a possible mix-up between two specific specimens (e.g., two bone marrow biopsies) if the two patients are known to be of

different blood types. Common fixatives do not change antigenicity, but decalcification can diminish immunoreactivity for H antigen.[9–11]

HLA typing using PCR can be used to identify very small tissue fragments microdissected from glass slides.[12,13]

Polymorphic microsatellite markers can be analyzed using PCR and can be used to provide a definite match (or mismatch) between a patient and a specimen.[14–18]

The Armed Forces DNA Identification Laboratory (AFDIL) can identify fixed specimens using a variety of techniques (see www.afip.org, for details).

Extraneous tissue ("floaters")

Extraneous tissue consists of fragments of tissue that are present on a slide but are derived from a different specimen. This becomes a significant problem if the extraneous tissue contains malignant cells because it may be impossible to determine definitively that the tissue is extraneous and does not belong to the specimen. Extraneous tissue may contaminate other tissue prior to its arrival in the pathology department, as it is being processed in the cutting room, from small pieces of loose tissue in a tissue processor (typically placental villi), or during slide preparation.

In a large study, extraneous tissue was found on 0.6% of slides in a prospective study and 2.9% of slides in a retrospective study.[19] Most of the extraneous tissue was introduced during preparation of the slide. In less than a third of the cases, the tissue was in the paraffin block. In 0.3% to 3.1% of cases with extraneous tissue, the extraneous tissue caused moderate to severe diagnostic difficulty.

Extraneous tissue can also cause problems when microdissection and sensitive molecular techniques are used. Special microtomes, water baths, and cleaning procedures may be required.

Extraneous tissue should be diligently avoided using the following precautions:

- All dissecting tools (forceps, scissors, scalpel) should be kept in a jar of water between uses. This will wash off small tissue fragments and avoid larger fragments adhering to dirty tools. Do not reuse a scalpel blade for more than one case. Tissue often sticks to one side of a blade (inevitably the side that is out of view).
- The dissection area should be kept clean. After cutting in any case with known malignancy, be especially fastidious in removing any soiled material on the cutting surface, gloves, or other surfaces.
- Small fragments and friable specimens should be wrapped in paper or placed in a bag to prevent tissue fragments escaping from a cassette.
- Solutions in tissue processors should be changed routinely.
- During embedding, tools and equipment must be cleaned between cases.
- Water baths (used when making glass slides) should be kept free of extraneous tissue between specimens.

The significance of extraneous tissue may range from the trivial to the diagnostically dangerous. Strategies for identifying tissue as extraneous include:

- Checking the block to see if the extra fragment is present. If it is not, or additional recuts do not reveal the fragment, this is evidence that the fragment may have been introduced during slide preparation.
- Checking other cases processed the same day to determine if the tissue in the fragment resembles another case.
- Looking for ink on the suspected extraneous tissue. If ink is present, and the correct specimen tissue was not inked, this is evidence that it is tissue from a different case.
- Submitting additional tissue from the specimen to determine if additional tissue fragments similar to the possible extraneous tissue are present.

There is no standard procedure for documenting extraneous tissue on a slide. Various methods used by pathologists include:

- Circling the extraneous tissue and writing "floater" or its equivalent on the glass slide.
- Making deeper levels that do not include the extraneous tissue. The deeper levels become the permanent slides and the initial slide(s) are discarded.
- If the extraneous tissue is in the paraffin block, the tissue may be removed from the block and new slides prepared. The initial slide(s) are discarded.
- Noting the presence of extraneous tissue in the pathology report.
- Keeping a separate logbook or computerized record of slides with extraneous tissue.

Very obvious cases of no diagnostic importance may not require documentation.

In exceptional cases in which it cannot be determined if important diagnostic tissue is intrinsic or extrinsic to a specimen, it may be necessary to type the tissue (see "Identification of tissue" above). If such methods fail to provide a definitive answer, the case must be signed out with extraneous tissue in the differential diagnosis. The clinician should be called and informed of the situation so that he or she can decide whether additional biopsies are warranted.

REFERENCES

1. Renshaw AA. Adequate tissue sampling of prostate core needle biopsies. Am J Clin Pathol 107:26-29, 1997.
2. Brat DJ, Wills ML, Lecksell KL, Epstein JI. How often are diagnostic features missed with less extensive histologic sampling of prostate needle biopsy specimens? Am J Surg Pathol 23:257-262, 1999.
3. Reyes AO, Humphrey PA. Diagnostic effect of complete histologic sampling of prostate needle biopsy specimens. Am J Clin Pathol 109:416-422, 1998.
4. Burke AP, Farb A, Robinowitz M, Virmani R. Serial sectioning and multiple level examination of endomyocardial biopsies for the diagnosis of myocarditis. Mod Pathol 4:690-693, 1991.
5. Li-cheng Wu M, Dry SM, Lassman CR. Deeper examination of negative colorectal biopsies. Am J Clin Pathol 117:424-428, 2002.
6. Nash JW, Niemann T, Marsh WL, et al. To step or not to step: an approach to clinically diagnosed polyps with no initial pathologic finding. Am J Clin Pathol 117:419-423, 2002.
7. Calhoun BC, Gomes F, Robert ME, Jain D. Sampling error in the standard evaluation of endoscopic colon biopsies. Am J Surg Pathol 27:254-257, 2003.
8. Renshaw AA. Adequate sampling of breast core needle biopsies. Arch Pathol Lab Med 125:1055-1057, 2001.
9. Adegboyega PA, Gokhale S. Effect of decalcification on the immunohistochemical expression of ABH blood group isoantigens. Appl Immunohistochem Mol Morphol 11:194-197, 2003.
10. Ota M, Fukushima H, Akamatsu T, Nakayama J, Katsuyama T, Hasekura H. Availability of immunostaining methods for identification of mixed up tissue specimens, Am J Clin Pathol 92:665-669, 1989.
11. Ritter JH, Sutton TD, Wick MR. Use of immunostains to ABH blood group antigens to resolve problems in identity of tissue specimens. Arch Pathol Lab Med 118:293-297, 1994.
12. Shibata D. Identification of mismatched fixed specimens with a commercially available kit based on the polymerase chain reaction. Am J Clin Pathol 100:666-670, 1993.
13. Bateman AC, Sage DA, Al-Talib RK, Theaker JM, Jones DB, Howell WM. Investigation of specimen mislabelling in paraffin-embedded tissue using a rapid, allele-specific, PCR-based HLA class II typing method. Histopathology 28:169-174, 1996.
14. Abeln EC, van Kemenade FD, van Krieken JH, Cornelisse CJ. Rapid identification of mixed up bladder biopsy specimens using polymorphic microsatellite markers. Diagn Mol Pathol 4:286-291, 1995.
15. Gras E, Matias-Guiu X, Catasus L, Arguelles R, Cardona D, Prat J. Application of microsatellite PCR techniques in the identification of mixed up tissue specimens in surgical pathology. J Clin Pathol 53:238-240, 2000.
16. O'Brian DS, Sheils O, McElwaine S, McCann SR, Lawler M. Sorting out mix-ups. The provenance of tissue sections may be confirmed by PCR using microsatellite markers. Am J Clin Pathol 106:758-764, 1996.
17. Kessis TD, Silberman MA, Sherman M, Hedrick L, Cho KR. Rapid identification of patient specimens with microsatellite DNA markers. Mod Pathol 9:183-188, 1996.
18. Hunt JL, Swalsky P, Sasatoni E, Niehouse L, Bakker A, Finkelstein D. A microdissection and molecular genotyping assay to confirm the identity of tissue floaters in paraffin-embedded tissue blocks. Am J Clin Pathol 127:213-217, 2003.
19. Gephardt GN, Zarbo RJ. Extraneous tissue in surgical pathology. A College of American Pathologists Q-Probes study of 275 laboratories. Arch Pathol Lab Med 120:1009-1014, 1996.

The surgical pathology report: from the glass slide to the final diagnosis

4

After the specimen has been processed and the glass slides made, the pathologist must render a diagnosis. Numerous large, multi-volume, multi-authored pathology texts are available to aid in diagnosis. Once the interpretation has been made, a surgical pathology report is issued and becomes part of the patient's medical record. The pathology report serves five main purposes, providing:

1. **Diagnostic and prognostic information** for the individual patient.
2. **Information to guide treatment** of the individual patient.
3. **Criteria for eligibility for clinical trials.** Since the results of these trials will affect the treatment of many other patients, the accuracy of information in the report affects not only the individual patient enrolled in a trial, but many other patients as well.
4. **Information for clinical databases** to be used in both clinical and basic research. The content of pathology reports is important for the understanding of disease processes as well as new investigations into the treatment and pathogenesis of disease.
5. **Quality assurance.** The contents of the pathology report may be reviewed to evaluate various indicators of quality care for pathology departments and for the overall care of patients.

■ ELEMENTS OF A SURGICAL PATHOLOGY REPORT

- Institution identifiers: Name, address, telephone number, FAX number.
- Patient identifiers: Name, date of birth, hospital identification number, gender.
- Name of the pathologist responsible for the report.
- Name of the clinician(s) submitting the specimen as well as other clinicians caring for the patient.
- Specimen number: A unique specimen identification number assigned by the pathology department. This number should be located prominently at the top portion of each page of the report for easy identification.
- Date of procedure and date the specimen was received.
- Date the report was issued.
- Clinical history.
- Type of specimen submitted, including a list of all specimens submitted.

- Operating room consultation reports: The specimen examined, type of examination (gross examination, frozen section, cytologic preparations), and intraoperative diagnosis are listed. The pathologist responsible for rendering the diagnosis is identified.
- Gross description: Include the disposition of all tissue (e.g., saved for EM, frozen, research) and any special techniques used (e.g., decalcification, inking of margins). Specify whether all or only a part of the specimen has been submitted.
- Other materials received, such as specimen radiographs (describe what they show) and peripheral blood smears.
- Description of tissue submitted for microscopic sections: Type of tissue, number of cassettes. It is preferable to provide each block of tissue with a unique identifier.
- Microscopic description: Provided when appropriate, as in unusual tumors or diseases. A microscopic description is not necessary for every specimen if important information is provided in the diagnosis.
- Specimen heading: The organ, site, and type of procedure are specified. In some cases, specific labeling provided by the surgeon may be required to identify the specimen (e.g., a specimen labeled "closest margin").
- Diagnosis: The type or types of pathologic processes present. Important information from the gross examination (e.g., tumor size) is included. The results of special studies are discussed. Discrepancies between the intraoperative diagnosis and the final diagnosis are discussed.
- A statement that the pathologist has examined gross and/or microscopic tissues before rendering the diagnosis may be required for billing purposes.
- Consultations: Intradepartmental consultations can be documented by including the names of the consulting pathologists. External consultations initiated by the pathologist can be documented by incorporating the consultant's report. External consultations not initiated by the pathologist may be incorporated at his or her discretion.
- Checklists for malignant tumors: Include all relevant information for prognosis and staging. Used in addition to, or sometimes in lieu of, a diagnosis in some institutions. The CAP (see www.cap.org) and the ADASP (see www.panix.com/~adasp/) have published suggested synoptic reporting forms (see Part 2).

- AJCC classification: For tumor resections, the pathologist should provide sufficient information for T and N classifications to be made. The actual T and N categories may be provided. Staging is not required as this often requires additional information (e.g., the results of the metastatic work-up) not available to the pathologist.
- Suggestions for clinicians: These are usually best discussed directly with the clinician. When incorporated into the report, they should, in general, be phrased as suggestions.
- Clinically significant unsuspected findings: It is preferable that such findings be conveyed immediately to the clinician(s) with a phone call. This may be documented in the report.
- Amended reports: An amended report should be clearly indicated, preferably on the first page of the report and the date of the amendment given. It should be stated if the new information is different from the original information.
- A list of prior surgical and cytologic specimens from the same institution. It is helpful to have available a list of all prior diagnoses pertaining to a patient at the time of final sign-out to aid in the interpretation of the current specimen and to avoid possible errors.

This list incorporates the recommendations of the Association of Directors of Anatomic and Surgical Pathology.[1]

■ DIAGNOSTIC HEADINGS

Headings need to be as accurate and as informative as possible and should include:

- Organ or tissue
- Site
- Surgical procedure
- Relevant gross descriptors (e.g., length of colon, weight of the spleen)
- Specific designations given by the clinician (e.g., "tissue closest to the margin")

Usually the headings are based on the label used for the specimen or the gross recognition of the type of specimen. If the type of specimen or type of surgery cannot be recognized, it is generally preferable to discuss the case with the surgeon as the type of specimen can affect the method of processing as well as how the specimen should be billed.

Specimen headings using "Specimen labeled" often do not provide useful information on the type of specimen examined. For example, [Specimen labeled "Right Lung"]

could be anything from a transbronchial biopsy to an extrapleural pneumonectomy. This type of heading forces the reader to search for this important information in the gross description.

Examples of appropriate headings include:

Colon resections	Right colectomy (ascending colon and cecum (44 cm), terminal ileum (4 cm), and appendix
	Sigmoid colon (30 cm), resection
	Abdominoperineal resection—rectum (35 cm) and anus (15 cm)
Breast resections	Left breast, modified radical mastectomy and axillary dissection
	right breast, simple mastectomy
	Left breast, reexcision
	Right breast excisional biopsy, wire localization for calcifications
	Left breast, stereotactic 14-gauge core needle biopsies for a spiculated mass
Lung resections	Left lung, pneumonectomy
	Right lower lobe of lung, lobectomy
	Right upper lobe of lung, wedge resection
Prostate	Prostate, radical prostatectomy (42 g)
	Prostate, suprapubic prostatectomy (150 g)
	Prostate, transurethral resection (33 g)
Skin	Skin of chest, excision
	Skin of right leg, 3-mm punch biopsy
	Skin of face, shave biopsy

Never use a label that may be misleading (e.g., one that may imply an incorrect diagnosis) as someone reading the report may easily mistake a heading for a diagnosis.

All separately submitted specimens are given separate diagnoses with separate headings. If multiple specimens have the same name and it is appropriate to combine two or more separately submitted specimens (i.e., they all clearly represent the same type of tissue from the same site and separating the specimens does not provide additional information), this may be indicated in the heading [Mesenteric mass (two specimens)].

If frozen sections were performed, they may be incorporated into the heading: [Inguinal lymph node (including frozen section A and touch preparation A)].

■ STANDARDIZED DIAGNOSIS FORMS

CAP (www.cap.org) and ADASP (www.panix.com/~adasp) have developed standardized reporting forms for most common tumors.

Advantages of a standardized synoptic (*synoptic* is Greek for an overall view of things, a summary or synopsis) report include:

- Uniform diagnostic terms, criteria, and style are established for a department or group of pathologists. Additional standard criteria can be included in each report (the basis of grading systems, definitions, etc.).

- Provides checklists to ensure that important diagnostic and prognostic features are always included. Some data elements are now required for accreditation as a cancer center. Additional information for AJCC classification and/or grading can be incorporated into the standard form for easy access by the pathologist.
- Facilitates preparation of the report by staff and residents.
- Facilitates typing of reports by secretaries as mnemonics can be used for many sentences or phrases. This can shorten turn-around time by providing finished reports more quickly.
- Important information is easily accessible for clinicians.
- Information is readily incorporated into computerized databases.
- As a teaching tool, the report provides important diagnostic features of the most common diagnoses for each organ system.

However, descriptions of unusual or complicated specimens should not be squeezed into a standard format but must be given an appropriate individualized pathology report. Any type of standardized report needs to be flexible enough to allow additional comments for unusual findings.

There are disadvantages of synoptic reporting:

- It may adversely affect resident training by stifling independent thinking. Residents may become dependent on checklists and templates.
- Pathologists may not be able to reach a consensus on the types of information to be provided or on specific diagnostic criteria.
- Errors may be more difficult to detect with the use of templates as complete sentences or parameters may be changed by typographical errors.

In most cases, however, it should be possible to develop a system with enough standardization to provide important information for clinical management and enough flexibility to provide additional information for unusual cases. The use of checklists has been shown to significantly improve the incorporation of important information into pathology reports.[2]

Part 2 includes sign-out checklists for all major tumor types and resections and can be the basis for synoptic reporting. The lists are based on published recommendations, departmental recommendations by subspecialists, and the local needs of surgeons and oncologists. The lists need to be modified for the specific requirements of each institution and will require modification over time.

■ TURN-AROUND TIME

For optimal patient care, surgical cases need to be signed out in a timely fashion and clinicians must be kept informed of the status of cases. Standards have been developed for different types of specimens[3]:

Routine cases: two working days
Complex cases: additional time is allowed if special procedures are required.

Turn-around time is measured from the time of specimen accession (day 0) to the day the report is signed by the pathologist. In the report cited above, 95% of routine biopsy cases and 91% of routine complex cases were signed out within two working days.

■ MODIFICATION OF AN EXISTING REPORT

Additional information

It is not infrequent that information needs to be added to a report. This can be done in an addendum. However, pathologists must be aware that, because clinicians do not know that an addendum has been issued, many addenda are never seen or are overlooked by clinicians because the addendum is added to the bottom of the report or may be on a second page. If important information is pending, it is preferable in most instances to wait for the information to incorporate it into the main report (see below). If that would create a substantial delay, it is helpful to indicate in the initial report that an addendum will be added in the future so that clinicians are alerted to its existence. If an addendum must be added that contains important information, it is preferable also to notify the clinician to alert him or her to its addition.

Revised diagnosis

On rare occasions a final diagnosis must be changed. In one survey, 0.74 per 1000 final reports underwent a change in a final diagnosis.[4] The most common reasons for changing a diagnosis were:

1. A review requested by a clinician
2. An extradepartmental review requested by the pathologist
3. Additional special stains or other studies
4. Additional clinical information was obtained
5. Intradepartmental consultation.

Given the potential harm an erroneous diagnosis can cause, it is usually preferable to delay issuing a report until all available information has been considered. Thus, it is advisable to seek intra- and extradepartmental consultations as well as special studies prior to rendering a final diagnosis in appropriate cases. In addition, clinicians play an important role in detecting pathology errors such as misidentification of patients or errors caused by failure to provide sufficient clinical information.

An issued final report is part of the medical record; changes to this report may be subject to institutional requirements and state laws regarding medical records. In general, changes must be made in a way that documents the change, and the date of the change, in a manner that does not alter or delete prior diagnoses.

An addendum may be added to the report explaining the change in diagnosis. However, it is helpful, if possible, to place a prominent message at the top of the main report to indicate that an important addendum has been added.

If the revised diagnosis replaces the original diagnosis in the main body of the report, it should be clearly labeled "revised diagnosis." The original report should be retained below with a heading to the effect "The following original diagnosis is retained for documentation purposes only."

Corrected reports

Occasionally, nondiagnostic errors are present in reports because of typographic mistakes or omissions, specimen misidentification, or the absence of important clinical information. The changes required can usually be made in an addendum. If the changes are significant, the clinician should be notified.

Change in patient identification

In the survey sited above, in 0.39 per 1000 reports there was a change in patient identification[4]. Unfortunately, most such errors are undetectable by the pathology laboratory if the specimen has been mislabeled. Original reports should be maintained for documentation purposes but corrections must be made. In rare cases, it may be necessary to use tissue identification techniques to determine the source of the specimen (see p. 32, "Identification of tissue").

■ DOCUMENTATION FOR BILLING

Some types of information must be documented in the gross description or final diagnosis in order to bill appropriately for the specimen. Failure to document this information could result in fines for over-billing.

Billing documentation in gross descriptions

- Type of specimen.
- Number of specimens.
- Decalcification of bone.
- Inking and sampling of margins (for breast biopsies).
- Lymph node evaluation (in some cases lymph nodes can be billed separately from the main resection).
- Intraoperative evaluation (gross or frozen sections, number of frozen sections).
- Specimen radiograph received and evaluated.

Billing documentation in final diagnosis

- Type of specimen.
- Number of specimens.
- Histochemical stains (types).
- Immunohistochemical studies (document each study).
- Microscopic evaluation of margins for breast biopsies.

Billing documentation for consultations

- Number of different accession numbers.
- Histochemical stains received and reviewed.
- Immunohistochemical studies received and reviewed.
- Immunoperoxidase studies performed.

REFERENCES

1. Association of Directors of Anatomic and Surgical Pathology. Standardization of the surgical pathology report. Am J Surg Pathol 16:84-86, 1992.
2. Zarbo RJ. Interinstitutional assessment of colorectal carcinoma surgical pathology report adequacy. Arch Pathol Lab Med 116:1113-1119, 1992.
3. Zarbo RJ, Gephardt GN, Howanitz PJ. Intralaboratory timeliness of surgical pathology reports. Arch Pathol Lab Med 120:234-244, 1996.
4. Nakhleh RE, Zarbo RJ. Amended reports in surgical pathology and implications for diagnostic error detection and avoidance. A College of American Pathologists Q-Probes Study of 1,667,547 accessioned cases in 359 laboratories. Arch Pathol Lab Med 122:303-309, 1998.

Consultation reports

5

■ TYPES OF CONSULTATION

Pathology consultations occur when slides are shown to a second pathologist and a second interpretation of the slides is documented. There are many types of consultation and each has different features. Types of consultation include:

- Intra-institutional consultations
- Specialist consultations
- Consultations for special studies
- Institutional consultations
- Medicolegal consultations
- Review of pathology slides or blocks for treatment protocols or research

The Association of Directors of Anatomic and Surgical Pathology has issued guidelines for consultations.[1-3]

■ INTRA-INSTITUTIONAL (IN-HOUSE) CONSULTATIONS

Pathologists within an institution or group often show slides to each other if the case is difficult or unusual. Some pathology groups have mandated review of certain types of case, and such review can reduce errors.[4] Daily or weekly "difficult case" conferences are used for this purpose.

The typical legal standard of care for pathologists is that the pathologist acts as another pathologist would in a similar situation. Thus, it is important to document that the case was shown to another pathologist should a legal issue arise. This can be accomplished by having two pathologists sign the report, by a note in the report (e.g., "This case was shown to Dr. Smith who concurs with the above diagnosis"), or documented as a record of a departmental conference. If the second pathologist only reviewed selected slides, this should be noted.

■ SPECIALIST CONSULTATIONS

The opinion of a specialist may be requested for difficult and unusual cases. A survey showed that 0.5% of cases,

on average, are sent for extradepartmental review.[5] Usually this type of consultation is initiated by the original pathologist. The referring pathologist should provide:

- **Selected representative slides.** Recuts that the specialist can keep for his or her files are often preferred. Special stains or immunoperoxidase studies should be included if they are important for diagnosis. Blocks or unstained (coated) slides should be included if it is anticipated that additional studies will be needed.
- **A letter explaining the reason for the consultation** and the difficulty as perceived by the referring pathologist. This letter should also document any specific issues that need to be addressed. In turn, the consultant should directly address these issues by direct communication with the referring pathologist, in a letter or in the consultation report. If the consult is sent to a specific pathologist, it is helpful to determine if the consultant is available to review the case in a timely fashion.
- **Clinical and demographic information on the patient.** This may include other reports as appropriate, such as radiologic reports of bone lesions or operative notes.
- **The pathology report, including the gross description and a description of the site of origin of each of the slides.** The report need not be signed out if it is being held for the opinion of the consultant. Pathology reports on other specimens should be included if they are relevant to the consultation.
- **The FAX number, telephone number, and address** of the requesting pathologist in order for the consultant to communicate the results in a timely fashion.
- **Reports of prior consultations on the same case.** If simultaneous consultations with other specialists have been requested, it is helpful to include this information.
- **Billing information.** The cost of the consultation is generally borne by the referring pathologist or his or her pathology group.

The specialist will generate a report and communicate the findings to the referring pathologist. Any irreplaceable materials (blocks, cytology slides, slides of lesions that are not seen on other levels, etc.) are returned to the original pathologist.

The results of the consultation should be incorporated into the original pathology report and communicated to the patient's physicians, if the referring pathologist agrees with the diagnosis. In unusual cases, if the referring pathologist does not agree with the diagnosis, it may be appropriate to seek consultation with other specialists. The referring pathologist may be held legally liable for errors made by the specialist and is responsible for the final diagnosis.

It is generally acknowledged that a specialist may use consultation cases as part of a larger series of cases for publication with acknowledgment of referring pathologists if possible. The authorship of specific case reports should be negotiated between the original pathologist and the specialist.

Information should not be withheld from the specialist. Cases involved in legal actions should be treated as legal consultations.

In some cases, a clinician or patient may initiate a second review by a specialist. In such cases the results are usually conveyed by the specialist to the patient's physician. In unusual cases, the patient may be contacted directly with the results. The results of the consultation should always be sent to the original pathologist as well. The cost is usually borne by the patient.

■ CONSULTATIONS FOR SPECIAL STUDIES

Special studies (most commonly immunoperoxidase studies but also EM or DNA analysis) are sometimes required for the evaluation of certain cases. Appropriate materials may be sent either to other pathology departments or to commercial laboratories that offer these services. In order to obtain the maximum benefit from such consultations the following should be sent:

- Appropriate materials for the study requested (e.g., paraffin blocks containing the lesion, fresh tissue, tissue fixed for EM)
- The diagnosis or differential diagnosis
- The specific studies requested
- Demographic information on the patient for identification
- Billing information

A report giving the results of the special studies is generated. The results should be incorporated into the original pathology report with an interpretation.

If an opinion on the diagnosis is also requested, the consultation is processed as for a specialist consultation.

■ INSTITUTIONAL CONSULTATIONS

Institutions often require pathology review for all patients seeking a second opinion or treatment, and this practice is recommended by the ADASP. These consultations provide the following:

- Confirmation of diagnosis prior to definitive treatment (e.g., chemotherapy or surgery)
- Provision of additional information that may be used at the second institution but is not routinely provided in all pathology reports (e.g., breast cancer lymphovascular invasion)
- Correlation with subsequent findings if the patient undergoes surgery at the second institution (e.g., evaluation of a re-excision for residual carcinoma).

Many studies have analyzed the results of institutional consultations[6–16]. The following general conclusions have been drawn:

- Pathologic diagnosis is very accurate and in more than 90% of cases the original diagnosis is confirmed. These reports may be used as part of the JCAHO-required quality assurance program.
- In approximately 5% of cases a significant change in diagnosis results in a change in patient treatment. The ADASP has suggested that an acceptable threshold for significant disagreement is 2%.[1–3]
- In a greater number of cases, additional information is provided by the second review and this information is useful to help guide treatment at the second institution.
- In most studies, when there is a discrepancy, the second reviewer's diagnosis is correct more often than the original diagnosis. In many cases, the discrepancy is the result of differences in criteria or interpretative opinions for lesions known to be subject to high degrees of interobserver disagreement. In some cases, the original diagnosis proves to be correct and the original pathologist may choose to seek additional opinions.
- The cost of reviewing pathology slides is minimal compared to the cost of treatment or the potential morbidity of inappropriate treatment. Therefore, a second review is generally recommended to improve patient care and reduce medical costs.

If a consultation results in a significant change in interpretation, it is recommended that the reviewing pathologist do the following:

- Contact the original pathologist to inform him or her of the change in diagnosis. Both pathologists should try to resolve any differences that might be caused by the review of different slides or levels, the performance of additional special studies, or knowledge of additional clinical information. The second pathologist may choose to seek additional opinions.
- Contact the treating physicians to ensure that the patient receives appropriate treatment.
- Provide a rationale for the change in diagnosis in the report, when possible. For example, rather than reporting on lymph nodes previously diagnosed as free of metastases as "Metastatic carcinoma present in a lymph node," it is more helpful and informative to report the findings as "Metastatic carcinoma present in a lymph node. The metastasis measures much less than

0.1 cm in size, is seen only in the deeper level prepared for the consultation, and is not seen in the original slide." If the discrepancy is in the interpretation of a difficult lesion, this can also be explained (e.g., "The differential diagnosis includes carcinoma in situ and high grade dysplasia, however the former diagnosis is favored due to the following...").

The following material should be sent for an inter-institutional consultation:

- Slides relevant to the consultation (see below). It is preferable that these slides be reviewed before being sent, particularly if recuts are performed, to ensure that the original findings are present and that there are no new additional findings.
- The original pathology report.
- The reports of other consultations.
- A letter stating what materials are being sent and requesting return of the materials after consultation. This letter includes the address and phone number of the institution to facilitate the return of materials.
- Other reports, if relevant (e.g., hormone receptor studies for breast carcinomas if not included in the original pathology report).

Blocks need not be sent unless specifically requested. In general, blocks and slides should not be sent together to avoid the possibility of losing all of the patient's materials. If the second institution requests blocks to perform special studies, only selected blocks should be sent or additional glass slides can be prepared and sent. If the lesion is small (i.e., seen in only one block), it may be preferable to have the original slides returned before the block is sent or to send unstained slides. In general, recuts and/or special studies performed by the consulting institution are not returned to the original institution.

It is preferable that only slides relevant to the consultation be sent. Due to the fact that second review is known to reveal errors in a small number of cases, it is important to focus such reviews on current medical treatment and not on potential medicolegal issues (see "Legal consultations" below). For example, review of prior prostate core needle biopsies after a diagnosis of prostatic carcinoma has been rendered may reveal a small focus of atypical ducts or carcinoma that had been missed. However, this is a legal and not a medical issue and would be better addressed as a legal consultation. Slides that need not be sent would include:

- Prior benign biopsies (unless specifically requested).
- Prior fine needle aspiration (FNA) or core needle biopsies if there has been a subsequent excision with a concordant diagnosis. For example, it would be appropriate to send an FNA with a suspicious or malignant diagnosis if the subsequent excision was diagnosed as benign, but not if it was diagnosed as malignant.
- Irrelevant specimens (e.g., a prior cholecystectomy in a patient with lung cancer).

- Irrelevant slides (e.g., slides that would not have findings that would change current evaluation or treatment).

The choice to review or not to review slides once they have been received by a second institution or pathologist is a controversial one, and clear guidelines have not been developed. If the pathology is unrelated to the current disease or currently affected organ system, it is generally agreed that these slides need not be reviewed at the discretion of the pathologist, due to lack of medical necessity. Prior cytologic diagnoses need not be reviewed if the diagnosis was subsequently confirmed by a biopsy.

Slides on specimens related to the patient's current disease should be reviewed. This is the current policy of Brigham and Women's Hospital. If certain types of specimens are not reviewed, there should be a general policy that applies to all such cases (e.g., all prostate core needle biopsies prior to a diagnosis of carcinoma or all lymph nodes from breast cancer patients excised more than one year prior to consultation).

A report is generated by the second hospital. The cost of the consultation is usually borne by the patient or the patient's insurance company.

All original slides, blocks, and the consultation report are returned to the original institution. If the reviewing pathologist wishes to keep original slides, the request must be approved by the referring institution.

■ LEGAL CONSULTATIONS

A request from lawyers for materials related to a legal action may be in the form of a subpoena that often includes a blanket request for all slides, reports, blocks, and wet tissue pertaining to the patient. The original slides are considered legal evidence. This material may be difficult for pathologists to provide, is often irrelevant to the case, and may also be requested by the opposing lawyers. Since these materials constitute the patient's medical record, it is not in the patient's best interest that the entire record becomes sequestered as legal evidence. Such materials may not be returned after the legal action is finished. In addition, pathologists can be held liable for the loss of such materials unless specifically ordered by a court to release them.

It is preferable for the pathologist to discuss the case with the lawyer to determine the material that is actually necessary for the legal evaluation of the case. In some cases, it may be arranged for the materials to be reviewed at the original institution. This is recommended in cases in which the material is irreplaceable (e.g., cytology slides).

Reimbursement can be requested for the cost of reviewing and retrieving slides and for making new slides if necessary. These requests may or may not be honored by the requesting law firm.

It may be advisable to contact the insurer of the pathologist or institution before sending out materials.

This is particularly true if the institution or physicians associated with the institution are named in the lawsuit.

A pathologist may be asked to be an expert consultant in a legal case. In general, a pathologist makes an agreement with a law firm to review slides and possibly offer testimony in court or as a deposition. The pathologist may be asked to offer an expert opinion on issues not generally addressed medically. For example, a typical issue in failure to diagnose breast cancer is "retrognosis" (trying to determine the probable size of the cancer in the past) as opposed to the typical medical issues of prognosis.

It is inappropriate for a patient, clinician, or pathologist to request review of a case for legal reasons as an institutional consultation. Such consultations are intended for review to guide patient care. Legal consultations are typically handled as personal consultations to a specific pathologist and billed to the legal firm.

■ REVIEW FOR RESEARCH OR TREATMENT PROTOCOLS

Pathology materials are sometimes requested as part of a research project or a treatment protocol into which a patient has been enrolled[17-18]. It is the pathologist's role to balance the best interests of the patient with the need for medical research.

Blanket requests for all slides and blocks, to be stored permanently as part of a research protocol, are generally not in the best interest of the patient and may also interfere with other equally valid research projects. It is usually not known how quickly such materials could be made available for patient care. In addition, if the project is terminated there may not be funds to ensure the return of all the materials collected, just as research projects rarely provide funds for the collection and sending of such materials.

The following guidelines are suggested:

- Recut selected glass slides are preferable to releasing original material. Slides appropriate for the proposed study (e.g., unstained tissue on coated slides for immunoperoxidase studies) can be sent. The researchers will need to address the appropriateness of such materials for their studies (e.g., possible loss of antigenicity in cut slides over time).
- If blocks are released, a time limit should be imposed for return of the block. The researchers may make recuts but should not exhaust the tissue in the block.
- Release of paraffin blocks for permanent storage for possible future studies is, in general, discouraged unless multiple blocks demonstrating the pathologic lesion are available. For example, new markers relevant to current treatment of the patient (e.g., HER-2/neu immunohistochemistry for eligibility for Herceptin treatment) may require the ready accessibility of paraffin blocks.

- It may be possible to take cores of tissue from a block for the preparation of tissue arrays, but to leave sufficient tumor tissue in the block should additional studies be required. The original pathology department should be contacted before using blocks for such a purpose.

There are also issues of patient confidentiality involved in their material being used in research protocols. It may become necessary in the future for such materials to be coded to prevent identification of the patient. It may be possible to remove patient identifiers from pathology reports.[19] In some cases, ethical issues may arise, such as whether to reveal or not reveal new information discovered during examination of cases as part of a research protocol (e.g., gene carrier status, previously undetected lymph node metastases). These issues should be addressed in conjunction with Human Studies Committees prior to the start of a research project.

■ RECEIVING CONSULTATION MATERIALS

All materials received for consultation must be documented. This is important both for evaluating possible discrepancies in diagnosis due to review of different materials and for appropriate return of the materials.

The materials received are checked against the letter listing the materials sent by the other institution. Any discrepancies should be resolved by calling the original pathology department.

All slides and blocks must be accompanied by the corresponding pathology report to ensure that the slides correspond to the correct patient. In unusual circumstances, if the original pathology report is unavailable (e.g., slides received from another country) the circumstances of how the slides were received and the name of the person confirming the identification of the slides should be documented.

The name and birth date or age of the patient is checked for each set of slides. Sometimes hospitals send all specimens from different patients with the same name. Failure to detect misidentified material can result in significant errors in diagnosis and treatment.

Gross descriptions of consult cases

A sample dictation is as follows:

1. The first statement is a summary listing all slides and blocks received as well as the name of the institution and the complete mailing address (not a PO Box) for US institutions. If the slides are from another country, the complete mailing address (not a PO box) and a telephone number must be included. This is necessary to ensure that the materials can be returned:

Received from Memorial Hospital, 52 Washington Street, Harvard, MA 02365, are five glass slides and two paraffin blocks.

Received from King Edward X Memorial Hospital, Department of Pathology, 12 Hollingsbrook Road, Hamilton DV-04, Bermuda, are five (5) glass slides and two (2) paraffin blocks.

If materials are received from more than one hospital, they are initially grouped together and later described separately:

Received from two different hospitals are 50 glass slides and 32 paraffin blocks.

2. The oldest specimen is described first, followed by each subsequent specimen in chronologic order. The number of slides and blocks, the main surgical number, subnumbers, and any labels (e.g., "iron stain") are listed. If slides were received broken, this is stated in the gross description. Each statement includes the type of specimen and the date of the procedure.

   If slides and blocks are received from more than one hospital, the oldest specimen is listed first, followed by the remaining specimens from that hospital. The specimens from the second hospital are then listed.

   If paraffin blocks are received, they are described along with the corresponding slides. If the blocks are to be recut, the recut slides corresponding to the consultation numbers are identified (e.g., block "C" is recut as block #1, block "E" is recut as block #2, etc.).

3. The surgical pathology report is stated as having been received. If the report is not available, obtain confirmation from the submitting physician.

   The original surgical pathology report is not received. According to Dr. H. Jones, the slide corresponds to a colon biopsy taken from the patient in June of 1993.

4. Describe any other material received with the case:
   Surgical pathology reports without slides (state the type of specimen, the date, and a brief summary of the outside diagnosis)
   Consult letters (from whom, to whom, on what date)
   Consultation reports (hospital, material, number, and date)
   X-rays (what type and on what date)
   Discharge summaries (number of pages, date).

Sample description

Received from Central Hospital, Someplace, NJ, are 16 glass slides and 2 paraffin blocks.

Eight of the slides and the two paraffin blocks are labeled S04-1261 and are described in an accompanying surgical pathology report as a bezoarectomy and pyloroplasty from a procedure on 3/10/04. The slides

are sublabeled "A," "B," "C," "D," "E," "F," "H," and "A-PAS," and the blocks are sublabeled "A" (recut as subnumber 1) and "B" (recut as subnumber 2). A report from Impox Incorporated, Smalltown, MA, numbered 04-50675 and dated 3/23/04, gives the results of BEZ-32 immunoperoxidase studies performed on paraffin blocks from this specimen (reported as "negative").

The remaining eight slides are labeled S04-2229 and sublabeled "1," "3," "4 Giemsa," "5," or not sublabeled (four slides, cytologic preparations), and are described in an accompanying surgical pathology report as core needle biopsies of a "liver tumor" from a procedure on 5/12/04.

Also received is an additional pathology report without accompanying slides numbered S04-3476, dated 5/3/04 describing a left supraclavicular lymph node biopsy (outside diagnosis: "Metastatic carcinoma").

Included is a consultation report from General Hospital, Elsewhere, MA, numbered S04-7661 and dated 4/15/04, on material from Central Hospital labeled S04-1261.

■ SENDING OUT SLIDES FOR CONSULTATION

Pathology departments frequently receive requests to send slides to other locations. The reason for the request must be clearly stated or determined as this will determine the types of material sent (see specific recommendations for the six types of consultations previously described).

When slides are sent, they should always be accompanied by the original pathology reports and other outside consultation reports on the same material. This should include information as to how the consultation should be billed. In some cases it may be appropriate to send additional information such as operative notes, radiologic reports, and electron micrographs. If the patient is seeking a second opinion, it is often preferable to have the clinician request the slides so that the slides can be forwarded to the consulting pathologist with the appropriate clinical history and the reason for consultation.

Slides must be sent in appropriate packaging, preferably in a plastic slide holder (packed so that the slides do not rattle) placed within a cardboard box or tube with supporting packing, to ensure their safe transfer to another institution. Dr. PP Rosen has published useful suggestions.[20]

■ SIGN-OUT OF CONSULT CASES

The headings give the name of the original hospital, the city, and the state. The specimen headings, in general, should be whatever the original hospital used. Include the surgical number and the date. Specify that slides were received and whether paraffin blocks were recut. For example:

Consult slides and paraffin blocks from Central Hospital, Someplace, NJ:

Bezoarectomy and pyloroplasty (S04-1261; dated 3/10/04):

In addition to the diagnosis of the tissue on the slides, the final report should also include the types of information listed below. Although the original surgical pathology reports should be kept on file, they are often more difficult to access than the consultation pathology report. In addition, the original report may not be readily available to clinicians or other pathologists later reviewing the case. Therefore, all information of pathologic importance should be abstracted from the original report and included in the consultation report (either in the gross description or the final diagnosis).

- Prognostic information from the gross description should be included (e.g., size of tumor, number of lymph nodes examined, etc.).
- If the slides are from a large resection, a brief description of the specimen (derived from the gross description) is helpful. For example:

According to the original surgical pathology report, the specimen consisted of an "ovoid tumor mass" (7 cm in greatest dimension) with focal areas of necrosis and hemorrhage which was covered by "a few strands of connective tissue and muscle."

- Information included in the original report, but not documented by the slides received, should be mentioned but with a disclaimer. For example:

According to the original surgical pathology report, four of five axillary lymph nodes were involved by metastatic carcinoma (slides not received for review).

- Any additional information of pathologic importance provided in the consultation material, such as results of electron microscopy or immunoperoxidase studies, is included with a statement as to whether or not they were reviewed as part of the consultation. For example:

According to the original surgical pathology report, the tumor cells were immunoreactive for S100 protein and melanoma specific antigen (HMB-45) and negative for keratin (CAM 5.2)(slides not received for review).

According to the original surgical pathology report, the tumor was sent for estrogen receptor analysis (positive at 100 fm/mg) and flow cytometric analysis (DNA index 1.9, S-phase fraction 22%).

- Review of special studies, such as histochemical stains and immunoperoxidase studies, that are interpreted as part of the consultation must be documented. For example:

Immunoperoxidase studies performed at the original institution on formalin-fixed tissue and reviewed here reveal that the malignant cells are immunoreactive for cytokeratin (AE1/AE3) and not immunoreactive for S100 and leukocyte common antigen, supporting the diagnosis of metastatic carcinoma.

- If there is a discrepancy with the original diagnosis (e.g., due to additional levels, special studies, or different diagnostic criteria), it is helpful to provide information as to why this occurred, (see "Institutional Consultations.")
- If unstained slides and/or paraffin blocks are received and additional studies are performed, this is specifically documented:

Immunoperoxidase studies on formalin-fixed tissue performed on recut sections reveal that the malignant cells are immunoreactive for S100 and HMB-45 and are not immunoreactive for cytokeratin (AE1/AE3) or leukocyte common antigen, supporting the diagnosis of metastatic melanoma.

REFERENCES

1. Association of Directors of Anatomic and Surgical Pathology. Consultations in surgical pathology. Am J Surg Pathol 17:743-745, 1993.
2. Association of Directors of Anatomic and Surgical Pathology. Consultations in surgical pathology. Am J Clin Pathol 102:152-153, 1994.
3. Association of Directors of Anatomic and Surgical Pathology. Consultations in surgical pathology. Hum Pathol 24:691-692, 1993.
4. Renshaw AA, Pinnar NE, Jiroutek MR, Young ML. Quantifying the value of in-house consultation in surgical pathology. Am J Clin Pathol 117:751-754, 2002.
5. Azam M, Nakhleh RE. Surgical pathology extradepartmental consultation practices, a College of American Pathologists Q-probes study of 2746 consultations from 180 laboratories. Arch Pathol Lab Med 126:405-412, 2002.
6. Abt AB, Abt LG, Olt GJ. The effect of interinstitution anatomic pathology consultation on patient care. Arch Pathol Lab Med 119:514-517, 1995.
7. Cooper K, Fitzgibbons PL. Surgical Pathology Committee of CAP, ADASP, Institutional consultations in surgical pathology. How should diagnostic discrepancies be handled? Arch Pathol Lab Med 126:650-651, 2002.
8. Epstein JI, Walsh PC, Sanfilioppos F. Clinical and cost impact of second-opinion pathology. Am J Surg Pathol 20:851-857, 1996.
9. Khalifa MA, Dodge J, Covens A, Osborne R, Ackerman I. Slide review in gynecologic oncology ensures completeness of reporting and diagnostic accuracy. Gynecol Oncol 90:425-430, 2003.
10. Kronz JD, Milord R, Wilentz R, Weir EG, Schreiner SR, Epstein JI. Lesions missed on prostate biopsies in cases sent in for consultation. Prostate 54:310-314, 2003.

11. Murphy WM, Rivera-Ramirez I, Luciani LG, Wajsman Z. Second opinion of anatomical pathology: a complex issue not easily reduced to matters of right and wrong. J Urol 165:1957-1959, 2001.

12. Staradub VL, Messenger KA, Hao N, Wiley EL, Morrow M. Changes in breast cancer therapy because of pathology second opinions. Ann Surg Oncol 9:982-987, 2002.

13. Tomaszewski JE, Bear HD, Connally JA, et al. Consensus conference on second opinions in diagnostic anatomic pathology. Who, what, and when. Am J Clin Pathol 114:329-335, 2000.

14. Tsung JS. Institutional pathology consultation. Am J Surg Pathol 28:399-402, 2004.

15. Weir MM, Jan E, Colgan TJ. Interinstitutional pathology consultations. A reassessment. Am J Clin Pathol 120:405-412, 2003.

16. Wurzer JC, Al-Saleem TI, Hanlon AL, Freedman GM, Patchefsky A, Hanks GE. Histopathologic review of prostate biopsies from patients referred to a comprehensive cancer center, correlation of pathologic findings, analysis of cost, and impact on treatment. Cancer 83:753-759, 1998.

17. Grody WW. Molecular pathology, informed consent, and the paraffin block. Diagn Mol Pathol 4:155-157, 1995.

18. Mills SE, Kempson RL, Fechner RE, et al. Guardians of the wax...and the patient [Editorial]. Mod Pathol 8:699-700, 1995.

19. Gupta D, Saul M, Gilbertson J. Evaluation of a deidentification (De-Id) software engine to share pathology reports and clinical documents for research. Am J Clin Pathol 121:169-171, 2004.

20. Rosen PP. Special report: Perils, problems, and minimum requirements in shipping pathology slides. Am J Clin Pathol 91:348-354, 1989.

Operating room consultations

6

■ PURPOSE OF OPERATING ROOM CONSULTATIONS

I wish you pathologists would find a way to tell us surgeons whether a growth is cancer or not while the patient is still on the table.

William Mayo, 1905

When cancer becomes a microscopic disease, there must be tissue diagnosis in the operating room.

Joseph Colt Bloodgood, 1927

There are three principal reasons for operating room (OR) consultations:

1. To provide rapid gross or microscopic diagnoses to guide intra- or perioperative patient management. The most common diagnoses requested include:
   - Identification of an unknown pathologic process
   - Evaluation of margins
   - Identification of lymph node metastases
   - Identification of tissues
2. So that tissue can be optimally processed for special studies to be used for diagnosis, treatment, or research.
3. To confirm that lesional tissue is present for diagnosis on permanent sections and/or after special studies.

■ FROZEN SECTIONS ARE NOT PERMANENT SECTIONS

The diagnostic information provided by frozen-section analysis is limited in comparison to the information based on permanent sections that can be provided in the final sign-out of a case:

- **Sampling.** Only minute portions of tissue can be frozen well. Thus, the amount of tissue that can be evaluated microscopically is only a small proportion of the tissue that is typically sampled for permanent sections.
- **Ice crystal artifact.** Freezing tissues can create artifacts that make diagnosis difficult or sometimes impossible. These tissue changes are permanent, and small lesions of primary diagnostic importance should not be frozen in their entirety. Other technical problems can also hinder intraoperative diagnosis.

- **Lack of special studies.** It is generally not possible to perform special histochemical or immunohistochemical studies in the timeframe of a surgical operation. Final diagnosis may require such studies and be altered according to the information gleaned from them.
- **Lack of consultation.** For some difficult or unusual lesions, the opinions of additional pathologists may be required for a final diagnosis.

For these reasons, the goals of intraoperative consultation must be limited to what is feasible and reliable under these conditions.[1] In most cases, the pathologist is able to provide the information needed by the surgeon to complete the operation.

■ INAPPROPRIATE FROZEN SECTIONS

The education of surgeons is the career-long task of the surgical pathologist. It must be a collegial process, never confrontational and never attempted when a patient is under anesthesia.

Virginia Li Volsi[2]

Potentially inappropriate frozen sections include the following:

1. **Unnecessary but not harmful to the patient.** An example is freezing a section of a large tumor for which further surgery or treatment is not anticipated until a diagnosis based on permanent section is obtained. Such cases may be avoided by discussion with the surgeon either during or after the procedure. Such practices result in increased charges without benefit to the patient.
2. **Unnecessary and potentially harmful to the patient.** These cases usually concern small primary lesions frozen in their entirety. Artifactual distortion or loss of tissue might prevent diagnosis. Although this applies to any site, frozen sections should especially be avoided in cases of pigmented skin lesions and small breast lesions. In such cases the pathologist must be an advocate for the patient and clearly explain that the patient's best interests (and ultimately the surgeon's) would not be served by performing a frozen section.
3. **Situations in which a frozen section has low sensitivity or specificity but could, rarely, be useful.** Examples of

this include frozen sections taken from a well-circumscribed follicular lesion of the thyroid to look for capsular invasion or the examination of a breast re-excision for DCIS at the margin. Pathologists, surgeons, and institutions usually have policies concerning the examination of such specimens. If a frozen section is performed, the surgeon must be aware of the possibility that there could be a change in diagnosis when permanent sections are studied.

The actual frequency of inappropriate frozen sections is reported to be less than 5% of all frozen sections.[3] However, in another study, frozen sections performed for apparently unnecessary reasons resulted in a change in patient outcome in 9% of cases.[4] Thus, when confronted with what appears to be an inappropriate request for frozen section, it would be advisable to enter into a discussion with the surgeon to determine what information is required by the surgeon and how he or she intends to use it. Such a dialogue can be an ideal forum for optimizing the use of intraoperative consultations.

■ PERFORMING OPERATING ROOM CONSULTATIONS

1. When the specimen is transported to the OR consultation room it must be accompanied by appropriate clinical information:
   - Patient identifiers (preferably a hospital or clinic number)
   - Relevant clinical history (e.g., results of a fine needle aspiration of a thyroid nodule prior to resection or prior history of malignancy)
   - Type of tissue or location of biopsy
   - Purpose of the consultation

   If the reason for examining the specimen is unclear, the surgeon must be contacted to avoid inappropriate specimen processing.

2. Examine the specimen and record a gross description (e.g., size and number of fragments, previously incised tumors, presence of localization wire). Information on what was done to the specimen (e.g., location of frozen sections, tissue removed for research, tissue taken for special studies) is recorded. A diagram can be invaluable to indicate the location of anatomic landmarks, lesions, margins, sites sampled, etc. If the orientation is unclear, call the surgeon to clarify.

3. Prepare cytologic preparations and/or frozen section(s) as appropriate.

4. An OR consultation diagnosis is rendered based on the gross and microscopic findings.

5. The results are communicated to the surgeon. The OR should be called first. If the surgeon is not present, page him or her, call the surgeon's office, or leave an e-mail message as necessary. If the surgeon cannot be contacted, document this in the report.

The optimal turn-around time for frozen sections is 15 minutes or less.

6. Record any relevant clinical information received from the surgeon or from the patient's chart, if it is provided. This information is often critical for the evaluation of the specimen and should be communicated to the pathologist responsible for the final diagnosis on permanent sections. This information can be recorded on the back of the OR consultation form.

7. All frozen-section remnants should be processed for permanent sections or saved frozen for special studies. The comparison of frozen sections to the permanent sections is an important quality control measure.

8. Tissue for special studies is allocated and taken to the appropriate laboratories.

Preparing frozen sections

Freezing is an imperfect but rapid method for solidifying small pieces of tissue in order to make thin sections for histologic examination. Ice crystals form within the tissue during freezing and can cause significant permanent artifacts. The secret to good frozen sections is in the preparation of the block.

There are many types of commercial cryostat and embedding techniques. However, the following general principles apply to most.

Tips for better frozen sections
Selecting the tissue

- Small, thin portions of tissue freeze best (generally not more than $0.5 \times 0.5 \times 0.3$ cm). Never try to freeze fragments larger than the diameter of the chuck. Tissues with little water (e.g., fat) do not freeze well and are extremely difficult to section. Avoid including fat in the specimen (e.g., around lymph nodes or breast lesions).
- Blot the outer surface of the specimen dry using a paper towel or gauze pad.
- If orientation is important (e.g., with en face sections), record how the specimen is oriented in the block.

Preparing the block (embedding medium frozen on a metal chuck)

- Embedding medium is placed on a metal chuck that has been pre-cooled in a cryostat. When partially frozen, the block can be inverted on the shelf to create a flat surface. Blocks with frozen embedding medium should be prepared prior to receipt of specimens to avoid wasting time waiting for the medium to freeze.
- If multiple small fragments must be sectioned, a special block may be prepared. After the embedding medium is frozen, pre-cut the block on the cryostat to create a flat surface in the plane of the blade. Tissue placed on this

block will all be in the same plane for cutting, which will maximize the amount of tissue on each glass slide.

- Do not use old blocks (e.g., those left overnight in a cryostat that goes through a freeze-thaw cycle) as they will be soft and crumbly.
- Embedding medium must be completely cleaned from the chuck (a toothbrush works well) before reuse. Crystals can be removed by dipping the chuck in methanol.

Freezing the tissue

- Place the tissue on the block, making sure the tissue is not folded. Cover the tissue rapidly with embedding medium. Activate a "quick freeze" option, if available, to cool the metal shelf holding the chucks.
- If positioning of a small fragment of tissue is important, add a drop of embedding medium to the top of the frozen block and place the tissue into this drop. The tissue can then be oriented before the embedding medium freezes.
- Different tissues require different freezing temperatures to cut well. For example, breast, skin, and fatty tissues must be kept very cold (i.e., –20°C) or they will be too soft to cut. Lymph nodes, spleen, brain, and liver cut better if the temperature is higher (i.e., –10°C) and may shatter during sectioning if too cold.
- When the embedding medium is partially frozen (i.e., begins to look opaque) the block may be rapidly cooled by turning it upside down on the metal shelf. Alternatively, a "heat extractor" (a plunger-shaped metal bar) can be placed on top of the tissue. However, this maneuver sometimes results in distortion of the tissue if it is performed before the embedding medium is sufficiently frozen. Wait until the center, as well as the outer rim, has had time to cool.

Commercially available aerosol sprays were used in the past to rapidly cool the block or parts of the cryostat. However, they are not necessary for the preparation of good quality frozen sections and their use is not recommended because of the danger of aerosolizing infectious agents. Three cases of conversion to a positive tuberculin skin test have been linked to aerosols produced by spraying a tissue block with a compressed gas coolant.[5,6]

The aerosol sprays should not be inhaled! Symptoms of overexposure include lightheadedness and shortness of breath. Inhalation is a possible cause of cardiac arrhythmias. Direct exposure of skin may cause frostbite. And if that isn't enough, the release of Freon contributes to the destruction of the ozone layer!

Cutting sections

- After the block is well frozen, the chuck is positioned in the cryostat for cutting. The block is manually moved forward until close to the blade.

- The blade and plate must be kept free of fragments of the embedding medium that can distort or wrinkle the frozen sections. Gauze firmly wrapped around a long swab can be kept cooled in the cryostat to be used for cleaning unused sections from the blade or chuck; this avoids changing the temperature and is also a much safer method of cleaning the blade. Avoid rubbing the gauze against the edge of the blade as this may dull the edge.
- As the blade cuts the tissue, the tissue must be gently anchored to prevent folding or curling. This can be accomplished with the anti-roll bar (a plastic plate attached to the cryostat) or by using a small pre-cooled paintbrush. After the section is cut, a glass slide is gently laid on top of the section. The tissue section will melt onto the slide. *The slide must immediately be placed in methanol.* Any delay in this step will introduce significant drying artifacts.
- If the specimen is too cold and is shattering, the block can be warmed slightly with a thumb.
- If true levels are desired (i.e., slides revealing deeper areas of the tissue), the block is moved forward manually, and another section taken at a deeper level. It would take over 100 passes of the knife to cut through a 1 mm thick specimen if the block was not advanced manually. Additional levels prepared without manual advancement rarely reveal additional histologic information.
- In general, two slides are sufficient for diagnosis and documentation. Additional slides may be made if the tissue is difficult to cut, true levels are made, or there are multiple pieces of tissue on the block at different levels that need to be evaluated.

Removing the block from the chuck

- *Never* cut blocks off chucks with a razor blade. The hardness of the embedding medium is highly variable and it is very easy to lose control of the blade and accidentally cut the fingers holding the chuck. Warm the chuck slightly by holding the stem for about 30 seconds; the block can then be removed with a finger. Alternatively the chuck can be dipped briefly in formalin or left on the counter for a minute or two.
- Excess embedding medium can be trimmed away from the tissue. The remaining tissue is placed in formalin to be submitted for permanent sections. Very small fragments should be wrapped in paper or placed in a small specimen bag.
- If tissue is to be saved frozen it should be transferred to another freezer. Most cryostats undergo freeze-thaw cycles that will damage tissue.
- The most representative frozen-section slide should be saved for filing with the permanent sections.

Staining slides

Fixed sections are stained with hematoxylin and eosin. The following procedure gives good results:

1. Stain in hematoxylin for a minimum of 90 seconds or 90 dips—agitation speeds the staining process. Cytology specimens can be stained for a shorter period of time (e.g., 30 seconds). Remove and blot excess dye on absorbent material.

   Stains nuclei blue.

2. Rinse slides in water with about 10 dips until gross stain is removed. Blot remaining water on a gauze pad. Change the water frequently between cases.

   Removes excess dye.

3. Dip three times, or for about 2 seconds, in acid alcohol (1% HCl in distilled water). Poor staining of nuclei could be due to too little hematoxylin staining or too long in HCl.

   Preferentially removes hematoxylin from non-nuclear components—"differentiation."

4. Dip three times, or for about 2 seconds, in ammonia water (2% sodium borate).

   This restores the basic pH to the dye and enhances the staining—"blueing."
   The color of the nuclei is changed from purple to blue. The time spent in the ammonia water does not alter staining.

5. Stain in eosin for 20 to 30 seconds, or with dips. Blot excess eosin on a gauze pad.

   Stains cytoplasm and other constituents pink to red.

6. Dehydrate the slide in successively increasing concentrations of alcohol, dipping approximately 10 times in each beaker. Let all the fluid drain off the slide.

   Removes excess eosin as well as water from the tissue.

   Poor staining can be due to prolonged time in alcohol.
7. Dip slides in xylene until the fluid runs clear on the slide (if there are streaks it means that there is water in the tissue). Slides are left in xylene until coverslipped to avoid drying artifact that can make interpretation difficult or impossible. Any water present in the xylene will result in cloudy sections.

   Xylene has a high index of refraction and renders tissues transparent.

8. Remove excess xylene from the slide by blotting on paper towels. Add one to two drops of mounting medium to the coverslip and gently place the slide on the coverslip. Avoid introducing bubbles. If bubbles are present, more xylene can be introduced under the edge of the coverslip to allow the slide to be read.

Slide holders should be rinsed it in a waste methanol container before replacing them in the methanol in the staining rack, to avoid carrying over xylene. Xylene in methanol produces almost unreadable cloudy slides with poor staining and bubble artifacts.

The staining racks should be kept covered to avoid evaporation and changes in pH.

Slides can be destained by going backwards through the solutions but skipping the eosin.

If slides need to be left in a solution for a period of time, the best choices are the ammonia water or the xylene. Prolonged time in HCl or alcohol will result in poor staining.

Performing frozen sections on fixed tissue

Formalin fixation denatures proteins; this adversely affects the adherence of tissues to glass slides. Formalin-fixed tissue therefore can be extremely difficult to examine by frozen section as the tissue tends to slide off the slide. If it is absolutely imperative to evaluate fixed tissue, the following modifications may be helpful:

- If the tissue is relatively large, and has not been in Formalin for a long time, tissue from the central portion of the specimen may have fewer changes due to fixation.
- Wash the tissue and blot dry prior to freezing. Formalin freezes at a lower temperature than water and can produce large ice crystals.
- Use coated slides (e.g., the type of slides used for immunohistochemistry).
- Allow the tissue to dry on the slide prior to staining.
- The HCl and ammonia water steps may be omitted.
- Perform all staining steps very gently and keep the slide at an angle to prevent the tissue from sliding off.

■ INTRAOPERATIVE CYTOLOGY

Cytologic examination can be as accurate as frozen sections for many specimens[7] and has the following advantages:

- It is rapid.
- There is no ice crystal artifact.
- It is easy to perform.
- All tissue is preserved for permanent sections or special studies.
- Large areas of tissue can be sampled.
- Cytologic information is provided, such as cell–cell cohesiveness (e.g., carcinoma versus lymphoma) and nuclear morphology (e.g., papillary thyroid carcinomas).
- It provides excellent teaching material with cytologic–histologic correlation.

Cytologic preparations are especially useful in the following situations:

- All suspected lymphoproliferative disorders
- Most CNS lesions
- Documentation of previously diagnosed malignancies before taking tissue for special studies or research

- Thyroid nodules
- Infectious cases (AIDS or hepatitis B) to avoid contaminating the cryostats or aerosolizing infectious agents (see Chapter 8, "Safety Precautions")
- Lung nodules with gross findings strongly suggesting infectious granulomas
- Minute specimens if additional material will not be available
- To sample tissue that would be difficult to cut in the cryostat (e.g., fatty tissue, necrotic tissue, bone specimens).

Preparation of cytology slides

1. Make a fresh cut through the tissue. The tissue should be free of gross blood. Lungs and other bloody tissues may require blotting of the surface with a paper towel.
2. **Touch preparations** are made by touching a glass slide to the tissue several times.

Smears are made by scraping the tissue with the edge of a glass slide. The material removed is evenly smeared onto a second glass slide.

Fine needle aspirations may be performed using a 23- or 25-gauge needle attached to a 10-mL syringe and making several passes through the lesion while pulling back on the plunger to create a vacuum. A small drop (approximately 2 to 3 mm in diameter) is expelled onto a glass slide and smeared with another glass slide.

3. **Hematoxylin and eosin staining.** The slides must be fixed *immediately* in methanol (without hesitation) to avoid drying artifacts. The slides are stained using the same protocol as for frozen sections. The appearance of the cells is similar to that seen on tissue sections and nuclear detail is well preserved.

Diff-Quik or Giemsa staining. The slides are air dried and then stained. The appearance of the cells is different from that seen in non-air-dried slides. Cytoplasmic features are well seen but nuclear detail is less distinct. Noncellular material is well seen (e.g., colloid, matrix in salivary gland lesions). This type of staining may be preferred for some specimens such as bone marrow aspirates, parathyroid glands, and salivary glands.

■ REPORTING THE RESULTS OF OPERATING ROOM CONSULTATIONS

A verbal report is given directly to the surgeon and a corresponding written report is generated.

Written reports

The OR consultation report should include the following:

- **Specimen heading** (type and number of specimens).
- **Type of examination** (gross examination, frozen section, cytologic examination).
- **Diagnosis.** The diagnosis should not include abbreviations that may not be well understood by other healthcare workers reading the report in the patient's chart.
- **Disposition of the tissue for special studies** (e.g., "Tissue saved for EM and sent for flow cytometry.").

An appropriate diagnosis can almost always be rendered by gross or microscopic examination. The annotation "diagnosis deferred" is used only when a decision is made not to provide a diagnosis (e.g., the tissue could not be cut or the block was lost inside the cryostat). It is not used to indicate that the final diagnosis will be based on permanent sections; this should be understood to be true for all cases examined by frozen section. In general, deferred diagnoses constitute less than 5% of all OR consultations.

Sample operating room consultation reports

Supraclavicular lymph node (frozen section A1 and touch preparation A2): Lymph node with no tumor seen.

Left breast biopsy, wire localization for a mass (frozen section A1): Invasive carcinoma (1.4 cm), present at the superior surgical resection margin.

Level 4 lymph nodes (frozen sections A1 and A2): Two lymph nodes with noncaseating granulomas.
Differential diagnosis includes sarcoidosis and infection.
Tissue is sent to microbiology for mycobacterial and fungal culture.

Left extrapleural pneumonectomy (frozen section B1): Tumor present as multiple foci involving both parietal and visceral pleura, grossly consistent with the patient's prior diagnosis of *malignant mesothelioma*.
The bronchial resection margin is free of tumor (frozen section B1).
Tumor is fixed in formalin and taken for cytogenetics, electron microscopy, and snap freezing.
Tumor (2 × 2 × 1 cm) and normal tissue (3 × 3 × 2 cm) taken for the tissue bank.

Verbal reports

The results of all OR consultations are communicated to the surgeon as soon as possible. Failure to reach the surgeon directly should be documented in the report and should include what was done to try to contact him or her.

When calling back the results to the operating room, the pathologist should identify him- or herself (e.g., "Dr. Smith from Pathology"), identify the patient, and identify the specimen. The diagnosis should be clear and concise, especially if the pathologist is not speaking to the surgeon directly (e.g., a circulating nurse is relaying the message). The pathologist should listen to what the nurse tells the surgeon in order to make corrections if necessary.

■ ACCURACY OF OPERATING ROOM CONSULTATIONS

The accuracy of frozen-section evaluation is reported to be 94% to 97% when compared to permanent-section evaluation. CAP has suggested that an acceptable rate of major discrepancies is 3%.[8] Discrepancies can be categorized for quality assurance analysis as:

Category A: Minor disagreement with no effect on patient care

Category B: Disagreement with some, but not significant, consequence for patient care

Category C: Major disagreement with serious impact on patient care

Accuracy varies according to the goal of the frozen section. For example, when performed for the purposes of evaluation of margins, lymph node metastases, or tissue identification, accuracy can approach 100%. However, when performed to evaluate an unknown pathologic process, accuracy is usually lower (e.g., 83.47%[9]).

Errors can be classified into the following:

- Sampling error (c. 40%)
- Interpretative error (c. 40%)
- Technical problems (c. 10%)
- Incorrect/incomplete clinical history (c. 10%)

Many of these errors are avoidable.

Sampling errors (block or specimen)

Sampling errors include failure to select the appropriate tissue after gross examination or to completely sample the tissue in the frozen-section block.

Such errors can be avoided or minimized:

Thoroughly dissect large specimens. Gross sampling errors can be minimized by processing specimens in the OR consultation room in the same way as one would during final processing. This includes inking and serially sectioning and dissecting large specimens. Although this is more time consuming, it allows for complete examination of all tissue and the ability to select the best tissue for frozen section.

Freeze small specimens in entirety, when appropriate. For example, if lymph nodes are being evaluated by frozen section to determine whether a definitive resection or complete lymph node dissection should be performed subsequently, it is preferable to freeze the entire node when possible. Failure to find a metastasis in the non-frozen tissue may lead to unnecessary resections of stage IV tumors (e.g., for lung carcinoma) or subsequent additional surgery (e.g., a later axillary dissection for a missed positive sentinel node).

Ensure that all tissue frozen is represented on the slide. Sampling error resulting from failure to examine all tissue frozen in the block can be minimized by careful block preparation. If multiple fragments are present, try to have all fragments at the same level in the block. Sections of all the fragments should be represented on the slides prepared. This may require preparing multiple slides and/or making true deeper levels through the frozen tissue.

Interpretative errors

Interpretative errors can be avoided or minimized:

1. **Limit interpretations to what is necessary for the surgeon to know at the time of surgery.** In some cases, "lesional tissue" is adequate. In others, "benign" versus "malignant" will suffice. Rarely is a specific histologic subtype or grade required at the time of frozen section, and such information is likely to change at final diagnosis.

2. **Review prior pathology slides, when relevant.** If the patient has had a prior diagnostic procedure, it is often helpful to review slides of prior resections, especially in cases of unusual malignancies or tumors difficult to diagnose by frozen section (e.g., signet ring cell carcinomas, angiosarcomas, tumors after treatment).

3. **Examine the tumor as well as its margins by frozen section, when appropriate.** In some cases it is extremely difficult to evaluate margins by frozen section if the type of tumor is unknown or has been previously treated. It is often very helpful to compare changes at the margin with the tumor itself.

4. **Insist on well-frozen and stained material.** If the technical quality is poor (see below) and cannot be improved, it may be preferable to defer a diagnosis.

5. **Insist on an adequate, relevant clinical history.** An accurate evaluation of the findings often cannot be made without knowledge of the clinical setting (e.g., prior diagnosis of malignancy, prior treatment, unusual gross appearance).

In some cases a definitive diagnosis cannot be made and it is appropriate to defer the diagnosis until permanent sections can be examined. In most institutions fewer than 5% of intraoperative diagnoses need to be deferred.

There are types of lesions that are well known to be subject to interpretative error: these should be either avoided completely or only attempted when the surgeon is aware of the likelihood of a change in diagnosis. The most common examples are the evaluation of malignancy in chronic pancreatitis, borderline lesions of the ovary, grossly benign breast tissue, and well-circumscribed follicular lesions of the thyroid.

Technical problems

The interpretation of frozen sections can be made more difficult by poor technique in freezing tissue or preparing slides. Ice crystal artifact, thick sections, folded tissue, and xylene artifact can render the most obvious lesions uninterpretable. Careful attention to technique can minimize these problems.

Some tissues are difficult to section and are best avoided. Adipose tissue freezes poorly due to the lower water content and it may not be possible to evaluate it. Large fragments of bone cannot be sectioned, although cytologic preparations of marrow or intermingled soft tissue may be attempted.

Incorrect or incomplete clinical history

The reason for performing a frozen section should be clear to the pathologist before proceeding. If not, it is better to delay processing the tissue and obtain the history rather than risk inappropriate tissue processing.

The pathologist must always have a high index of suspicion for prior procedures. If a prior biopsy site or atypical cells are present, then a history of possible radiation therapy or chemotherapy should be queried.

It may be helpful to have the patient's chart brought to the OR consultation room along with the tissue for examination. The pathologist can then abstract the information required for pathologic evaluation and include this as clinical information on the pathology report.

■ QUALITY CONTROL OF OPERATING ROOM CONSULTATIONS

Pathology departments usually review the accuracy of operating room consultations. Tissue used for the frozen section is fixed and a permanent section prepared. The final diagnosis, based on all tissue submitted, is compared to the intraoperative diagnosis. The original frozen section must be reviewed if there is a discrepancy. In such cases the reason for the discordance may be one of the following[10-12]:

- 1. Interpretation
- 2. Block sampling
- 3. Specimen sampling
- 4. Technical inadequacy
- 5. Lack of essential clinical or pathologic data
- 6. Other (indicate)

When there is a significant discrepancy between a frozen-section diagnosis and a final diagnosis, the reason for the discrepancy should be documented in the final report and the surgeon notified of the change.

■ COMMON OPERATING ROOM CONSULTATIONS

Operating room consultations mostly fall into a few general categories, and the objectives of the consultation are well known to the pathologist and surgeon. If the reason for the consultation is unclear, it is advisable to contact the surgeon before processing the tissue.

Bone biopsies

Before a bone lesion is approached surgically, a presumptive diagnosis will be made based on the radiographic appearance, the location, and the patient's age. Because the approach to evaluation varies depending on the most likely diagnosis and planned intraoperative treatment, the clinical and radiologic differential diagnosis must be provided before processing the specimen. Cancellous bone can be cut on a cryostat. Portions of cortical bone are thicker and should not be cut.

Presumptively benign lesions

Reason for consultation. To confirm that a lesion is benign before continuing with a procedure that could preclude limb preservation if malignancy were present (e.g., curettage and packing).

Change in surgery. A definitive procedure will be completed if a malignancy is not present. If a benign diagnosis is confirmed on the small initial biopsy, the surgeon will often perform curettage of the lesion, which will provide abundant material for later permanent sections. If a malignancy is found, the surgeon will stop after the biopsy. If a malignant tumor is missed on frozen section, the curettage will contaminate the entire bone and may result in the need for an amputation.

Evaluation. In general, all the tissue initially provided should be used for frozen section.

Presumptively malignant lesions

Reason for consultation. To confirm that sufficient tissue is present for diagnosis.

Change in surgery. Additional tissue may be taken if necessary for diagnosis. Most patients will then undergo radiation and chemotherapy before a definitive resection.

Evaluation. A frozen section or cytologic preparation is performed on only a small portion of the tissue to confirm that diagnostic tissue is present and to guide apportionment of tissue, for example for cytogenetics if Ewing's/PNET is a possibility.

Margins on large resections

Reason for consultation. To determine if the margins are free of a known malignant tumor.

Change in surgery. Additional tissue may be resected to obtain clean margins.

Evaluation. In general, the resected bone must be bisected in order to identify the distance of the tumor grossly from the margin. A frozen section can be taken of the cancellous bone at the margin or a cytologic preparation may be prepared from the marrow space.

Frozen section of cancellous bone removed with a curette from a mandibular margin has been reported to be an accurate determination of final margin status.[13]

Revision total joint arthroplasty

Reason for consultation. To determine if infection is present.

Change in surgery. It may be difficult to distinguish mechanical from septic loosening of a prosthetic joint. If infection is present, drainage or removal of the prosthesis may be indicated and replacement of a prosthesis may be delayed until after treatment.

Evaluation. At least two representative sections of a biopsy of periprosthetic tissue (considered to be the most grossly suspicious area by the surgeon) are examined and the number of polymorphonuclear leukocytes (PMNs) per high-power field (HPF) ($\times$40—the field size is not further specified) is assessed.[14] At least 5 HPFs should be counted in the most cellular areas of the section.

10 PMNs per HPF has an 89% positive predictive value (PPV) for infection

5 to 9 PMNs per HPF has a 70% PPV

Less than 5 PMNs has a 98% negative predictive value

Pitfalls. False positives (3% of cases) and false negatives (6% of cases) can occur.[15] Surgical management should be based on the preoperative and intraoperative clinical assessment as well as on frozen-section results.

False positives: PMNs seen only in surface fibrin should not be included. Patients with rheumatoid arthritis may have acute inflammation not related to sepsis. Perivascular PMNs are usually the result of prolonged surgery.

False negatives: These usually result from sampling error. At least two blocks of tissue should be frozen. Additional blocks should be frozen if tissue from different sites is provided by the surgeon. Tan/pink tissue should be

chosen for examination. White fibrous tissue or fibrin is unlikely to yield useful material for diagnosis.

Dermatopathology

Carcinoma

Reason for consultation. Evaluation of margins of basal cell carcinomas or squamous cell carcinomas from the face. The surgeon may want to take as little skin as possible in order to achieve a satisfactory cosmetic result.

The use of frozen sections for the diagnosis or margin evaluation of melanocytic lesions is strongly discouraged. If a clinician requests such an evaluation, the pathologist should inform him or her that frozen section often compromises definitive diagnosis and that the evaluation should be made on well-fixed and oriented permanent sections.

Change in surgery. Additional tissue may be taken to ensure clean margins.

Evaluation. The specimen is usually an oriented ellipse. Because the main lesion has almost always been biopsied, it is often difficult to determine the location of the closest margin. If the paperwork does not indicate which margin is to be frozen, contact the surgeon before proceeding.

Draw a diagram showing the orienting suture, ink colors, and site of frozen sections. For small ellipses, it is useful to ink the two margins to be evaluated by frozen section in two different colors. Both margins can be evaluated in a single section. Take perpendicular sections at the margins indicated as "close" by the surgeon. Make sure the sections are thin, but full thickness, and include the deep margin.

Skin exfoliation

Reason for consultation. It is sometimes necessary to distinguish between staphylococcal scalded skin syndrome (SSSS) and toxic epidermal necrolysis (TEN) to guide treatment. Both can present with areas of exfoliated skin and can be difficult to differentiate on clinical grounds. This is one of the true dermatopathologic emergencies.

Change in treatment. SSSS is treated with antibiotics. TEN may require steroids or withdrawal of possible sensitizing medications.

Evaluation. The specimen is a fragment of the exfoliated skin. The skin is rolled as tightly as possible using a forceps. Cross-sections are taken for frozen section in order to evaluate a perpendicular section.

- **TEN:** The cleavage plane occurs at the dermal–epidermal junction. The presence of full-thickness epidermal cell necrosis is supportive of TEN.
- **SSSS:** The cleavage plane occurs near the granular cell layer. Therefore, only the most superficial aspect of the epidermis and keratin layer are seen.

Fasciitis

Reason for consultation. To establish the diagnosis of necrotizing fasciitis, a rapidly progressive infection that causes death in 25% to 33% of patients. Streptococci are the causative bacteria in about one third of cases, but polymicrobial infections are common and include staphylococci, enterococci, enterobacteriaceae (*E. coli, Acinetobacter, Pseudomonas, Klebsiella*), *Bacteroides*, and *Clostridium*. The initial symptoms (the triad of exquisite pain disproportionate to physical findings, swelling, and fever) are difficult to distinguish from those of cellulitis or an abscess. Initially spread is horizontal, and small bullae frequently form on the skin. In later stages, large hemorrhagic bullae occur and necrosis of skin and deep tissues ensues.

Change in treatment. A definitive diagnosis can help to guide rapid wide surgical debridement and/or amputation, resulting in a much better prognosis. Useful biopsies must be obtained within 4 days of the onset of symptoms. The advantage of early diagnosis is lost once skin and muscle become necrotic and the need for debridement is obvious.

Evaluation. An excisional biopsy including skin, subcutaneous tissue, and muscle is optimal.

Features favoring necrotizing fasciitis[16,17]:

- Liquefactive necrosis of superficial fascia
- PMN infiltration of the deep dermis and fascia
- Fibrinous thrombi in arteries and veins passing through the fascia
- Angiitis with fibrinoid necrosis of arterial and venous walls
- Microorganisms within the destroyed fascia and dermis (Gram stain)
- Absence of muscle involvement

The usual differential diagnosis is with cellulitis or erysipelas. In these conditions, inflammation is present but it occurs in superficial tissue without significant involvement of deep soft tissue and fascia.

Breast biopsies

Carcinoma

Reason for consultation. Diagnosis of invasive carcinoma.

Change in surgery or processing. Additional tissue may be taken for clear margins and/or an axillary dissection may be performed. Fresh tumor tissue may be taken for flow cytometric analysis, if requested. Intraoperative consultation is unnecessary if the result will not lead to a change in procedure.

Evaluation. The most important objective in examining breast biopsies is to make a definitive diagnosis. Therefore, tissue must not be used for frozen

sections if the final diagnosis could be compromised. Only grossly evident masses of sufficient size (the recommendation is over 1 cm[18]) should be examined by frozen section. Smaller masses, grossly benign tissue, or tissue removed for the evaluation of calcifications should *never* be frozen as freezing can introduce artifacts in small lesions, precluding a diagnosis on permanent sections.

If the specimen has been oriented, care must be taken in inking the margins and processing the tissue in order to be able to submit tissue according to this orientation (see Chapter 15, "Breast").

Note the location of any palpable masses. If the mass is larger than 1 cm and suspicious for invasive carcinoma, a frozen section may be performed. If a definitive diagnosis of invasive carcinoma is made, tumor may be taken for flow cytometric analysis if requested or for tumor banking. Make a careful measurement of the maximal tumor size to the nearest 0.1 cm. The important sizes for staging are 0.5 cm, 1 cm, 2 cm, and 5 cm. Do not round to the nearest 1 cm. A gross evaluation of margins for the proximity of invasive carcinoma may also be provided (see below).

If a definitive diagnosis cannot be made (e.g., the differential diagnosis includes a complex sclerosing lesion and tubular carcinoma), all lesional tissue must be submitted for histologic evaluation. Do not take tissue for flow cytometric analysis or other studies.

Pitfalls. False positive rates are low (<1%) but can occur.[19] Thus definitive surgery may best be deferred for small or questionable lesions.

False negative rates are higher, but reported to be less than 10%. The rate is lower if restricted to lesions grossly suspicious for invasive carcinoma.

In general, frozen-section evaluation is not useful to either diagnose DCIS or exclude its presence.

Margins

Reason for consultation. To grossly evaluate the adequacy of margins for invasive carcinoma.

Change in surgery. Additional tissue may be taken at a margin deemed to be close.

Evaluation. Most invasive carcinomas can be detected as grossly palpable masses. Very few cases of DCIS can be detected grossly and are difficult to diagnose by frozen section.

If there is no prior diagnosis, process the specimen as described above.

If a diagnosis of invasive carcinoma has been made previously, it is generally unnecessary to perform a frozen section, and the margins are evaluated grossly for involvement. If the carcinoma is present (e.g., after a core biopsy), the distance to each margin is determined and reported to the surgeon. If the carcinoma has been excised (e.g., after excisional biopsy), the rim of the biopsy cavity is examined for areas suspicious for residual invasive carcinoma at the margin. Selected frozen sections of grossly suspicious areas may be helpful.

Margin involvement by DCIS is difficult to assess by frozen section:

- The marginal tissue usually consists of grossly benign adipose tissue, which is difficult to freeze and section adequately.
- It may be difficult to distinguish hyperplastic lesions from DCIS on frozen sections.
- Not all marginal tissue can be evaluated by frozen section. Additional tissue examined by permanent sections may later be shown to be involved.

However, some institutions do evaluate margins by either cytologic means[20,21] or frozen section.[22] The majority of the cases evaluated have been invasive carcinomas and not DCIS alone. The value of such margin evaluation depends on the definition of a "positive" margin, and institutional criteria for the necessity of further surgical procedures based on margin evaluation.

Sentinel lymph nodes

Reason for consultation. To determine whether a metastasis is present in the node.

Change in surgery. If a metastasis is found in the sentinel lymph node, a completion axillary dissection will be performed.

Evaluation. On average, there will be two sentinel lymph nodes. The nodes should be grossly dissected from the tissue received. Separate the fat, and ink each node a different color. It is very important to be able to keep track of the number of involved nodes as this is an important prognostic factor and is used to classify women for clinical trials.

Slice each node into 0.2 to 0.3 cm slices.

If there is a grossly evident metastasis, only one representative section need be frozen.

If the nodes are grossly normal, freeze *all* of the slices. All macrometastases (>0.2 cm) should be identified using this method. If there are multiple nodes, it may be prudent to discuss with the surgeon before proceeding.

Touch preparations can also be used to evaluate the nodes. Each node should be scraped and evaluated separately. Make sure the work area is clean and distant from any other specimens with malignancies to avoid contamination.

Pitfalls. False negatives for macrometastases can occur if the entire node is not frozen. Micrometastases (<0.2 cm) will often be missed due to sampling, but there is no practical method to find all such small metastatic deposits. Metastases from lobular carcinomas can be very subtle on frozen section and it is helpful to know if the patient has this type of cancer. If a definite diagnosis cannot be made, it is better to defer the diagnosis. A completion dissection

can be performed at a later time.

Gastrointestinal specimens

Esophagectomies and gastrectomies

Reason for consultation. To determine if the resection margins are free of malignancy or dysplasia and to ensure that the lesion has been resected.

Change in surgery. Additional esophagus or stomach may be resected to achieve clean margins.

Evaluation. Gross inspection of the opened specimen is often sufficient to establish clear margins. However, tumors (particularly diffuse-type gastric carcinomas or esophageal adenocarcinomas) located close to the resection margins may infiltrate beneath grossly normal mucosa. Therefore, complete inspection of the margins and selection of appropriate frozen sections is essential.

Ink the serosa and adventitia along the area to be opened.

Open the proximal and distal margins by cutting as close as possible to the staple line.

Open the specimen longitudinally, but avoid cutting through the lesion. Esophagectomy and gastrectomy specimens are best opened by following the greater curvature of the stomach, unless a lesion is present there.

Record the size and location of any lesions and the distance from the proximal and distal margins. Patients have often had prior radiation and/or chemotherapy, and the residual tumor may not be grossly evident or quite subtle (e.g., a shallow mucosal ulceration). Avoid touching the mucosa, which is fragile and easily abraded. If necessary, the mucosa can be gently rinsed with saline.

Esophagectomies are often involved by Barrett's esophagus, which is recognizable as granular pink mucosa. Record the length of this segment and its closest approach to the proximal margin. If Barrett's mucosa is present at the proximal margin, a frozen section is essential as dysplasia may be present and additional resection may be necessary.

Take the margins en face, unless a gross lesion is very close to the margin and a perpendicular section can include both the lesion and margin. The margin section should be taken from the area closest to the site of the tumor. It is important that the en face section is full thickness, including mucosa, submucosa, and muscularis, as carcinoma may involve any of these layers. Because the overlying mucosa may curl over the edge of the cut margin, it may be necessary to gently pull back this mucosa to line it up over the muscularis before taking the section.

Colonic malignancy or polyps

Reason for consultation. To determine whether the margins are free of malignancy or polyps, to measure accurately the length of the margin, and to ensure that the lesion has been resected.

Change in surgery. Additional colon may be resected.

Evaluation. In the majority of cases, gross evaluation of the margins is sufficient to ensure clear margins. However, since these patients are at risk for multiple lesions, the margins must be completely opened and inspected to establish that they are clear.

Examine the segment of bowel externally to determine if there is evidence of invasive tumor at the serosal surface or puckering of the serosa (indicative of invasion into the muscularis). If the segment is from the recto-sigmoid, examine the mesentery to determine the location of the recto-sigmoid junction.

Completely open any stapled ends by cutting as close as possible to the staple line. Cut along the antimesenteric surface with blunt scissors to open the bowel. However, adjust the line of opening to avoid transecting any lesions. The bowel lumen may be rinsed clean with a small amount of saline, if necessary. Tap water is hypotonic and will damage tissue.

The lesions present are described and the distance from the proximal and distal margins is measured and recorded on the OR consultation report. The bowel is often returned to the OR for the surgeon to view.

Bowel segments can contract up to 40% within 10 to 20 minutes after excision.[23] Because close margins may be an indication for postoperative radiation therapy for rectal carcinomas, margin lengths are best measured as soon as possible after excision.

Frozen sections are rarely necessary for margin evaluation if the uninvolved mucosa is grossly normal. In cases of malignancy arising in inflammatory bowel disease (see below), frozen-section evaluation may be indicated in selected cases. Evaluation of margins after treatment (typically radiation) or for certain histologic types (i.e., signet ring cell carcinomas) can also be difficult and may require frozen section.

If it is unclear why a segment of bowel was removed (e.g., no lesion is apparent), contact the surgeon. For example, if the surgery was performed for a previously biopsied polyp with invasive carcinoma, the "lesion" may be a subtle prior biopsy site consisting of mucosal ulceration that must be found and sampled for permanent sections to ensure that a complete resection has been performed. Alternatively, it is possible that a lesion has been missed and additional surgery must be performed.

Sample OR consultation report

Specimen no. 2, rectosigmoid resection (33 cm) (gross examination): Ulcerated lesion (4.4 cm) grossly consistent with adenocarcinoma, located 3 cm proximal to the rectosigmoid junction. The tumor is 5 cm from the distal margin and 24 cm from the proximal margin.
The specimen is returned to the operating room per the surgeon's request.

Inflammatory bowel disease (IBD)

Reason for consultation. In cases of Crohn's disease the bowel may be inspected for gross ulceration at the margin.

Change in surgery. The intent is to resect grossly involved bowel. Additional bowel may be resected if gross changes are present at the margin. The evaluation of margins in Crohn's disease is very controversial: some studies have found that the length of uninvolved mucosa or the presence of microscopic findings at the margin affect recurrence rates.[24,25]

Evaluation. The outer surface of the bowel is inspected for creeping fat or fistulas indicative of IBD.

Open the bowel as described above. Inspect the mucosa for changes of IBD. Look carefully for any areas suspicious for malignancy. In cases of Crohn's disease, margins should be inspected for gross ulceration. The typical operation for ulcerative colitis is a total colectomy with removal of all colonic mucosa, and margins are not important.

Frozen sections are not needed for the evaluation of inflammatory changes. Frozen sections may be helpful in cases of suspected malignancy arising in IBD.

Sample OR consultation report

Sigmoid colon (28 cm) (gross examination): Thickened bowel wall with linear mucosal ulcerations and fistula tract, consistent with prior diagnosis of *Crohn's disease*.
Gross ulceration present at the proximal resection margin.
The distal resection margin is free of ulceration. Surgeon informed.
The specimen is returned to the operating room per the surgeon's request.

Liver biopsies prior to transplant[26-28]

Reason for consultation. Biopsies may be performed to assess donor organ status prior to liver transplant.[26–28] Unlike kidney allografts, there is no alternative treatment should the transplanted liver fail.

Change in surgery. The liver may not be used for transplantation.

Evaluation. Either a wedge biopsy (at least 1.5 cm^2) or a cutting needle biopsy (at least 2 cm in length) may be performed. Wedge biopsies may be misleading, since fibrous tissue from Glisson's capsule penetrates into the parenchyma for 0.5 cm or more. There also may be superficial contusion and inflammation to the liver if the cause of the donor's demise was trauma. Therefore, a cutting needle biopsy is a more reliable method of assessing liver status.

The biopsy must be processed rapidly as fat is diminished after even a few minutes in air. Placing the biopsy in saline can cause distortion (chromatin clumping and edema of extracellular spaces), making the evaluation of necrosis difficult.

The entire needle or wedge biopsy specimen is frozen. Assess:

1. The absence or presence of fatty change and the percent of hepatocytes affected. The fatty change is characteristically microvesicular. However, special stains for microvesicular fat are not required, since the amount of fatty change needed to "reject" the donor liver for transplant must be obvious on H&E sections. Minimal or mild (up to 25% of hepatocytes) fatty change is still acceptable for transplantation. Severe fatty change (>60% of hepatocytes) is associated with a nonfunctioning graft.
2. The extent of inflammation and/or hepatocyte necrosis. Mild focal necrosis may occur during harvesting of the organ. More severe or extensive necrosis indicates a high likelihood of graft failure.
3. The presence or absence of fibrosis.
4. Any indication of alcohol-induced injury: fibrosis, moderate to severe fatty change, "alcoholic hepatitis" (neutrophils in parenchyma, hepatocyte necrosis, cholestasis), and Mallory's hyaline/ballooning degeneration.

The decision to use the organ is based on the following considerations:

Extensive, moderate to severe, fatty change in the donor liver indicates substantial hepatic damage prior to the time of harvest and is correlated with a poor outcome following transplantation of the donor liver. A liver with only minimal to mild fatty damage may be declined if serum liver enzymes are also increased.

Extensive, severe hepatocellular necrosis also presages a stormy outcome, usually related to primary graft failure following implantation. Such necrosis is usually attributable to cellular injury occurring during the agonal period.

Mild preexisting liver disease is not usually a contraindication to liver transplantation. However, its presence must be documented, so as not to misinterpret post-transplantation biopsies. Thus, mild fibrosis or portal tract inflammation from previous viral hepatitis, assuming the patient also has serologic evidence of infection by the same virus, has been accepted.

The exception is:

Evidence of alcohol-induced liver disease, which is correlated with potential compromise of the graft weeks, months, or even a year or two later.

Pitfalls:
- Lipofuscin in older patients (in a centrilobular location) can be mistaken for cholestasis (bile located in canaliculi) or iron deposits (in a periportal location).

- Fat can be difficult to evaluate in air-dried specimens.
- Necrosis can be difficult to evaluate in specimens sent in saline.

Pancreas

Reason for consultation. To determine whether malignancy is present.

Change in surgery. If malignancy is present a major resection may be carried out (e.g., a Whipple resection) and/or staging biopsies may be performed.

Evaluation. Pancreatic carcinomas can be very difficult to detect grossly and microscopically in a background of chronic pancreatitis, which results in a dense, firm, nodular gland. Biopsies are usually small wedge or needle biopsies that are associated with a significant risk of complications. Useful diagnostic criteria for pancreatic carcinoma on frozen section have been published[29] (see box on next page):

Pitfalls. False positive diagnoses are rare, but false negatives have been reported in more than 30% of cases. These latter cases are due in equal part to sampling error (i.e., the area of carcinoma was not biopsied for frozen section) and to interpretation error.[30] Sampling error can be reduced by examining multiple biopsies. Interpretation error can be minimized by using the criteria described above and paying attention to the following histologic findings:

- Accessory pancreatic ducts can be found in smooth muscle of the duodenum, but consist of groups of glands surrounded by loose connective tissue. Malignant glands invading muscle are present singly and are in contact with muscle cells.
- The distribution of ducts can become irregular in cases of severe pancreatitis. Other criteria of malignancy should be searched for as well.
- Islets become prominent in chronic pancreatitis and may mimic clusters of epithelial cells with marked nuclear variation in size.
- Atrophic acini and ductules can appear to have incomplete lumens.
- Normal ducts can occasionally be seen adjacent to nerves and simulate perineural invasion.

Genitourinary specimens

Sperm identification

Reason for consultation. To determine whether spermatozoa are being produced by the testis.

Change in surgery. Men with azoospermia may have primary failure of spermatogenesis or an obstructed vas deferens. Urologists may send fluid milked from the proximal vas deferens for identification of spermatozoa before performing anastomotic surgery to correct an obstruction.

Major criteria (present in all cases of carcinoma)

1. Nuclear size variation equal to, or greater than, 4:1
2. Incomplete glandular lumens
3. Disorganized duct distribution

Minor criteria (present in 28% to 70% of cases of carcinoma)

1. Huge, irregular epithelial nucleoli
2. Necrotic glandular debris
3. Glandular mitoses
4. Glands unaccompanied by stroma in smooth muscle fascicles
5. Perineural invasion

Evaluation. The fluid is placed on a slide and coverslipped. Without staining the slide, the preparation is examined for the presence of spermatozoa. The OR consultation report notes whether spermatozoa are present or absent.

Motility depends on temperature and time elapsed since preparation of the slide and thus is not a very accurate predictor of true motility, if absent.

After the diagnosis is rendered, the coverslip is removed and the slide placed in 95% ethanol. The slide can be stained with H&E and permanently coverslipped.

Donor renal biopsies prior to transplant

Reason for consultation. Evaluation of wedge or core biopsies of donor kidneys before transplantation if the patient has a medical condition that could affect the kidney (e.g., hypertension or older age) or if a gross lesion is noted.

Change in surgery. The organ may not be used for transplantation.

Evaluation. Frozen sections are prepared (usually one from each kidney). Evaluate the following:

1. Number of glomeruli in the sample.
2. The number and percent of sclerosed glomeruli (e.g., "5 out of 40 glomeruli show global glomerulosclerosis").
3. The level of tubular atrophy and interstitial fibrosis (percentage of sample involved).
4. The degree of vascular scarring (mild, moderate, or severe).
5. Any other relevant findings (tumors, acute inflammation, cysts, etc.).

The use of frozen sections for this purpose is being evaluated, and criteria for not using an organ for transplantation are not yet established.[28] Greater than 20% glomerulosclerosis is associated with poor allograft survival and function.

Nephrectomy, cystectomy, or ureterectomy for transitional cell carcinoma

Reason for consultation. To evaluate the ureteral margins for the presence of transitional cell carcinoma.

Change in surgery. The surgeon may take an additional portion of the ureter to achieve margins free of carcinoma.

Evaluation. A length of ureter is usually provided separate from the main excision. A suture may mark the true margin. A complete cross-section of the ureter is taken for frozen section. The true margin may be embedded so that the first frozen section is the true margin.

Partial nephrectomy

Reason for consultation. To evaluate the margin of a partial nephrectomy. Usually, the patient has compromised function of the contralateral kidney.

Change in surgery. Additional kidney tissue may be taken or a complete nephrectomy may be performed.

Evaluation. Ink the kidney over the open area of transection. Serially section the kidney perpendicular to the margin and evaluate grossly for any lesions present. The margin closest to the tumor is frozen. Approximately 17% of cases have positive margins.[31] Frozen section is generally reliable for diagnosis of carcinomas, but diagnosis of unusual tumors can be difficult.[32]

Gynecologic pathology

Ovary

Reason for consultation. Evaluation of malignancy of an ovarian tumor.

Change in surgery. If a malignancy is identified, appropriate staging biopsies (e.g., omental biopsies, biopsies of other suspicious areas, peritoneal washings, lymph node biopsies) and either total abdominal hysterectomy (TAH) or bilateral salpingo-oophorectomy (BSO) will be performed. If extensive disease is present, and a metastatic carcinoma is identified, the appropriate surgery may be performed. Fertility may be preserved if a benign diagnosis is rendered.

Evaluation. All cysts and solid tumors are opened and serially sectioned. See page 437 for appropriate procedures for opening cysts. In general, ovarian tumors in women over the age of 40 are more commonly borderline or malignant whereas those in women under the age of 40 are more commonly benign.

Unilocular cysts with a smooth inner lining. Almost always benign. Gross examination is sufficient. "Endometriomas" are unusual in postmenopausal women and should be examined by frozen section to exclude carcinoma in this age group.

Mature teratomas (dermoid cysts). These cysts are filled with sebaceous material and hair, and are almost always benign. Gross examination is sufficient unless substantial solid areas are present or the tumor has spontaneously ruptured.

Unilocular or multilocular cysts with irregular linings. Visually inspect the lining for any areas of irregularity (e.g., minute papillary excrescences) or solid areas. Do not touch the inner surface as this may remove diagnostic lining cells. Multilocular cysts or cysts with solid areas are more suspicious for malignancy. Frozen sections may be performed on the most suspicious areas.

Solid masses. Examine the surface for involvement as this could affect staging. Multiple nodules may signify metastatic disease. Frozen sections are generally performed unless the gross appearance is characteristic of a fibroma or leiomyoma.

Pitfalls. If tumors are divided into benign, malignant, and borderline, frozen sections and permanent sections are concordant in more than 90% of cases.[33] The following types of tumor are the most difficult to evaluate by frozen section:

Large tumors (>10 cm). Additional sections may be helpful to look for focal invasive carcinoma.

Mucinous carcinomas. These carcinomas are often heterogeneous and can require extensive sampling for correct classification.

Borderline tumors. Approximately 20% of tumors classified as borderline on frozen section will be reclassified as malignant after more extensive sampling for permanent sections.

Uterus
Endometrial carcinoma

Reason for consultation. Evaluation for presence or absence of endometrial carcinoma. If present, the grade, depth of invasion, and involvement of the cervix (stage II) is determined.

Change in surgery. If carcinoma invades deeply into the myometrium (usually the outer half or outer third), and/or the carcinoma is grade II or III, and/or the cervix or isthmus are involved, the surgeon may decide to perform pelvic and paraaortic lymphadenectomy.

Evaluation. The serosa is carefully inspected for areas suspicious for direct tumor invasion or serosal implants. Suspicious areas on the serosa are inked. Open the uterus along the lateral edges using scissors (see p. 423). Carefully inspect (but do not touch!) the endometrial lining for gross evidence of tumor (usually pale yellow heaped-up areas). Make serial transverse incisions from the mucosal surface to, but not through, the serosa (leaving the specimen intact) at 0.5 cm intervals.

Myometrial invasion by tumor grossly appears as effacement of the normal myometrial texture. Depth of invasion can be determined grossly in many cases. A frozen section should be performed in the area most suspicious for the deepest extent of myometrial invasion. The surface of the fallopian tubes and ovaries is also carefully inspected, and the ovaries are cross-sectioned and examined for areas suspicious for malignancy.

Pitfalls. False positive and false negative frozen-section diagnoses are reported for all three prognostic factors.[34] Overall, grade is accurately determined in 67% to 96% of cases, depth of invasion in 85% to 95%, and cervical involvement in 65% to 96%.

Leiomyoma

Reason for consultation. Evaluation of presumed leiomyomata for possible malignancy. Clinical features suspicious for malignancy include such ultrasound findings as an irregular border or cystic areas, large size, soft consistency, and difficulty in removing the lesion from the uterine wall. However, this last finding is more commonly associated with adenomyosis than with malignant invasion.

Change in surgery. If the initial procedure is a myomectomy, a total hysterectomy may be performed if a malignancy is present. Additional biopsies may be taken of any suspicious peritoneal lesions.

Evaluation. All masses are sectioned at 1 to 2 cm intervals. Typical leiomyomas are white, whorled, firm, and without necrosis or hemorrhage. Degenerative changes are common and include a carneous (fleshy) appearance or cystic mucoid areas. Features suggestive of malignancy include a soft consistency, necrosis, hemorrhage, infiltrative borders, and vascular invasion. Frozen sections may be performed on grossly suspicious lesions.

Pitfalls. Infertile premenopausal women undergoing myomectomy to improve uterine function may be receiving hormonal treatments. An increased mitotic rate and necrosis can be present in benign leiomyomas. A definitive diagnosis of malignancy should not be made on frozen section unless obvious features of malignancy are present.

If there has been a recent surgical procedure (e.g., a partial myomectomy or endometrial curettings), increased mitoses and necrosis may be seen in benign leiomyomas.

Vulvectomy

Reason for consultation. To evaluate the resection margins for carcinoma or dysplasia.

Change in management. Additional vulvar skin may be resected.

False positive: >50% myometrial invasion (c. 9% of cases); carcinomatous involvement of adenomyosis or deep lymphovascular invasion mistaken for invasion.
False negative: Myometrial invasion (c. 10% of cases); diffusely invasive carcinomas with widely spaced glands and a minimal desmoplastic response may not be seen grossly or on frozen section.

Evaluation. If a gross lesion or biopsy site is present, the closest margin may be frozen as a perpendicular section. If no gross lesion is evident, it is useful to determine the location of the clinical lesion (often previously excised) and to sample the margin at this site.

Products of conception

Reason for consultation. Pregnant women (positive hCG) who present with vaginal bleeding or pelvic pain and who do not have an obvious intrauterine pregnancy by ultrasound are at risk for an ectopic pregnancy and its associated complications (e.g., fatal hemorrhage). Endometrial curettings or tissue from the vaginal vault are submitted to determine the presence of placental villi and/or a recent implantation site: their presence would confirm that the pregnancy was intrauterine. Rarely, a gestational sac may be present.

Change in management. If an intrauterine pregnancy cannot be documented, the patient may require pelviscopy.

Evaluation. Such specimens are best examined with a dissecting microscope. Float the specimen in saline in a Petri dish. It may be necessary to rinse the specimen free of blood. Frozen sections should be performed on the tissue most likely to be villi (Table 6-1).

Pitfalls. In a study in which all tissue was frozen, the correct diagnosis was made in 93% of cases.[35] There was a 5.7% false negative rate; this resulted from villi being present in deeper sections of the tissue that were not seen on frozen section. There was one false positive case (1.1%

of the total) resulting from misinterpretation of edematous endocervix as villi. Frozen sections of an avillous intrauterine pregnancy are difficult to interpret and the diagnosis requires verification of trophoblast (placental site or isolated). The diagnosis is often missed.

Head and neck resections

Reason for consultation. To determine the adequacy of margins.

Change in surgery. Additional tissue may be taken to achieve clean margins. A reconstructive procedure is often performed immediately, so the opportunity to resect more tissue in the future may not be an option. Postoperative radiation therapy may compromise the reconstruction and is avoided if possible.

Evaluation. It is preferable to review any complicated specimens with the surgeon prior to inking to identify anatomic structures, the location of probable tumor, and surgical margins. Perpendicular sections are taken at the closest margins. A very narrow margin (e.g., less than 0.1 cm) may be considered to be adequate.

En face margins are sometimes used to sample a larger area if the mucosa appears grossly normal. The en face margin is embedded so that the first full-thickness frozen section represents the "true" mucosal margin. Multiple sections may be made, but must be numbered to identify the first section. If tumor is found only on deeper sections (e.g., in deeper levels of the frozen section or in the permanent sections), the tumor is not present at the true margin.

Pitfalls. Radiation changes, particularly in minor salivary glands, may be difficult to distinguish from invasive carcinoma. Establish whether or not the patient has received radiation therapy. Look for squamous metaplasia and a lobular arrangement, which favor benign changes.

Perineural invasion is common in these tumors and, if present, can be responsible for local recurrence. The juxtaoral organ of Chievitz is found at the angle of the mandible and consists of epithelial nests in close proximity to nerves. This normal structure can be mistaken for perineural invasion on frozen section.[36]

Table 6-1 Differentiation of placental villi from decidualized endometrium

	COLOR	STRUCTURE	BRANCHING	CONSISTENCY
Villi	White (or pink)	Complex three-dimensional architecture (like a shrub or sea anemone)	Acute-angle branching	Springy (rapidly re-expand after being gently squeezed)
Decidualized endometrium	Pink (but may be white) More opaque than villi	Glandular and vascular structures may mimic villi	Structures run in parallel and are not branched	Not springy

Lung and pleura

Mediastinal staging of lung carcinomas

Reason for consultation. To determine whether a lung carcinoma is resectable (stage I, stage II, or stage IIIA lung carcinomas with involvement of ipsilateral but not contralateral mediastinal lymph nodes) or to terminate lymph node sampling once a positive lymph node is found.

Change in surgery. Patients without lymph node metastases may proceed to definitive resection in the same procedure. Patients with metastatic disease may have a curtailed procedure as additional nodes are not necessary for staging, and resection may not be indicated.

If positive nodes are found at frozen section, the patient may be kept in the hospital longer for oncologic planning and consultation and possibly other radiologic examinations. If the nodes are negative, the patient is usually discharged the same day.

Evaluation. The purpose of the node biopsy must be known, as this will alter the processing of the specimen:

Staging of lung carcinoma: The entire node or nodes are frozen. Patients are generally older and have a lung mass.

Evaluation of lymphadenopathy: The differential diagnosis includes lymphoma, infection, and sarcoidosis. Only a portion of the specimen should be frozen or touch preparations used. Tissue should be preserved for possible special studies, including microbiological culture, frozen tissue, and flow cytometry (see p. 517, "Lymph Nodes, Spleen and Bone Marrow"). Patients are usually younger and generally do not have lung involvement.

Pitfalls. In one study, 30% of patients undergoing mediastinal staging had metastatic disease.[37]

False positive results: Not reported.

False negative (1.6% of patients): Macrometastases (>0.2 cm) can be missed if the entire node is not frozen. Small metastatic deposits may be missed due to sampling, but there is no practical method to find all micrometastases.

Pulmonary resections for lung masses

Reason for consultation. To identify malignancy in lung masses.

Change in surgery. If malignancy is present, additional surgery may be indicated to ensure clean margins and/or complete staging.

Evaluation. Lung masses may be resected by wedge resection, lobectomy, or pneumonectomy.

Wedge resections

Wedge resection is often the initial procedure for the evaluation of small masses. The pleura is inspected for involvement by tumor or adherence to the underlying mass. The mass is bisected, avoiding any area of possible pleural involvement (which should be preserved for evaluation by permanent sections). A representative section of the mass is frozen for diagnosis. In cases of malignancy, the margins of a wedge resection are taken by cutting away the staple line as close to the staples as possible. The exposed lung parenchyma is blotted dry and then inked. A perpendicular or en face section of lung tissue in the area closest to the tumor can be used as the margin. However, check with the surgeon first to determine whether a more extensive resection is going to be performed (e.g., lobectomy), in which case margins on the wedge resection are irrelevant. Only parenchymal involvement by tumor should be reported as a positive margin. Loose tumor cells in air spaces are most likely artifacts and are usually not considered a true positive margin.

Lobectomies

The mass is evaluated as described above. The distance to the bronchial margin is determined. Carcinomas can extend into the bronchus for varying distances beyond the gross tumor (adenocarcinomas c. 2 cm, squamous cell carcinomas c. 1.5 cm). In one study, no carcinoma further than 3 cm from the bronchial margin had a positive margin.[38] Margins can also appear falsely positive grossly because of fibrous or lymphoid tissue.

The margin is taken as an en face section of the bronchus.

Grossly normal and >3 cm from the tumor: Embed the bronchial ring with the proximal (i.e., "true") margin down. This cut surface is usually flatter and yields a complete section of the margin. Positive margins are rare. In the rare case of an initial section positive for tumor, deeper levels into the block can be made to determine whether the carcinoma is present at the true margin.

Grossly suspicious margin or tumor <3 cm from the margin: Embed with the true margin upward. The first frozen section will be the "true" margin.

Care should be taken not to include pulmonary parenchyma away from the bronchial ring in the frozen section, as tumor in this area will not be present at the bronchial stump in the patient.

If tumor is present in the frozen section, the location and nature of the tumor must be specified:

- In situ carcinoma in the bronchial mucosa
- Submucosal invasive carcinoma
- Parabronchial invasive carcinoma
- Carcinoma in lymphatics or peribronchial lymph nodes.

Carcinomas with salivary gland morphology are rare but have a high incidence of positive margins. Carcinoid tumors may undermine the bronchial mucosa and be difficult to see grossly.

Pitfalls. Overall, more than 95% of margins can be accurately diagnosed. True positive margins are rare (approximately 6% of cases).

False positive (c. 2%):

- Squamous metaplasia mistaken for carcinoma in situ
- Radiation changes mistaken for carcinoma
- Peribronchial lymphocytes mistaken for small cell carcinoma (in such cases it is helpful to know the histologic type of the primary)

False negative (c. 2%):

- Sampling errors
- Carcinoma in situ mistaken for squamous metaplasia
- Carcinoma mistaken for submucosal glands

Open lung biopsies

Reason for consultation. Open lung biopsies are usually performed on critically ill patients with a wide differential diagnosis. Frozen sections are performed to provide a preliminary diagnosis (e.g., tumor versus infection) and to guide apportionment of tissue. Culture and special stains on histologic sections are complementary studies for the identification of infectious disease.[39]

Change in management. A preliminary diagnosis may aid in selection of treatment of critically ill patients before permanent sections are available.

Evaluation. Apportioning tissue is done with the clinical differential in mind and according to the histologic appearance. The specimen is kept sterile until a block of tissue can be removed for cultures. Evaluation and processing includes:

1. Determine whether the specimen is adequate for the studies required: 1 cm^3 is marginal, 2 cm^3 is optimal. If the specimen is too small for all studies required, call the surgeon and request more tissue.
2. Using sterile technique, serially section through the specimen looking for focal lesions. Transfer a block of tissue to a sterile container for microbiology. Each requisition form must be labeled with the date and the collection time to conform to JCAHO guidelines. The type of specimen should also be described. Each microbiology laboratory has individualized guidelines for the submission of specimens.
3. The two major indications for frozen-section evaluation are:
   - To determine whether a malignancy is present in order to perform a more definitive procedure or to initiate treatment.
   - In lung transplant patients, to guide therapy for possible rejection or infection (e.g., a virus).
   - In other cases, valuable diagnostic material is better examined by permanent sections. Smears should be used if possible because of the high rate of infection in these patients.
4. The remaining tissue is apportioned for:
   - B5 fixation and snap freezing if lymphoma or leukemia is suspected.
   - Fixation in formalin.
5. Special stains on smears for infectious organisms may be helpful if they would be available prior to special stains on permanent sections. Smears should be fixed in methanol. Air-dried slides are potentially infectious and should not be submitted to the laboratory.

Lymph nodes for suspected lymphoproliferative disorders

Reason for consultation. To determine whether sufficient tissue is present for eventual diagnosis and special studies.

Change in surgery. Additional tissue may be provided if the initial specimen does not contain a lesion or is inadequate.

Evaluation. *Never freeze an entire specimen.* Cytologic preparations are often very helpful for evaluating small specimens and are usually superior to frozen sections for the diagnosis of lymphoproliferative diseases. Frozen sections may be performed on larger specimens if cytologic preparations are not adequate.

If a lymphoproliferative disorder is suspected, tissue should be saved for:

1. **B5 fixation:** best for morphology and immunoperoxidase markers for hematopathology.
2. **Snap freezing** (some markers are only available for frozen tissue). This tissue can also be used for DNA or RNA analysis.
3. **Formalin fixation** if the differential diagnosis includes carcinoma (keratins are not preserved well in B5), infectious disease (staining is better in formalin), or if Hodgkin's disease (HD) is suspected (lacunar cells in nodular sclerosis HD are seen only in formalin-fixed tissue).
4. **Flow cytometry:** Can be helpful in selected cases.
5. **Microbiologic culture:** Tissue may be sent for culture if the differential diagnosis includes an infectious process.

The intention of the frozen section is not to provide a definitive diagnosis. Usually "lesional tissue present" or "suspicious for a lymphoproliferative disorder" are sufficient intraoperative diagnoses.

Neuropathology: Stereotactic brain biopsies

Reason for consultation. Stereotactic biopsies are performed for deep-seated (i.e., thalamic) brain lesions not amenable to open surgical biopsy or resection or in patients with AIDS who have not responded to empiric treatment for presumed toxoplasmosis or primary CNS lymphoma. OR consultation is requested to determine whether the specimen is adequate for eventual diagnosis, including apportioning tissue for special studies (e.g., EM, cytogenetics, microbiologic culture).

Change in surgery. If the specimen is nondiagnostic, additional passes with the stereotactic needle should be done (if considered safe by the surgeon), and repeat frozen sections and/or smear preparations should be examined until diagnostic material is obtained.

Evaluation. The pathologist should be aware of the clinical setting and neuroimaging characteristics of the lesion, as these factors can aid in the differential diagnosis under consideration. Both smears and frozen sections should be performed for maximum accuracy.[40] Smears should be made from 0.5 mm samples from each end of the core biopsy specimen (or from one end of each core biopsy if more than one core is provided). If possible, some of the core (or cores) should be preserved unfrozen (i.e., free of frozen artifact) for permanent sections or ancillary studies.

Pitfalls. The major pitfall is inadequate sampling.[41] Since gliomas can be heterogeneous in cellularity, with the edges of high-grade tumors often mimicking diffuse, low-grade tumors, multiple biopsies are required for accurate diagnosis. Correlation with the neuroimaging is therefore crucial to be sure that the intraoperative diagnosis "makes sense." Intraoperative bleeding is a grave danger, so that the surgeon may be reluctant to provide additional material in the event of an initial nondiagnostic pass. Nevertheless, the pathologist must not be tempted to "overcall" minimal abnormalities on minute specimens, lest the surgeon believe there is adequate diagnostic material when there is not.

Soft tissue tumors and mesotheliomas

Biopsies

Reason for consultation. To determine whether sufficient lesional tissue is present in a diagnostic biopsy for eventual diagnosis on permanent sections and for special studies.

Change in surgery. The surgeon may remove additional tissue if the tissue is nondiagnostic or is insufficient for needed studies.

Evaluation. A frozen section or touch preparation may be performed to determine whether lesional tissue is present, to give a preliminary diagnosis, and to guide apportionment of tissue for special studies. A definitive diagnosis is not necessary, as final classification of such lesions often requires examination of multiple sections of the lesion and special studies. Often a diagnosis of "lesional tissue present" is sufficient. *Do not freeze the entire specimen.* If only a small amount of tissue is available (i.e., the surgeon cannot provide more tissue), then the entire specimen should be saved for permanent sections. If the tissue does not appear lesional or is necrotic, additional tissue may be requested from the surgeon.

These tumors often require special studies for their correct classification. For mesotheliomas, see also Chapter 26, "Extrapleural pneumonectomies," and page 513, "Pleural biopsies." Tumors are serially sectioned and representative sections taken for special studies:

1. **Quick-fix formalin:** Thin sections of the tumor are placed in a sufficient volume of formalin for rapid fixation. The fixation of the main tumor mass may be delayed while tissue is taken for other studies, photography, dissection, etc. These sections must be thin enough to not require recutting before submission.

2. **Electron microscopy:** A small portion of tumor is cut into small cubes (<1 mm per side) using a sharp blade and fixed for possible EM examination.

3. **Cytogenetics.** Cytogenetic studies can be helpful for classification or diagnosis in some cases. The tumor submitted must be viable and sterile.

4. **Snap freezing.** Small sections of tumor (similar to the size used for a frozen section) can be saved frozen. Such tissue may be useful for molecular diagnostic studies (DNA and RNA analysis) as indicated.

   If the specimen is small, and additional fresh tissue is not available for snap freezing, a frozen-section remnant can be saved frozen. Cool the surface of the block by turning the block upside down on the shelf and using the "quick cool" option on the cryostat. When cooled, add embedding medium and allow it to freeze. This will protect the tissue surface from thawing during transfer to permanent storage in a freezer.

5. **B5.** If lymphoma is in the differential diagnosis, tissue should also be fixed in B5 and possibly sent for flow cytometry (see p. 517, "Lymph Nodes, Bone Marrow and Spleen").

The remainder of the specimen is saved for possible photography and routine fixation in formalin.

Resections

Reason for consultation. To evaluate the adequacy of margins.

Change in surgery. Additional tissue may be taken at close or positive margins.

Evaluation. Resections of sarcomas and mesotheliomas are often large and complicated. If the orientation is unclear, seek clarification from the surgeon. The specimen is inked and serially sectioned. With occasional exceptions, it is generally inappropriate to freeze margins for sarcomas, since any margin less than 2 cm is usually an indication for radiotherapy. If margins are frozen, they are taken as perpendicular margins and not en face margins.

In extrapleural pneumonectomies, all tissue possible has usually been removed from the thoracic cavity and these margins are not evaluated except on specific request by the surgeon. The bronchial resection margin is usually evaluated by frozen section.

Thyroid nodules

Lobectomies

Reason for consultation. To determine whether a carcinoma is present.

Change in surgery. Additional surgery may be performed if a carcinoma is present:

- **Papillary carcinoma:** Complete thyroidectomy and possible lymph node dissection.
- **Follicular carcinoma:** Complete thyroidectomy.
- **Medullary carcinoma:** Complete thyroidectomy, and possible lymph node dissection and evaluation of parathyroids. If medullary carcinoma was not previously suspected, the operative team should be aware that there is a 10% to 15% chance the patient has a pheochromocytoma.

Evaluation. The use of intraoperative frozen section is controversial and varies among institutions. FNA and frozen sections can both be used effectively to guide management if the local accuracy rates for both techniques are known.

FNA positive for papillary carcinoma: FNA can have a greater than 95% accuracy rate for this diagnosis. There is only a small probability that frozen section will yield a definitive benign diagnosis. The diagnosis of papillary carcinoma can usually be easily corroborated by either frozen section or touch preparations, if requested.

FNA suspicious for papillary carcinoma: 30% to 50% of these lesions prove to be malignant. Frozen section or touch preparations can be helpful in establishing a definite diagnosis at surgery.

FNA suggestive of a follicular neoplasm: Approximately 20% to 30% of these lesions prove malignant. The determination of malignancy of follicular lesions is difficult and the probability of detecting capsular or vascular invasion on a frozen section is low. In one study, frozen-section evaluation correctly modified the surgical procedure in 3.3% of such cases but led to an incorrect procedure in 5% of cases.[42] If frozen-section evaluation is undertaken, the surgeon must be aware that few cancers are detected by this technique and that false positives can occur.

FNA interpreted as benign: The risk of carcinoma in this group is less than 10%. In one study, frozen-section evaluation identified only a third of the carcinomas missed by FNA in this group and produced an equal number of false positive cases.[43]

FNA inadequate or not performed: Frozen-section evaluation can be helpful in these cases. If follicular lesions are excluded, the sensitivity is over 95% and the specificity approaches 100%.

Before the specimen is examined, any previous FNA reports and thyroid ultrasound examinations should be reviewed to determine the likely type and site of lesions present.

The thyroid is inked, serially sectioned, and grossly evaluated for the presence of a single nodule or multiple nodules. Whenever possible, the location of nodules previously sampled by FNA should be identified to facilitate the correlation between histologic and cytologic findings.

A multinodular gland is more likely to be benign whereas a solitary lesion may be an adenoma or carcinoma.

Frozen sections should be taken from the edge of the lesion, including capsule if present.

Cytologic preparations are useful to look for the nuclear features of papillary carcinoma (intranuclear inclusions, grooves, large hypochromatic nuclei, and small nucleoli).

Pitfalls. The likelihood of not detecting capsular or vascular invasion in follicular carcinomas due to sampling error is high. In addition, distortion introduced by freezing artifact may make the evaluation of capsular and vascular invasion difficult. The follicular variant of papillary carcinoma may be mistaken for a follicular lesion. Cytologic preparations are very helpful for evaluating the nuclear features in such lesions.

Lymph node biopsy

Reason for consultation. Evaluation of a cervical lymph node in a patient with known or suspected thyroid carcinoma.

Change in surgery. If metastatic thyroid carcinoma is diagnosed, a total thyroidectomy may be performed or additional lymph nodes taken.

Evaluation. The lymph node is serially sectioned and the most abnormal area frozen.

Pitfalls. Multinodular thyroid glands may have parasitic nodules that appear to be lymph nodes to the surgeon. If the gland is involved by thyroiditis and germinal centers are present, it is possible to mistake such a nodule for metastatic thyroid carcinoma. However, the nuclear features of papillary carcinoma are not present.

The presence of normal thyroid inclusions in cervical nodes is controversial: some pathologists interpret these cases as metastatic thyroid carcinoma. In order to be interpreted as "benign inclusions," such inclusions should be limited to a few follicles found beneath the capsule in a single lymph node. Cytologic features of papillary carcinoma must be absent.

Parathyroid surgery

Reason for consultation.
Parathyroid surgery is undertaken either for primary hyperparathyroidism (usually caused by a solitary adenoma) or for secondary hyperparathyroidism (almost

always resulting from chronic renal failure). The distinction between primary and secondary hyperparathyroidism is best made on clinical grounds (i.e., elevated serum calcium versus low serum calcium), and the distinction between an adenoma (a single enlarged gland) and primary hyperplasia (two or more enlarged glands) is best made by surgical evaluation of all four glands.

Some institutions use rapid serum parathyroid hormone assays to guide surgery for adenomas. If the serum level drops after removal of an adenoma, further surgical exploration and frozen-section evaluation may not be necessary.[44] Serum calcium also drops rapidly after the removal of a hyperfunctioning adenoma.

Change in surgery. If parathyroid tissue is not demonstrated, the surgeon may continue to search for additional parathyroid glands.

Evaluation. The role of the pathologist is to determine whether parathyroid tissue is present in each specimen submitted. Although normal glands usually have more than 25% adipose tissue and adenomas usually have less than 5%, this is not an absolutely reliable diagnostic feature.

Adenomas: The adenoma will have been removed in entirety and have a smooth, ovoid appearance. Both the size and weight are important diagnostic features. Document parathyroid parenchyma by frozen section. The three remaining normal glands are visually inspected and one to three of them may be biopsied. These biopsies are small and are frozen in entirety to document the presence of parathyroid parenchyma.

Secondary hyperplasia: Three glands will have been removed and the fourth gland partially resected. All glands are markedly enlarged: their size and weights should be documented. Freeze a representative section of each to confirm the presence of parathyroid parenchyma.

Pitfalls. The identification of parathyroid tissue can be made with 99% accuracy.[45] The most frequent problem in the study of Westra et al was distinguishing between thyroid and parathyroid tissue.

Parathyroid tissue mistaken for thyroid: Pseudofollicular and trabecular structures may be present, containing material that looks like colloid, and resemble normal thyroid. Parathyroid tissue can also resemble a Hürthle cell nodule if comprised of oxyphilic cells. Thyroid follicles frequently contain calcium oxalate crystals, which are easily seen with polarization. These crystals are not seen in parathyroid tissue.

Thyroid tissue mistaken for normal parathyroid tissue: Stromal edema or frozen-section artifact can mimic adipose tissue. Rarely, adipose metaplasia may be present. In some cases, immunohistochemistry is necessary to discriminate between the two tissues. This

problem most frequently arises when there is a multinodular thyroid gland with small parasitic nodules or an intrathyroidal parathyroid gland.

Lymph node mistaken for parathyroid tissue: Frozen-section artifact can mimic adipose tissue within a lymph node, and it can be mistaken for parathyroid tissue.

Sampling error: Small diagnostic areas of parathyroid tissue may be missed.

■ PRECAUTIONS AGAINST INFECTION IN THE OR CONSULTATION ROOM

Pathology personnel handle potentially infectious material every day. It is estimated that 50% of the patients who are HIV positive are undiagnosed at the time of admission to the hospital, and this is undoubtedly also true of other patients with infectious diseases. Pathologists therefore must do their best to limit the risk of infection to themselves and to the people they work with by handling *all* specimens with universal precautions.

OR consultations on tissues from patients with known infectious diseases may be performed *if* this information is important for immediate patient management. If the purpose of the examination is unclear, the surgeon should be contacted to clarify what information would be useful to the clinicians. Frozen sections are avoided if possible.

Three cases of conversion to a positive tuberculin skin test have been linked to aerosol produced by spraying a tissue block with a compressed gas coolant,[5,6] demonstrating that, although rare, exposure can occur. These sprays are no longer recommended for use. Cytologic preparations are not as hazardous for infectious specimens and often are as good or better than frozen sections for diagnosis. If a frozen section is performed on tissue from a patient known or suspected to be positive for HIV, hepatitis B or C, or have mycobacterial infection, the cryostat must be clearly marked as contaminated and should be decontaminated before further use.

Guidelines—infection precautions

- Always wear gloves when handling specimens. Double gloving (as well as the use of aprons, face masks, and eye protection) is recommended for known infectious cases or for bloody specimens. An OSHA-approved TB respirator must be worn for known or suspected cases of TB.
- After working on a specimen with known or potential pathogens, *immediately remove your gloves*. Do not touch anything else in the room (e.g., the cryostats, staining rack, microscopes, telephones) with contaminated gloves. If you want to protect your hands from these surfaces, use a pair of clean gloves.
- Clean the workstation by removing all blood, tissue, and sharps (razor blades, scalpels, syringe needles). Tissue is placed in appropriately labeled containers in

formalin or stored in the refrigerator in sealed bags or specimen containers. Make sure the containers are tightly sealed and leak proof. Sharps and glass slides must be discarded in the appropriate designated containers. Used tools (forceps, rulers, scalpel handles, etc.) should be rinsed free of gross blood and disinfected.

- Before removing the scalpel blade from the handle, all gross tissue and blood should be cleaned off in a disinfectant solution. A forceps is used for this procedure.
- Always leave the workstation ready for the next frozen-section examination.
- Always wash your hands before leaving the OR consultation room.
- Disposable gowns, aprons, face masks, and eye protection are recommended whenever exposure to blood or tissue is expected.
- Do not eat or drink in the OR consultation room, bring food into the room, or dispose of empty food containers in the room. The presence of food or former food containers is against OSHA rules and may result in penalties or closure.

See Chapter 8, "Safety precautions," for more information, or if a significant exposure should occur.

REFERENCES

1. Ranchod M, ed. Intraoperative Consultations in Surgical Pathology, State of the Art Reviews. Vol 3, No 2 Philadelphia. Hanley & Belfus, 1996.
2. Li Volsi V. A surgical pathologist views practice parameters. Am J Clin Pathol 103:1-2, 1995.
3. Weiss SW, Willis J, Jansen J, Goldblum J, Greenfield L. Frozen section consultation, utilization patterns and knowledge base of surgical faculty at a university hospital. Am J Clin Pathol 104:294-298, 1995.
4. Zarbo RJ, Schmidt WA, Bachner P, et al. Indications and immediate patient outcomes of pathology intraoperative consultations, a College of American Pathologists/Centers for Disease Control and Prevention Outcomes Working Group Study. Arch Pathol Lab Med 120:19-25, 1996.
5. Tuberculosis infection associated with tissue processing. MMWR Morb Mortal Wkly Rep 30:73-74, 1981.
6. Duray PH, Flannery B, Brown S. Tuberculosis infection from preparation of frozen sections. N Engl J Med 305:167, 1981.
7. Sidawy MK, Silverberg SG. Intraoperative cytology. Am J Clin Pathol 96:1-3, 1991.
8. CAP Quality Improvement Manual in Anatomic Pathology. Illinois, College of American Pathologists, 1993.
9. Sawady J, Berner JJ, Siegler EE. Accuracy of and reasons for frozen sections: A correlative, retrospective study. Hum Pathol 19:1019-1023, 1988.
10. Association of Directors of Anatomic and Surgical Pathology. Recommendations on Quality Control and Quality Assurance in Anatomic Pathology. Hum Pathol 22:1099, 1991.
11. Association of Directors of Anatomic and Surgical Pathology. Recommendations on Quality Control and

Quality Assurance in Anatomic Pathology. Am J Surg Pathol 15:1007-1009, 1991.
12. Association of Directors of Anatomic and Surgical Pathology. Recommendations on Quality Control and Quality Assurance in Anatomic Pathology. Mod Pathol 5:567-568, 1992.
13. Forrest LA, Schuller DE, Lucas JG, Sullivan MJ. Rapid analysis of mandibular margins. Laryngoscope 105:475-477, 1995.
14. Lonner JH, Desai P, Dicesare PE, Steiner G, Zuckerman JD. The reliability of analysis of intraoperative frozen sections for identifying active infection during revision hip or knee arthroplasty. J Bone Joint Surg Am 78:1553-1558, 1996.
15. Abdul-Karim FW, McGinnis MG, Kraay M, Emancipator SN, Goldberg V. Frozen section biopsy assessment for the presence of polymorphonuclear leukocytes in patients undergoing revision of arthroplasties. Mod Pathol 11:427-431, 1998.
16. Stamenkovic I, Lew D. Early recognition of potentially fatal necrotizing fasciitis; the use of frozen-section biopsy. N Engl J Med 310:1689-1693, 1984.
17. Majeski J, Majeski E. Necrotizing fasciitis: improved survival with early recognition by tissue biopsy and aggressive surgical treatment. South Med J 90:1065-1068, 1997.
18. Fechner RE. Frozen section examination of breast biopsies. Practice parameter. Am J Clin Pathol 103:6-7, 1995.
19. Bianchi S, Palli D, Ciatto S, et al. Accuracy and reliability of frozen section diagnosis in a series of 672 nonpalpable breast lesions. Am J Clin Pathol 103:199-205, 1995.
20. Cox CE, Ku NN, Reintgen DS, Greenberg HM, Nicosia SV, Wangensteen S. Touch preparation cytology of breast lumpectomy margins with histologic correlation. Arch Surg 126:490-493, 1991.
21. England DW, Chan SY, Stonelake PS, Lee MJR. Assessment of excision margins following wide local excision for breast carcinoma using specimen scrape cytology and tumour bed biopsy. Eur J Surg Oncol 20:425-429, 1994.
22. Sauter ER, Hoffman JP, Ottery FD, Kowalyshyn MJ, Litwin S, Eisenberg BL. Is frozen section analysis of reexcision lumpectomy margins worthwhile? Margin analysis in breast reexcisions. Cancer 73:2607-2612, 1994.
23. Goldstein JS, Soman A, Sacksner J. Disparate surgical margin lengths of colorectal resection specimens between in vivo and in vitro measurements. The effects of surgical resection and formalin fixation on organ shrinkage. Am J Clin Pathol 111:349-351, 1999.
24. McLeod RS. Resection margins and recurrent Crohn's disease. Hepatogastroenterology 37:63-66, 1990.
25. Fazio VW, Marchetti F, Church M, et al. Effect of resection margins on the recurrence of Crohn's disease in the small bowel. A randomized controlled trial. Ann Surg 224:563-571, 1996.
26. Hertzler GL, Millikan WJ. The surgical pathologist's role in liver transplantation. Arch Pathol Lab Med 115:273, 1991.
27. Markin RS, Wood RP, Stratta RJ, et al. Predictive value of intraoperative liver biopsies of donor organs in patients undergoing orthotopic liver transplantation. Transplant Proc 22:418, 1990.
28. University of Pittsburgh Transplant Web site (http://tpis.upmc.edu/).
29. Hyland C, Kheir SM, Kashlan MB. Frozen section diagnosis of pancreatic carcinoma, a prospective study of

64 biopsies. Am J Surg Pathol 5:179-191, 1981.

30. Campanale RP, Frey CF, Farias R, Twomey PL, Guernsey JM, Keehn R, Higgins G. Reliability and sensitivity of frozen-section pancreatic biopsy. Arch Surg 120:283-288, 1985.

31. Brown JA, Hubosky SG, Gomella LG, Strup SE. Hand assisted laparoscopic partial nephrectomy for peripheral and central lesions: a review of 30 consecutive cases. J Urol 171:1443-1446, 2004.

32. Krishnan B, Lechago J, Ayala G, Truong L. Intraoperative consultation for renal lesions. Implications and diagnostic pitfalls in 324 cases. Am J Clin Pathol 120:528-535, 2003.

33. Tangjitgamol S, Jesadapatrakul S, Manusirivithaya S, Sheanakul C. Accuracy of frozen section in diagnosis of ovarian mass. Int J Gynecol Cancer 14:212-219, 2004.

34. Kir G, Kir M, Cetiner H, Karateke A, Gurbuz A. Diagnostic problems on frozen section examination of myometrial invasion in patients with endometrial carcinoma with special emphasis on the pitfalls of deep adenomyosis with carcinomatous involvement. Eur J Gynaecol Oncol 25:211-214, 2004.

35. Spandorfer SD, Menzin AW, Barnhart KT, LiVolsi VA, Pfeifer SM. Efficacy of frozen-section evaluation of uterine curettings in the diagnosis of ectopic pregnancy. Am J Obstet Gynecol 175:603, 1996.

36. Tschen JA, Fechner RE. The juxtaoral organ of Chievitz. Am J Surg Pathol 3:147-150, 1979.

37. Gephardt GN, Rice TW. Utility of frozen-section evaluation of lymph nodes in the staging of bronchogenic carcinoma at mediastinoscopy and thoracotomy. J Thorac Cardiovasc Surg 100:853-859, 1990.

38. Maygarden SJ, Detterbeck FC, Funkhouser WK. Bronchial margins in lung cancer resection specimens: utility of frozen section and gross evaluation. Mod Pathol 17:1080-1086, 2004.

39. Renshaw AA. The relative sensitivity of special stains and cultures in open lung biopsies. Am J Clin Pathol 102:736-740, 1994.

40. Folkerth RD. Smears and frozen sections in the intraoperative diagnosis of central nervous system lesions. Neurosurg Clin N Am 5:1-18, 1994.

41. Brainard JA, Prayson RA, Barnett GH. Frozen section evaluation of stereotactic brain biopsies. Diagnostic yield at the stereotactic target position in 188 cases. Arch Pathol Lab Med 121:481-484, 1997.

42. Chen H, Nicol TL, Udelsman R. Follicular lesions of the thyroid, Does frozen section evaluation alter operative management? Ann Surg 222:101-106, 1995.

43. Hamburger JI, Hamburger SW. Declining role of frozen section in surgical planning for thyroid nodules. Surgery 98:307-312, 1985.).

44. Carter AB, Howanitz PJ. Intraoperative testing for parathyroid hormone: a comprehensive review of the use of the assay and the relevant literature. Arch Pathol Lab Med 127:1424-1442, 2003.

45. Westra WH, Pritchett DD, Udelsman R. Intraoperative confirmation of parathyroid tissue during parathyroid exploration, a retrospective evaluation of the frozen section. Am J Surg Pathol 22:538-544, 1998.

Special studies

7

The pathologist's H&E is like the clinician's H&P (history and physical)—basic examinations that are performed on every specimen or patient to form the cornerstone of diagnosis. However, the pathologist is no longer limited to H&E: a wide variety of special studies are available to evaluate pathologic processes, from simple histochemical stains to global gene expression patterns. Pathologists are now clinical cell biologists. Familiarity with the types of special studies available is important as the initial processing of the gross specimen may limit the types of studies that can be performed.

■ HISTOCHEMISTRY

Almost all histochemical stains are suitable for use on formalin-fixed tissues. Common stains and their uses are listed in Table 7-1. However, numerous other types of stains and modifications are used and pathologists must be aware of individual laboratory practices.

Table 7-1 Histochemical stains		
STAIN	COMPONENTS STAINED	POSSIBLE USES AND COMMENTS
AFOG (acid fuchsin orange G; modified Masson's trichrome)	Nuclei: brown Connective tissue: blue Basement membrane: blue Proteins, fibrin, readsorption droplets in cells, immune complexes: red/orange/yellow RBCs: yellow	Evaluation of renal biopsies
Alcian blue	Acid mucins: blue (e.g., normal intestinal glands) Nuclei: red Cytoplasm: pink	Sometimes used to identify mucosubstances in mesotheliomas or intestinal metaplasia; affected by pH; hyaluronidase digestion can be used to identify hyaluronic acid
Alcian blue–PAS	Intestinal metaplasia: dark purple Normal stomach: pink	Demonstrates both acid and neutral mucins
Alcian yellow	Free mucus: yellow Bacteria: dark blue	Identification of *H. pylori* in gastric biopsies
Acid-fast bacilli stains (Fite–Faraco, Ziehl–Neelsen, Kinyoun)	TB: red and beaded MAI: red *Nocardia*: pink Tissue: blue	Identification of mycobacteria; modifications are used to demonstrate *M. leprae* or *Nocardia*; tissues fixed in Carnoy's cannot be used, and B5 is suboptimal; slides must be examined under oil

Table 7-1 Histochemical stains—*cont'd*

STAIN	COMPONENTS STAINED	POSSIBLE USES AND COMMENTS
Alizarin red S	Calcium: orange red, polarizes	Identifies calcium in tissues
Bile	Bile: dark green on a yellow background	Identification of bile
Bodian's	Nerve fibers and neurofibrils: black Nuclei: black Tissue: blue	Neural tumors, identification of axons
Chloroacetate esterase (CAE; Leder)	Mature myeloid cells, mast cells: red granules Nuclei: blue	Evaluation of leukemias; identification of mast cells; cannot be used for tissue fixed in Zenker's or B5
Congo red	Amyloid: orange-red with apple-green birefringence after polarization Nuclei: blue	Detection of amyloid; immunoperoxidase studies can be used to identify specific types; overstaining can result in false positives
Dieterle	Spirochetes, *Legionella*, other bacteria: brown to black Tissue: pale yellow or tan	Infectious lesions; melanin, chromatin, formalin pigment, and foreign material may also stain
Diff-Quik® (a modified Giemsa stain)	*H. pylori*: dark blue Other bacteria: blue Nuclei: dark blue Cytoplasm: pink	Evaluation of chronic gastritis
Elastic stains (Verhoeff–van Gieson) (= ET)	Elastic fibers: blue black to black Nuclei: blue to black Collagen: red Other tissue: yellow	Identification of arteries and veins, vasculitis, invasion of lung tumors into visceral pleura, abnormal elastic fibers in elastofibromas
Fibrin (see phosphotungistic acid–hematoxylin [Mallory's PTAH])		To demonstrate fibrin in renal biopsies
Fontana–Masson	Melanin, argentaffin granules, chromaffin granules, some lipofuscin: black Nuclei: red	Identification of melanin in melanomas and secretory granules in neuroendocrine tumors; use of this stain has largely been replaced by immunohistochemistry
Giemsa (May–Grünwald)	Bacteria (e.g., *H. pylori*): blue Parasites (*Leishmania, Plasmodium*) Mast cells: red to purple granules Nuclei: blue Cytoplasm of leukocytes: pink to blue depending on cell type and differentiation	Lymphoproliferative disorders (good nuclear and cytoplasmic detail); identification of bacteria, rickettsias, and *Toxoplasma gondii*
Gram (Brown–Hopps, Brown–Brenn)	Gram-positive bacteria: blue Gram-negative bacteria: red Nuclei: red Tissue: variable	Identification of bacteria, some cases of actinomycetes, *Nocardia*, coccidioidomycosis, blastomycosis, cryptococcosis, aspergillosis, rhinosporidiosis, and amebiasis
Grimelius	Argentaffin and argyrophil granules: dark brown to black Nuclei: red Background: pale yellow-brown	Evaluation of neuroendocrine tumors (largely replaced by the use of immunohistochemistry for chromogranin)
Hematoxylin and eosin (H&E)	Nuclei: dark blue or purple Cytoplasm: pink to red	Standard stain for the routine evaluation of tissues
Iron (colloidal iron)	Ferric iron (e.g., hemosiderin): blue Nuclei: red Background: pink	Bone marrow (iron stores, myelodysplasias), liver (hemochromatosis); chromophobe renal cell carcinomas are positive

Table 7-1 Histochemical stains—*cont'd*

STAIN	COMPONENTS STAINED	POSSIBLE USES AND COMMENTS
Melanin bleach		Removes melanin from tissue, usually for IHC; melanin can be difficult to distinguish from IHC positivity
Methyl green–pyronin Y	DNA (nuclei): green to blue-green RNA: red Goblet cells: mint green Plasma cell and immunoblast cytoplasm: pink to red Mast cells: orange Background: pale pink to colorless	Plasma cell lesions (largely replaced by immunohistochemistry); does not work well on tissues decalcified with formic acid
Mucicarmine (Mayer)	Mucin: deep rose to red Capsule of cryptococcus: deep rose to red Nuclei: black Tissue: blue or yellow	Identification of adenocarcinomas, identification of cryptococcus
Oil red O	Fat: red Nuclei: blue	Requires frozen sections (lipids are dissolved by most fixatives or during processing); tissue fixed in formalin can be used if tissue is frozen
Periodic acid–Schiff (PAS)	Glycogen: red Basement membranes (BM): red Mucins: red Colloid: red Fungi: red	Classification of tumors with glycogen (e.g., Ewing's/PNET, rhabdomyosarcoma, renal cell carcinoma), glomerular diseases (BM), identification of adenocarcinomas (mucin), fungal diseases (especially in argentophilic areas: neutrophils and debris), spironolactone bodies in adrenal adenomas treated with this drug
Periodic acid–Schiff with diastase digestion (PAS-D)	As above, except glycogen has been digested and will not be stained	Identification of glycogen in tumors; identification of fungus in glycogen-rich tissue (e.g., skin); PAS-D resistant deposits in liver are present in α_1-antitrypsin deficiency
Phosphotungistic acid–hematoxylin (Mallory's PTAH)	Glial fibers: blue Nuclei: blue Neurons: salmon pink Myelin: blue Skeletal muscle cross-striations: blue Fibrin: blue Collagen: red-brown	Identification of neural lesions; skeletal muscle differentiation (Zenker's fixative is preferred); this stain has been replaced by IHC for muscle markers
Reticular fibers (Gomori, Gordon and Sweets, Snook) (RETIC)	Reticulin: black Mature collagen, type 1: brown Immature collagen, types 3 and 4: black	Bone marrow (myelophthisis), liver (fibrosis, veno-occlusive disease), carcinoma versus sarcoma (reticular network); largely replaced by IHC
Silver stain (Grocott methenamine–silver nitrate—GMS) (GMS or MMS)	Fungi: black *Pneumocystis carinii*: black Mucin: taupe to gray Tissue: green	Evaluation of infectious diseases; bacteria will also stain black
Steiner	Spirochetes, *H. pylori*, *Legionella*, other bacteria: dark brown to black Tissue: light yellow	Evaluation of infectious diseases
Toluidine blue	Mast cells: deep violet Background: blue	Mast cell diseases, chronic cystitis

Table 7-1 Histochemical stains—cont'd

STAIN	COMPONENTS STAINED	POSSIBLE USES AND COMMENTS
Trichrome (Gomori's trichrome, Masson) (= TRI)	Mature collagen, type 1: dark blue Immature collagen, types 3 and 4: light blue Mucin: green or blue Nuclei: black Cytoplasm, keratin, muscle fibers: red	Liver (fibrosis)
Von Kossa calcium	Calcium: black Tissue: red	Demonstration of phosphate and carbonate radicals with calcium in tissues, identification of malakoplakia (Michaelis–Gutmann bodies)
Warthin–Starry	Spirochetes: black Cat scratch bacillus and *Bartonella henselae* (bacillary angiomatosis): black Other bacteria: black Tissue: pale yellow to light brown	Infectious lesions
Wright's	Eosinophilic granules: pink Neutrophilic granules: purple Lymphocytic cytoplasm: blue Nuclei: blue to purple	Blood smears

The WebPath section of the University of Utah site (http://medlib.med.utah.edu) has useful descriptions of special stains and illustrative photographs.

■ IMMUNOPEROXIDASE STUDIES

The development of methods to detect antigens on tissue sections with antibodies was a major advance in surgical pathology. Immunohistochemical (IHC) studies are most frequently used for the following purposes:

- Classification of tumors (e.g., carcinoma versus lymphoma, B-cell versus T-cell lymphoma)
- Identification of in situ lesions versus invasion (e.g., myoepithelial markers in breast cancers, basal cell markers in prostate)
- Prognostic factors (e.g., Ki-67 in glioblastomas)
- Predictive factors to guide specific therapy (e.g., c-kit, estrogen and progesterone receptors, HER2/neu)
- Identification of extracellular material (e.g., β_2-microglobulin amyloid)
- Identification of infectious agents (e.g., cytomegalovirus).

Use of immunohistochemistry

A differential diagnosis is generated after examination of the H&E stained slides. Immunohistochemistry is then used to gain evidence for or against diagnostic possibilities. "Trolling" cases through an immunohistochemistry laboratory by ordering numerous antibody studies without a clear reason in mind is more likely to lead to misguided diagnosis due to aberrant immunoreactivity than to provide an unexpected correct diagnosis.

A very useful website has been developed by Dr. Dennis M. Frisman (http://www.immunoquery.com): it tabulates published literature on the immunoreactivity profiles for numerous tumors. There is also a comprehensive list of the included references with web links.

Panels

There are no absolute rules for immunoreactivity in cells and tissues. Aberrant positive immunoreactivity (or absence of immunoreactivity) is occasionally observed for all antibodies, either due to biologic variability (e.g., occasional keratin-positive melanomas) or technical factors (impure antibodies, cross-reaction with other antigens, failure to preserve antigenicity). Thus, immunohistochemical markers are used most effectively as panels of markers, with interpretation based on an immunohistochemical profile.

Slides for immunohistochemistry

Tissue is often dislodged from normal glass slides during the treatments required for IHC. Slides must be coated (e.g., with glue, poly-L-lysine, gelatin, albumin) or special commercial slides must be used. If slides are being prepared by another laboratory, the type of glass slide to be used must be specified.

Factors affecting immunogenicity

Numerous variables can affect antigenicity. The most common are described below. Each laboratory must optimize its procedures for each antibody used. Studies on tissues or slides not prepared in the routine fashion for a laboratory must be interpreted with caution.

Type of fixative.

Some fixatives destroy some antigens (e.g., Bouin's diminishes ER immunoreactivity, keratins are not well preserved in B5).[1] Most studies are based on formalin-fixed tissue. Results cannot be assumed to be equivalent for other fixatives.

Length of time of fixation in formalin.

Protein cross-linking and antigenicity generally decrease with fixation times over 24 hours. To some extent, this effect can be reversed using antigen-retrieval methods.

Prior decalcification in hydrochloric acid.

This decreases the antigenicity of some epitopes (predominantly nuclear) but not others (predominantly cytoplasmic).[2] Decalcifying agents using EDTA do not alter immunogenicity.

Decreased: ER, PR, Ki-67, p53, Ber-EP4 (tumor cells).
Not affected: calcitonin, chromogranin, GCDFP-15, HMB-45, thyroglobulin, S100, PSA, keratins (CK 20, CAM 5.2, AE1/AE3), others.

Length of time since the glass slide was cut.[3–6] The immunoreactivity of the majority of antigens declines over days to weeks and may be lost completely at 1 month.[3–6] The loss may be due to oxidation of amino acids with exposure of tissue to air, as the immunogenicity of tissue deeper in the block can be preserved for many years. Antigen-retrieval methods do not completely restore the antigenicity of old slides. Coating slides with paraffin, storing the slides in a nitrogen desiccator, and/or storing at lower temperatures can partially preserve antigenicity. However, studies should be performed on newly cut slides, if possible.

Antigen-retrieval procedures. These include proteolysis, heating (microwave, steam), and special incubation fluids. To some extent these methods reverse the effects of formalin fixation. Variable effects are observed for different antibodies.

Type of antibody (polyclonal versus monoclonal versus mixture of different monoclonals), epitope detected. Very different results can be obtained with different antibodies to the same protein or different commercial sources of the same antibody.

Incubation time, incubation temperature, dilution of antibody.

Methods of signal amplification.

Temperature of baking the slide.

Controls

Controls are essential for the appropriate interpretation of immunohistochemical studies and to ensure that all steps of this complicated procedure have been adequately performed.

Positive controls. Tissues known to be immunoreactive should be included each time an antibody is used for a test case. Internal positive controls should always be

evaluated when present as they control not only for the technique used but also for the antigenicity of the tissue under investigation. Table 7-30 (see pp. 103) lists normal cells that are generally immunoreactive for each antibody. Some laboratories have used vimentin as a control for immunogenicity as almost all tissue should demonstrate positivity.[7] Given the wide and nonspecific distribution of vimentin, smooth muscle α-actin may be more useful in this context as pericytes, vascular smooth muscle, and myoepithelial cells present in most tissues are immunoreactive.

Examples of internal controls are:

- S100: Normal nerves, melanocytes and Langerhans' cells in epidermis, cartilage, some myoepithelial cells, skin adnexa
- Estrogen and progesterone receptors: Normal luminal cells in ducts and lobules of the breast
- CD31, FVIII: Vascular endothelium
- c-kit: Mast cells
- Smooth muscle α-actin: Blood vessel walls, myoepithelial cells in the breast
- Vimentin: Blood vessels, stromal cells
- High-molecular-weight keratin: Squamous epithelium
- Low-molecular-weight keratin: Glandular epithelium
- CD15: polymorphonuclear leukocytes.

Negative controls. The primary antibody is replaced with non-immune animal serum diluted to the same concentration as the primary antibody for a negative control. No positive reaction should be present. If multiple primary antibodies that are reactive with different target antigens are used, then they may serve as negative controls for each other. Although the best negative control would be to use antibody preabsorbed against the target antigen, this is rarely practical in a diagnostic laboratory. Diagnostic slides should also be evaluated for internal negative controls. Aberrant immunoreactivity of tissues that should not be immunoreactive indicates that the immunoreactivity is nonspecific and should not be used for interpretation.

Evaluation of immunoperoxidase studies

The following features must be taken into consideration when evaluating immunoperoxidase studies:

Examples:
Nuclear: ER, TTF-1, P63, Myf4, Ki-67 (MIB-1)
Membranous: EMA, HER2/neu, e-cadherin, EGFR
Cytoplasmic: actin, keratin
Stromal: amyloid (β_2-microglobulin, calcitonin, lambda chain)

In rare cases, immunoreactivity in an unusual location is of diagnostic importance:

- TTF-1: Cytoplasmic (instead of nuclear) positivity in hepatocellular carcinomas.
- Ki-67 (MIB-1): Cytoplasmic and membrane (instead of nuclear) positivity in trabecular hyalinizing

adenomas of the thyroid and sclerosing hemangiomas of the lung.

- Beta-catenin: Nuclear (instead of cytoplasmic) positivity in solid-pseudopapillary tumors of the pancreas and pancreaticoblastomas. Both nuclear and cytoplasmic positivity is seen in the majority of colon carcinomas. Nuclear positivity is present in approximately 20% of endometrioid endometrial carcinomas.

Identification of immunoreactive cells. Immunoreactivity of tumor cells must be distinguished from immunoreactivity of normal entrapped cells (e.g., desmin-positive skeletal muscle cells infiltrated by tumor, S100-positive Langerhans' cells in tumors, smooth muscle α-actin-positive blood vessels, etc.). Plasma cells have large amounts of cytoplasmic immunoglobulin and can react nonspecifically with many antibodies.

Intensity of immunoreactivity. Some weak immunoreactivity may be present as a nonspecific finding. It is important to compare positive cells with control slides and with normally non-immunoreactive cells to determine whether the immunoreactivity is significant.

Number of immunoreactive cells. In some cases, the number of positive cells may be important as a criterion for positivity or as a prognostic marker (e.g., markers of proliferation such as Ki-67). In other cases, rare weakly positive cells must be distinguished from intermingled normal cells or just nonspecific immunoreactivity.

Criteria for a "positive" result. Specific criteria for evaluating IHC have been developed for a few antibodies (see Tables 15-3, 15-4, and 7-28). However, criteria do not exist for most antibodies or are not universally used by all pathologists. The significance of immunoreactivity varies with the type of lesion, the antibody, and the specific assay. Strong positivity in the majority of cells is easily interpreted as a positive result. As the number of positive cells decreases, and the intensity of immunoreactivity weakens, the lower threshold of a "positive" result becomes more difficult to determine.

Time. Alkaline phosphatase chromogens (red color) fade over time. DAB (brown color) is more permanent. This is not a problem in evaluating current pathology specimens. However, if immunoperoxidase slides are reviewed after a period of time, some chromogens may have faded and once-positive results may appear to be negative.

Location of immunoreactivity (Fig. 7-1). Antigens are present in specific sites. Some antigens may be present in more than one location or be extracellular.

Artifacts. Nonspecific positivity should be suspected when immunoreactivity is present in atypical locations:

Background: Suspect nonspecific positivity if normal cells or stroma are positive. This can occur with suboptimal performance of the assay or suboptimal antibodies.

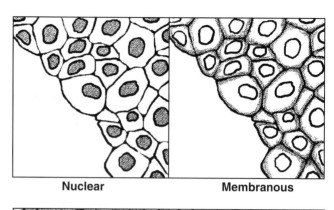
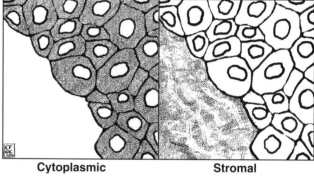

Figure 7-1 Location of immunoreactivity.

Edge artifact: Antibodies can pool at edges or in holes in tissue. True positivity should also be present in the center of the tissue.

Necrosis or crushing of cells: Nonspecific positivity can be seen in disrupted cells. Although keratin is generally reliable in necrotic tumors, other markers generally should not be interpreted.

Inappropriate location (e.g., cytoplasm instead of nucleus): Occasionally ER or PR is present in the cytoplasm instead of the nucleus. This is not interpreted as a positive result.

Common panels for immunohistochemical studies

Tables 7-3 to 7-30 include information from the literature as well as the personal experiences of the staff at Brigham and Women's Hospital. Because of the many differences in specific antibodies, laboratory assays, and criteria for considering a result "positive," results may vary among institutions. The results have been divided into five categories for general markers and four categories for hematopathology markers (Table 7-2). Note that "%" refers to the number of tumors reported to be positive, not the number of cells positive within a tumor.

The actual markers used to evaluate a case depend upon the differential diagnosis based on the H&E appearance. In some cases, an initial panel that is often used for typical cases has been suggested. Not all markers listed would be used for all cases, and some markers are

Table 7-2 Evaluation of positivity of immunohistochemical studies

CATEGORY	GENERAL MARKERS % OF TUMORS	INTERPRETATION	CATEGORY	HEMATOPATHOLOGY MARKERS % OF TUMORS	INTERPRETATION
Positive (POS)	>90%	Almost always positive; a negative result would be unusual	+	>90%	Almost always positive
High	60–90%	Most tumors are positive	+/–	>50%	Majority positive
Moderate (Mod)	40–60%	May or may not be positive – usually the least useful type of marker	–/+	<50%	Minority positive
Low	10–40%	Most tumors are negative	–	<10%	Rarely positive
Negative (neg) or rare	<10%	Almost all tumors are negative; a positive result would be unusual	Blank		Results unknown or too few cases to quantify
Blank		Results unknown or too few cases to quantify ? = Results based on very few cases (e.g., <10)			

included to indicate when they would not be useful for distinguishing the tumors listed in the table.

Cytokeratin 7 and Cytokeratin

The combination of these two cytokeratins has been found to be useful to divide carcinomas into four main groups (Ck7+/Ck20+, Ck7+/Ck20–, Ck7–/Ck20+, Ck7–/Ck20–).[8–10]

In Tables 7-3 to 7-7, other commonly used antibodies have been included to show differences within each group. The most useful additional antibodies depend on the specific differential diagnosis.

Spindle cell lesions, soft tissue lesions, and sarcomas See Table 7-8.

Small blue cell tumors See Table 7-9.

Myoepithelial markers in breast cancer
See Table 7-10.

Epidermal lesions of the nipple See Table 7-11.

Endocervical carcinoma versus endometrial carcinoma See Table 7-12.

Endometrial stromal sarcoma versus leiomyosarcoma See Table 7-13.

Primary ovarian carcinoma versus metastatic carcinomas See Table 7-14.

Ovarian carcinoma versus mesothelioma
See Table 7-15.

Trophoblastic lesions See Table 7-16.

Tumors of germ cells and sex-cord stromal tumors See Table 7-17.

Adrenal and kidney tumors See Table 7-18.

Tumors of bladder, prostatic, or renal origin
See Table-7.19.

Prostate carcinoma versus other lesions
See Table 7-20.

Hepatic tumors See Table 7-21.

Thyroid and parathyroid lesions See Table 7-22.

B-cell neoplasms See Table 7-23.

T-cell neoplasms See Table 7-24.

Hodgkin's lymphoma See Table 7.25.

Metastatic tumors of unknown origin
See Table 7-26.

Poorly differentiated tumors See Table 7-27.

Estrogen and progesterone receptor evaluation and HER2/neu score
See Chapter 15, pages 240-243.

EGFR (HER1) score See Table 7-28.

Differential diagnosis of epithelial mesothelioma and lung adenocarcinoma[13]
See Table 7-29.

Table 7-3 Predominantly CK7+/CK20+

TUMOR	CK7+ CK20+	CK7+ CK20−	CK7− CK20+	CK7− CK20−	34β E12	CAM 5.2	CK 5/6	EMA	BER-EP4	CEA m	CEA p	TTF-1	P63	WT-1	S100	CHRO	HEP	OTHER
Cholangiocarcinoma	High	Low	Low	neg	High	POS	Low	POS	POS	High	POS	neg	Low				rare	
Transitional cell carcinoma	POS	Low	neg	neg	Mod	POS	High	POS		Mod	Mod	neg	High	neg	neg	neg	neg	
Pancreas	High	Low	Low	neg		POS	Low	POS	POS	High	POS	neg	Mod		neg	neg	Low	DPC4 lost in 55%
Ovarian mucinous	POS	Low	neg	neg		POS	neg	POS		Mod	Low			neg			Low	
Esophageal adenocarcinoma	POS	neg	neg	neg								neg	Low	neg			Mod	

Table 7-4 CK7−/CK20+

TUMOR	CK7+ CK20+	CK7+ CK20−	CK7− CK20+	CK7− CK20−	34β E12	CAM 5.2	CK 5/6	EMA	BER-EP4	CEA m	CEA p	TTF-1	P63	WT-1	S100	CHRO	HEP	OTHER
Merkel cell carcinoma	Rare	neg	High	Low	Low	High	neg	High	POS	POS	POS	neg		neg	Low	High	neg?	NSE High
Colon adenocarcinoma	Low	neg	High	Low	neg	POS	neg	High	POS	POS	POS	neg	Low	neg	Low	neg	neg	CDX2 POS

Table 7-5 Predominantly CK7+/CK20−

TUMOR	CK7+ CK20+	CK7+ CK20−	CK7− CK20+	CK7− CK20−	34β E12	CAM 5.2	CK 5/6	EMA	BER-EP4	CEA m	CEA p	TTF-1	P63	WT-1	S100	CHRO	HEP	OTHER
Acinic cell carcinoma	neg	POS	neg	neg	POS	POS		Mod			Low				POS	Low		
Adenoid cystic carcinoma	neg	POS	neg	neg	POS	High	POS	Mod		POS	Low		POS		Mod	neg	neg	GFAP Low
Breast ductal carcinoma	Low	High	neg	neg	neg[a] Mod	POS	Low	POS	High	High	Mod	neg	Low[a]	High	Mod	Low	neg	ER/PR[b] GCDP Mod
Breast lobular carcinoma	Low	POS	neg	neg		POS	neg	POS	Mod	Mod	Mod	neg	Low			Low	neg	ER/PR[b] GCDP Mod E-cadherin neg
Brenner tumor	neg	POS	neg	neg				POS			High			Low	neg?	POS		Calretinin Low NSE POS
Cervical squamous cell carcinoma	neg	High	Low	neg	POS	neg	POS	POS		POS	Low	neg	POS			neg	neg	HPV POS p16 High
Choroid plexus	neg	High	Low	neg		POS		Low	neg	neg	neg				Mod			GFAP High
Chordoma	neg	POS	neg	neg	Mod	POS		POS	neg	neg	neg				POS	neg		GFAP neg
Craniopharyngioma	neg	POS	neg	neg	POS		POS											
Embryonal carcinoma	neg	POS	neg	neg	neg	POS		Low	POS	Low	Low		neg		neg	neg	neg	PLAP High CD30 High
Endometrial carcinoma	Low	High	neg	neg		POS	Low	POS	POS	High	High	High	High?	neg?	High	neg	neg	Vimentin POS ER High
Lung: adenocarcinoma	Low	High	Low	neg	Mod	POS	neg	POS	POS	High	High	High	High?	Low	Low	neg	Low	
Lung: BAL[c] non-mucinous	neg	POS	neg	neg	POS	POS	High	POS		High	High	High	Mod	neg	Mod	neg	neg	
Meningioma: secretory type[d]	neg	POS	neg	neg		neg	High	POS	neg	POS	POS			High	Low	Low	neg	PR Mod ER neg
Mesothelioma	neg	High	neg	Low	High	POS	High	High	neg	neg	neg	neg	neg	High	neg	Low	neg	Calretinin High

Table 7-5 Predominantly CK7+/CK20——cont'd

TUMOR	CK7+ CK20+	CK7+ CK20−	CK7− CK20+	CK7− CK20−	34β E12	CAM 5.2	CK 5/6	EMA	BER-EP4	CEA m	CEA p	TTF-1	P63	WT-1	S100	CHRO	HEP	OTHER
Mixed tumor[e]	neg	POS	neg	neg		POS	POS	Low		Low	neg?		POS		POS		neg	GFAP High SMA POS Calponin POS
Ovarian: endometrioid	neg	POS	neg	neg		POS	Low	POS	POS	Low	Low	neg?	Low	High	Low		neg	ER Mod
Ovarian: serous carcinoma	neg	POS	neg	neg		POS	Low	POS	POS	neg	neg	neg?	Low	POS	High		neg	ER High Calretinin Low
Renal cell: papillary and chromophobe	neg	POS	neg	neg	POS			POS		neg				Mod[f]				
Thyroid: papillary	neg	POS	neg	neg	POS	POS	Mod	High		neg	Mod	POS	High		High	neg	neg	Thy POS Calci neg
Thyroid: follicular	neg	POS	neg	neg	neg		neg	Mod		neg	Low	POS	Low		Mod	neg	neg	Thy POS Calci neg
Thyroid: medullary	neg	POS	neg	neg	neg		neg	neg		POS	Mod	POS				POS	neg	Thy rare Calci POS

[a] p63 may be positive in breast "basal like" carcinomas, some spindle cell metaplastic carcinomas, squamous cell carcinomas, and some papillary carcinomas. These subtypes may also have less typical keratin subsets such as CK14 (detected by 34β E12), CK17 (detected by MNF-116), or CK5/6.

[b] Most well and moderately differentiated ductal carcinomas, and carcinomas of special type (except for medullary) will be positive for hormone receptors. Poorly differentiated carcinomas, metaplastic carcinomas, and medullary carcinomas are usually negative. Well and moderately differentiated lobular carcinomas are almost always positive for ER, and usually positive for PR. Poorly differentiated lobular carcinomas may be negative for these markers.

[c] Non-mucinous bronchiolo-alveolar carcinomas (BAL) have an immunophenotype similar to lung adenocarcinomas. Mucinous BALs are more likely to be CK20 positive (approximately 70% positive) and less likely to be TTF-1 positive (approximately 30% positive).

[d] Secretory meningiomas are frequently positive for CK7 and CEA, whereas other subtypes are usually negative for CK7 and CEA. The majority of all types of meningiomas are positive for PR (including meningiomas in males).

[e] Mixed tumors (pleomorphic adenomas) occur most frequently in the salivary glands, but can also arise in soft tissues (myoepithelial tumors of soft tissue). These tumors have a similar immunophenotype with keratin (AE1/AE3 77%) or PANK (68%) or EMA (63%) present in the majority of tumors and frequent expression of markers associated with myoepithelial cells (e.g., calponin, GFAP, SMA, S100, p63). However, p63 is seen less frequently (23%) as compared to salivary tumors (100%).

[f] Chromophobe renal cell carcinomas may be positive for WT-1. Other types are negative.

Table 7-6 Predominantly CK7–/CK20–

TUMOR	CK7+ CK20+	CK7+ CK20–	CK7– CK20+	CK7– CK20–	34β E12	CAM 5.2	CK 5/6	EMA	BER-EP4	CEA m	CEA p	TTF-1	P63	WT-1	S100	CHRO	HEP	OTHER
Adrenal cortical adenoma	neg	neg	neg	POS		neg	neg	neg		neg	Low	neg			neg	neg	Low	Melan-A103 POS Inhibin POS
Carcinoid	neg	Low	Low	High	neg	POS	Low	Low		Mod	Mod	VAR[a]	neg		VAR[b]	POS	Low	
Epithelioid sarcoma	neg	Low	neg	POS	Mod	High	Low (focal)	POS (focal)					Low (foc)		neg	neg	neg	
Esophageal squamous cell carcinoma	neg	Low	neg	High	POS	High?	POS	POS	High?	Low?	Low	neg	POS		neg	neg	neg?	
Seminoma	neg	Low	neg	High	neg	Low	Low	neg		neg	neg				neg	neg	neg	PLAP POS CD117 POS
Head and neck squamous cell carcinoma	neg	Low	Low	High	POS	neg	POS	POS		neg	neg	neg	POS		neg	neg	neg	
Hepatocellular carcinoma	Low	Low	Low	High	Low	POS	neg	Low	Low	neg	High[c]	High[d] (cyt)	Low		neg	neg	High	AFP Mod
Lung: squamous cell carcinoma	neg	Low	Low	High	POS	High	POS	Low		Mod	Low	neg	POS		neg	neg	Low	
Lung: small cell carcinoma	neg	Low	neg	High	neg	High	neg	POS	POS	Mod	High	POS	rare	neg	neg?	Mod	neg	
Pheo/paraganglioma	Rare	Rare	Rare	POS	neg	neg	neg	neg		neg		neg			High	POS		Inhibin neg Melan-A103 rare
Prostatic carcinoma	neg	neg	Low	High	neg	POS	neg	Low	POS	neg	Mod	neg	neg	neg	neg	Low	neg	PSA POS
Renal cell carcinoma: clear cell	neg	Low	neg	High	neg	High	neg	POS	Low	Low	neg	neg	Low	neg?	Low	neg	neg	Vime POS

Table 7-6 Predominantly CK7–/CK20– —cont'd

TUMOR	CK7+ CK20+	CK7+ CK20–	CK7– CK20+	CK7– CK20–	34βE12	CAM 5.2	CK 5/6	EMA	BER-EP4	CEA m	CEA p	TTF-1	P63	WT-1	S100	CHRO	HEP	OTHER
Squamous cell carcinoma	neg	Low	Low	High	POS	Low	POS	POS	neg	Mod	Low	Low	POS		neg	neg	neg	
Thymic carcinoma					POS	POS	POS	Mod	High	Low	neg?	neg	POS	neg	neg	Low	neg?	CD5 Mod
Thymoma	neg	Low	neg	High	POS	High	High	Mod		Low	neg?	neg	POS	neg	neg	neg?	neg?	CD5 neg

a Non-pulmonary carcinoid tumors are negative for TTF-1. Some pulmonary carcinoids may be positive.
b Sustentacular cells may be positive for S100 and positivity can vary with site.
c CEA has a canalicular pattern in hepatocellular carcinoma, a diffuse cytoplasmic pattern in other carcinomas.
d TTF-1 immunoreactivity in hepatocellular carcinoma is cytoplasmic (not nuclear as in lung and thyroid carcinomas). Positivity can vary with the antibody used to detect TTF-1.

Table 7-7 No dominant CK7/CK20 pattern or pattern unknown

TUMOR	CK7+ CK20+	CK7+ CK20–	CK7– CK20+	CK7– CK20–	34βE12	CAM 5.2	CK 5/6	EMA	BER-EP4	CEA m	CEA p	TTF-1	P63	WT-1	S100	CHRO	HEP	OTHER
Gastric adenocarcinoma	Low	Low	Low	Low	neg	POS	neg	High	POS	High	High	neg	Low	neg?	Low	neg	Low	
Ameloblastoma/ Adamantinoma[a]					POS	neg	neg	neg							neg?	neg?		
Lymphoepithelial carcinoma[b]					POS			High		Mod?	Mod?		POS		neg[c]			

a Approximately 15% of ameloblastomas are positive for CK7.
b Approximately 50% of nasopharyngeal carcinomas are positive for CK7. Many cases in Asian and North African patients (less commonly in US patients) are associated with EBV. EBV can be demonstrated by in situ hybridization, PCR, or occasionally by immunohistochemistry. These carcinomas are also positive for broad-spectrum keratins (AE1/AE3 and PANK).
c S100-positive dendritic cells are present.

Table 7-8 Spindle-cell/soft-tissue lesions and sarcomas

	AE1/AE3	CAM 5.2	EMA	S100	HMB-45	HHF-35	SMA	DESMIN	H-CALDESMON	CD34	CD31	FVIII	c-kit CD117	CD99	OTHER
Neural															
Perineurioma	neg	neg	POS	Low	neg	Mod	Low	neg		neg	neg	neg	neg	Mod	CLAUD-1 POS[a]
Neurofibroma	neg	neg	POS[b]	POS	neg	neg	neg	neg		High	neg	neg	neg	neg	
MPNST	Low	Low	Low	Mod	neg	Low	Low	neg	neg	Low	neg	neg	neg		GFAP Mod
Schwannoma	Low	neg	Neg[c]	POS	neg	neg	neg	neg		Mod	neg	neg	neg		CD68 POS
Granular cell tumor[d]	neg	neg	neg	POS	neg	neg	neg	neg		neg					CD68 POS Calretinin POS Inhibin POS
Melanoma	rare	rare	neg	POS	High[e]		neg	neg	neg	neg	neg	neg	Mod	Low	Melan-A High FLI-1 neg
Clear cell sarcoma	neg	neg	neg	High	POS	Low	neg	neg		neg	neg	neg	Low	Low	Melan-A Mod
PEComa[f]	neg	neg	neg	Low	POS	POS	POS	High	Mod	Low	neg	neg	VAR[g]		Melan-A POS
Gastrointestinal stromal tumor	neg	neg	neg	Low		Mod	Low	neg	High	High	neg	neg	POS	POS	
Muscle															
Rhabdomyosarcoma	Low	Low	Low	neg	neg	High	Mod	High	neg	Low	neg	neg	neg	Low	Myf4 POS WT-1 Mod FLI-1 neg
Glomus tumor	neg	neg	neg	neg	neg	POS	POS	Low	High	Low	neg	neg	neg		
Leiomyoma or leiomyosarcoma	Low	Low	Mod	neg	neg	POS	POS	High	POS	Low	neg	neg	neg	Low	ER/PR High CD10 Low
Endometrial stromal sarcoma	Mod (focal)	Low (focal)			neg		High	Mod	neg	neg				neg	ER/PR High CD10 High
Vascular															
Angiosarcoma	Low[h]	Low[h]	rare	neg	neg	Low	Low	neg		High	High	High	Low		FLI-1 POS
Kaposi's sarcoma	neg	neg	neg	neg		neg	POS	neg		POS	High	Mod	neg		FLI-1 POS HHV 8 POS

Table 7-8 Spindle-cell/soft-tissue lesions and sarcomas—cont'd

	AE1/AE3	CAM 5.2	EMA	S100	HMB-45	HHF-35	SMA	DESMIN	H-CALDESMON	CD34	CD31	FVIII	c-kit CD117	CD99	OTHER
Epithelioid hemangioendothelioma	High	neg	neg	neg	neg	neg	Low	neg		High	High	POS	neg		FLI-1 POS
"Fibrous"															
Fibrosarcoma	neg	Low	neg	neg	neg	neg	neg	neg		neg				Low	
Solitary fibrous tumor	neg	neg	Low	neg		neg	Low	neg	neg	POS	neg	neg	neg	High	
DFSP	neg	neg	neg	neg	neg	High	Low	neg	neg	POS	neg	neg	neg		
Dermatofibroma	neg	neg	neg	neg	neg	High	High	Mod	neg	neg	neg		neg	neg	ER Low
Fibromatosis	neg	neg	neg	Mod		High	High	Mod	neg	neg					
Postoperative spindle cell nodule	Mod	Mod	Low	neg		High	High	Mod	neg	neg					
Myofibroblastic tumors		neg	neg	neg		POS	High	Mod	neg	Mod		neg			ER High PR POS
Atypical fibroxanthoma	neg	neg	neg	neg	neg		Low	neg	neg	Low					CD68 Mod
Other															
Osteosarcoma	neg	neg	Low	Low	neg	Mod	High	neg	neg					Low	
Chondrosarcoma	neg	neg	Low	POS	neg	neg	neg	neg		neg				Low	
Chondroblastoma	neg	neg	neg	POS		Mod	Low	neg	neg?					POS	
Mesenchymal chondrosarcoma	neg	neg	neg	POS	neg		rare	Low						POS	My4 neg
Extraskeletal myxoid chondrosarcoma	neg	neg	Low	Low	neg	neg	neg	neg		Low	neg	neg	Low	neg	
Alveolar soft part sarcoma	neg	neg	neg	Low	neg	Low	Low	Low		Low	neg	neg	neg	Low	myoD1 neg myogenin neg TFE3 POS^j
Epithelioid sarcoma	POS	POS	POS	neg	neg	Low	Low	neg		Mod	neg	neg	neg	Low	FLI-1 neg
Synovial sarcoma^k	High	High	High	Mod	neg	neg	Low	neg	neg	neg	neg	neg	neg	High	WT-1 neg

Table 7-8 Spindle-cell/soft-tissue lesions and sarcomas—cont'd

	AE1/AE3	CAM 5.2	EMA	S100	HMB-45	HHF-35	SMA	DESMIN	H-CALDESMON	CD34	CD31	FVIII	c-kit CD117	CD99	OTHER
Adenomatoid tumor	POS	POS	POS							neg	neg			neg	Ber-EP4 High Calretinin POS
Mesothelioma sarcomatoid type[m]	High	POS	Low			POS	High	Low		neg	neg			Low	WT-1[n] Calretinin Low
Meningioma	neg[o]	neg[o]	High	Low	neg	Low	Low	neg		Low	neg	neg		POS	ER neg PR POS PANK Low
Carcinoma: spindle cell[p]	VAR	VAR	VAR	VAR	neg	rare	rare	neg		neg	neg	neg			

[a] Some claudin-1-positive perineurial cells can be present in neurofibromas and schwannomas.

[b] Perineural cells are positive for EMA in neurofibromas.

[c] EMA may be positive in capsule and perineural cells of schwannomas.

[d] Congenital granular cell tumors are positive for CD68 but negative for S100 and NSE.

[e] HMB-45 is less frequently present in spindle cell melanomas and usually negative in classic desmoplastic melanomas. Other markers for melanoma are also less frequently positive in these subsets.

[f] PEComas (perivascular epithelioid cell tumors) include angiomyolipoma, lymphangioleiomyomatosis, clear cell sugar tumor of the lung, clear cell myomelanocytic tumor of ligamentum teres/falciform ligament, and abdominopelvic sarcoma of perivascular epithelioid cells.

[g] Results in the literature are conflicting. Angiomyolipomas are likely not positive for CD117.

[h] Keratin positivity in angiosarcomas is more common in epithelioid types.

[i] Cellular dermatofibroma may show focal desmin immunoreactivity.

[j] Alveolar soft-part sarcomas are characterized by a translocation that fuses the TFE3 transcription factor gene at Xp11 to a novel gene at 17q25 called ASPL. These sarcomas demonstrate nuclear immunoreactivity for TFE3 (as do rare pediatric renal tumors with the same translocation) and this immunoreactivity is not present in other tumors or normal tissues. The characteristic cytoplasmic crystals are composed of monocarboxylate transporter 1 (MCT1) and its chaperone CD147. However, these proteins are found in many other cell types and are not specific for this tumor.

[k] Keratin and EMA positivity are usually only focal in monophasic synovial sarcomas.

[l] Claudin-1 is positive in glandular areas of synovial sarcoma but less so in spindle cell areas.

[m] The immunohistochemical pattern for epithelioid mesotheliomas is given in Table 7-30.

[n] WT-1 may be positive in a minor epithelioid component of sarcomatoid mesotheliomas, but is generally negative in the spindle cells.

[o] Secretory meningiomas are typically cytokeratin 7 positive (CK20 negative) and also positive for CEA. Other subtypes are generally negative for keratin. However, malignant meningiomas may be positive for keratin.

[p] Squamous cell carcinomas with a spindle cell morphology are generally strongly positive for AE1/AE3 (less commonly for CAM 5.2), EMA, and p63. Spindle cell carcinomas of the breast often express markers expressed by myoepithelial cells such as "basal keratins" (including cytokeratin 14 which is included in the group detected by PANK or MNF-116), smooth muscle α-actin, and p63. Poorly differentiated carcinomas with spindle cell morphology may only show focal positivity for keratins and EMA.

Table 7-9 Small blue cell tumors

TUMOR	PANK	CAM 5.2	CK20	EMA	S100	HMB-45	NSE	SYN	CHRO	CD99	SMA	HHF 35	DES MIN	MYF-4	LCA	NFP	WT-1[a]	PAS[b]
Melanoma	rare	rare	neg	neg	POS	High[c]	High	Low	neg	Low	Low	neg	neg	neg	neg	neg		
Esthesioneuroblastoma	Low	Mod	neg	Low	POS		POS	High	Mod	Low		neg	neg	neg?	neg	Mod		
Neuroblastoma	neg	neg	neg	Low	Mod	neg	POS	High	High	neg	neg	neg	neg		neg	High	Low	neg
Small cell carcinoma[d]	POS	Mod	neg	POS	neg	neg	High	Mod	Mod	Low		neg			neg	neg		neg
Merkel cell carcinoma[e]	POS	POS	POS	POS	neg	neg	High	Mod	High	Low		neg	neg?		neg	Mod		neg
Desmoplastic small round cell tumor	POS	POS	neg	POS	Low	neg	High	Low	Low	Mod	Low	Low	POS	neg		neg	POS	POS
Ewing's sarcoma (PNET)	Low	Low	neg	Low	Low	neg	Mod	Low	neg	POS[f]	neg	Low	neg		neg	Low	neg	POS
Medulloblastoma	neg		neg	neg?	Low		POS	POS		Low			Low		neg	neg		
Rhabdomyosarcoma	neg	Mod	neg	neg	Low	neg	Mod	neg	neg	Low	Low	POS	POS	POS	neg	Low	Mod	POS
AML	neg	neg	neg	neg	Low	neg	POS?	neg	neg	Mod					High			
Lymphoma	neg	neg	neg	neg	neg	neg	neg	neg	neg	Var	neg	neg	neg	neg	POS			neg[g]

[a] Polyclonal WT-1.
[b] PAS is a histochemical stain for glycogen. A PAS-D stain confirms the presence of glycogen by treatment of the tissue with diastase, which digests the glycogen and eliminates the positivity. Although used for these tumors in the past, these studies are currently not usually performed.
[c] MART-I is also frequently positive in melanomas.
[d] Small cell carcinomas of the lung are positive for TTF-I.
[e] Merkel cell carcinomas demonstrate a dot-like perinuclear pattern for most markers.
[f] Significant immunoreactivity is a membrane pattern in the majority of the cells.
[g] Some plasma cell lymphomas may be positive.
Ewing's sarcoma (PNET), desmoplastic small round cell tumor, rhabdomyosarcoma, neuroblastoma, and medulloblastoma have characteristic cytogenetic changes (see Table 7-33).
EM has some advantages over immunohistochemistry in the evaluation of childhood small round blue cell tumors.[11]
Initial panel. Keratin, S100, LCA.
Additional studies may be helpful depending on the histologic appearance and the results of the initial studies.

Table 7-10 Myoepithelial markers in breast carcinoma

MARKER	LOCATION	NORMAL LUMINAL CELLS	MYOEPITHELIAL CELLS	BLOOD VESSELS	MYOFIBROBLASTS	CARCINOMAS[a]	COMMENT
p63	Nucleus	neg	POS	neg	neg	rare	Only nuclear marker Clean background
SMA	Cytoplasm	neg	POS	POS	POS	rare	Positive in most myoepithelial cells
CD10	Membrane	neg	POS	neg	POS	rare	
SMM-HC	Cytoplasm	neg	POS	POS	High	rare	
Calponin	Cytoplasm	neg	POS	POS	Mod	rare	

[a] Rare carcinomas with myoepithelial features (adenoid cystic carcinomas, some spindle cell carcinomas, some basal-like carcinomas, some carcinomas associated with *BRCA1* mutations) can show focal to diffuse positivity for myoepithelial markers.

Myoepithelial markers can be useful for the evaluation of breast lesions:
- Invasive carcinoma versus sclerosing adenosis (frequently involved by DCIS, LCIS, or apocrine metaplasia).
- DCIS versus DCIS with microinvasion. Double immunolabeling with p63 (brown nucleus) and cytokeratin (AE1/AE3—red cytoplasm) can be useful to highlight small nests of tumor cells lacking myoepithelial cells.
- DCIS versus carcinoma invading as circumscribed tumor nests versus lymphovascular invasion.

S100 protein and cytokeratins (e.g. 34β E12) are not recommended for this purpose, as fewer myoepithelial cells are positive and luminal cells are also sometimes positive.

p63 is a good general marker for myoepithelial cells and is particularly helpful in cases with prominent myofibroblasts (e.g., sclerosing lesions) or with blood vessels closely apposed to tumor cells (e.g., papillary fronds in papillary DCIS). In some cases, SMA may be positive in more cells than p63.

Table 7-11 Epidermal lesions of the nipple

	AE1/AE3	CAM 5.2 OR CK7	CK20	EMA	S100	HMB-45	GCDFP-15	CEA p	CEA m	HER2	ER OR PR	MUCICARMINE STAIN
Paget's disease of the nipple	POS	POS	neg	POS	Mod	neg	Mod	Mod	Low	POS	Low	High
Squamous cell carcinoma	POS	Low	Low	POS	Low	neg	neg	Low	Mod	Low	neg	neg
Melanoma	Low	Low	neg	Low	POS	POS	neg	Mod	neg	neg	neg	neg

Most cases of Paget's disease of the nipple are associated with DCIS deeper in the breast and involve the lactiferous sinuses, and approximately half will also have areas of invasion. Rare cases may be difficult to interpret due to the absence of associated disease in the breast or if the initial biopsy is shallow. In some cases, Paget cells may take up melanin and may be difficult to distinguish from melanoma. Toker cells in nipple epidermis are CAM 5.2 and CK7 positive but negative for HER2/neu.

Initial panel. CAM 5.2 (or CK7), HER2, and S100 with additional antibody studies based on these findings, if necessary.

Cases of extramammary Paget's disease are more likely to be CK20 positive and less likely to be positive for HER2/neu (less than 40%).

Table 7-12 Endocervical carcinoma versus endometrial carcinoma

	CK7	CK20	VIM	CEA m	CEA p	P16	HPV (IN SITU)	ER	PR
Endocervical carcinoma	POS	rare	rare	POS	High	POS (difffuse, strong)	High	Low (focal)	Low
Endometrial carcinoma	POS	rare	POS	Low[a]	Mod	Low (patchy, weak)	neg	High (diffuse)	High

[a] 27% of cases have some positivity but primarily in squamous areas and only focally in glandular areas.

Table 7-13 Endometrial stromal sarcoma versus leiomyosarcoma

	CD10	DESMIN	H-CALDESMON	ER/PR
Endometrial stromal sarcoma	High	Mod	neg	High
Leiomyosarcoma	Low	High	POS	High

Table 7-14 Primary ovarian carcinoma versus metastatic carcinomas

	CK7	CK20	DPC4 (SMAD4)	CDX2	ER	CEA m	CEA p
Endometrioid ovarian carcinoma	POS	neg		Low	Mod	Mod	Low
Clear cell ovarian carcinoma	POS	neg		Mod?	Mod		neg
Mucinous ovarian carcinoma	POS (diffuse)	High (patchy)	POS	Mod	Low	Mod	Low
Mucinous breast carcinoma	POS	Low	POS	neg[a]	POS	Mod	Low
Pancreatic carcinoma	POS	High	Mod	Mod	neg	High	POS
Appendiceal carcinoma	Low (patchy)	POS	POS			High	Low
Mucinous colon carcinoma	Low (patchy)	POS (diffuse)	High	POS	neg	POS	POS

[a] Breast cancers, in general, are negative for CDX2. Results for mucinous breast carcinomas have not been reported.

Table 7-15 Ovarian carcinoma versus mesothelioma

	CK7	CK20	CK5/6	CEA m	CEA p	CD15 (LEUM1)	ER	WT-1	CALRET	BER-EP4
Peritoneal mesothelioma	High	neg	POS	neg	neg	rare	rare	High	High	neg
Ovarian serous carcinoma	POS	Low	neg	neg	neg	Mod	POS	POS	Low	POS
Ovarian endometrioid carcinoma	POS	neg	Low	Mod	Low		High	High	Low	POS
Ovarian mucinous carcinoma	POS	High	neg	Mod	Low		Low	neg	Low	

Table 7-16 Trophoblastic lesions

	KERATIN	ALPHA-INHIBIN	HPL[a]	HCG[a]	CD146 (MELCAM)	KI-67[b]	P57[c]	DNA PLOIDY[d]
Choriocarcinoma	POS	POS	Weak (focal)	Strong (diffuse)	POS	69%		
Placental site trophoblastic tumor	POS	POS	Mod (greater than hCG)	Focal (less than HhPL)	POS	>14%		
Epithelioid trophoblastic tumor	POS	POS	Focal	Focal	Focal	>14%		
Placental site nodule	POS	POS	Weak (focal)	Focal	Focal	<1%		
Exaggerated placental site			POS (diffuse)	Focal	POS	0%		
Partial mole	POS	POS	Weak[e] (diffuse)	Weak (diffuse)			POS	Triploid
Complete mole	POS	POS	Weak[e] (focal)	Strong (diffuse)			rare[f]	Diploid (paternal)
Hydropic fetus	POS	POS					POS	Diploid (60%) Triploid (40%)

[a] Evaluated in syncytiotrophoblast.
[b] Implantation-site intermediate trophoblastic cells are evaluated for the number of Ki-67-positive cells. CD146 can be used to help identify these cells using a double label technique. Lymphocytes can also be positive for Ki-67 and should not be counted.
[c] p57 is a paternally imprinted gene, expressed from the maternal gene, which shows decreased expression in complete moles, whose DNA is completely derived from paternal DNA.
[d] Ploidy is usually determined by flow cytometry.
[e] Increases with advancing pregnancy.
[f] In complete moles, p57 positivity is present in villous stromal cells and extravillous trophoblast but absent in intermediate trophoblast lining the villi.
Cytokeratin and alpha-inhibin (present in syncytiotrophoblastic cells and some intermediate trophoblastic cells) are not useful for the differential diagnosis of these lesions, but may be helpful if other types of tumors are in the differential diagnosis.

Table 7-17 Tumors of germ cells and sex-cord stromal tumors

	CK7	CK20	AE1/AE3	CAM5.2	NSE	EMA	PLAP[a] (mem)	AFP	CD30 (Ki-1, Ber-H2)	CD117 (c-kit)	VIM	hCG	HPL	INHIBIN	MELAN-A103	OTHER
Seminoma	Mod	neg	Mod	Low[b]	High	neg	POS	neg	Low	POS	Mod	Low[c]	neg	neg	neg	
Embryonal carcinoma	High	neg	POS	POS	High	Low	High	Low	High[d]	neg	Low	Low	neg	neg	neg	
Yolk sac tumor			POS	POS	High	neg	Mod	High	Low		Low	neg	neg	neg	neg	
Choriocarcinoma			POS	POS	Mod	Mod	Mod	neg	neg		neg	POS	POS	POS	neg	
Intratubular germ cell neoplasia				neg			POS			POS	neg					
Spermatocytic seminoma				Mod (focal)			neg		Mod							
Leydig cell tumor	Mod	Mod	Mod	Mod		Low	Low	neg			POS			POS	High	
Granulosa cell tumor	Mod	Low	Low	Mod	Low	neg	neg	neg		neg	POS			POS	High	WT-1 High HHF35 High S100 Mod
Sertoli cell tumor			Mod	Mod		POS	neg				High			POS		

[a] PLAP is expressed in embryonic germ cells, but not in normal spermatogonia, spermatocytes, and spermatids.

[b] CAM5.2 is present as a strong dot-like paranuclear positivity. 80% of mediastinal seminomas are positive for CAM5.2 compared to 20% to 30% of testicular seminomas.

[c] hCG may be positive in trophoblasts in seminomas.

[d] Only 35% of embryonal carcinomas metastatic to lymph nodes after chemotherapy are positive for CD30.

Table 7-18 Adrenal and kidney tumors

	AE1/AE3	CK7	CK20	PANK	CAM5.2	MUC-1 (EMA)	S100	CHROM	SYN	MELAN-A103[a]	INHIBIN	NSE	NFP	AMACR	VIM	OTHER	IRON STAIN
Adrenal tumors[b]																	
Cortical adenoma	neg	neg	neg	Low	Low	neg	neg	neg	POS	POS	High	High	neg	neg	High	TTF-1 neg CD10 neg	
Cortical carcinoma					neg		neg	neg	High	POS	POS		neg				
Pheo/paraganglioma		neg	neg	neg	neg	neg	High[c]	POS	POS	neg	neg	POS	POS		Mod	GFAP mod	
Kidney tumors																	
Renal cell carcinoma: clear cell	High	Low	neg	High	High	High (diff)	Low	neg	neg	neg	neg	Mod	neg		High	p63 neg TTF-1 neg GFAP low RCC POS CD10 POS	Focal, course
Papillary	POS	High	Low	POS		Mod (mem)								POS		RCC POS CD10 POS	Focal, coarse
Chromophobe	High	High	neg	POS		POS (mem)								neg	neg	RCC Mod CD10 neg	Diff, strong
Oncocytoma[d]	Mod	High	neg	POS												RCC neg CD10 low	Focal, weak
Transitional cell carcinoma	Mod	POS	High	POS	POS	POS	neg	neg	neg	neg		Low		Low	Low	p63 POS CD10 mod	

diff, diffuse positivity; mem, positivity located on membrane.
[a] Positivity is also present with MART-1.
[b] Clear cell renal cell carcinoma (RCC) metastatic to the adrenal can sometimes be confused with an adrenal cortical tumor (thus, the older term for "clear cell carcinoma of "hypernephroma"). RCC has clear cytoplasm (compared to the bubbly cytoplasm of the adrenal cortex) and blood lakes are typically present. Glycogen is present in RCC and absent in adrenal lesions (demonstrated by PAS with and without diastase). Cytokeratin and EMA are useful IHC markers.
[c] Positivity is present in sustentacular cells. These cells may be absent in malignant tumors.
[d] 50% of oncocytomas have a punctate/dot-like pattern for CK8 or CK18 which is not seen in RCC. EM may be helpful to distinguish oncocytoma from chromophobe RCC (see Table 7-33).
Renal cell carcinoma subtypes have typical cytogenetic abnormalities (see Table 7-33).
CD117 (c-kit) has been reported to be positive in almost all papillary renal cell carcinomas (cytoplasmic) and chromophobe carcinomas (membrane) but is not present in clear cell carcinomas. Mutations in c-kit were only found in papillary carcinomas.

Table 7-19 Tumors of bladder, prostatic, or renal origin

	CK7	CK20	KERATIN HMW	PSA	PAP	AMACR	CEA m	CEA p	P63	CA125	MUCI
Prostatic carcinoma	Low	Low	neg	High	POS	POS	neg	Mod	neg	neg	neg
Transitional cell carcinoma	POS	High	Mod	neg	neg	Low	Mod	Mod	High	neg	neg
Bladder adenocarcinoma	High	High	neg	neg	neg		Mod	High		Low	POS
Renal cell carcinoma: clear cell	Low	neg	neg	neg			Low	neg	Low	neg	neg
Rectal adenocarcinoma	Low	POS	neg	neg	neg		POS	POS			neg	POS
Seminal vesicle carcinoma	High	neg		neg	neg		VAR	POS		High	

Table 7-20 Prostate carcinoma versus other lesions

	34β E12 (BASAL CELLS)	P63 (BASAL CELLS)	AMACR (504S) (GLANDULAR CELLS)
Benign glands	POS	POS	neg
PIN	POS	POS	High
Invasive carcinoma	neg	neg	POS

Antibody cocktails. These antibodies can be combined to facilitate the evaluation of small lesions:
34β E12 + p63 labels a greater number of basal cells than either marker alone
AMACR + p63 and/or 34β E12 facilitates the identification of small foci of invasive carcinoma.

Table 7-21 Hepatic tumors

	CK7	CK20	AE1/ AE3	CAM 5.2	KERATIN HMW	CEA m	CEA p	TTF-1	HEP	AFP	CD10	CHROM	MUCI	BILE	CIRRHOSIS	HBV
Hepatocellular carcinoma (HCC)	Low	neg	Low	POS	neg	neg	High[a]	High[b] (cyt)	High	Mod	High[a]	neg	rare	May be present	65–90%	50%
Hepatoblastoma			Low	POS		Low	High[a]		POS	High		Low			absent	rare
HCC: fibrolamellar	Mod ?	neg					POS[a]		POS	neg ?			neg	May be present	absent	rare
Cholangiocarcinoma	POS	Mod	POS	POS	High	High	POS	neg	neg	neg	neg		75–100	neg	rare	rare
Metastatic carcinoid tumor	Low	Low	High	POS		Mod	Mod	Low[c] (nuc)	neg		Low	POS		neg	absent	absent

cyt = cytoplasmic immunoreactivity; nuc = nuclear immunoreactivity.

[a] Bile canalicular pattern. Other carcinomas have a membrane or cytoplasmic pattern.

[b] TTF-I is seen in the cytoplasm (unlike the nuclear pattern seen in lung and thyroid carcinomas).

[c] Carcinoids arising at sites other than lung are very unlikely to be positive for TTF-I. Lung carcinoids may be positive and are more likely to express CK7. Sinusoids of HCC show diffuse CD34 positivity in 80% to 90% of cases, but this is not seen in normal liver. CD34 positivity can also be seen in focal nodular hyperplasia. Metastatic carcinomas can show diffuse positivity in 20% of cases, but the positive endothelial cells are present throughout the tumor and the cells do not surround nests of tumor cells, as is seen in HCC. Reticulin stains can be helpful in the evaluation of fine needle aspirates or core needle biopsies of liver lesions. HCC has an abnormal pattern of absent, decreased, or expanded trabecula, whereas benign lesions show a normal trabecular pattern.

Metastatic carcinomas can usually be distinguished from HCC by frequent expression of CK7, only rare expression of HepPar1, the absence of a bile canalicular pattern for CEA p and CD10, and the absence of cytoplasmic positivity for TTF-I.

Metastatic carcinomas to the liver often cannot be reliably distinguished from cholangiocarcinomas by histologic appearance or immunohistochemical pattern, with the exception of colorectal carcinomas. If the patient has a known primary carcinoma, it is most helpful to compare the two tumors.

Table 7-22 Thyroid and parathyroid lesions

	KER HMW	CK19	HBME[a]	GALECTIN-3	CALCITONIN	SYN	CHRO	RET	P27	PPAR GAMMA	THY	TTF-1	S100[b]	CEA M	CEA P	CD57	RB PROTEIN	VIM	OTHER
Thyroid lesions																			
Hyperplastic nodule		Mod	Low	Low	neg				POS	neg	POS	POS				Low	POS		
Follicular adenoma	neg	Mod	Low	Low	neg	Mod	neg	neg	POS	Low 10%	POS	POS	Low			Low	POS	POS	
Follicular carcinoma	neg	Mod	Mod	Low	neg	High	neg	neg	POS	Low 30%	POS	POS	Mod	neg	Low	Mod	neg?	POS	
Papillary carcinoma: follicular variant	POS	POS	POS	Mod	neg			Low	Low Mod	Low 10%	POS	POS				High	neg		
Papillary carcinoma	POS	POS	High	POS	neg	High	neg	Low	POS	Low 10%	POS	POS	High	neg	Mod	POS	neg	POS	p63 POS
Medullary carcinoma	neg			Mod	POS	POS	POS			neg	Low	POS		POS	Mod	Mod	Mod	High[c]	
Anaplastic carcinoma[d]		Mod									rare	rare							
Parathyroid lesions																			
Parathyroid adenomas and carcinomas					Low	Low	POS		High[e]	neg	neg	neg	Low				POS	neg/weak	PTh POS RCC POS Cyclin D1 POS

[a] Tumors with Hürthle cell changes may be negative for HBME.
[b] Hürthle cells (both benign and neoplastic) are positive for S100 (nuclear and cytoplasmic).
[c] Spindle cells may be positive for vimentin.
[d] Anaplastic thyroid carcinomas are frequently negative for TTF-1, thyroglobulin, and CK20.
[e] p27 is low in parathyroid carcinomas.
Thyroid adenomas, follicular carcinomas, papillary carcinomas, and medullary carcinomas are CK7 positive and CK20 negative. Variable immunoreactivity has been reported for CK7 in anaplastic carcinomas.
Metastatic carcinomas to the thyroid will be negative for thyroglobulin, TTF-1 (except for lung carcinomas), and calcitonin.
DDIT3 and ARG2 are new markers that may prove helpful for distinguishing follicular carcinoma (approximately 70% to 80% positive) from adenoma (90% negative).

Table 7-23 B-cell neoplasms

B cell markers

	CD45 LCA	CD19 B4	CD20 L26	CD22	CD79a	sIg	cIg	CD5 Leu1	CD10 CALLA	CD23	CD43 Leu 22	CD34	bcl-2	bcl-6	CD138 SYNDECAN	CYCLIN D1	OTHER
Precursor lymphoblastic lymphoma/leukemia	+/–	+	+/–	+/–	+ cyt	–	+M	–	+[a]	–	+/–	+/–	–	–	–	–	TdT + CD99 +
Small lymphocytic lymphoma/CLL	+	+	+ wk	+ wk	+	+M/D wk	–/+	+	–	+	+/–	–	+	–	–	–	CD11c+ wk CD79b – FMC7 –
Mantle cell lymphoma	+	+	+	+	+	+M/D	–	+	–	–	+	–	+	–	–	+	CyclinD + FMC +
Marginal zone lymphoma (MALT)	+	+	+	+	+	+	+/–	–	–	–	+/–	–	+	–	–/+[b]	–	CD11c +/– CD21+ CD35+
Follicular lymphoma	+	+	+	+	+	+M	–	–	+	–/+	–/+	–	+/–	+	–	–	CDw75 +
Burkitt lymphoma and Burkitt-like lymphoma	+	+	+	+	+	+M	+/–	–	+	–	+/–	–	–	+	–	–	TdT- MIB-1 100% EBER in situ in 52% MYC[c]
Mediastinal large B-cell lymphoma	+	+	+	+	+/–	–	–	–	–	–	–	–	–	+	–	–	CD30+/– wk
Large B-cell lymphoma	+/–	+	+	+	+	+/–	+/–	–/+	–/+	–	–/+	–	–/+	+/–	–	–	CD30 +/– MIB-1 >40%
Lymphoplasmacytic lymphoma	+/–	+	+	+	+	+M/D	+M/G st	–	–	–	+/–	–			–/+[b]	–	

Table 7-23 B-cell neoplasms—cont'd

B cell markers

	CD45 LCA	CD19 B4	CD20 L26	CD22	CD79a	sIg	cIg	CD5 Leu 1	CD10 CALLA	CD23	CD43 Leu 22	CD34	bcl-2	bcl-6	CD138 SYNDECAN	CYCLIN D1	OTHER
Hairy cell leukemia	+	+	+	+	+	+		–	–	–	–	–	–	–	–	–/+	DBA.44+ CD79b– CD11c+ CD103+ CD25+ st FMC7+
Primary effusion lymphoma	+	–	–	–	–	–	–	–	–	–		–		–	+	–	CD30 (Ki-1)+ HHV8+ EBER +/–
Plasmacytoma/ myeloma	–/+	–	–/+	–	+	–	+G/A st	–	–/+	–	+/–	–	–		+	–/+	CD56+ CD38 + EMA +

cyt = cytoplasmic immunoreactivity; M, D, G, A, type of heavy Ig chain present; st = strong immunoreactivity; wk = weak immunoreactivity.
a Lymphoblasts in t(4;11)(q21;q23) ALL are CD10 negative and frequently CD24 negative.
b Positive in plasma cell component.
c The myc gene (8q24) is translocated to Ig genes:
t(8;14) (heavy chains) 85% of cases
t(2;8) (kappa light chain)
t(8;22) (lambda light chain).

Table 7-24 T-cell neoplasms

	CD45 LCA	TCR	CD2 TE/T11	CD3 T3	CD43 Leu 22	CD5 Leu 1	CD7 LEU 9	CD4 T4	CD8 T8	CD25 IL2R	TIA-1	Granzyme B	CD56 NCAM	CD30 Ki-1	TdT	ALK	OTHER
Precursor lymphoblastic lymphoma/leukemia	+	−	+/−	+	+/−	+/−	+	+/−	+/−	+/−	−	−	−	−	+	−	CD34+ CD99+ CD1a +/−
T-cell prolymphocytic leukemia	+	+	+	+wk	+	+	+	+/−	−/+	+/−	−	−	−	−	−	−	CD1a−
Adult T-cell lymphoma/leukemia	+	+	+	+	+	+	−/+	+	−/+	+	−	−	−	+/−	−	−	
Mycosis fungoides and Sézary syndrome	+	TCRβ+	+	+	+	+	−/+	+	−/+	−/+	−/+	+/−	−	−	−	−	HECA+
Peripheral T-cell lymphoma, NOS	+	+	+/−	+/−	+	+/−	−/+	+/−	−/+	−/+	+	+/−	−/+	+ (large cells)	−	−	
Hepatosplenic T-cell lymphoma	+	TCRδ1+ TCRαβ−	+	+	+	−	+/−	−	−	−	+	−	+/−	−	−	−	CD57− CD16−/+ LMP-1− Perforin −
Panniculitis-like T-cell lymphoma CD56+	−	−	CD3ε	+	+	−	+	+	+	−	+	+	+	−	−	−	CD95+
CD56−	+	+	CD3ε	−	+	−	+	−	+	−	−/+	+	−	−	−	−	CD95−
Angioimmunoblastic lymphoma	+	+	+	+	+	+	+	+	−/+	−	+	+	−	−	−	−	CD10+/− CD57+ bcl-6+−
Enteropathy-type T-cell lymphoma	+	+		+	+	−	+	−	−/+	−	+/−	+/−	+ (small cells)	+ (large cells)	−	−	CD103+

Table 7-24 T-cell neoplasms—cont'd

	CD45 LCA	TCR	CD2 TE/T11	CD3 T3	CD43 Leu 22	CD5 Leu 1	CD7 LEU 9	CD4 T4	CD8 T8	CD25 IL2R	TIA-1	Granzyme B	CD56 NCAM	CD30 Ki-1	TdT	ALK	OTHER
Anaplastic large cell lymphoma (Ki-1 lymphoma)	+/-	+/-	+/-	-/+	+/-	-/+	-/+	+/-	-/+	+/-	+/-	+/-	-/+	+ (mem, Golgi)	-	+/-[a] (cyt, nuc)	Clusterin+[b] EMA+/- Perforin +/- EBER- BSAP-
Extranodal NK/ T-cell lymphoma, nasal type	+	-	+	- CD3ε+ (cyt)	+	-	-/+	-	-	-	+	+	+	-/+	-	-	EBER+ CD16+ CD57-
Blastic NK-cell lymphoma	-	-	-/+	-	+/-	-	-/+	+/-		-			+	-	+/-	-	CD33- Myelo-

cyt = cytoplasmic; nuc = nuclear; wk = weak immunoreactivity.
[a] Only positive in systemic ALCL (subset); negative in primary cutaneous ALCL.
[b] Expressed in all cases of systemic ALCL but less commonly in primary cutaneous ALCL and very rarely in diffuse large B-cell lymphoma, peripheral T cell lymphoma, and NS HD.

Table 7.25 Hodgkin's lymphoma

	CD45 LCA	CD20 L26	CD3 T3	CD15 LEUM1	CD30 Ki-1	EMA	slg	CD79a	CDw75	Oct2	BOB.1	BSAP	LMP1	OTHER
Classical Hodgkin lymphoma (HL)	–	–/+	–	+/–	+	– Rare	–	–/+	–	–	–/+	+	+/–	traf-1 + bcl-2 +
Nodular sclerosis HL	–	–/+	–	+/–	+	– Rare	–	–/+	–	–	–/+	+	–/+	
Lymphocyte-rich HL	–	–/+	–	+/–	+	– Rare	–	–/+	–	–	+/–	+	+/–	
Mixed cellularity HL	–	–/+	–	+/–	+	– Rare	–	–/+	–	–	–/+	+	+/–	
Lymphocyte-depleted HL	–	–/+	–	+/–	+	– Rare	–	–/+	–	–	–/+	+	+ (if HIV +)	
Nodular lymphocyte predominant HL	+	+	–	–	–/+	+/–	+	+ wk	+/–	+	+	+	–	bcl-6 + bcl-2 –

wk = weak.

Table 7-26 Markers for tumors of unknown origin

TYPE OF TUMOR	IMMUNOHISTOCHEMICAL MARKER(S)	POTENTIAL TREATMENT AND COMMENTS
Breast	ER/PR HER-2/neu GCDFP-15	ER/PR+ tumors can be palliated with hormonal treatment. HER-2/neu+ carcinomas can be treated with Herceptin[a]. GCDFP-15 is not very sensitive, as many breast carcinomas are negative. The most common type of breast carcinoma to present as an occult primary is invasive lobular carcinoma. Rare women will present with positive axillary nodes with no known primary. Most of these women will have breast cancer. The prognosis is the same, whether or not the primary is detected
Carcinoid tumor	Chromogranin	Chromogranin positivity should be strong and diffuse. Focal and/or weak positivity can be seen in many carcinomas. Metastatic breast cancer and prostate cancer can closely resemble carcinoid tumor and both can be positive for chromogranin. Carcinoid tumors can be palliated with tumor-directed pharmaceuticals
Germ cell tumors	PLAP	PLAP is not specific but a germ cell tumor is unlikely if it is negative. Inhibin is more likely to be positive in choriocarcinomas. Chemotherapy for possible cure
GIST	c-kit (CD117)	Treatment with Gleevec[b]
Lung adenocarcinoma	TTF-1	10% to 20% of patients will have specific activating mutations in EGFR (detected by PCR) and these patients may respond well to treatment with gefitinib[c]
Lymphoma	LCA, B- and T-cell markers	Treatment for cure or long-term palliation
Prostate	PSA or PrAP	Hormonal therapy effective for palliation
Small cell carcinoma	TTF-1 (if of lung origin)	Diagnosis made by H&E appearance. Neuroendocrine markers are often positive. p63 is usually negative. Chemotherapy for palliation

Table 7-26 Markers for tumors of unknown origin—*cont'd*

TYPE OF TUMOR	IMMUNOHISTOCHEMICAL MARKER(S)	POTENTIAL TREATMENT AND COMMENTS
Squamous cell carcinomas	CK5/6, p63	Not specific, but characteristic. H&E appearance usually sufficient to reveal keratin production or intercellular bridges Radiation therapy often effective
	p16 or HPV	HPV or p16 is most commonly present in carcinoma of the cervix, but may be seen in carcinomas at other sites (e.g., basaloid carcinomas of the tonsil) Approximately 26–38% of patients with a cervical lymph node metastasis of unknown primary will have an occult tonsillar carcinoma. Complete sampling of the tonsil may be necessary to identify these small carcinomas
Thyroid: papillary or follicular carcinoma	Thyroglobulin and TTF-1	Lung carcinomas are also TTF-1 positive, but will be thyroglobulin negative Highly effective treatment for cure with radioactive iodine
Thyroid: medullary carcinoma	Calcitonin	Palliative treatment with tumor-directed radionucleotides If familial, important for counseling other family members
Trophoblastic tumors	Inhibin	Inhibin is not specific, but a trophoblastic tumor is unlikely if it is negative Chemotherapy for possible cure

[a] Trastuzumab (Herceptin) is a monoclonal antibody directed against the HER-2/neu receptor.
[b] Imatinib mesylate (STI571, Gleevec™, Glivec™) is a small molecule tyrosine kinase inhibitor used for CML, ALL (Ph+), and GIST. The KIT protein is encoded by the *c-KIT* proto-oncogene and is a transmembrane receptor protein with tyrosine kinase activity. Mutated proteins may or may not respond to therapy with Imatinib. Mutations that render KIT independent of its ligand, SCF (stem cell factor), have been found in GIST, AML, germ cell tumors and systemic mastocytosis. Wild-type KIT and KIT with mutations in the juxtamembrane domain (the intracellular segment between the transmembrane and tyrosine kinase domains) are found in GISTs and are sensitive to imatinib. Other tumor types are associated with mutations in the enzymatic domain and the altered protein is generally not sensitive to imatinib.
[c] Gefitinib (Iressa) is a tyrosine kinase inhibitor that is effective against a small subset of lung adenocarcinomas with specific activating mutations.
Pathologists frequently receive specimens with metastatic tumors.[12] Often, the site of origin is known to the clinician but this information is not provided to the pathologist. A good clinical history is frequently more successful for correct classification than a battery of immunoperoxidase studies. The CK7/CK20 pattern is generally helpful to narrow down the potential site of origin of carcinomas (see Tables 7-3 to 7-7). Additional studies can then be used to identify specific types of carcinoma. The most important tumors to identify are those with specific therapeutic treatments for cure or palliation.

Table 7-27 Markers for poorly differentiated tumors

TYPE OF TUMOR	IMMUNOHISTOCHEMICAL MARKER	COMMENTS
Carcinoma	Broad-spectrum keratins AE1/AE3 or PANK (MNF-116)	Some carcinomas may express unusual keratin subtypes. If negative, try other keratin types (e.g., CAM 5.2). The CK7/CK20 pattern may be helpful in determining the likely site of origin Some non-carcinomas can have an epithelioid appearance and strongly express keratins (e.g., epithelioid angiosarcoma, epithelioid sarcoma, mesothelioma)
Melanoma	S100 protein	S100 is strongly positive in the vast majority of melanomas Some carcinomas (esp. breast) and sarcomas are also positive for S100 and additional markers may be required HMB-45 and MART-1 are expressed by most epithelioid melanomas but may be focal or absent in non-epithelioid melanomas (e.g., spindle cell or desmoplastic melanomas)
Lymphoma	Leukocyte common antigen (LCA)	Present in almost all non-Hodgkin's lymphomas. May be absent in 30% of anaplastic (Ki-1) large cell lymphomas. These lymphomas are keratin negative but may express EMA. These tumors will be positive for CD30 (Ki-1) and ALK

Table 7-28 Scoring of the EGFR (HER 1) test

SCORE	INTENSITY OF MEMBRANE STAINING	% OF CELLS POSITIVE
0	No staining	0
1+ (Positive)	Weak	≥1%
2+ (Positive)	Moderate	≥1%
3+ (Positive)	Strong	≥1%

The EGFR pharmDx™ assay has been approved by the FDA to select patients with colorectal carcinoma for treatment with a monoclonal antibody to EGFR (cetuximab or Erbitux). This test has not been shown to be superior to other comparable tests.

Unlike HER2/neu, the mechanism of overexpression of EGFR does not appear to be gene overexpression.

Table 7-28 illustrates the suggested method for scoring this test.

Immunoreactivity can be membrane or cytoplasmic. Only membrane immunoreactivity is scored, but can be partial or complete.

In clinical trials, 75% to 85% of colorectal carcinomas have been positive (1+ to 3+). Patients with positive results treated with cetuximab alone or in combination with other agents have shown clinical responses (11% to 23%). Patients with carcinomas with scores of 0 for EGFR were not treated.

No correlation has been found between the degree of tumor response and the percentage of EGFR-positive cells or the intensity of staining.

Note: Many normal cells are also positive for EGFR (notably hepatocytes and basal squamous cells).

Table 7-29 Differential diagnosis of epithelial mesothelioma and lung adenocarcinoma

	EPITHELIAL MESOTHELIOMA	LUNG ADENOCARCINOMA
Immunohistochemistry		
AE1/AE3 keratin	POS (perinuclear)[a]	POS (membrane)[b]
Calretinin	POS	neg
WT1 (clone 6F-H2)	POS (nuclear)[c]	neg[d]
CEA (polyclonal)	neg	High[e]
LeuM1 (CD15)	neg	High
TTF-1	neg	High
Mucins		
Mucicarmine	3–4%	60%
PAS-D	<3%	65%
Alcian blue	30%	POS
Alcian blue + hyaluronidase	Staining lost	Staining preserved
Ultrastructure (EM)		
Microvilli	Elongated, serpiginous, and branched	Short, blunt, rigid appearing
Length to diameter ratio	10 to 16:1	4 to 7:1
Cytogenetics		
	Deletions of 1p, 3p, 17p, loss of 9 and 22	Deletions of 3p, highly variable changes

[a] Keratin immunoreactivity is accentuated around the nucleus and is present in the cytoplasm, without prominent membrane accentuation.
[b] Keratin immunoreactivity is diffusely present in the cytoplasm with membrane accentuation in some cells.
[c] WT1 immunoreactivity is nuclear.
[d] Metastatic adenocarcinomas are generally negative for WT1 except for ovarian serous carcinomas and some renal carcinomas (see Table 7-5).
[e] Most metastatic adenocarcinomas will be positive for CEA, but there are some exceptions (see Table 7-5).
Tissue should be obtained for EM and cytogenetics, if possible.
Initial panel. AE1/AE3, calretinin, WT-1 (clone 6F-H2), CEA, Leu-M1, and TTF-1 with additional studies ordered in difficult cases.
Other antibodies generally reported as negative in epithelial mesotheliomas and positive in lung adenocarcinomas include the following: MOC-1, B72.3, Ber-EP4, and BG-8. Cytokeratins 5 and 6 are reported to be positive in mesotheliomas and negative in lung carcinomas. However, in our experience, these markers have proven less useful than those listed above. The use of EMA is controversial. Strong membrane positivity is characteristic of epithelial mesothelioma, whereas cytoplasmic positivity is characteristic of adenocarcinomas.
Less is known about the immunophenotype of pure sarcomatoid mesotheliomas. The spindle cells are positive for cytokeratin, but are less frequently positive for the other markers as compared to the epithelioid cells. Tumors that can, on occasion, resemble mesotheliomas are generally negative for cytokeratins, with the notable exceptions of some cases of angiosarcoma, epithelioid hemangioendothelioma, synovial sarcoma, epithelioid sarcoma, and leiomyosarcoma (see Table 7-8).

Table 7-30 Antibodies for immunohistochemistry

General markers

NAME (ALTERNATE NAME)	ANTIGEN (LOCATION)	NORMAL CELLS AND TISSUES	TUMORS	USES	COMMENTS
Alpha fetoprotein* (AFP, α₁-fetoprotein)	Glycoprotein present in fetal liver (cytoplasm, granular)	Fetal liver, regenerating liver cells	HCC (but not the fibrolamellar variant), hepatoblastomas, yolk sac tumors, embryonal carcinoma (but less commonly)	HCC (+/−) versus other cell types (however, AFP is rarely present in other carcinomas such as breast and ovary) Yolk sac tumors (+) versus other germ cell tumors (−/+).	Correlates with extracellular hyaline eosinophilic globules in yolk sac tumors
Alpha-1-antitrypsin (AAT, α₁-AT)	Glycoprotein inhibiting proteolytic enzymes produced in the liver (cytoplasm)	Histiocytes, reticulum cells, mast cells, Paneth cells, salivary gland	HCC, germ cell tumors, true histiocytic neoplasms, colon and lung carcinoma, others	Accumulates in liver cells in AAT deficiency	Not specific for tumor type. CD68 is somewhat more specific for macrophages
Alpha smooth muscle actin* (SMA, SM-ACT)	Smooth muscle isoform of actin (cytoplasm)	Smooth muscle, myoepithelial cells, blood vessel walls, pericytes, some stromal cells of intestine, testis, and ovary, myofibroblasts in desmoplastic stroma Not in striated muscle or myocardium	Smooth muscle tumors, myofibroblastic tumors, PEComas, glomus tumors, KS, some spindle cell carcinomas (e.g., with features of myoepithelial cells)	Identification of smooth muscle differentiation (muscle or myofibroblasts) in tumors Sclerosing lesions (myoepithelial cells present) versus invasive carcinoma, in the breast	Good marker for myoepithelial cells of the breast but also positive in myofibroblasts in stroma. p63 is only positive in myoepithelial cells
AMACR* (P504S, alpha-methylacyl-CoA racemase)	Mitochondrial and peroxisomal enzyme involved in the metabolism of branched-chain fatty acid and bile acid intermediates (cytoplasm)	Not present in normal tissues	Colorectal carcinoma (92%), colonic adenomas (75%), prostate carcinoma (83%), PIN (64%), breast cancer (44%), ovarian carcinoma, TCC, lung carcinoma, RCC, lymphoma, melanoma	Can be combined with p63 to distinguish prostate carcinoma (AMACR +, p63 absent in basal cells) from benign mimics (AMACR −, p63 present in basal cells)	
Androgen receptor (AR)	Mediates the function of androgens (nucleus)	Prostate, skin, oral mucosa	Osteosarcoma, prostatic carcinoma, breast carcinoma, ovarian carcinomas, others		
B72.3 (Tumor-associated glycoprotein 72, TAG-72, CA 72-4)	Oncofetal glycoprotein, may be a precursor of the MN blood group system, sialosyl-Tn antigen (cytoplasm, membrane)	Not present in most benign adult epithelial cells (may be present in secretory endometrium), apocrine metaplasia, and fetal GI tract	Adenocarcinomas (esp. ovary, colon, breast)	Adenocarcinoma (+ >90%) versus mesothelioma (5%) or mesothelial cells (−)	Other markers are more useful for this purpose

Table 7-30 Antibodies for immunohistochemistry—cont'd

NAME (ALTERNATE NAME)	ANTIGEN (LOCATION)	NORMAL CELLS AND TISSUES	TUMORS	USES	COMMENTS
bcl-2*	Protein involved in inhibition of apoptosis (membrane, cytoplasm)	Medullary lymphocytes and epithelial cells of the normal thymus, mantle and T zone small lymphocytes	Synovial sarcoma, solitary fibrous tumor, myofibroblastic tumors, schwannoma, neurofibroma, granular cell tumor, GIST, KS, melanoma Small lymphocytic lymphoma/ CLL, mantle cell lymphoma, follicular lymphoma, marginal zone lymphoma (MALT), some large B-cell lymphoma	Synovial sarcoma (+/−) versus mesothelioma (−) Thymic carcinomas strongly express bcl-2 compared to thymomas Small lymphocytic lymphoma, mantle cell lymphoma, and marginal zone lymphoma (MALT) (+) vs reactive follicles (−)	The bcl-2 gene is involved in the t(14;18) found in follicular lymphomas
Ber-EP4 (Epithelial specific antigen (ESA), Ep-CAM)	Glycoprotein (membrane)	All epithelial cells except superficial layers of epidermis	Most carcinomas	Adenocarcinoma (+; strong and diffuse in 60–100%) versus mesothelioma (− or focal in 26%)	Other markers are better for distinguishing adenocarcinoma from mesothelioma
Beta-amyloid (6F/3D)	Amyloid present in Alzheimer's disease (AD) and in cerebral amyloid angiopathy (extracellular)	None	Senile plaque core in AD, amyloid cores, neuritic plaques, neurofibrillary tangles	Diagnosis of AD, other diseases	Found in AD, Lewy body dementia, Down's syndrome, hereditary cerebral amyloidosis (Dutch type)
Beta-catenin	Component of the adherens junction that binds to e-cadherin and functions in cell adhesion and anchoring the cytoskeleton; signaling molecule of the Wnt/ wingless pathway (membrane, cytoplasm)	Urothelium, breast epithelium, colon, esophagus, stomach, thyroid	TCC, colonic adenocarcinomas and adenomas, breast carcinoma, esophageal squamous cell carcinoma, head and neck squamous cell carcinomas, gastric carcinoma, ovarian carcinoma, thyroid carcinoma, prostate carcinoma, HCC, brain neoplasms	Aberrant nuclear expression in solid-pseudopapillary tumors of the pancreas (95%) and pancreatoblastomas (78%)	
Beta-2 micro-globulin	Immunoglobulin associated protein (extracellular deposits of amyloid)	Plasma cells		Identification of amyloid in patients on dialysis	Amyloid tends to accumulate around joints and in the GI tract

Table 7-30 Antibodies for immunohistochemistry—cont'd

NAME (ALTERNATE NAME)	ANTIGEN (LOCATION)	NORMAL CELLS AND TISSUES	TUMORS	USES	COMMENTS
BG8	Lewis blood group y antigen (cytoplasm)	Red blood cells, endothelial cells	Adenocarcinomas (95%), rare mesotheliomas (about 5%)		Other markers are better for distinguishing adenocarcinoma from mesothelioma
Blood group antigens	A, B, and H antigens (membrane)	Epithelial cells and red blood cells, endothelial cells	Lost or abnormally expressed in many carcinomas	Can be helpful to identify potentially misidentified specimens	
CA125* (OC125)	Mucin-like glycoprotein, antibody to ovarian carcinoma antigen (luminal surface)	Epithelial cells, mesothelial cells	Adenocarcinomas of ovary, breast, lung (bronchioloalveolar), and others (rarely colon), TCC, the uterus, squamous cell carcinoma, seminal vesicle carcinoma, anaplastic lymphoma	Seminal vesicle carcinoma (+) versus prostate carcinoma (−)	Used as a serum marker for monitoring ovarian cancer
CA19-9 (Carbohydrate antigen 19-9)	Antigen of sialyl Lewis[a]-containing glycoprotein; antibody to colon carcinoma (cytoplasm)	Epithelial cells of breast, colon, kidney, liver, lung, pancreas, salivary gland, others	Adenocarcinomas of GI tract, pancreas, ovary, lung, and bladder, rare in mesotheliomas Chronic pancreatitis		Used as a serum marker for monitoring gastrointestinal and pancreatic carcinomas
Calcitonin*	Peptide hormone produced by C cells (cytoplasm and extracellular amyloid)	C cells of the thyroid	Medullary carcinoma of the thyroid (within tumor cells and in amyloid)	ID of C-cell hyperplasia ID of medullary thyroid carcinoma	Used as a serum marker for medullary carcinoma
Caldesmon* (h-caldesmon)	Actin and calmodulin binding protein in smooth muscle (cytoplasm)	Vascular and visceral smooth muscle cells, some myoepithelial cells of the breast	Smooth muscle tumors, PEComa, GIST	Smooth muscle tumors (+) vs myofibroblastic lesions (−) or endometrial stromal tumors (−)	
Calponin (CALP)*	Protein that binds to calmodulin, F-actin, and tropomyosin to regulate smooth muscle contraction (cytoplasm)	Vascular and visceral smooth muscle cells, myoepithelial cells of the breast, periacinar and periductal myoepithelial cells of the salivary gland	Myoepithelioma, some smooth muscle tumors, myofibroblastic lesions	May be helpful to identify myoepithelial cells in breast lesions	SMA is a better marker of myofibroblasts

Table 7-30 Antibodies for immunohistochemistry—*cont'd*

NAME (ALTERNATE NAME)	ANTIGEN (LOCATION)	NORMAL CELLS AND TISSUES	TUMORS	USES	COMMENTS
Calretinin*	Intracellular calcium-binding protein of the troponin C superfamily with an EF-hand domain (*cytoplasm, nucleus*)	Subsets of neurons, pineal cells, germinal epithelium of ovary, mesothelial cells, keratinocytes, breast, sweat glands, neuroendocrine cells, thymus	Epithelial mesotheliomas (less + in sarcomatoid type), adenomatoid tumor, some lung squamous cell carcinomas, rare adenocarcinomas, mesenchymal tumors (e.g., synovial sarcoma), granular cell tumor, Leydig cell tumor, granulosa cell tumor	Epithelial mesotheliomas (>90%) versus adenocarcinoma (<10%)	Useful marker in that it is positive in mesothelioma and usually negative in carcinomas
Carcinoembryonic antigen* (*CEA, CD66e*)	Glycoproteins with immunoglobulin-like regions found in fetal tissues (*cytoplasm*)	Fetal tissues	Adenocarcinomas (liver, colon, pancreas, bile duct, and lung more than breast, liver, ovary), TCC, medullary carcinoma of the thyroid Usually absent in RCC, prostate carcinoma, and papillary or follicular thyroid carcinomas	Adenocarcinoma (+) versus mesothelioma (−) HCC: polyclonal CEA has a canalicular pattern	Different reactivity patterns occur with different antibodies and with polyclonal versus monoclonal antibodies
CD5* (*Leu 1*)	Transmembrane glycoprotein (*membrane*)	T cells and B-cell subsets (mantle zone)	Thymic carcinoma, adenocarcinomas, mesothelioma (cytoplasmic). T-cell leukemias and lymphomas, aberrantly expressed in low-grade B-cell lymphomas (CLL or mantle cell lymphoma)	Thymic carcinoma (+/−) versus thymoma (−). Thymic carcinoma (+/−) versus metastatic squamous carcinoma (−) Classification of low-grade B-cell lymphomas. Evaluation of T-cell lymphomas (this marker is frequently lost)	
CD10* (*CALLA [common acute leukemia antigen], J5*)	Cell surface metalloendopeptidase that inactivates peptides (*membrane*)	Precursor B cells, granulocytes, rare cells in reactive follicles, myoepithelial cells of breast, bile canaliculi, fibroblasts, brush border of kidney and gut	Endometrial stromal sarcoma, RCC (clear cell and papillary types), HCC, TCC, rhabdomyosarcoma, pancreatic carcinoma, schwannoma, melanoma Precursor lymphoblastic lymphoma/leukemia, follicular lymphoma, Burkitt's lymphoma, CML, angioimmunoblastic lymphoma	Myoepithelial cell marker in breast Endometrial stromal sarcoma (+) versus leiomyosarcoma (−/+) (but caldesmon is preferred for this purpose) Evaluation of low-grade lymphomas Evaluation of leukemias	Not specific for nonlymphoid neoplasms

Table 7-30 Antibodies for immunohistochemistry—cont'd

NAME (ALTERNATE NAME)	ANTIGEN (LOCATION)	NORMAL CELLS AND TISSUES	TUMORS	USES	COMMENTS
CD15* (LeuM1)	3-fucosyl-N-acetyllactosamine, X-hapten—CHO moiety linked to cell membrane protein (membrane and cytoplasm)	Granulocytes, monocytes	Adenocarcinomas CMV-infected cells RS cells (not LP HD) in a membranous and Golgi pattern, some large T-cell lymphomas, MF, some leukemias	Adenocarcinomas (+) versus mesotheliomas (−) Evaluation of HD	
CD30* (Ber-H2, Ki-1)	Single chain transmembrane glycoprotein homologous to the nerve growth factor superfamily (cytoplasm, membrane, and Golgi)	Activated B and T cells, some plasma cells, immunoblasts, interdigitating cells, histiocytes, follicular center cells, decidualized endometrium, reactive mesothelial cells, most other tissues negative	Embryonal carcinoma, some vascular tumors (not KS), some mesotheliomas Anaplastic large cell (CD30+) lymphomas, mediastinal large B-cell lymphoma, primary effusion lymphoma, HD (but not LP HD), some other B- and T-cell lymphomas, EBV-transformed B cells	Evaluation of anaplastic large cell (CD30+) lymphomas Evaluation of HD (RS cells are positive except in LP HD) Evaluation of peripheral T-cell lymphoma (large cells may be positive)	
CD31* (PECAM-1, platelet-endothelial cell adhesion molecule)	Transmembrane glycoprotein functioning in cell adhesion (cytoplasm, membrane)	Endothelial cells, platelets, megakaryocytes, plasma cells, histiocytes, other hematopoietic cells	Vascular tumors (>80% of angiosarcomas), KS, histiocytic neoplasms, PEComa, very rarely other tumors	ID of endothelial differentiation in tumors Evaluation of angiogenesis	Most sensitive and specific marker for endothelial cells
CD34* (HPCA-1, hematopoietic progenitor cell, class I, QBEnd10)	Single chain transmembrane glycoprotein, leukocyte differentiation antigen (cytoplasm, membrane)	Hematopoietic progenitor cells (decreases with maturation), endothelial cells, fixed connective tissue cells (e.g., in skin), fibroblasts	Acute leukemia, sarcomas of vascular origin, KS, epithelioid sarcoma, GIST, DFSP, solitary fibrous tumor, neurofibroma, schwannoma, spindle cell lipoma	Identification of endothelial or fibroblastic differentiation in tumors Evaluation of angiogenesis Evaluation of the number of blasts in bone marrow in acute leukemia Solitary fibrous tumor (+) versus sarcomatoid mesothelioma (−) DFSP (+) versus dermatofibroma (−)	Not specific but can be useful in context with other features
CD44v3 (CD44 variant 3, H-CAM)	Transmembrane glycoprotein that mediates cell adhesion (membrane)	Many, including myometrium	Many, including endometrial carcinomas	Possibly helpful to distinguish cellular leiomyoma (+) from endometrial stromal sarcoma (−)	Many splice variants of CD44 are present in normal and malignant cells

Table 7-30 Antibodies for immunohistochemistry—cont'd

NAME (ALTERNATE NAME)	ANTIGEN (LOCATION)	NORMAL CELLS AND TISSUES	TUMORS	USES	COMMENTS
CD57* (Leu 7, HNK-1)	Lymphocyte antigen that cross reacts with a myelin-associated glycoprotein (membrane)	T-cell subsets, NK cells, myelinized nerves, neuroendocrine cells, prostate, pancreatic islets, adrenal medulla	Nerve sheath tumors (occasional), leiomyosarcoma, synovial sarcoma, rhabdomyosarcoma, neuroblastoma, neuroendocrine gliomas, neuroendocrine carcinomas, neurofibromas, some prostate carcinomas Angioimmunoblastic lymphoma, T gamma lymphoproliferative disorder (large granular cell lymphocytic leukemia)	ID of neuroendocrine differentiation in tumors ID of angioimmunoblastic T-cell lymphoma Evaluation of NK neoplasms	Not very specific for solid tumors
CD63 (NKI/C3, melanoma-associated antigen, ME491)	Member of the tetraspanin or transmembrane 4 superfamily (TM4SF) found on lysosomes (cytoplasm or membrane)	Melanocytes, mast cells, histiocytes, salivary gland cells, sweat gland cells, pancreatic cells, islets of Langerhans, prostatic cells, Paneth cells, peribronchial glands, pituitary	Nevi, melanomas, carcinoids, medullary carcinomas of the thyroid, some adenocarcinomas	Cellular neurothekoma (NKI/C3 + and S100 −) versus melanocytic lesions (NKI/C3 and S100 +) ID of melanocytic lesions	May be negative in desmoplastic melanomas
CD68* (KP1, CD68-PGM1, Mac-M)	Intracellular glycoprotein associated with lysosomes (cytoplasm, membrane)	Macrophages, monocytes, neutrophils, basophils, large lymphocytes, Kupffer cells, mast cells, osteoclasts	Neurofibroma, schwannoma, MPNST, granular cell tumors, PEComa, melanomas, atypical fibroxanthoma, RCC Some lymphomas, histiocytic sarcomas, APML, Langerhans proliferative disorders	Best general marker for macrophages, although not specific to this cell type	The antibody PG-M1 does not react with granulocytes Not very specific for solid tumors

Table 7-30 Antibodies for immunohistochemistry—cont'd

NAME (ALTERNATE NAME)	ANTIGEN (LOCATION)	NORMAL CELLS AND TISSUES	TUMORS	USES	COMMENTS
CD99* (MIC-2, 12E7, Ewing's sarcoma marker, E2 antigen, HuLy-m6, FMC 29, O13 [different epitope])	MIC2 gene product—glycoproteins (p30 and p32) involved in rosette formation with erythrocytes (membrane) Membrane immunoreactivity is more specific than cytoplasmic	Cortical thymocytes, T lymphocytes, granulosa cells of ovary, pancreatic islet cells, Sertoli cells, some endothelial cells, urothelium, ependymal cells, squamous cells	PNET/Ewing's sarcoma, chondroblastoma, mesenchymal chondrosarcoma, synovial sarcoma, solitary fibrous tumors, GIST, some alveolar rhabdomyosarcomas, desmoplastic small cell tumors, small cell carcinomas, granulosa cell tumors, yolk sac components of germ cell tumors, Sertoli–Leydig cell tumors, atypical fibroxanthoma, meningioma B- and T-cell precursor lymphoblastic lymphoma/leukemia	Thymic carcinomas (lymphocytes +) versus other carcinomas. ID of PNET/Ewing's sarcoma (immunoreactivity should be clearly membranous in the majority of the cells) Evaluation of lymphoblastic lymphoma/leukemia	O13 is the most commonly used antibody Immunoreactivity is highly dependent upon the antigen retrieval system used
CD117* (c-kit, stem cell factor receptor)	Transmembrane tyrosine kinase receptor (ligand is stem cell factor)—apoptosis is inhibited when the ligand is bound (cytoplasm, membrane)	Mast cells, interstitial cells of Cajal (ICC—pacemaker cells of the GI tract found throughout the muscle layers and in the myenteric plexus), epidermal melanocytes, mononuclear bone marrow cells (4%), Leydig cells, early spermatogenic cells, trophoblast, breast epithelium	GIST (>95%), seminomas (>70%), intratubular germ cell neoplasia, mature teratomas (>70%), papillary RCC (cytoplasmic—associated with mutations), chromophobe RCC (membrane —not associated with mutations), some melanomas (focal), mast cell tumors, some carcinomas, some brain tumors, some PNET/Ewing's sarcoma, some angiosarcomas AML (>50%), CML in myeloid blast crisis	ID of GIST (+) versus leiomyomas (−) and schwannomas (−) ID of seminomas ID of mast cells (mastocytosis)	Mast cells are an excellent internal control CD117 positivity does not correlate with mutations and/or oncoprotein activity in tumors not known to have activating mutations and is, in general, not of clinical or therapeutic significance in this setting (e.g., to detect tumors likely to respond to therapy directed against the protein, e.g. Gleevec).

Table 7-30 Antibodies for immunohistochemistry—cont'd

NAME (ALTERNATE NAME)	ANTIGEN (LOCATION)	NORMAL CELLS AND TISSUES	TUMORS	USES	COMMENTS
CD141 (Thrombomodulin, TM)	Transmembrane glycoprotein, receptor for thrombin (cytoplasm [epithelial cells], membrane [mesothelial cells])	Endothelium, platelets, monocytes, synovial cells, syncytiotrophoblast, mesothelial cells, dermal keratinocytes, islet cells, peripheral nerves	Mesotheliomas, TCC, KS, squamous cell carcinomas, choriocarcinomas, rarely adenocarcinomas, benign and malignant vascular tumors	Mesothelioma (+ 80%) versus adenocarcinoma (+ 10%) (but variable results have been reported in other studies)	Other markers are better for distinguishing adenocarcinoma from mesothelioma
CD146* (melanoma cell adherin molecule, MELCAM, MCAM, MN-4, MUC18, A32 antigen, S-Endo-1)	Membrane cell adhesion glycoprotein of the Ig gene superfamily (membrane)	Implantation site intermediate trophoblast, myofibroblasts, endothelium, pericytes, Schwann cells, ganglion cells, smooth muscle, cerebellar cortex, breast luminal and myoepithelial cells, external root sheath of hair follicle, subcapsular epithelium of thymus, follicular dendritic cells, basal cells of bronchus and parathyroid, subpopulations of activated T cells	Melanoma, angiosarcoma, KS, leiomyosarcoma, placental site trophoblastic tumor, choriocarcinoma. May be focally positive in squamous cell carcinoma and small cell carcinoma of the lung, mucoepidermoid carcinoma, breast carcinoma, some leukemias, neuroblastoma	ID of placental site trophoblastic tumors	
CDX2* **(CDX-88)**	Homeobox nuclear transcription factor specific for the intestinal tract that regulates MUC1 expression (nucleus)	Small intestine, colon, and endocrine pancreas	Colon carcinomas (usually strong and diffuse), small intestine carcinomas, mucinous ovarian carcinomas, bladder adenocarcinomas, some gastric, esophageal, pancreatic, and bile duct carcinomas. HCC, breast, lung, and head and neck carcinomas are usually negative	ID of colon carcinomas and other carcinomas of the gastrointestinal tract. However, other carcinomas (e.g., mucinous ovarian carcinoma) can also be positive	

Table 7-30 Antibodies for immunohistochemistry—cont'd

NAME (ALTERNATE NAME)	ANTIGEN (LOCATION)	NORMAL CELLS AND TISSUES	TUMORS	USES	COMMENTS
Chromogranin A*	Acidic glycoprotein in neurosecretory granules (*cytoplasm, granular*)	Islet cells of pancreas, bronchial Kulchitsky cells, parathyroid, adrenal medulla, anterior pituitary, C cells of thyroid	Pheochromocytoma, carcinoids (not rectal), small cell carcinoma, neuroblastoma, some breast and prostatic carcinomas, Merkel cell tumors, islet cell tumors, medullary carcinoma of the thyroid, parathyroid lesions, Brenner tumor	ID of neuroendocrine differentiation in tumors Not present in pituitary prolactinomas Pheochromocytoma (+) versus adrenal cortical carcinoma (−) Parathyroid (+) versus thyroid (−)	Most specific marker of neuroendocrine differentiation Also can be detected in serum Bouin's solution or B5 fixation may increase immunogenicity
Claudin-1 (*CLDN1*)	Protein component of the tight junction complex (*membrane—not cytoplasmic*)	Epithelial cells, perineurial cells, some endothelial cells (venules)	Perineurioma, synovial sarcoma (epithelioid areas, lower in spindle cell areas) carcinomas Some perineurial cells may be present in neurofibromas and schwannomas	Perineurioma (+) versus DFSP (−), fibromatosis (−), low-grade fibromyxoid sarcoma (−)	
Collagen IV	Major constituent of basement membranes (*basement membrane*)	Mesangial cells within glomeruli, basement membranes, basal lamina of capillaries	Tumors with external lamina (schwannomas, smooth muscle tumors)	Absence or loss may be associated with stromal invasion by carcinomas	
Desmin*	Intermediate filament in muscle (*cytoplasm*)	All striated muscle (Z bands) and many smooth muscle cells, myofibroblasts, smooth muscle of some blood vessels	Rhabdomyosarcoma (80% +), leiomyosarcoma (50–70% +), PEComa, desmoplastic small round cell tumors (usually dot-like), some myofibroblastic tumors, endometrial stromal sarcoma	ID of muscle differentiation in tumors	
DPC4* (*homozygously deleted in pancreatic carcinoma, locus 4, Smad4*)	Transcriptional regulator interacting with the TGF-beta signaling pathway (*nucleus*)	Normal tissues	Expressed in most carcinomas Lost in 31% of Pan IN-3, 55% of pancreatic carcinomas, and 22% of stage IV colon carcinomas	Mucinous ovarian carcinoma (+) versus metastatic pancreatic carcinoma (− in 55%)	Mutated in familial juvenile polyposis in 25–60% of cases

Table 7-30 Antibodies for immunohistochemistry—cont'd

NAME (ALTERNATE NAME)	ANTIGEN (LOCATION)	NORMAL CELLS AND TISSUES	TUMORS	USES	COMMENTS
E-cadherin	Transmembrane cell adhesion molecule that binds to catenins for cell polarization, glandular differentiation, and stratification *(membrane)*	Epithelial cells	Most carcinomas—may be lost in poorly differentiated carcinomas Not present in LCIS and invasive lobular carcinoma of breast or gastric signet ring cell carcinomas	Ductal (+) versus lobular (–) lesions of the breast	Diagnostic importance in the breast has not been established
EGFR *(Epidermal growth factor receptor, HER1)*	Transmembrane protein receptor of the type 1 growth factor family with tyrosine kinase activity *(membrane positivity scored, cytoplasmic positivity is not scored)*	Many types of epithelium, skin eccrine and sebaceous glands, mesenchymal cells, perineurium. The strongest membrane positivity is present in hepatocytes, bile ducts, basilar squamous cells, pancreatic ducts, breast epithelium, lung alveolar lining cells, mesothelial cells, prostate epithelium, endometrial glands and stroma	Adenocarcinomas (esp. colon), squamous cell carcinomas, TCC, neural tumors, sarcomas	Expression is increased in tumors of higher grade and poorer prognosis Colon carcinomas (80–90% positive): response to cetuximab does not appear to be related to IHC score (see Table 7-29)	Patients with colon carcinomas expressing EGFR are eligible for trials of targeted therapy (cetuximab).
Epithelial membrane antigen* *(EMA, MUC1, HMFG, DF3, CA 15-3, CA 27.29, PEM, many others)*	Episialin, glycoprotein found in human milk fat globule membranes *(cytoplasm [more common in malignant cells], membrane [more common in benign cells])*	Epithelial cells, perineurial cells, meningeal cells, plasma cells, usually negative in non-neoplastic mesothelial cells	Carcinomas, mesotheliomas (thick membrane pattern), some sarcomas (synovial sarcoma, epithelioid sarcoma, leiomyosarcoma, some osteosarcomas), adenomatoid tumor, chordoma, perineurioma, neurofibroma, meningioma, desmoplastic small round cell tumor, Sertoli cell tumor Some anaplastic large cell lymphomas (CD30 +), plasma cell neoplasms	ID of epithelial differentiation in tumors; however, keratin is more specific for this purpose Synovial sarcoma (typically focal positivity) versus other sarcomas	There are over 50 monoclonal antibodies recognizing different glycosylation patterns in normal tissues and tumors[16]

Table 7-30 Antibodies for immunohistochemistry—cont'd

NAME (ALTERNATE NAME)	ANTIGEN (LOCATION)	NORMAL CELLS AND TISSUES	TUMORS	USES	COMMENTS
Epstein-Barr virus* **EBV-encoded nonpolyadenylated early RNAs** (*EBERS*)	RNA produced by EBV (*nucleus*)	EBV-infected B cells	All EBV-related tumors	Most sensitive marker for EBV	Detected by in situ hybridization for RNA on paraffin sections
LMP-1	Latent membrane protein (*membrane*)	EBV-infected B cells	Nasopharyngeal carcinomas, RS cells (not LP HD), transplant lymphomas, AIDS related lymphomas, endemic Burkitt's lymphoma (rare in sporadic cases)	Evaluation of EBV related neoplasms	
EBNA 2 (*nuclear antigen 2*)	Nuclear protein (*Nucleus*)	EBV-infected B cells	Transplant-related lymphomas, AIDS-related lymphomas. Not present in Burkitt's lymphoma, nasopharyngeal carcinomas, or HD	Evaluation of transplant- and AIDS-related lymphomas	
Estrogen receptor* (*ER, 1D5, H222, others*)	Steroid binding protein (*nucleus*)	Breast epithelial cells (not myoepithelial cells), epithelial and myometrial cells of the uterus	Breast carcinomas (>70%), gynecologic carcinomas, some skin appendage tumors, rare in other carcinomas, present in some meningiomas, smooth muscle tumors, some melanomas, some thyroid tumors, desmoid tumors, myofibroblastomas of breast, vulvovaginal stromal tumor	Prognosis and prediction of response to hormonal therapy of breast cancer Only nuclear positivity is scored ID of metastatic breast cancer	Antibodies recognize different epitopes and have varying sensitivities in formalin-fixed tissue. Antigenicity may be diminished after decalcification or exposure to heat during surgery
Factor VIII-related antigen* (*VWF, FVIII:RAg, von Willebrand's factor*)	Glycoprotein involved in coagulation, part of FVIII complex (*cytoplasm*)	Endothelial cells, megakaryocytes, platelets, and mast cells, endocardium	Vascular tumors (often absent in angiosarcomas) Not present in KS, PEComa Megakaryocytic AML (M7) is positive	ID of endothelial differentiation in tumors (specific but not very sensitive) Evaluation of angiogenesis Evaluation of M7 (megakaryocytic) leukemias	May not detect smaller blood vessels (see CD 31 and 34). Present in Weibel–Palade bodies. Not a sensitive marker for vascular neoplasms

Table 7-30 Antibodies for immunohistochemistry—cont'd

NAME (ALTERNATE NAME)	ANTIGEN (LOCATION)	NORMAL CELLS AND TISSUES	TUMORS	USES	COMMENTS
Factor XIIIa (*Factor XIII subunit A*)	Transglutaminase involved in the coagulation pathway (*cytoplasm*)	Fibroblasts, dendritic reticulum cells in reactive follicles, dermal dendrocytes, liver, placenta, platelets, megakaryocytes, monocytes, macrophages	Fibroblastic neoplasms, dermatofibroma		Not very specific
Fascin	Actin binding protein thought to be involved in the formation of micro-filament bundles (*cytoplasm*)	Interdigitating reticulum cells in lymph nodes, dendritic cells of lymph node, thymus, spleen and peripheral blood, histiocytes, smooth muscle, endothelial cells, squamous mucosal cells, lining cells of splenic sinuses	RS cells and their variants (but not LP HD), rare non HD lymphomas Reticulum cell tumors Some sarcomas Some high-grade breast carcinomas		Not very specific
Fibronectin	Glycoproteins found in BMs and extracellular matrix, bind to integrins (*extracellular*)		Stroma of many tumors		
Fli-1* (*Friend leukemia integrin-site 1*)	Transcription factor (ETS family)—translocation in Ewing's can result in an EWS–Fli-1 fusion protein (*nucleus*)	Endothelial cells (hemangioblasts, angioblasts), small lymphocytes	Ewing's sarcoma/PNET, vascular tumors (including KS), Merkel cell carcinoma, melanoma Can also be weakly present in lymphomas, synovial sarcoma, some carcinomas	ID of vascular tumors (unlike other vascular markers, Fli-1 is nuclear) ID of Ewing's sarcoma/PNET	Reactivity can be variable with high background and may be difficult to interpret
Galectin-3* (*Gal-3*)	Lectin with anti-apoptosis function (galactoside-binding protein) (*nucleus, cytoplasm, membrane, extracellular matrix*)	Many epithelial cells, lymphocytes, mesenchymal cells, macrophages, activated endothelial cells	Many carcinomas, adenomas, lymphomas, soft tissue tumors	Thyroid carcinomas (papillary and to a lesser extent follicular) show higher expression than benign lesions In some carcinomas, expression is diminished in higher-grade lesions	

Table 7-30 Antibodies for immunohistochemistry—cont'd

NAME (ALTERNATE NAME)	ANTIGEN (LOCATION)	NORMAL CELLS AND TISSUES	TUMORS	USES	COMMENTS
Glial fibrillary acidic protein (GFAP)	Intermediate filament (cytoplasm)	Normal and reactive astrocytes, developing and reactive ependymal cells, developing oligodendrocytes, choroid plexus, Schwann cells, enteric glial cells, pituitary cells, chondrocytes	Tumors of astrocytes, ependymal cells, and oligodendrocytes, MPNST, myoepitheliomas (salivary glands and soft tissue), sweat gland tumors, Merkel cell carcinomas, chordomas	ID of neural differentiation in tumors (30% of MPNSTs are +) Neuroblastomas are negative, schwannomas may be focally + Merkel cell carcinoma (+) versus small cell carcinoma (−) (but CK20 is a better marker for this purpose) ID of myoepithelial neoplasms	
GLUT-1 (glucose transporter 1)	Component of trans-membrane glucose transport (membrane)	Erythrocytes, perineurium, blood vessels, tropho-blasts, renal tubules, germinal center cells	TCC, lung carcinoma, squamous cell carcinoma, adenocarcinomas of colon, lung, bile ducts, kidney, ovary, pancreas, stomach, and endometrium, germ cell tumors		Not very specific
Gross cystic disease fluid protein-15* (GCDFP, CDP, BR-2, BRST-2)	Protein found in breast fluid (cytoplasm)	Apocrine sweat glands, apocrine metaplasia of the breast	Breast carcinomas (60%), sweat gland carcinomas, some salivary gland tumors, some prostate carcinomas	ID of apocrine differentiation in tumors ID of breast metastases (however, only positive in about 60%)	
HepPar-1* (hepatocyte paraffin-1, HP1)	Mitochondrial protein (cytoplasm, coarsely granular)	Liver	HCC, some cases of gastric adenocarcinoma, esophageal adenocarcinoma, others negative or rarely positive	HCC (80–95%) versus metastatic carcinomas to the liver	
HBME-1*	Antigen to microvilli on mesothelioma cells (membrane and cytoplasm)	Mesothelial cells, epithelial cells	Mesotheliomas (epithelial type—thick, membrane staining), adenocarcinomas, chordomas, chondrosarcomas	Positivity higher in thyroid carcinomas than in adenomas May be absent in thyroid carcinomas with Hürthle cell features	Not a specific marker for mesotheliomas

Table 7-30 Antibodies for immunohistochemistry—cont'd

NAME (ALTERNATE NAME)	ANTIGEN (LOCATION)	NORMAL CELLS AND TISSUES	TUMORS	USES	COMMENTS
HER-2/neu (c-erbB2)	Growth factor receptor (tyrosine kinase) homologous to epidermal growth factor receptor (membrane, some cytoplasm)	Absent or rare in normal cells	Breast carcinomas (20–30%), Paget's disease of nipple (>90%), less frequently in other carcinomas (ovary, uterus, GI, pancreas), some synovial sarcomas	Poor prognostic factor in breast cancer Positivity used to select patients for treatment with Herceptin (scored from 0 to 3+) (see Chapter 15)	Only membrane positivity is scored Gene amplification (detected by FISH) correlates with strong complete membrane immunoreactivity in >90% of cases
HHF-35* (Muscle-specific actin, MSA, muscle common actin, EM ACT)	Alpha and gamma smooth muscle actins, recognizes a common epitope of alpha skeletal, cardiac, and smooth muscle (cytoplasm)	Smooth, striated, and cardiac muscle, smooth muscle of blood vessels, pericytes, myoepithelial cells, myofibroblasts	Numerous tumors including tumors of muscle, glomus tumor, PEComa, GIST, DFSP, dermatofibroma, myofibroblastic tumors, spindle cell carcinomas, salivary gland tumors, mesothelioma, others	ID of muscle differentiation in tumors	Sensitive but not specific. Present in tumors not of muscle origin
HHV8*	Latent nuclear antigen of human herpesvirus type 8 (nucleus)	Absent in normal tissue	KS (endothelial cells and some perivascular cells) Primary effusion lymphoma (PEL), AIDS-associated multicentric Castleman's disease	Evaluation of KS and PEL	
HMB-45* (E-MEL, melanoma-specific antigen)	Oligosaccharide side-chain of a melanosomal antigen, gp100/pmel17 (cytoplasm)	Fetal melanocytes and some normal adult superficial melanocytes, retinal pigment epithelium	Melanoma (epithelioid but not spindle cell or desmoplastic type), clear cell sarcoma, PEComa, tumors associated with tuberous sclerosis, melanotic schwannoma, others	ID of metastatic melanoma. Melanophages can also be positive Melan-A may be more specific ID of PEComa	NKI-betab detects the same protein Tissues fixed in B5 may have high background staining

Table 7-30 Antibodies for immunohistochemistry—cont'd

NAME (ALTERNATE NAME)	ANTIGEN (LOCATION)	NORMAL CELLS AND TISSUES	TUMORS	USES	COMMENTS
hMLHI (*human mutS homologue 2*) **and hMSH2** (*human mutL homologue 1*)	Proteins involved in mismatch repair of DNA (these genes account for 95% of HNPCC) (*nucleus*)	Most normal tissues May be lost in areas of chronic inflammation	Expression (or non-expression) is not specific for tumor type	Absence is associated with germline mutations in HNPCC patients and with gene silencing by methylation in 15% of sporadic colon carcinomas —correlated with characteristic clinical, pathologic, and treatment response features IHC will not detect the 5% of patients with mutations in other genes or rare patients with mutated gene products that are immunoreactive	Other assays for microsatellite instability utilize PCR (90% sensitive for microsatellite instability (MSI)
Hormones (ER and PR are listed separately)	Insulin, gastrin, glucagon, somatostatin, calcitonin, ACTH, FSH, LH, PRL, TSH, others (*cytoplasm*)	Hormone-producing cells	Hormone-producing tumors	ID of hormone products in tumors	May not correlate well with serum levels of the same markers May not correlate with response to hormonal therapies (e.g., ER in tumors other than breast and tamoxifen)
Human chorionic gonadotropin* (*hCG, β-hCG*)	Beta chain of the hormone (*cytoplasm*)	Syncytiotrophoblasts	Choriocarcinoma, giant cells in seminomas, placental site tumors (weak)	ID of trophoblastic differentiation in tumors	
Human placental lactogen* (*HPL, hPL*)	Hormone (*cytoplasm*)	Trophoblast	Choriocarcinoma (may be weak), complete moles (strong), partial moles (weak), some lung and stomach carcinomas	ID of trophoblastic differentiation in tumors	
Inhibin*: **alpha subunit**	Hormone produced by ovarian granulosa cells and prostate, inhibits FSH production (*cytoplasm*)	Ovarian granulosa cells, Sertoli cells, pregnancy luteomas, ovarian follicles, syncytiotrophoblast, adrenal cortex, hepatocytes	Granulosa cell tumors, juvenile granulosa cell tumors, Sertoli and Leydig cell tumors, ovarian stromal cells around other tumors, hydatidiform moles, choriocarcinoma, thecofibroma, adrenal cortical tumor, granular cell tumor	ID of sex cord stromal differentiation in ovarian tumors Distinguishes adrenal cortical tumors (>70% +) versus HCC (<5% +) and RCC (<5% +)	

Table 7-30 Antibodies for immunohistochemistry—cont'd

NAME (ALTERNATE NAME)	ANTIGEN (LOCATION)	NORMAL CELLS AND TISSUES	TUMORS	USES	COMMENTS
Keratins*	Intermediate filaments *(cytoplasm)*	Epithelial cells	Carcinomas, mesotheliomas, desmoplastic small round cell tumors (dot-like pattern), thymomas, chordomas, synovial sarcomas, epithelioid sarcoma, leiomyosarcoma, trophoblastic tumors, some other sarcomas, rarely melanomas	ID of poorly differentiated carcinomas Site of origin of carcinomas	
AE1/AE3*	Two monoclonal antibodies. AE1 detects 10, 15, 16, and 19. AE3 detects 1 to 8. *(Cytoplasm)*		Most carcinomas. The only common carcinomas that are frequently negative are HCC (70% negative) and RCC, clear cell type (20% negative) Epithelioid hemangio-endothelioma, epithelioid sarcoma, synovial sarcoma, mesothelioma, adenomatoid tumor	ID of epithelial differentiation in tumors. HCC (−/+) versus cholangio-carcinoma and metastatic carcinomas (+)	Good broad-spectrum keratin
CAM 5.2*	8, 18 *(cytoplasm)*	Simple and glandular epithelium	Most carcinomas including those usually negative for CK7 and 20: HCC, prostatic carcinoma, thymic carcinoma, gastric carcinoma, RCC small cell carcinoma Carcinoid tumor, thymoma, germ cell tumors, mesothelioma, dendritic cells Synovial sarcoma, epithelioid sarcoma Many squamous cell carcinomas are negative	ID of carcinomas that may be negative for CK7 and CK20 Paget's disease (+) versus squamous cell carcinoma (−) Positivity for dendritic cells in lymph nodes and elsewhere may be confused for micrometastases	May be positive when other keratins are negative

Table 7-30 Antibodies for immunohistochemistry—cont'd

NAME (ALTERNATE NAME)	ANTIGEN (LOCATION)	NORMAL CELLS AND TISSUES	TUMORS	USES	COMMENTS
Keratin 5/6*	5/6 (cytoplasm)	Basal cells, stratum spinosum of epidermis, mesothelial cells	Squamous cell carcinomas, TCC, mesotheliomas, squamous metaplasia in adenocarcinomas, thymic carcinoma	Less frequently present in non-squamous cell carcinomas	Has limited use in routine practice
Keratin 7*	7 (cytoplasm)	Simple epithelia, respiratory epithelium, transitional epithelium, endothelial cells of small veins and lymphatics Not present in squamous epithelium	Most adenocarcinomas of glandular epithelial origin, TCC, mesothelioma, neuroendocrine neoplasms Not Merkel cell carcinoma or colon carcinoma Rare in clear cell RCC (but present in other variants), prostate carcinoma, HCC, lung small cell carcinoma, thymoma, carcinoid Not present in squamous cell carcinomas of the skin, but may be present in squamous cell carcinomas arising from non-keratinizing epithelium (e.g., cervical carcinoma)	The combination of CK7 and CK20 is used to distinguish carcinomas arising at different sites (see Tables 7-3 to 7-7)	
Keratin 20*	20 (cytoplasm)	Gastric foveolar epithelium, intestinal villi and crypt epithelium, Merkel cells, taste buds, umbrella cells of urothelium, subsets of epithelial cells Not present in non-epithelial cells	Colon carcinoma, Merkel cell carcinoma, TCC, adenocarcinoma of the bladder, pancreatic carcinoma, cholangio-carcinoma, mucinous ovarian carcinoma, esophageal adenocarcinoma	Merkel cell carcinomas CK20 positive, whereas most similar tumors are negative ID of metastatic colon carcinomas (the pattern of CK7−, CK20 + is most frequently seen in this carcinoma, but can rarely be seen in other types)	

Table 7-30 Antibodies for immunohistochemistry—cont'd

NAME (ALTERNATE NAME)	ANTIGEN (LOCATION)	NORMAL CELLS AND TISSUES	TUMORS	USES	COMMENTS
PAN-K* (MNF-116)	Broad spectrum detection of keratins including 5, 6, 8, 17, and 18 (cytoplasm)	Simple and squamous epithelial cells		Detection of keratin in all carcinomas, including poorly differentiated carcinomas (esp. spindle cell squamous cell carcinomas) May be more sensitive than AE1/AE3 for carcinomas with myoepithelial ("basal") features due to inclusion of the "basal" keratin CK17	
34βE12* (903)	High-molecular-weight keratins including 1, 5, 10, 14 (cytoplasm)	Complex epithelia, basal cells, myoepithelial cells	TCC, cholangiocarcinoma, squamous cell carcinoma, non-mucinous bronchiolo-alveolar lung carcinoma, RCC (papillary and chromophobe types), mesothelioma, papillary thyroid carcinoma, thymic carcinoma, lympho-epithelial carcinoma	TCC (+) versus prostate carcinoma (–) or RCC (–) Prostate carcinoma (no basal cells) versus benign lesions (with some + basal cells present). Can be combined with p63 for this use	
Ki-67* (MIB-1)	Protein found during the entire cell cycle but not in G0 (nucleus)	Any cycling cell	Any cycling tumor	Used as a prognostic marker for some tumors Detects number of cycling cells in Burkitt's lymphoma and large B-cell lymphoma Aberrant membrane and cytoplasmic immuno-reactivity is present in trabecular hyalinizing adenoma of the thyroid and sclerosing hemangioma of the lung	MIB-1 recognizes an epitope preserved in formalin-fixed tissue
Laminin	Component of basement membranes (basement membrane)	Basement membranes	Nerve sheath tumors, smooth muscle tumors	Loss associated with stromal invasion by carcinoma Present in microglandular adenosis of the breast	

Table 7-30 Antibodies for immunohistochemistry—cont'd

NAME (ALTERNATE NAME)	ANTIGEN (LOCATION)	NORMAL CELLS AND TISSUES	TUMORS	USES	COMMENTS
Lysozyme (Ly)	Muramidase (mucolytic enzyme) (cytoplasm)	Circulating monocytes, some tissue macrophages, granulocytes, salivary gland, lacrimal gland, stomach and colon epithelial cells (inflamed or regenerative), apocrine glands, Paneth cells, some other epithelial cells	Salivary gland tumors, stomach and colon carcinomas AML with monocytic differentiation	Marker for histiocytes but not specific. May mark activated phagocytic macrophages Evaluation of myeloid leukemias	Not specific for identification of solid tumors
MAC 387 (L1 antigen, calprotectin, calgranulin, cystic fibrosis antigen)	Three polypeptide chains released with activation or death of neutrophils (cytoplasm)	Neutrophils, monocytes, some tissue macrophages, eosinophils, squamous mucosa, reactive skin, synovial lining cells	Lung carcinomas (not small cell or carcinoid), squamous cell carcinomas Histiocytic neoplasms (but not Langerhans cells)	Marker for macrophages (but not as specific as CD68)	Belongs to the S100 protein family Cells can passively take up antigen resulting in false positive results
Melan-A or MART-1* (melanoma antigen recognized by T cells), A103	Melanocyte differentiation antigen (cytoplasm) Melan-A (clone A103) and MART-1 are two different antibodies	Melanocytes of skin, uvea, and retina Melan-A is also positive in adrenal cortex, granulosa and theca cells of the ovary, Leydig cells	Melanomas (but <50% of spindle cell or desmoplastic melanomas), PEComas Melan-A is also positive in adrenocortical tumors, Leydig cell tumor, granulosa cell tumor	ID of melanomas. Melan-A is not positive in melanophages and may be more specific for the detection of micrometastases in lymph nodes Melan-A distinguishes adrenocortical tumors (–) (≥50% +) versus HCC and RCC (–)	More sensitive than HMB45 Peptides are used for melanoma immunotherapy Melan-A has a broader spectrum of immunoreactivity than MART-1
Myf-4* (MRF4, myogenin)	Human homologue of myogenin— muscle regulatory protein (nucleus)	Striated muscle	Rhabdomyosarcoma	ID of skeletal muscle differentiation in tumors	Better than MyoD1
MyoD1	Nuclear phosphoprotein, role in myogenic regulation (nucleus)	Developing muscle tissues (myoblasts), adult muscle is negative	Rhabdomyosarcoma (esp. poorly differentiated tumors), mixed mullerian tumors	ID of skeletal muscle differentiation in tumors	Background positivity is often high, making interpretation difficult

Table 7-30 Antibodies for immunohistochemistry—cont'd

NAME (ALTERNATE NAME)	ANTIGEN (LOCATION)	NORMAL CELLS AND TISSUES	TUMORS	USES	COMMENTS
Myoglobin	Oxygen binding protein (*cytoplasm*)	Striated muscle (including cardiac muscle), not smooth muscle	Tumors of striated muscle (rhabdomyosarcoma + 50%), but often negative in poorly differentiated tumors	ID of skeletal muscle differentiation in tumors	More specific but less sensitive than actin and desmin
Myosin Heavy Chain (fast) (*SM-MHC, Fast myosin*)	Contractile protein with 2 heavy and 4 light chains and many isoforms (*cytoplasm*)	Visceral and vascular smooth muscle, myoepithelial cells of the breast Striated muscle: type 2 fibers	Tumors with myoepithelial cells Rhabdomyosarcoma (some)	Marker for myoepithelial cells in the breast—may have less positivity in vascular endothelial cells and myofibroblasts ID of skeletal muscle differentiation in tumors	Antibodies to different isoforms will detect different types of muscle fibers
NEU N	(*Neuronal nuclei*)	Neuronal cells including cerebellum, cerebral cortex, peripheral ganglion cells			
Neurofilaments (*70 + 200 kD, NFP*)	Intermediate filaments with three subunits (*cytoplasm*)	Neuronal cells, adrenal medulla	Tumors of neuronal origin or with neuronal differentiation, neuroblastoma, medulloblastoma, retinoblastoma, Ewing's/PNET, esthesioneuroblastoma, Merkel cell carcinoma, some endocrine tumors (carcinoids, pheochromocytomas)	ID of neuronal differentiation in tumors ID of Merkel cell carcinomas	
Neuron-specific enolase* (*NSE—do not confuse with the enzyme non-specific esterase*)	Gamma-gamma enolase isoenzyme (*cytoplasm*)	Neuroectodermal and neuroendocrine cells, more weakly striated and smooth muscle, megakaryocytes, T cells, some platelets, neurons, pituitary cells, hepatocytes	Neuroectodermal and neuroendocrine tumors, melanomas (including desmoplastic melanomas), many breast carcinomas, germ cell tumors, alveolar soft part sarcoma	ID of neuronal or neuroendocrine differentiation in tumors	Lacks specificity

Table 7-30 Antibodies for immunohistochemistry—cont'd

NAME (ALTERNATE NAME)	ANTIGEN (LOCATION)	NORMAL CELLS AND TISSUES	TUMORS	USES	COMMENTS
p16 (MTS1, CDKN2)	Binds to and inhibits the cyclin-dependent kinases cdk4 and cdk6 (cytoplasm and nuclear)	Absent	Cervical squamous cell carcinomas and adenocarcinomas (both in situ and invasive), endocervical carcinoma, endometrial carcinoma. Some basaloid squamous cell carcinomas of the tonsil in young patients that are associated with HPV16	Evaluation of cervical lesions. Possible use predicting tonsillar site for metastatic squamous cell carcinoma of the head and neck	Overexpression is due to HPV-induced cell cycle dysregulation
p27kip1	A cyclin-dependent kinase inhibitor that regulates progression from G1 to S phase	Proliferating cells			
p53* (Multiple antibodies to wild-type and mutant forms)	Tumor suppressor gene product—probably most frequently mutated gene in malignancy (nucleus)	Overexpression uncommon or absent in normal cells or benign tumors	Many malignant tumors, but not specific for malignancy	Overexpression may be used as a prognostic factor	Different antibodies recognize different wild type and mutant forms of the protein and will give different results
p57 (kip2, p57KIP2)	Cyclin-dependent kinase inhibitor (CDKI) acting to inhibit cell proliferation, paternally imprinted (nucleus)	Cytotrophoblast, intermediate trophoblast, villous stromal cells, decidual stromal cells, absent in syncytiotrophoblast		Diploid complete moles show absent or low expression in cytotrophoblast and villous stromal cells (may be present in villous intermediate trophoblast and decidual stromal cells), partial moles and hydropic abortions have normal expression	

Table 7-30 Antibodies for immunohistochemistry—cont'd

NAME (ALTERNATE NAME)	ANTIGEN (LOCATION)	NORMAL CELLS AND TISSUES	TUMORS	USES	COMMENTS
p63*	Protein with at least six major isotypes, including deltaNp63, member of the p53 family (nucleus)	Proliferating basal cells of cervix, urothelium, prostate, and myo-epithelial cells of breast, basal squamous cells, squamous metaplasia	Squamous cell carcinomas, TCC, adenomyo-epithelioma, adenoid cystic carcinoma, nasopharyngeal carcinoma, "basal type" breast carcinomas, papillary carcinoma of the thyroid, others	ID of myoepithelial cells in sclerosing breast lesions Diagnosis of prostatic carcinoma by showing absence of basal cells (more sensitive when combined with 34βE12). Basaloid squamous lung cancer (+) versus small cell (−). ID of metastatic poorly differentiated squamous cell carcinomas	Easier to interpret than SMA as myofibroblasts are negative
Placental alkaline phosphatase* (PLAP)	Alkaline phosphatase secreted by trophoblast (cytoplasm)	Placenta (trophoblast)	Germ cell tumors (but not spermatocytic seminoma), intratubular germ cell neoplasia, partial moles, some carcinomas of breast, ovary, lung, stomach, and pancreas, some rhabdomyosarcomas (esp. alveolar type)	Absence of immunoreactivity makes a germ cell tumor unlikely. However, spermatocytic seminomas and immature teratomas are negative ID of intratubular germ cell neoplasia	
Progesterone receptor* (PR, PgR)	Steroid binding protein (nuclear)	Normal breast epithelial cells, endometrial cells, many smooth muscle cells, breast lobular stroma	Breast carcinomas, gynecologic carcinomas, some skin adnexal tumors, secretory meningiomas, endometrial stromal sarcomas, some leiomyomas, myofibro-blastic tumors, rarely other tumors	Prognosis and treatment of breast cancer ID of metastatic breast cancer	
Prealbumin (Transthyretin, TTR)	Plasma transport protein for retinol and thyroxine (cytoplasm)	Pancreatic islet cells, choroid plexus, retinal pigment epithelium, liver	Pancreatic islet cell tumors, carcinoid tumors, choroid plexus papillomas, choroid plexus carcinomas (may be focal or absent)	ID of choroid plexus neoplasms Evaluation of some forms of amyloidosis	Major subunit protein in some forms of inherited systemic amyloidosis

Table 7-30 Antibodies for immunohistochemistry—cont'd

NAME (ALTERNATE NAME)	ANTIGEN (LOCATION)	NORMAL CELLS AND TISSUES	TUMORS	USES	COMMENTS
Prostate-specific antigen* (PSA)	Member of kallikrein family of serine protease isolated from human seminal plasma (cytoplasm)	Normal prostatic epithelium, urachal remnants, endometrium, transitional cells of bladder	Prostatic carcinomas, some breast carcinomas	ID of prostatic carcinomas (may be lost in some poorly differentiated carcinomas). Seminal vesicle carcinomas are negative	More specific than PAP Used as a serum screening test for prostate cancer
Prostate acid phosphatase* (PrAP, PAP)	Isoenzyme of acid phosphatase (cytoplasm)	Normal prostatic epithelium, periurethral glands, anal glands, macrophages	Prostatic carcinomas, TCC, rectal carcinoids	ID of prostatic carcinomas (may be lost in some poorly differentiated carcinomas)	
RCC* (Renal cell carcinoma marker, gp200)	Glycoprotein on surface of renal tubules, breast epithelial cells, epididymis (cytoplasm, membrane)	Renal tubules, breast, epididymis	Clear cell and papillary RCC, breast carcinoma, embryonal carcinoma	Clear cell and papillary RCC (+) versus chromophobe carcinoma (−/+) and oncocytoma (−)	
RET* (Rearranged during transfection)	RET proto-oncogene. Surface glycoprotein of the receptor tyrosine kinase family (cytoplasm)	Neurons, embryonic kidney	Papillary thyroid carcinomas (78%), follicular variant of papillary carcinoma (63%), Hürthle cell carcinoma (57%), insular carcinoma (50%), medullary carcinoma, not present in follicular carcinomas or benign lesions Neuroblastoma (+), pheochromocytoma (+)	Evaluation of thyroid tumors	Germline mutations occur in MEN2A and 2B (10q11.2), familial medullary thyroid carcinoma, and some cases of Hirschsprung's disease
S100 protein*	Calcium binding protein isolated from the CNS (member of the EF hand family) (nucleus and cytoplasm)	Glial and Schwann cells, melanocytes, chondrocytes, adipocytes, myoepithelial cells, Langerhans cells, macrophages, reticulum cells of lymph nodes, eccrine glands, others	Melanoma (including spindle cell and desmoplastic types), clear cell sarcoma, schwannoma, chordoma, ependymoma, astroglioma, Langerhans proliferative disorders, some carcinomas (e.g., breast, ovary endometrial, thyroid), granular cell tumor, histiocytic sarcoma, myoepithelioma	ID of melanoma (if negative, melanoma is highly unlikely) ID of Langerhans proliferative disorders Sustentacular cells in pheochromocytomas (loss may be poor prognostic factor) ID of neural tumors ID of cellular schwannomas (more strongly and diffuselypositive than in MPNST)	Langerhans cells and macrophages in tumors may be misinterpreted as positivity in the tumor itself S100 is very soluble and may be eluted from frozen tissues

Table 7-30 Antibodies for immunohistochemistry—cont'd

NAME (ALTERNATE NAME)	ANTIGEN (LOCATION)	NORMAL CELLS AND TISSUES	TUMORS	USES	COMMENTS
Synaptophysin*	Transmembrane glycoprotein found in presynaptic vesicles (cytoplasm)	Neuroectodermal and neuroendocrine cells, neurons	Medulloblastoma, neuroblastoma, pheochromocytoma, paragangliomas, carcinoids, small cell carcinoma, medullary carcinoma of the thyroid, neural neoplasms, pancreatic islet cell tumors	ID of neuroendocrine differentiation in tumors ID of neuronal differentiation in CNS tumors	
Synuclein-I	Neuron-specific protein associated with synaptosomes (Lewy bodies)	Brain	Present in Lewy bodies (Lewy body dementia and Parkinson's disease)		
Tau	Microtubule-associated protein (cytoplasm, extracellular)	Normal neuronal cell bodies and dendrites, neuropil, glial cells	Abnormal amounts in Alzheimer's disease in neurofibrillary tangles and senile plaques	Evaluation of Alzheimer's disease, Pick's disease, supranuclear palsy corticobasal degeneration, others	
Thyroglobulin*	Glycoprotein produced by thyroid follicular cells (cytoplasm)	Thyroid follicles	Thyroid carcinomas (papillary, follicular, and Hürthle cell types, rarely present in medullary carcinomas)	ID of metastatic thyroid carcinoma Loss may be a poor prognostic factor	Thyroglobulin can diffuse into metastatic tumors to the thyroid
TTF-I* (Thyroid transcription factor I)	Transcription factor for thyroglobulin, thyroid peroxidase, Clara cell secretory protein, and surfactant proteins (nucleus; aberrant cytoplasm positivity in HCC)	Thyroid, lung, and some brain tissues	Thyroid carcinomas (including medullary carcinoma; may be negative in anaplastic carcinoma), lung adenocarcinomas (75%, but lower in mucinous bronchioloalveolar carcinomas), small cell carcinoma of lung (>90%), HCC (cytoplasmic), absent or focal in most other adenocarcinomas	Mesothelioma (−) versus adenocarcinoma (+/−) Lung adenocarcinoma (+/−) versus metastatic breast carcinoma (−) Small cell carcinoma of lung (+) versus metastasis from other sites (−), but some extrapulmonary small cell carcinomas can also be + HCC (cytoplasmic 71%), rare in other tumor types	The detection of cytoplasmic TTF-I may depend on the specific antibody used and the antigen-retrieval method

Table 7-30 Antibodies for immunohistochemistry—cont'd

NAME (ALTERNATE NAME)	ANTIGEN (LOCATION)	NORMAL CELLS AND TISSUES	TUMORS	USES	COMMENTS
Ulex (Ulex europaeus I lectin, UEA I)	Lectin, fucose residues on blood group H (cytoplasm)	Endothelial cells	Vascular tumors, some carcinomas	Evaluation of angiogenesis	Not very specific
Vimentin*	Intermediate filament (cytoplasm)	Mesenchymal cells, fibroblasts, endothelial cells, chondrocytes, histiocytes, lymphocytes, many glial cells, myoepithelial cells, smooth muscle	All mesenchymal tumors, neural tumors, melanomas, meningiomas, chordoma, Leydig cell tumor, granulosa cell tumor, Sertoli cell tumor, adrenal cortical adenoma. May be co-expressed with keratin in carcinomas of endometrium, thyroid, kidney (clear cell), adrenal cortex, lung, salivary gland, ovary, and liver	May be poor prognostic factor if co-expressed with keratin or GFAP	Can be used as an internal control for immunogenicity. Not a specific marker for tumor type or line of differentiation
WT1* (Wilms' tumor I protein)	Zinc finger transcription factor (cytoplasm, nucleus)	Sertoli cells, decidual cells of uterus, granulosa cells of ovary, blood vessels, myelocytic cells	Wilms' tumors (epithelial and blastemal components), epithelial mesotheliomas (nuclei—80–90%), acute leukemia (nuclei), adenocarcinomas (cytoplasmic; esp. breast, ovary), desmoplastic small cell tumors (nuclear and cytoplasmic), rhabdomyosarcoma	Mesothelioma (+, nuclear) versus adenocarcinoma (adenocarcinoma usually negative for nuclear positivity except for ovarian)—monoclonal antibody used. Desmoplastic small cell tumors—use polyclonal antibody	The gene is located on 11p13 and is inactivated in 5–10% of sporadic Wilms' tumors and nearly 100% of Denys–Drash syndrome patients. Antibodies detect epitopes at different ends of the protein and may give different results. Not very specific

Table 7-30 Antibodies for immunohistochemistry—cont'd

Hematopathology markers

NAME (ALTERNATE NAME)	ANTIGEN (LOCATION)	NORMAL CELLS AND TISSUES	TUMORS	USES	COMMENTS
ALK Protein* (Anaplastic lymphoma kinase, ALK-1, p80)	The ALK gene (2p23) is translocated to part of the nucleophosmin (NPM) gene (5q35) to form the fusion protein p80 and is overexpressed (cytoplasm, nucleus)	Nervous system	Anaplastic (CD30+) large cell lymphomas—approximately one third have t(2:5)(p23:q35) Some inflammatory myofibroblastic tumors	ID of anaplastic large cell lymphomas	The pattern of immunoreactivity varies with the translocation present
Alpha-1-antichymotrypsin (ACH)	Serine protease inhibitor (cytoplasm)	Histiocytes, granulocytes, others	Histiocytic tumors, many adenocarcinomas, melanomas, many sarcomas	Marker for histiocytes but CD68 is more specific	Not specific for tumor type
Alpha-1-antitrypsin (AAT, α₁-AT)	Glycoprotein synthesized in the liver that inhibits proteolytic enzymes (esp. elastase) (cytoplasm)	Histiocytes, reticulum cells, mast cells, Paneth cells, salivary gland	HCC, germ cell tumors, histiocytic neoplasms, colon and lung carcinomas, others	Accumulates in liver cells in AAT deficiency	Not specific for tumor type CD68 is a more specific marker for macrophages
bcl-2*	Protein involved in inhibition of apoptosis (membrane, cytoplasm)	Medullary lymphocytes and epithelial cells of the normal thymus, mantle and T zone small lymphocytes	CLL, mantle cell lymphoma, follicular lymphoma, marginal zone lymphoma Synovial sarcoma, other soft tissue tumors	Follicular center cell lymphomas (+) versus reactive follicles (−). Hyperplastic marginal zones of the spleen, abdominal lymph nodes, and ilial lymphoid tissue are + Malignant thymomas may have greater reactivity than other thymomas Synovial sarcoma is more frequently positive compared to mesothelioma	Involved in the t(14:18) found in 90% of FCC lymphomas Not specific for ID of solid tumors

Table 7-30 Antibodies for immunohistochemistry—cont'd

NAME (ALTERNATE NAME)	ANTIGEN (LOCATION)	NORMAL CELLS AND TISSUES	TUMORS	USES	COMMENTS
Bcl-6*	Proto-oncogene—Kruppel-type zinc finger protein with homology to transcription factors *(nucleus)*	Normal germinal center B cells	Follicular lymphomas, diffuse large B-cell lymphomas, Burkitt lymphoma, mediastinal large B-cell lymphoma, LP HD Not present in B-CLL, hairy cell leukemia, mantle cell lymphoma, and marginal zone lymphomas	Evaluation of B-cell lymphomas	Involved in gene rearrangements at 3q27 in lymphomas
Blood group antigens	A, B, and H antigens *(membrane)*	Epithelial cells, endothelial cells, erythrocytes	Abnormally expressed or lost in many carcinomas	Sometimes helpful in identifying specimens	
BOB.1* *(B-cell Oct-binding protein 1)*	Coactivator that interacts with Oct transcription factors in B cells *(cytoplasm)*	B cells (including plasma cells)	B-cell lymphomas and leukemias, Reed–Sternberg cells in LP HD, usually absent in other HD types	Evaluation of HD	BOB.1 and Oct2 are necessary (but not sufficient) for Ig expression
BSAP* *(B-cell specific activator protein)*	Transcription factor encoded by the *Pax-5* gene that regulates B-lineage specific genes	B cells	All B-cell neoplasms and HD		Not reliable in Zenker's fixed tissue
CD1a* *(T6)*	Membrane glycoprotein *(membrane)*	Cortical thymocytes (immature T cells), Langerhans cells, dendritic cells	Langerhans proliferative disorders, lymphoblastic lymphoma	Evaluation of Langerhans proliferative disorders Evaluation of lymphoblastic lymphoma	
CD2* *(TE,T11, rT3, Leu 5a + b, LFA-2)*	Glycoprotein mediating adhesion of activated T cells and thymocytes with antigen-presenting cells and target cells, functions in E rosette formation *(membrane)*	T cells, NK cells, cortical thymocytes	T-cell neoplasms, may be aberrantly lost in peripheral T-cell neoplasms	Pan T cell marker	
CD3* *(T3)*	C3 antigen (five polypeptide chains) *(membrane, cytoplasm)*	T cells, cortical thymocytes	T-cell neoplasms, may be aberrantly lost in peripheral T-cell neoplasms Anaplastic large cell lymphoma is often negative	Best pan T cell marker	In paraffin sections, NK cells may also be positive

Table 7-30 Antibodies for immunohistochemistry—cont'd

NAME (ALTERNATE NAME)	ANTIGEN (LOCATION)	NORMAL CELLS AND TISSUES	TUMORS	USES	COMMENTS
CD4* (TH, T4, Leu 3)	Transmembrane glycoprotein, HIV receptor (membrane)	T helper/inducer cells, macrophages, Langerhans cells	MF, other T-cell neoplasms	Evaluation of MF Evaluation of T-cell neoplasms	
CD5* (Leu 1)	Transmembrane glycoprotein (membrane)	T cells and B-cell subsets (mantle zone)	T-cell leukemias and lymphomas, aberrantly expressed in low grade B-cell lymphomas (CLL or mantle cell lymphoma Thymic carcinoma, adenocarcinomas, mesothelioma (cytoplasmic)	Classification of low-grade B-cell lymphoma Evaluation of T-cell lymphomas (this marker is frequently lost) Thymic carcinoma (~40%) versus pulmonary squamous cell carcinoma (<5%)	
CD7* (Leu 9)	Membrane-bound glycoprotein (membrane)	Precursor T cells, T-cell subsets, NK cells, thymocytes	T-cell lymphomas and leukemias	Frequently (50%) lost in T-cell lymphomas versus reactive T cells (+) Evaluation of T-cell leukemias	
CD8* (T8, Leu 2)	Two glycoprotein chains (membrane)	T-cell subsets, NK cells, T cytotoxic/suppressor cells	T-cell lymphomas and leukemias	Evaluation of MF and T-cell lymphomas (this marker is frequently lost)	
CD10* (CALLA [common acute leukemia antigen], J5, neprilysin)	Cell surface metalloendopeptidase that inactivates peptides (membrane)	Precursor B cells, granulocytes, rare cells in reactive follicles, myoepithelial cells of breast, bile canaliculi, fibroblasts, brush border of kidney and gut	Follicular lymphoma, preB-ALL, Burkitt's lymphoma, CML, angioimmunoblastic lymphoma RCC (clear cell and papillary), HCC, rhabdomyosarcoma, endometrial stromal sarcoma	Evaluation of follicular center cell lymphoma Evaluation of leukemias Myoepithelial cell marker in breast Endometrial stromal sarcoma (+) versus leiomyosarcoma (–) (but caldesmon is preferred for this purpose)	
CD11b (Mac-1)	Cell surface receptor for the C3bi complement fragment (membrane)	Granulocytes, monocytes, macrophages	Myelomonocytic leukemias		
CD11c*	Member of the beta(2) integrin family that mediates adhesion to vascular endothelium, transendothelial migration, chemotaxis, and phagocytosis (membrane)	Myeloid cells, NK cells, dendritic cells, activated lymphoid cells	Hairy cell leukemia, B-cell prolymphocytic leukemia, some B-CLL, marginal zone lymphoma (MALT)		

Table 7-30 Antibodies for immunohistochemistry—cont'd

NAME (ALTERNATE NAME)	ANTIGEN (LOCATION)	NORMAL CELLS AND TISSUES	TUMORS	USES	COMMENTS
CD13 (My 7)	Aminopeptidase-N, a type II integral membrane metalloprotease functioning in cell surface antigen presentation, receptor for coronaviruses (membrane, cytoplasm)	Granulocytes, macrophages, bone marrow stromal cells, osteoclasts, renal tubules, intestinal brush border, cells lining bile duct canaliculi, endothelial cells, fibroblasts, brain cells	AML, CML with blast crisis, some ALL	Classification of leukemias	Requires frozen tissue
CD15* (Leu-M1)	3-fucosyl-N-acetyllactosamine, X-hapten—CHO moiety linked to cell membrane protein (membrane and granular perinuclear)	Granulocytes, monocytes	Reed–Sternberg cells (not LP HD), some large T-cell lymphomas, MF, some leukemias (adenocarcinomas), CMV-infected cells	Adenocarcinomas (+) versus mesotheliomas (–) Evaluation of HD	
CD16*	Low-affinity transmembrane Fc receptor for IgG (membrane)	NK cells, granulocytes, activated macrophages, subsets of T cells	Extranodal NK/T-cell lymphoma, some hepatosplenic T-cell lymphomas		
CD19 (B4)	B-cell type I integral membrane glycoprotein (membrane)	B cells, follicular dendritic cells, early myelomonocytic cells	pre-B-ALL and B-cell neoplasms (but not plasma cell lesions)	Good pan B cell marker	Fresh or frozen tissue required
CD20* (L26, B1, Leu 16)	B-cell non-glycosylated phosphoprotein functioning as a receptor during B-cell activation and differentiation (membrane, cytoplasmic)	B cells, monocytes, not plasma cells	B-cell lymphomas, Reed–Sternberg cells in LP HD, not plasmacytomas	Best pan B cell marker. Evaluation of B-cell lymphomas Evaluation of HD	Under investigation as a target for clinical treatment of B-cell lymphomas L26 is best for formalin-fixed tissue May be preserved in necrotic tissue
CD21* (B2)	Type I integral membrane glycoprotein functioning as the receptor for the C3d fragment of complement C3, CR2, receptor for EBV (membrane)	Follicular dendritic cells, mature B cells	Marginal zone (MALT) lymphomas, CLL (B cell), some T cell ALL, follicular dendritic cell tumors	ID of residual follicular structure in LP HD and other diseases Evaluation of low-grade B-cell lymphomas ID of follicular dendritic cell sarcoma	
CD22* (BL-CAM)	Type I integral membrane glycoprotein (membrane, cytoplasm)	B cells, precursor B cells	B-cell neoplasms (but not plasma cell lesions)	Pan B cell marker	

Table 7-30 Antibodies for immunohistochemistry—cont'd

NAME (ALTERNATE NAME)	ANTIGEN (LOCATION)	NORMAL CELLS AND TISSUES	TUMORS	USES	COMMENTS
CD23*	Membrane glycoprotein, low-affinity IgE receptor (membrane)	Subpopulation of peripheral B cells, follicular dendritic cells	CLL, but usually not mantle zone lymphoma, MALTomas, or follicular lymphomas	Evaluation of low-grade B-cell lymphomas	
CD25* (IL-2 receptor)	Interleukin-2 receptor (membrane, cytoplasm)	Subpopulation of T cells, myeloid precursors, oligodendrocytes HTLV-1 transformed T and B cells	Hairy cell leukemia, adult T-cell lymphoma/leukemia, some T-cell prolympho-cytic leukemia, precursor lymphoblastic lymphoma, and anaplastic large cell lymphoma	Evaluation of cutaneous T-cell lymphomas for potential anti-CD25 therapy	
CD30* (Ki-1, BERH2)	Single chain transmembrane glycoprotein, homologous to the nerve growth factor superfamily (cytoplasm, membrane and Golgi)	Activated B and T cells, some plasma cells, immuno-blasts, interdigitating cells, histiocytes, follicular center cells, decidualized endometrium, reactive mesothelial cells, most other tissues negative	Anaplastic (CD30+) large cell lymphomas, large B-cell lymphoma, primary effusion lymphoma, mediastinal large B-cell lymphoma, Reed–Sternberg cells (not LP HD), enteropathy T-cell lymphoma, peripheral T-cell lymphoma, EBV-transformed B cells Embryonal carcinoma, vascular tumors (not KS), some mesotheliomas, rarely carcinomas are positive	Evaluation of anaplastic (CD30+) lymphomas. Evaluation of HD (Reed–Sternberg cells are positive except in LP HD) Evaluation of peripheral T-cell lymphoma (large cells may be positive)	
CD33* (My 9)	Myeloid-specific receptor (sialic acid-binding immunoglobulin-like lectin or Siglec-3) (membrane)	Granulocytes, monocytes	AML	Evaluation of leukemias	Gemtuzumab ozogamicin is a humanized CD33 antibody linked to an antitumor antibiotic calicheaminin for the treatment of AML
CD34* (HPCA-1, QBEnd10)	Single chain transmembrane glycoprotein (cytoplasm, membrane)	Lymphoid and myeloid hematopoietic progenitor cells, endothelial cells, some skin cells, myofibroblasts	Acute leukemia Neurofibroma, angiosarcoma, KS, epithelioid hemangio-endothelioma, solitary fibrous tumor, DFSP, epithelioid sarcoma, GIST, myofibroblastic tumors	ID of endothelial or myofibroblastic differ-entiation in tumors Evaluation of angiogenesis Evaluation of the number of blasts in bone marrow in acute leukemia.	Not specific for endothelial cells

Table 7-30 Antibodies for immunohistochemistry—cont'd

NAME (ALTERNATE NAME)	ANTIGEN (LOCATION)	NORMAL CELLS AND TISSUES	TUMORS	USES	COMMENTS
CD35* (CR1, C3b/C4b R)	Transmembrane protein t that binds complement components C3b and C4b and mediates phagocytosis (membrane)	Erythrocytes, B cells, a subset of T cells, monocytes, neutrophils, eosinophils, glomerular podocytes, follicular dendritic cells	Marginal zone (MALT) lymphoma, follicular dendritic cell tumors	Detects follicular dendritic cells. ID of follicular dendritic cell sarcomas	
CD38*	Type II transmembrane glycoprotein with enzymatic action for the formation and hydrolysis of cADPR (membrane)	Immature B and T lymphocytes, thymocytes, mitogen-activated T cells, Ig-secreting plasma cells, monocytes, NK cells, erythroid and myeloid progenitors, brain cells	Acute leukemias, plasma cell lesions. Neurofibrillary tangles in Alzheimer's disease	ID of plasma cell lesions	Immunoreactivity may be a poor prognostic marker for patients with CLL
CD43* (Leu 22, L60)	Cell surface glycoprotein (membrane)	T cells, macrophages, granulocytes	AML (chloromas), T-cell neoplasms, aberrant expression in some low grade B-cell neoplasms (e.g. mantle cell lymphoma, SLL/CLL, marginal zone lymphoma), some MALT lymphomas	Evaluation of T-cell lymphomas and leukemias. Evaluation of low-grade B-cell lymphomas	Less specific than UCHL-1 for T cells
CD45, Leukocyte common antigen* (LCA, CLA) Note: CLA also refers to a different antigen, HECA-452	Five or more membrane glycoproteins (membrane, cytoplasm)	Lymphocytes, leukocytes, histiocytes, not plasma cells, erythrocytes, platelets	Non-Hodgkin's lymphomas, some anaplastic (CD30+) large cell lymphomas, Reed–Sternberg cells in LP HD (but not other types)	ID of poorly differentiated neoplasms as lymphomas. However, some anaplastic lymphomas and plasma-cytomas may be negative	Preserved in necrotic tissue. Best general marker for hematologic neoplasms
CD45RA (DPB)	Restricted form of leuko-cyte common antigen (membrane, cytoplasm)	B cells, monocytes, some T cells	B-cell neoplasms, hairy cells (not specific)	Pan B cell marker that can be used in Zenker's fixed tissue	Not completely specific—other B-cell markers are preferred
CD45RO (UCHL-1)	Isoform of CD45 (leukocyte common antigen) (membrane, cytoplasm)	T cells, granulocytes, monocytes	T-cell neoplasms, histiocytic sarcoma	Good pan T cell marker (CD3 is more specific)	
CD56* (NCAM)	Neural cell adhesion molecule—cell surface glycoprotein (membrane)	Neurons, astrocytes, Schwann cells, NK cells, subset of activated T cells	Some T/NK cell lymphomas, plasmacytomas. Neuroblastoma	Evaluation of panniculitis-like T-cell lymphoma (both CD56+ and CD56−) and T/NK lymphomas	

Table 7-30 Antibodies for immunohistochemistry—cont'd

NAME (ALTERNATE NAME)	ANTIGEN (LOCATION)	NORMAL CELLS AND TISSUES	TUMORS	USES	COMMENTS
CD57* (Leu 7, HNK-1)	Lymphocyte antigen that cross-reacts with a myelin-associated glycoprotein (membrane)	T-cell subsets, NK cells, myelinized nerves, neuroendocrine cells, prostate, pancreatic islets, adrenal medulla	Angioimmunoblastic T-cell lymphoma Nerve sheath tumors (occasional), leiomyosarcoma, synovial sarcoma, rhabdomyosarcoma, neuroblastoma, gliomas, neuroendocrine carcinomas, neurofibromas, some prostate carcinomas	ID of T gamma lymphoproliferative disorder (large granular cell lymphocytic leukemia) ID of neuroendocrine differentiation in tumors Evaluation of NK neoplasms	Not very specific for solid tumors
CD61 (GPIIIa, platelet glycoprotein IIIa)	Glycoprotein, receptor for fibrinogen, fibronectin, von Willebrand factor, and vitronectin (cytoplasm)	Megakaryocytes, platelets	Megakaryocytic leukemias	ID of megakaryocytic differentiation	
CD68* (KP1, CD68-PGM1, Mac-M)	Intracellular glycoprotein associated with lysosomes (cytoplasm, membrane)	Macrophages, monocytes, neutrophils, basophils, large lymphocytes, Kupffer cells, mast cells, osteoclasts	Some lymphomas, histiocytic sarcomas, APML, Langerhans proliferative disorders Neurofibroma, schwannoma, MPNST, granular cell tumors, PEComa, melanomas, atypical fibroxanthoma, RCC	Best general marker for macrophages, although not specific to this cell type	The antibody PG-M1 does not react with granulocytes
CD74 (LN2)	Subunit of MHC II-associated invariant chain (membrane)	B cells, monocytes, histiocytes	B-cell neoplasms, hairy cell leukemia, plasma cell lesions	Pan B cell marker	
CDw75* (LN1)	Sialylated glycoconjugate present in surface Ig-positive B cells (membrane, mytoplasm)	Mature B cells, T-cell subsets, fetal colon, epithelial cells	Reed–Sternberg cells of LP HD (not other types), follicular lymphomas Colon carcinomas (50%), gastric carcinomas	Evaluation of HD	
CD77 (BLA.36, PK antigen)	Globotriaosylceramide, glycolipic membrane from Burkitt's lymphoma cell line (cytoplasm, membrane)	Tonsillar B cells, dendritic reticulum cells, sinus-lining cells, macrophages, endothelial cell, epithelial cells	HD, Burkitt's lymphoma, rarely other B- and T-cell lymphomas	Evaluation of RS cells	

Table 7-30 Antibodies for immunohistochemistry—cont'd

NAME (ALTERNATE NAME)	ANTIGEN (LOCATION)	NORMAL CELLS AND TISSUES	TUMORS	USES	COMMENTS
CD79a (mb-1 protein)	Heterodimer of mb-1 (CD79a) and B29 (CD79b) polypeptides, B-cell antigen receptor (membrane)	B cells, plasma cells	Precursor B-cell ALL, B-cell lymphomas, plasma cell lesions, but not primary effusion lymphoma	Evaluation of B-cell neoplasms (may be the only B-cell marker present)	
CD79b*	See above (membrane)			Absent from CLL, hairy cell leukemia	
CD95* (Fas)	Transmembrane glycoprotein member of the nerve growth factor receptor/ tumor necrosis factor superfamily—mediates apoptosis (membrane)	Activated T and B cells, epithelial cells	Panniculitis-like T-cell lymphoma (if CD56+)		
CD99* (MIC-2, 12E7, Ewing's sarcoma marker, E2 antigen, HuLy-m6, FMC 29, O13 [different epitope])	MIC2 gene product— glycoproteins (p30 and p32) involved in rosette formation with erythrocytes (membrane) Membrane immunoreactivity is more specific than cytoplasmic	Cortical thymocytes, T lymphocytes, granulosa cells of ovary, pancreatic islet cells, Sertoli cells, some endothelial cells, urothelium, ependymal cells, squamous cells	B- and T-cell precursor lymphoblastic lymphoma/ leukemia PNET/Ewing's sarcoma, chondroblastoma, synovial sarcoma, solitary fibrous tumors, GIST, some alveolar rhabdomyosar- comas, desmoplastic small cell tumors, small cell carcinomas, granulosa cell tumors, yolk sac components of germ cell tumors, Sertoli–Leydig cell tumors, atypical fibroxanthoma, meningioma	Evaluation of lymphoblastic lymphoma/leukemia Thymic carcinomas (lymphocytes +) versus other carcinomas. ID of PNET/Ewing's sarcoma (immunoreactivity should be clearly membranous in the majority of the cells)	O13 is the most commonly used antibody Immunoreactivity is highly dependent upon the antigen retrieval system used
CD103*	Mucosal integrin αEβ7 with specificity for e-cadherin (cytoplasm)	T cells	Enteropathy-type T-cell lymphoma, hairy cell leukemia		Requires frozen tissue or cell suspension

Table 7-30 Antibodies for immunohistochemistry—cont'd

NAME (ALTERNATE NAME)	ANTIGEN (LOCATION)	NORMAL CELLS AND TISSUES	TUMORS	USES	COMMENTS
CD117* (c-kit, stem cell factor receptor)	Transmembrane tyrosine kinase receptor (ligand is stem cell factor)—apoptosis is inhibited when the ligand is bound (cytoplasm, membrane)	Mast cells, interstitial cells of Cajal (ICC—pacemaker cells of the GI tract found throughout the muscle layers and in the myemteroc plexus), epidermal melanocytes, mononuclear bone marrow cells (4%), Leydig cells, early spermatogenic cells, trophoblast, breast epithelium	GIST (>95%), seminomas (>70%), intratubular germ cell neoplasia, mature teratomas (>70%), some melanomas (focal), mast cell tumors, some carcinomas, some brain tumors, some PNET/Ewing's sarcoma, some angiosarcomas AML (>50%), CML in myeloid blast crisis	ID of GIST (+) versus leiomyomas (−) and schwannomas (−) ID of seminomas ID of mast cells (mastocytosis)	Mast cells are an excellent internal control CD117 positivity does not correlate with mutations and/or oncoprotein activity in tumors not known to have activating mutations and is, in general, not of clinical or therapeutic significance in this setting (e.g., to detect tumors likely to respond to therapy directed against the protein, e.g., Gleevec)
CD138* (Syndecan-1)	Transmembrane heparin sulphate glycoprotein that interacts with extracellular matrix and growth factors (membrane)	Pre-B cells, immature B cells, Ig-producing plasma cells, basolateral surface of epithelial cells, vascular smooth muscle, endothelium, neural cells	Plasma cell lesions, primary effusion lymphoma, plasma cell component of other B cell lymphomas Squamous cell carcinomas, other carcinomas	ID of plasma cells and their neoplasms Expression may be diminished or lost in poorly differentiated carcinomas	
CD207 (Langerin)	Langerhans cell specific C-type lectin (cytoplasm)	Langerhans cells of epidermis and epithelia	Langerhans cell histiocytosis		Induces formation of Birbeck granules
Clusterin* (Apolipoprotein J, complement lysis inhibitor, gp80, SGP-2, SP40, TRPM2, T64, ApoJ)	Multifunctional protein involved in lipid transport, complement regulation, immune regulation, cell adhesion, other functions (membrane, cytoplasm, nucleus)	Many tissues	Anaplastic large cell lymphoma (Golgi pattern) Alzheimer's disease—present in amyloid plaques and cerebrovascular deposits Many types of carcinomas		

Table 7-30 Antibodies for immunohistochemistry—cont'd

NAME (ALTERNATE NAME)	ANTIGEN (LOCATION)	NORMAL CELLS AND TISSUES	TUMORS	USES	COMMENTS
Cyclin D1* (*PRAD1, bcl-1*)	Cyclin-regulating cyclin-dependent kinases during G1 in the cell cycle, phosphorylates and inactivates the retinoblastoma tumor suppressor protein (*nucleus*)	Cycling cells (however, lymphocytes usually express only cyclins D2 and D3)	Mantle cell lymphoma Breast cancer (esp. lobular carcinomas and other ER positive carcinomas), esophageal cancer, bladder cancer, lung cancer, HCC, colon carcinoma, pancreatic carcinoma, head and neck squamous cell carcinomas, pituitary tumors, sarcomas Parathyroid adenomas (inversion involving cyclin D1 gene and the parathormone receptor)	ID of mantle cell lymphoma	Involved in t(11;14)(q13;q32) translocation in mantle cell lymphoma
DBA.44* (*HCL*)	B-cell antigen (*cytoplasm, membrane*)	Mantle zone B cells, some immunoblasts	Hairy cell leukemia (>95%), B-cell lymphomas (30%)	Evaluation of hairy cell leukemia	
Epithelial membrane antigen* (*EMA, MUC1, HMFG, DF3, CA 15-3, CA 27.29, PEM, many others*)	Episialin, glycoprotein found in human milk fat globule membranes (*cytoplasm [more common in malignant cells], membrane [more common in benign cells]*)	Epithelial cells, perineurial cells, meningeal cells, plasma cells, usually negative in mesothelial cells, monocytes	Some anaplastic large cell lymphomas (CD30+), plasma cell neoplasms, malignant histiocytosis, AML (M4 and M5), LP HD erythroleukemia, Carcinomas, mesotheliomas, some sarcomas (synovial sarcoma, epithelioid sarcoma), adenomatoid tumor; chordomas, perineurioma, neurofibroma, meningiomas, desmoplastic small round cell tumor; Sertoli cell tumor	ID of epithelial differentiation in tumors—however, keratin is more specific for this purpose. Beware of EMA in some large cell lymphomas Synovial sarcoma typically shows focal positivity	There are over 50 monoclonal antibodies recognizing different glycosylation patterns in normal tissues and tumors[16]
Epstein-Barr virus EBV-encoded nonpolyadenylated early RNAs (*EBERS*)	RNA produced by EBV (*nucleus*)	EBV-infected B cells	All EBV-related tumors	Most sensitive marker for EBV	Detected by in situ hybridization for RNA on paraffin sections

Table 7-30 Antibodies for immunohistochemistry—cont'd

NAME (ALTERNATE NAME)	ANTIGEN (LOCATION)	NORMAL CELLS AND TISSUES	TUMORS	USES	COMMENTS
LMP-1*	Latent membrane protein (*membrane*)	EBV-infected B cells	Nasopharyngeal carcinomas, Reed–Sternberg cells (not LP HD), transplant lymphomas, AIDS-related lymphomas, endemic Burkitt's lymphoma (rare in sporadic cases)	Evaluation of EBV-related neoplasms	
EBNA 2 (*nuclear antigen 2*)	Nuclear protein (*nucleus*)	EBV-infected B cells	Transplant-related lymphomas, AIDS-related lymphomas. Not present in Burkitt's lymphoma or nasopharyngeal carcinomas	Evaluation of transplant- and AIDS-related lymphomas	
Fascin	Actin bundling protein regulated by phosphorylation (*cytoplasm*)	Interdigitating reticulin cells from the T-cell zones, dendritic cells, reticular network, histiocytes, smooth muscle, endothelium, squamous cells, splenic sinuses	Reed–Sternberg cells (but not in LP HD) High-grade breast carcinomas	ID of Reed–Sternberg cells in classical HD Fascin positivity has also been reported in anaplastic large cell lymphoma	
FMC7	Antigen on subgroups of mature B cells, epitope of CD20 (*cytoplasm*)	B cells	B-cell lymphomas	Not expressed by CLL	Pan B cell marker Epitope of CD20 but reactivity low in cells with low cholesterol
Glycophorin A (*GPA*)	A glycosylated erythrocyte membrane protein (*membrane*)	Erythroid elements at all stages	Erythroleukemia	ID of erythroid elements (normal and neoplastic)	
Granzyme B*	Neutral serine proteases stored in granules in cytotoxic T cells and in NK cells involved in target cell apoptosis by exocytosis (*cytoplasm*)	Cytotoxic T cells and NK cells	Some T-cell lymphomas, Reed–Sternberg cells of some cases of EBV-positive HD		
Heavy immunoglobulin chains* (*G, A, M, D*)	Heavy chain of immunoglobulins (*Cytoplasm [plasma cells], membrane [lymphocytes]*)	Plasma cells (G>A>M>D)	Plasma cell tumors (monotypic expression of usually G or A), mantle zone lymphomas and WDLL/CLL may co-express M and D, lymphoplasmacytic lymphoma (M)	ID of monoclonal populations of plasma or plasmacytoid cells	

Table 7-30 Antibodies for immunohistochemistry—cont'd

NAME (ALTERNATE NAME)	ANTIGEN (LOCATION)	NORMAL CELLS AND TISSUES	TUMORS	USES	COMMENTS
HECA-452* (Endothelial cell antigen, cutaneous lymphocyte-associated antigen, CLA)	Cell surface glycoprotein (membrane)	T cells, more common in cutaneous T cells	Mycosis fungoides and other cutaneous T-cell lymphomas		Note: CLA is also used to refer to CD45
Hemoglobin (Hb)	Hemoglobin (cytoplasm)	Erythroid cells	Some leukemias	Marker for erythroid cells	
HHV8*	Latent nuclear antigen of human herpesvirus type 8 (nucleus)	Absent in normal tissue	Primary effusion lymphoma (PEL), AIDS-associated multicentric Castleman's disease; Kaposi's sarcoma (endothelial cells and some perivascular cells)	Evaluation of Kaposi's sarcoma and primary effusion lymphoma	
HLA-DR	Major histocompatibility complex Class II gene	B lymphocytes, macrophages, Langerhans cells, dendritic cells, activated T cells, some endothelial and epithelial cells	Leukemic myoblasts		Not very specific for cell type.
Light immunoglobulin chains* (lambda [L], kappa [K])	Light chain of immunoglobulins (cytoplasm)	Plasma cells (normally K>L), B cells	Plasma cell tumors, B-cell lymphomas	ID of monoclonal populations of plasma cells and B cells; ID of some types of amyloid	May require frozen tissue for assessment of B lymphoid cells; Excellent Ig preservation in plasma cells in B5 or Zenker's fixed tissue
Lysozyme (Ly)	Muramidase (cytoplasm)	Circulating monocytes, some tissue macrophages, granulocytes, salivary gland, lacrimal gland, stomach and colon epithelial cells (inflamed or regenerative), apocrine glands, some other epithelial cells	AML with monocytic differentiation, salivary gland tumors, stomach and colon carcinomas.	Marker for histiocytes but not specific. May mark activated phagocytic macrophages; Evaluation of myeloid leukemias; Strongly positive in monocytoid leukemias	Not specific for solid tumor identification
Mast cell tryptase	Serine protease (cytoplasm)	Mast cells	Mast cell neoplasms	ID of mast cell differentiation	
Myeloperoxidase* (MPO)	Enzyme in primary granules of myeloid cells (cytoplasm)	Myeloid cells, monocytes	AML, chloromas	Classification of leukemias	Can be used with tissue fixed in Zenker's fixative

Table 7-30 Antibodies for immunohistochemistry—cont'd

NAME (ALTERNATE NAME)	ANTIGEN (LOCATION)	NORMAL CELLS AND TISSUES	TUMORS	USES	COMMENTS
Oct2* (Octomer transcription factor)	Transcription factor of the POU homeo-domain family binding to the Ig gene octomer sites regulating B-specific genes (nucleus)	B cells	B-cell lymphomas and leukemias Reed–Sternberg cells in LP HD (but not other types)	Evaluation of HD	Interacts with the transcriptional coactivator BOB.I BOB.I and Oct are necessary (but not sufficient) for Ig expression
Perforin*	Pore-forming protein in cytoplasmic granules of cytotoxic T cells (cytoplasm)	NK cells, large granular lymphocytes, gamma/delta T cells	NK cell lymphomas, anaplastic large cell lymphoma	Evaluation of T-cell lymphomas	
TCR* (T-cell antigen receptor, JOVI I)	Two polypeptide chains (alpha and beta)	Peripheral T cells	Many T-cell lymphomas	Evaluation of T-cell lymphomas	Alpha/beta and gamma/delta T cell receptors can be evaluated in frozen tissue
Terminal deoxytransferase* (TdT)	Enzyme that catalyzes addition of nucleotides to ss DNA (nucleus)	Immature T and B cells	Lymphoblastic lymphoma/ ALL	Lymphoblastic lymphoma (+) versus Burkitt lymphoma (−)	
TIA-1 (T-cell intracellular antigen)	A cytolytic granule associated protein expressed in some CD8+ T cells (cytoplasm)	T cells, mast cells, polymorphonuclear leukocytes, eosinophils	Many T-cell lymphomas	Evaluation of T-cell lymphomas	

Table 7-30 Antibodies for immunohistochemistry—cont'd

NAME (ALTERNATE NAME)	ANTIGEN (LOCATION)	NORMAL CELLS AND TISSUES	TUMORS	USES	COMMENTS
traf-1* *(Tumor necrosis factor receptor-associated factor)*	Membrane-bound proteins that activate the nuclear factor-(kappa)B (NF-(kappa)B) transcription factor resulting in cell proliferation *(cCytoplasm)*		Hodgkin's lymphoma		May interact with LMP1

Abbreviations: AD, Alzheimer's disease; AIDS, acquired immunodeficiency syndrome; ALL, acute lymphocytic leukemia; AML, acute myelogenous leukemia; APML, acute promyelogenous leukemia; BM, basement membrane; CML, chronic myelogenous leukemia; CMV, cytomegalovirus; DFSP, dermatofibrosarcoma protuberans; EBV, Epstein–Barr virus; FISH, fluorescence in situ hybridization; GIST, gastrointestinal stromal tumor; HCC, hepatocellular carcinoma; HD, Hodgkin's disease; HNPCC, hereditary non-polyposis colorectal cancer; ID, identification; KS, Kaposi's sarcoma; LP HD, lymphocyte predominant Hodgkin's disease; MF, mycosis fungoides; MPNST, malignant peripheral nerve sheath tumor; NK, natural killer; PIN, prostatic intraepithelial neoplasia; PNET, primitive neuroectodermal tumor; RCC, renal cell carcinoma; RS, Reed–Sternberg cells; TCC, transitional cell carcinoma.

Notes:

NAME: The most common name used to refer to the marker; see also Box 7-1. The name may refer to the antigen, a CD number, or a specific antibody raised to the antigen. In some cases more than one name is commonly used. Antibodies with asterisks appear in the Tables. Most CD numbers correspond to a specific gene product. However, some correspond to antigens from post-translational modifications. For example, CD15 (LeuM1) is a carbohydrate side chain linked to a protein.

ALTERNATE NAME: This list includes abbreviations, antibody names (sometimes recognizing different epitopes), or other terms for the marker.

ANTIGEN: The antigen recognized by the antibody.

LOCATION: The normal location of the antigen. In some cases, only certain locations of the antigen are considered a positive result (e.g., nuclear immunoreactivity for estrogen receptor, membrane immunoreactivity for HER-2/neu).

NORMAL CELLS AND TISSUES: The presence of the marker in normal cells and tissues. These cells serve as important internal positive controls. Abnormal positive immunoreactivity is also an important control for the specificity of the study.

TUMORS: The tumors in which immunoreactivity is typically expected. Refer to the Tables for additional information.

USES: The most common uses for the marker. Different pathologists and institutions often have preferences for the use of certain markers.

COMMENTS: Additional comments regarding the marker.

Additional information on CD antigens can be found at http://www.ncbi.nlm.nih.gov/prow/guide/45277084.htm

Box 7-1 Alternative names for antigens

Looking for?	Find it under:
1D5	Estrogen receptor (G)
6F/3D	Beta-amyloid
12E7	CD99 (G, H)
34βE12	Keratins (G)
38.13	CD77 (H)
70 kD NF	Neurofilaments (G)
200 kD NF	Neurofilaments (G)
903	Keratins—34βE12 (G)
A (blood group antigen)	Blood group antigens (G)
A (Ig heavy chain α)	Heavy chain immunoglobulins (H)
A32 antigen	CD146 (G)
A103	MELAN-A (G)
AAT	Alpha 1-antitrypsin (G, H)
ACH	Alpha-1 antichymotrypsin (H)
AE1/AE3	Keratins (G)
AFP	Alpha-fetoprotein (G)
Alpha 1-antitrypsin	Alpha 1-antitrypsin (G, H)
Alpha 1-antichymotrypsin	Alpha 1-antichymotrypsin (H)
Alpha 1-fetoprotein	Alpha fetoprotein (G)
Alpha fetoprotein	Alpha fetoprotein (G)
Alpha-methylacyl-CoA racemase	AMACR (G)
Alpha smooth muscle actin	Alpha smooth muscle actin (G)
AMACR	AMACR (G)
Amyloid	Beta-amyloid (G)
Androgen receptor	Androgen receptor (G)
Apolipoprotein J	Clusterin (H)
AR	Androgen receptor (G)
B (blood group antigen)	Blood group antigens (G)
B1	CD20 (H)
B2	CD21 (H)
B4	CD19 (H)
B72.3	B72.3 (G)
bcl-1	Cyclin D1 (H)
bcl-2	bcl-2 (H, G)
B-cell specific activator protein	BSAP (H)
BER-EP4	BER-EP4 (G)
BERH2	CD30 (G, H)
Beta-amyloid	Beta-amyloid (G)
Beta-catenin	Beta-catenin (G)
Beta-2 microglobulin	Beta-2 microglobulin (G)
BG8	BG8 (G)
β-hCG	Human chorionic gonadotropin (G)
BLA.36	CD77 (H)
BL-CAM	CD22 (H)
Blood group antigens	Blood group antigens (G, H)

Looking for?	Find it under:
BR-2	Gross cystic disease fluid protein-15 (G)
BRST-2	Gross cystic disease fluid protein-15 (G)
C3b/C4bR	CD35 (H)
C5b-9	C5b-9 (G)
c-kit	CD117 (G)
CA 15-3	Epithelial membrane antigen (G, H)
CA 19-9	CA 19-9 (G)
CA 27.28	Epithelial membrane antigen (G, H)
CA 72-4	B72.3 (G)
CA125	CA125 (G)
CA19-9	CA19-9 (G)
Calcitonin	Calcitonin (G), Hormones (G)
Caldesmon	Caldesmon (G)
Calgranulin	MAC 387 (G)
CALLA	CD10 (G, H)
CALP	Calponin (G)
Calponin	Calponin (G)
Calprotectin	MAC 387 (G)
Calretinin	Calretinin (G)
CAM5.2	Keratins (G)
Carbohydrate antigen 19-9	CA19-9 (G)
Carcinoembryonic antigen	Carcinoembryonic antigen (G)
CD1a	CD1a (H)
CD2	CD2 (H)
CD3	CD3 (H)
CD4	CD4 (H)
CD5	CD5 (G, H)
CD7	CD7 (H)
CD8	CD8 (H)
CD10	CD10 (G, H)
CD11b	CD11b (H)
CD11c	CD11c (H)
CD13	CD13 (H)
CD15	CD15 (G, H)
CD16	CD16 (H)
CD19	CD19 (H)
CD20	CD20 (H)
CD21	CD21 (H)
CD22	CD22 (H)
CD23	CD23 (H)
CD25	CD25 (H)
CD30	CD30 (G, H)
CD31	CD31 (G)
CD33	CD33 (H)
CD34	CD34 (G, H)
CD35	CD35 (H)
CD38	CD38 (H)
CD43	CD43 (H)

Looking for?	Find it under:
CD44v3	CD44v3 (G)
CD45	CD45 (H)
CD45RA	CD45RA (H)
CD45Ro	CD45Ro (H)
CD56	CD56 (H)
CD 57	CD57 (G)
CD61	CD68 (G, H)
CD68	CD68 (G, H)
CD74	CD74 (H)
CDw75	CDw75 (H)
CD77	CD77 (H)
CD79a	CD79a (H)
CD79b	CD79b (H)
CD95	CD95 (H)
CD99	CD99 (G, H)
CD117	CD117 (G)
CD141	CD141 (G)
CDX	CDX (G)
CDKN2	p16 (G)
CDP	Gross cystic disease fluid protein-15 (G)
CEA	Carcinoembryonic antigen (G)
c-erbB2	HER-2/neu (G)
Chromogranin A	Chromogranin A (G)
c-kit	CD117 (G)
CLA	CD45 (H) or HECA-452 (H)
CLDN1	Claudin (G)
Clusterin	Clusterin (H)
Collagen IV	Collagen IV (G)
Common acute leukemia antigen	CD10 (G, H)
Complement lysis inhibitor	Clusterin (H)
CR1	CD35 (H)
Cyclin D1	Cyclin D1 (H)
Cystic fibrosis antigen	MAC 387 (G)
D (Ig heavy chain δ)	Heavy chain immunoglobulins (H)
DBA.44	DBA.44 (H)
Desmin	Desmin (G)
DF3	Epithelial membrane antigen (G, H)
DPB	CD45RA (H)
E2 antigen	CD99 (G, H)
EBERS	Epstein–Barr virus (G, H)
EBNA	Epstein-Barr virus (G, H)
E-cadherin	E-cadherin (G)
EGFR	EGFR (G)
EM ACT	HHF-35 (G)
EMA	Epithelial membrane antigen (G)
E-MEL	HMB-45 (G)
Endothelial cell antigen	HECA-452 (H)

Looking for?	Find it under:
Ep-CAM	BER-EP4 (G)
Epidermal growth factor receptor	EGFR (G)
Epithelial membrane antigen	Epithelial membrane antigen (G, H)
Epithelial specific antigen	BER-EP4 (G)
Epstein–Barr virus	Epstein–Barr virus (G, H)
ER	Estrogen receptor (G)
erbB2	HER-2/neu (G)
ESA	BER-EP4 (G)
Estrogen receptor	Estrogen receptor (G)
Ewing's sarcoma marker	CD99 (G, H)
Factor VIII related antigen	Factor VIII (G)
FVIII:RAg	Factor VIII (G)
Factor XIIIa	Factor XIIIa (G)
Fascin	Fascin (H)
Fast myosin	Myosin Heavy Chain (G)
Fibronectin	Fibronectin (G)
Fli-1	Fli-1 (G)
FMC7	FMC7 (H)
FMC 29	CD99 (G, H)
Friend leukemia integrin-site 1	Fli-1 (G)
FVIII:g	Factor VIII (G)
G (Ig heavy chain gamma)	Heavy chain immunoglobulins (H)
Gal-3	Galectin-3 (G)
Galectin-3	Galectin-3 (G)
Gastrin	Hormones (G)
GCDFP	Gross cystic disease fluid protein-15 (G)
GFAP	Glial fibrillary acidic protein (G)
Glial fibrillary acidic protein	Glial fibrillary acidic protein (G)
Glucagon	Hormones (G)
Glucose transporter 1	GLUT-1 (G)
GLUT-1	GLUT-1 (G)
GPIIIa	CD61 (H)
gp80	Clusterin (H)
gp200	RCC (G)
GPA	Glycophorin A (H)
Granzyme B	Granzyme B (H)
Gross cystic disease fluid disease-15	Gross cystic disease fluid protein-15 (G)
H (blood group antigen)	Blood group antigens (G)
H222	Estrogen receptor (G)
Hb	Hemoglobin (H)
HBME-1	HBME-1 (G)
h-caldesmon	Caldesmon (G)
H-CAM	CD44v3 (G)

Looking for?	*Find it under:*
hCG	Human chorionic gonadotropin (G)
HCL	DBA.44 (H)
HBME-1	HBME-1 (G)
Heavy chain immunoglobulins	Heavy chain immunoglobulins (H)
HECA-452	HECA-452 (H)
Hematopoietic progenitor cell, class 1	CD34
Hemoglobin	Hemoglobin (H)
HepPar-1	HepPar-1 (G)
Hepatocyte paraffin-1	HepPar-1 (G)
HER-2/neu	HER-2/neu (G)
HHF-35	HHF-35 (G)
HHV8	HHV8 (H)
HLA-DR	HLA-DR (H)
HMB-45	HMB-45 (G)
HMFG	Epithelial membrane antigen (G, H)
HNK-1	CD57 (G, H)
hMLH1	hMLH1 (G)
hMSH2	hMLH1 (G)
HNK-1	CD57 (G)
HP1	HepPar-1 (G)
HPCA-1	CD34 (G, H)
HPL	Human placental lactogen (G)
HuLy-m6	CD99 (G, H)
Human chorionic gonadotropin	Human chorionic gonadotropin (G)
Human herpesvirus 8	HHV8 (G, H)
Human mutL homologue 1	hMLH1 (G)
Human mutS homologue 2	hMLH1 (G)
Human placental lactogen	Human placental lactogen (G)
IL-2 receptor	CD25 (H)
Inhibin-alpha subunit	Inhibin-alpha subunit (G)
Insulin	Hormones (G)
J5	CD10 (G, H)
JOVI 1	TCR (H)
K (Ig light chain κ)	Light chain immunoglobulins (H)
Keratin 5/6	Keratins (G)
Keratin 7	Keratins (G)
Keratin 20	Keratins (G)
Keratins	Keratins (G)
Ki-1	CD30 (G, H)
Ki-67	Ki-67 (G)
kip2	p57 (G)
Kit	CD117 (G)
KP-1	CD68 (G, H)

Looking for?	*Find it under:*
L (Ig light chain lambda)	Light chain immunoglobulins (H)
L1 antigen	MAC 387 (G)
L26	CD20 (H)
L60	CD43 (H)
Laminin	Laminin (G)
LCA	CD45 (H)
Leu 1	CD5 (H)
Leu 2	CD8 (H)
Leu 3	CD4 (H)
Leu 5a + b	CD2 (H)
Leu 7	CD57 (G, H)
Leu 9	CD7 (H)
Leu 16	CD20 (H)
Leu 22	CD43 (H)
Leukocyte common antigen	CD45 (H)
LeuM1	CD15 (G, H)
Light chain immunoglobulins	Light chain immunoglobulins (H)
LFA-2	CD2 (H)
LMP-1	Epstein–Barr virus (G, H)
LN1	CDw75 (H)
LN2	CD74 (H)
Lysozyme	Lysozyme (H, G)
M (Ig heavy chain μ)	Heavy chain immunoglobulins (H)
Mac-1	CD11b (H)
MAC 387	MAC 387 (G)
Mac-M	CD68 (G, H)
MART-1	MELAN-A (G)
Mast cell tryptase	Mast cell tryptase (H)
mb-1	CD79a (H)
MCAM	CD146 (G)
ME491	CD63 (G)
MELAN-A	MELAN-A (G)
Melanoma antigen recognized by T cells	MELAN-A (G)
Melanoma-associated antigen	CD63 (G)
Melanoma cell adhesion molecule	CD146 (G)
Melanoma-specific antigen	HMB-45 (G)
MELCAM (or Mel-CAM)	CD146 (G)
MIB-1	Ki-67 (G)
MIC-2	CD99 (G, H)
MN-4	CD146 (G)
MNF-116	Keratin—Pan-K (G)
MPO	Myeloperoxidase (H)
MRF4	Myf-4 (G)
MSA	HHF-35 (G)
MTS1	p16 (G)

Looking for?	Find it under:
MUC1	Epithelial membrane antigen (G, H)
MUC18	CD146 (G)
Muscle common actin	HHF-35 (G)
Muscle-specific actin	HHF-35 (G)
My 7	CD13 (H)
My 9	CD33 (H)
Myeloperoxidase	Myeloperoxidase (H)
Myf-4	Myf-4 (G)
MyoD1	MyoD1 (G)
Myogenin	Myf-4 (G)
Myoglobin	Myoglobin (G)
Myosin Heavy Chain	Myosin Heavy Chain (G)
NCAM	CD56 (H)
Neprilysin	CD10 (G, H)
NEU N	NEU N (G)
Neurofilaments	Neurofilaments (G)
Neuron-specific enolase	Neuron-specific enolase (G)
NFP	Neurofilaments (G)
NKI-betab	HMB-45 (G)
NKI/C3	CD63 (G)
NSE	Neuron-specific enolase (G)
O13	CD99 (G, H)
OC125	CA125 (G)
Oct2	Oct2 (H)
Octomer transcription factor	Oct2 (H)
p16	p16 (G)
$p27^{kip1}$	$p27^{kip1}$ (G)
p53	p53 (G)
p57	p57 (G)
p63	p63 (G)
P504S	AMACR (G)
PAN-K	Keratins (G)
PAP	Prostate acid phosphatase (G)
PECAM-1	CD31 (G)
PEM	Epithelial membrane antigen (G, H)
Perforin	Perforin (H)
PGM1	CD68 (G, H)
PgR	Progesterone receptor (G)
PK antigen	CD77 (H)
Placental alkaline phosphatase	Placental alkaline phosphatase (G)
PLAP	Placental alkaline phosphatase (G)
Platelet glycoprotein IIIa	CD61 (H)
PR	Progesterone receptor (G)
PRAD1	Cyclin D1 (H)
PrAP	Prostate acid phosphatase (G)
Prealbumin	Prealbumin (G)
Progesterone receptor	Progesterone receptor (G)

Looking for?	Find it under:
Prostate acid phosphatase	Prostate acid phosphatase (G)
Prostate specific antigen	Prostate-specific antigen (G)
PSA	Prostate-specific antigen (G)
QBEnd10	CD34 (G, H)
Renal cell carcinoma marker	RCC (G)
ret	ret (G)
RCC	RCC (G)
rT3	CD2 (H)
S100	S100 (G)
S-Endo-1	CD146 (G)
SGP-2	Clusterin (H)
SMA	Alpha smooth muscle actin (G)
SM-ACT	Alpha smooth muscle actin (G)
Smad4	DPC4 (G)
SM-MHC	Myosin Heavy Chain (G)
Somatostatin	Hormones (G)
SP40	Clusterin (H)
Stem cell factor receptor	CD117 (G)
Synaptophysin	Synaptophysin (G)
Syndecan-1	CD138 (H)
Synuclein-1	Synuclein-1 (G)
T3	CD3 (H)
T4	CD4 (H)
T6	CD1a (H)
T8	CD8 (H)
T11	CD2 (H)
T64	Clusterin (H)
TAG-72	B72.3 (G)
Tau	Tau (G)
T cell antigen receptor	TCR (H)
T cell intracellular antigen	TIA-1 (H)
TCR	TCR (H)
TdT	Terminal deoxytransferase (H)
TE	CD2 (H)
Terminal deoxytransferase	Terminal deoxytransferase (H)
TH	CD4 (H)
Thrombomodulin	CD141 (G)
Thyroglobulin	Thyroglobulin (G)
Thyroid transcription factor 1	TTF-1 (G)
TIA-1	TIA-1 (H)
TM	CD141 (G)
traf-1	traf-1 (H)
Transthyretin	Prealbumin (G)
TRPM2	Clusterin (H)
TTF-1	TTF-1 (G)

Looking for?	Find it under:
TTR	Prealbumin (G)
Tumor-associated glycoprotein 72	B72.3 (G)
Tumor necrosis factor receptor-associated factor	traf-1 (H)
UCHL-1	CD45Ro (H)
UEA 1	Ulex (G)

Looking for?	Find it under:
Ulex	Ulex (G)
Vimentin	Vimentin (G)
von Willebrand's factor	Factor VIII (G)
VWF	Factor VIII (G)
Wilms' tumor 1 protein	WT1 (G)
WT1	WT1 (G)

G, General markers; H, hematopathology markers.

Results

The results of immunoperoxidase studies are incorporated into the surgical pathology report.[14] The following information is included:

- The type of tissue studied: formalin-fixed (or other fixatives) tissue, cryostat sections, cytology preparations, etc.
- The type of immunoagents used, being as specific as possible. For example, do not just list "keratin" but specify the type of keratin (e.g., AE1/AE3).
- The results of the studies in sufficient detail to allow interpretation: for example, the type of cell that is immunoreactive (e.g., tumor versus nontumor), intensity of immunoreactivity (e.g. weak, strong), and/or the number of cells immunoreactive (e.g., focal versus diffuse).
- Integration of the results into the final diagnosis, specifying whether they confirm or support a diagnosis, make one diagnosis more likely than others, or exclude one or more diagnoses.

■ ELECTRON MICROSCOPY

EM continues to have an important role in surgical pathology.[15]

Indications for EM studies

- Diagnostic renal biopsies for glomerular disease
- Adenocarcinoma versus mesothelioma (see Table 7-29)
- Difficult to classify tumors (Table 7-31)
- Nerve (e.g., toxic or drug-induced neuropathy) and muscle biopsies (e.g., inclusion body or nemaline myopathy)
- Bullous skin diseases (e.g., epidermolysis bullosa)
- Ciliary dysmorphology (primary ciliary dyskinesia or Kartagener's syndrome)
- Endomyocardial biopsies (e.g., Adriamycin toxicity, amyloid, nemaline)
- Liver biopsies for microvesicular fat in acute fatty liver of pregnancy
- Small bowel biopsies to look for pathogens (e.g., Whipple's disease)
- Congenital, inherited, and metabolic diseases (e.g., ceroid lipofuscinoses)
- Prion diseases.

Method

Ultrastructural details of tissues are rapidly lost; therefore fresh tissue must be fixed rapidly and well for EM. Tissues are usually fixed in special fixatives for EM to preserve lipids and glycogen (e.g., 2% paraformaldehyde and 2.5% glutaraldehyde in 0.1 M cacodylate buffer, pH 7.4).

1. Place a small fragment of tissue in a drop of fixative on a cutting surface.
2. Cut the tissue into multiple tiny fragments, each no greater than 0.1 cm in any dimension.
3. Place the tissue into the vial of fixative. Shake the vial to make sure all the tissue fragments are covered by fixative.

Note. If tissue from a small biopsy is found to be nondiagnostic on H&E, any tissue saved for EM should be retrieved for examination by light microscopy.

Results

A separate EM report is usually issued. The results should be incorporated into the final diagnosis.

■ SNAP-FROZEN TISSUE

Frozen tissue is useful for immunoperoxidase staining (some antibodies only detect antigens in frozen tissue), enzyme studies (muscle biopsies), and to save tissue for DNA or RNA studies.

Indications

Frozen tissue is useful for all specimens in which there is a question of a lymphoproliferative disorder, sarcomas, unusual tumors, and muscle biopsies.

Methods

Small (approximately $0.5 \times 0.5 \times 0.3$ cm^3) portions of tissue are placed in a clean specimen container moistened with a small amount of normal saline until they can be frozen.

Table 7-31 Electron microscopic features of poorly differentiated tumors

TUMOR	ULTRASTRUCTURE	ADDITIONAL TESTS	COMMENTS
Carcinoma	Well-developed desmosomes (pentalayered with a dense central line in the intracellular space) with intermediate filament attachment Tonofilaments and bundles of filaments (keratin) Adenocarcinomas: Intercellular lumina (but also present in vascular tumors) Microvilli Intracellular lumina (mucin vacuoles in signet ring cells) Squamous cell carcinomas Numerous intermediate filaments (keratin) and desmosomes	IHC: Cytokeratins are present in almost all carcinomas if broad-spectrum antibodies are used EMA is present in almost all carcinomas, but is less specific and sensitive Additional markers can be used to identify specific carcinomas	Other tumors can also be keratin positive and have desmosomes, filaments, and cytokeratin (mesothelioma, meningioma, synovial sarcoma, and epithelioid sarcoma)
Melanoma	Melanosomes in various stages of development, indicative of a melanin-forming cell type Abnormal pleomorphic melanosomes may be present in melanomas Desmoplastic melanomas lack melanosomes	IHC: S100, HMB-45, MART-1 HMB-45 and MART-1 may be absent in non-epithelioid melanomas The HMB-45 epitope (gp100) is present in immature melanosomes or premelanosomes, but is not specific to these structures	Melanosomes are also seen in clear cell sarcoma, pigmented schwannomas, PEComa, and other rare tumors. Mature forms can be taken up by melanophages, keratinocytes, and carcinomas
Lymphoma	No specific features are present. The cells lack cellular junctions and there is a paucity of cytoplasmic organelles	IHC: LCA	LCA may be absent in 30% of anaplastic (ALK1) lymphomas. These tumors can be EMA (+) but are keratin (−)
Sarcoma	Some types have specific diagnostic features of cell type (e.g., neural, smooth muscle, striated muscle) No well developed desmosomes	IHC: May be helpful for identifying specific types	Keratin negative except for synovial sarcoma and epithelioid sarcoma (or rarely in other types)

Protocol for freezing tissue

Equipment needed:

- Flask
- Labeled self-seal bag
- Pyrex beaker
- Liquid nitrogen
- Tin foil
- Isopentane (2-methylbutane).

Technique

1. Fill a flask half full with liquid nitrogen. Always wear protective gloves and a face shield. Dry ice can also be used. The liquid nitrogen is kept in a canister in the Reproductive Endocrinology Laboratory. Gloves and a face shield are stored nearby.

2. Work in a safety cabinet and wear surgical gloves and goggles. Label a freezer bag with the following:

- Date
- Patient's name in full
- Histology reference number
- Diagnosis/type of tissue.

3. Place 2 cm ($^{3}/_{4}$ inch) of isopentane (2-methylbutane) into a glass beaker. *Lower it gently* into the flask containing liquid nitrogen. The isopentane is ready to use when the liquid base is frozen solid (white particles will appear) and the remaining liquid is viscous. Remove the beaker from the flask carefully.

4. Using the forceps, drop small pieces of tissue directly into the isopentane. Freeze the tissue for approximately 30 seconds.

5. Remove the tissue with the forceps and quickly wrap in aluminum foil. Place the tissue in a labeled freezer bag and place in the flask containing the liquid nitrogen.

6. Transfer the specimen bag from the flask to a −20°C freezer.

Table 7-32 Cells, tumors, and structures with characteristic findings by electron microscopy

TUMOR	EM FINDINGS	CORRELATIONS AND OTHER DIAGNOSTIC TESTS
Alveolar soft part sarcoma	Rhomboid, rod-shaped, or spiculated crystals in a regular lattice pattern	The characteristic cytoplasmic crystals are composed of monocarboxylate transporter 1 (MCT1) and its chaperone CD147. These proteins are found in many other cell types and are not specific for this tumor Cytogenetics: t(X;17) creates a ASPL–TFE3 fusion protein IHC: TFE3 positive (as well as rare pediatric renal tumors with the same translocation). Immunoreactivity is not present in other tumors or normal tissues Histo: The crystals are PAS with diastase positive
Amyloid	Non-branching fibrils, 7.5 to 10 nm in width and up to 1 μm in length	May be present associated with plasma cell tumors, medullary carcinoma of the thyroid, Alzheimer's disease, or as an isolated finding (primary amyloidosis) IHC: Can be used to identify specific types of amyloid (e.g., lambda or kappa chains, β2-microglobulin, calcitonin, tau)
Bronchioloalveolar carcinoma of the lung (BAL)	Lamellar (surfactant) "myelin-like" granules in the supranuclear cytoplasm (typical of type II pneumocytes) Clara-like electron-dense granules in supranuclear cytoplasm. Intranuclear inclusions comprised of parallel microtubular arrays These features can also be seen in metastatic BAL	Cytogenetics: These carcinomas are less likely to be associated with smoking and have fewer cytogenetic changes Bronchioloalveolar carcinomas or adenocarcinomas with features of BAL are more likely to respond to Iressa (38%) as compared to other lung carcinomas (14%) due to specific mutations in EGFR Mucinous BAL has intranuclear inclusions but generally lacks the other EM features
Chordoma	Desmosomes, large vacuoles, glycogen, dilated ER, cytoplasmic invaginations, and intermediate filaments The physaliphorous (having bubbles or vacuoles) appearance is due to dilated ER, glycogen, and cytoplasmic invaginations	IHC: keratin (corresponds to intermediate filaments), EMA, S100
Clear cell sarcoma	Melanosomes in various stages of development Glycogen (resulting in clear cytoplasm)	Cytogenetics: t(12;22) EWS–ATF1 fusion protein IHC: S100, HMB-45

Dense core granules	Dense core granules (vesicle bound by a single membrane with a dense center—60 to 300 nm), cytoplasmic organelles involved in regulated exocytosis of cell products
	Examples:
	Pancreatic beta cells (insulin): angular crystalline inclusions
	Pheochromocytoma (epinephrine and norepine-phrine): large, pleomorphic, often clear or only partially filled
	Carcinoid:
	  Foregut—small, round
	  Midgut—larger, pleomorphic
	  Hindgut—mixed
		Found in tumors of neuronal or neuroendocrine origin
		Vesicles are comprised of granins (predominantly chromogranin A, chromogranin B, and secretogranin II) and various peptide hormones and transmitters, ATP, and biogenic amines
		IHC: chromogranin A (most specific). Specific products of tumors can also be detected
		Note: Prostate cancers and breast cancers can also show strong chromogranin positivity and can be mistaken for neuroendocrine tumors, particularly at metastatic sites

Desmoplastic small round cell tumor	Numerous desmosomes and tight junctions, numerous cell processes, large number of organelles (mitochondria and RER), microfilaments, small neurosecretory granules	Cytogenetics: t(11;22) EWS–WT1 fusion protein IHC: keratin, desmin, WT1, actin, EMA, NSE

Table 7-32 Cells, tumors, and structures with characteristic findings by electron microscopy—cont'd

TUMOR	EM FINDINGS	CORRELATIONS AND OTHER DIAGNOSTIC TESTS
Endothelial cells	Weibel–Palade bodies (cigar-shaped membrane bound structures filled with tubules in parallel arrays) Intracytoplasmic lumina may be present in normal cells and in epithelioid vascular neoplasms	Weibel–Palade bodies are frequently absent in tumors arising from endothelial cells (e.g., angiosarcomas). IHC markers are more sensitive to detect endothelial derivation The membranes are formed by P-selectin and the tubules contain FVIII IHC: Vascular markers (CD34, CD31, FVIII)
Ewing's sarcoma (PNET)	Homogeneous cell population characterized by the lack of specialized features, large pools of glycogen, no organelles, no extracellular matrix, variable numbers of neurosecretory granules and cell processes	Cytogenetics: t(11;22) EWS–FLI1 fusion protein (and other less common variants) IHC: CD99. FLI1 is also present, but is less specific Histo: PAS +/– diastase can detect glycogen, but is not currently used for diagnosis
Granular cell tumor	Numerous lysosomes (filled with tubular, vesicular, and amorphous material), phagosomes, and granules (correlating with the "granular" cytoplasm), reduplicated basal lamina surrounding groups of cells	IHC: S100, inhibin, CD68, calretinin
Langerhans cell histiocytosis	Birbeck granules (rod or tennis racket shaped) structures of variable length with a central periodically striated lamella	May serve as a reservoir for Langerin (a transmembrane type II Ca^{2+}-dependent lectin) and CD1a in the endosomal recycling compartment IHC: CD1a, Langerin, S100
Mast cells	Lamellar or scroll-like membrane pattern, granules of variable size	IHC: CD117 (c-kit), mast cell tryptase
Medullary carcinoma of the thyroid	Numerous neurosecretory granules (calcitonin) associated with stromal amyloid (calcitonin)	Cytogenetics: mutations in the *RET* gene (sporadic and germline) IHC: Calcitonin (in tumor cells and amyloid), chromogranin
Merkel cell carcinoma	Neurosecretory granules in processes or along cell membranes (subplasmalemmal)	IHC: chromogranin, NSE, cytokeratin 20
Mesothelioma	Elongated, serpiginous, and branched microvilli (generally 10 to 16 length: 1 width) apical without a glycocalyx or actin rootlets	Cytogenetics: Characteristic chromosome deletions and loss of 9 and 22 IHC: Calretinin, WT1
Neuroblastoma	Cellular processes with microtubules (neuropil), dense core granules, Homer–Wright rosettes (the center is comprised of a tangle of cell processes), synaptic vesicles, no glycogen	Cytogenetics: Changes are linked to prognosis IHC: chromogranin, NSE, NFP, synaptophysin
Oncocytoma	Numerous mitochondria packed in the cytoplasm (correlating with the granular appearance of the cytoplasm). In contrast, chromophobe renal cell carcinoma has fewer mitochondria and more microvesicles	Cytogenetics: Monosomy with loss of X or Y, 11q13. Chromophobe carcinomas have different cytogenetic changes IHC: RCC is negative in oncocytomas but positive in 45–50% of chromophobe renal cell carcinomas
Perineurioma	Long cell processes wrapping around adjacent cells	IHC: Claudin-1 (a component of tight junctions), EMA
Rhabdoid tumor of the kidney	Large paranuclear whorls of intermediate filaments (corresponding to cytokeratin and vimentin) and occasional tonofilaments	Cytogenetics: hSNF5/INI1 deletions and mutations IHC: Cytokeratin, vimentin

Table 7-32 Cells, tumors, and structures with characteristic findings by electron microscopy—*cont'd*

TUMOR	EM FINDINGS	CORRELATIONS AND OTHER DIAGNOSTIC TESTS
Rhabdomyosarcoma	Parallel thick (12 to 15 cm) and thin (6 to 8 nm) myosin-actin filaments, Z bands, filament ribosomal complexes Spider cells may be seen in cardiac tumors (clear cytoplasm divided by cytoplasmic processes and cross striations formed by leptofibrils)	Cytogenetics: Characteristic changes in alveolar and embryonal types IHC: Muscle markers (HHF-35, desmin, myf4)
Schwannoma	Basal lamina prominent, often reduplicated. Luse bodies (long spacing collagen, extracellular), myelin figures, long cell processes wrapping around collagen, may rarely have melanosomes (melanotic schwannoma)	Cytogenetics: Deletion of 2q (NF2 inactivation) IHC: S100

For additional information see also Tables 7-8, 7-9, 7-15, 7-33.

7. Discard the isopentane in a waste bottle. Liquid nitrogen can be allowed to evaporate.
8. Sterilize the beaker and forceps with 10% formalin.
9. Dispose of contaminated sharps and specimen containers in appropriate impervious biohazard containers. Wash your hands after removal of gloves.

If there is insufficient tissue for snap freezing, a frozen section from the OR Consultation Room may be saved frozen for potential studies. Many cryostats undergo an automatic defrost cycle and tissue left as a block in the cryostat will thaw and refreeze. Thus tissue to be saved frozen should be transferred to a freezer.

Results

The results of immunoperoxidase studies on frozen tissue are usually incorporated into the surgical pathology report.

■ IMMUNOFLUORESCENCE

Like immunoperoxidase studies, immunofluorescence detects antigens in tissues. However, because amplification of the signal is not used, it is better suited for precise localization of antigen/antibody complexes in tissues or for determining the deposition pattern of immune complexes (e.g., linear versus granular). Thus, it is most useful for the investigation of diseases related to immune complex deposition such as glomerular diseases and bullous diseases of the skin.

Tissue for immunofluorescence may be snap frozen (see instructions above) or stored in special fixatives for IF. If the specimen is not frozen, special care must be taken to ensure that the biopsy is kept moist in a sealed container.

Direct IF uses antibodies to detect antigens in the patient's *tissues*.

Indirect IF uses control tissues to detect antibodies (e.g., anti-BM) in the patient's *serum*.

Indications

Biopsies of some skin diseases (e.g., lupus, pemphigus, pemphigoid, and dermatitis herpetiformis), all diagnostic non-transplant renal biopsies, some transplant renal biopsies, and the evaluation of vasculitis in nerve biopsies.

Method

Tissue must be submitted fresh.

Results

The results of the examination are usually incorporated into the surgical pathology report.

Immunofluorescence of skin lesions

SLE (lupus band test). There is linear or granular staining along the dermal–epidermal junction for multiple immunoreactants (most commonly IgG and less often IgM or C3) in approximately 80% of cases. The specificity increases with the number of positive immunoreactants. Uninvolved sun-exposed skin shows positivity in most patients with active systemic lupus. Uninvolved skin in patients with discoid lupus is usually negative for this test.

Herpes gestationis. Perilesional skin shows linear basement membrane zone C3 and sometimes IgG.

Dermatitis herpetiformis. Granular IgA is seen at the tips of dermal papillae of uninvolved skin.

Pemphigus. IgG and C3 between epidermal cells create a net-like pattern. In pemphigus vulgaris, a split just above the basal cell layer creates a "tombstone" appearance to the row of basal cells at the base of the vesicle. In pemphigus foliaceus and related disorders, the split occurs near the granular cell layer.

Pemphigoid. Ig and C3 are present along the basement membrane but not between cells. Indirect IF reveals an anti-BM antibody.

MOLECULAR GENETIC PATHOLOGY

Molecular genetic pathology is the newest subspeciality in pathology with board certification. Molecular diagnostics incorporates many types of techniques for the investigation of genetic alterations in cells and viruses (e.g., Southern blotting, PCR analysis, FISH). It has applications in three main areas:

1. Inherited diseases:
   - Identification of inherited diseases (e.g., cystic fibrosis, hemochromatosis, factor V Leiden, prothrombin 20210A, fragile X syndrome)
   - Identification of genes conferring susceptibility to diseases (e.g., *BRCA1*).
2. Infectious diseases:
   - Detection of organisms
   - Identification of specific organisms
   - Quantitation of viral infection (e.g., HIV viral load).
3. Cancer
   - Identification of specific genetic alterations associated with tumors (Table 7-33)
   - Identification of clonality in hematolymphoid proliferations (Table 7-34)
   - Detection of minimal residual disease after treatment.

Molecular genetic studies are especially helpful for difficult-to-classify hematolymphoid proliferations because of the frequent and characteristic rearrangements that occur in many of these disorders. Unlike cytogenetics, the cells need not be viable; however, it is preferable that the nucleic acids are relatively intact. Southern blot and RNA based PCR (RT-PCR) assays are best performed on fresh or frozen tissues. Formalin-fixed, paraffin-embedded tissue is amenable to DNA-based PCR assays. Some fixatives (e.g., Bouin's) cause extensive breakage of DNA and may preclude genetic analysis of the tissue.

Indications

- B-cell proliferations: clonal rearrangements of the immunoglobulin heavy and light chain genes; specific translocations (see Table 7-34).
- T-cell proliferations: rearrangements of the γ and β T-cell receptor genes.
- Leukemias (see Table 7-34).
- Post-transplant lymphoproliferative disorders: clonal populations of EBV-infected cells.
- Oligodendrogliomas: PCR-based LOH analysis for 1p/19q deletions.

Method of submitting tissue

Fresh or frozen tissue (e.g., snap-frozen tissue) as well as fluids may be used. Cytologic preparations can be used for FISH.

Results

The results are usually either reported separately or incorporated into the surgical pathology report.

CYTOGENETICS

Cytogenetic studies have been demonstrated to be useful in several areas important to pathology:

Tumor classification, particularly sarcomas, lymphomas, brain tumors, and other unusual tumors (Ewing's sarcoma, synovial sarcoma).
Benign versus malignant lesions, for example:
   - Reactive mesothelial cells versus mesothelioma
   - Lipoma versus liposarcoma.
Prognosis, for example in neuroblastoma and multiple myeloma.
Research: Translocations are common to many tumors and usually identify genes important to the pathogenesis of the tumor.

Cells may be cultured to perform complete karyotype analysis or tissues can be analyzed for specific chromosomal alterations by fluorescence in situ hybridization (FISH). FISH studies can be performed on cultured cells, cytology preparations, and fixed and embedded tissues.

Indications

Cytogenetic studies are indicated for soft tissue tumors, mesotheliomas (tissue or pleural fluid), unusual tumors, poorly differentiated tumors, all subcutaneous lipomas larger than 5 cm, all subfascial lipomas (for karyotype), and oligodendrogliomas (for FISH).

Method for submitting tissue

Tissue for karyotyping must be fresh, viable, and relatively sterile. However, tissue may be submitted even if it has not been handled under strictly sterile conditions (contamination is not usually a problem). If specimens are to be held overnight, the tissue should be minced (into 1-mm cubes) in a sterile specimen container, covered with culture medium, and held overnight in the refrigerator. Fluids may also be submitted for analysis (especially pleural effusions with a suspicion of mesothelioma).

Results

The results of the cytogenetic analysis should be incorporated into the final diagnosis.

Table 7-33 Common cytogenetic and genetic changes in solid tumors of diagnostic or therapeutic significance

TUMOR TYPE	CHARACTERISTIC CYTOGENETIC CHANGES	GENETIC CHANGES	FREQUENCY	COMMENTS
Adenoid cystic carcinomas	6q translocations and deletions	>50%		
Adrenal cortical carcinomas		2p16 loss	>90%	This area is close to the region associated with Carney complex type 2
		17p13 LOH	85%	These changes are less common in localized tumors (25–35%) but, if present, such tumors are more likely to metastasize. The 11p15 imprinted region is also involved in Beckwith–Wiedemann syndrome
		11p15 LOH with duplication of the active paternal allele leading to IGF-II overexpression	85%	
Alveolar soft part sarcoma	der(X)(X;17)(p11;q25)	ASPL–TFE3 fusion	>90%	TFE3 can be detected by IHC. This translocation is also present in rare papillary-like renal tumors in young adults (see "Renal tumors" below)
Aneurysmal bone cyst	t(16;17)(q22;p13)	CDH11–USP6 fusion	>50%	
Angiomatoid fibrous histiocytoma	t(12;16)(q13;p11)	FUS–ATF fusion		
Breast carcinoma		HER-2/neu amplification	20–30%	Detected by FISH (gene amplification) or IHC (protein overexpression). Positive carcinomas are more likely to respond to Herceptin
		BRCA1 and BRCA2 germline mutations	<5%	Patients are more likely to be young and have multiple carcinomas. BRCA1 carcinomas are frequently high grade, have "medullary" features, and lack ER, PR, HER-2. BRCA2 carcinomas have no specific pathologic features
Carcinoma of the upper aerodigestive tract in children	t(15;19)(q13;p13.2)	BRD4–NUT fusion		Patients with this translocation have a poor prognosis
Chondromyxoid fibroma	Deletion of 6q		>75%	
Clear cell sarcoma	t(12;22)(q13;q12)	EWS–ATF1 fusion	>75%	
Colon carcinoma		hMLH1 and hMSH2 mutations	15% of sporadic carcinomas	95% of HNPCC patients have germline mutations in these genes. Absence can be detected by IHC or by PCR assays for microsatellite instability. Mutations are correlated with characteristic clinical, pathologic, and treatment response features
		EGFR (HER1) overexpression	82% of all carcinomas	Approximately 23% of patients treated with cetuximab[b] and chemotherapy respond. IHC for EGFR may be used to select eligible patients

Table 7-33 Common cytogenetic and genetic changes in solid tumors of diagnostic or therapeutic significance—*cont'd*

TUMOR TYPE	CHARACTERISTIC CYTOGENETIC CHANGES	GENETIC CHANGES	FREQUENCY	COMMENTS
Colon carcinoma (Continued)		*APC* mutations	80% of all carcinomas	Also present as a germline mutation in familial adenomatous polyposis syndrome
		LKB1/STK11 LOH	~15%	Germline mutations occur in some cases of Peutz–Jeghers syndrome. Mutations appear to be rare in sporadic colon carcinoma but LOH is observed in some
		DPC4 (*Smad4* or *MADH4*) mutations (18q21.1)	10–20%	Germline mutations occur in some cases of juvenile polyposis syndrome. Mutations in sporadic carcinomas are uncommon
Desmoplastic small round cell tumor	t(11;22)(p13;q12)	*EWS–WT1* fusion	>75%	WT1 can be detected by IHC
Dermatofibrosarcoma protuberans	t(17;22)(q21;q13) resulting in a ring chromosome	*COL1A1–PDGFB* fusion	>75%	The same translocation is present in giant cell fibroblastoma, but without formation of a ring chromosome
Endometrial stromal tumor	t(7;17)(p15;q21)	*JAZF1–JJAZ1* fusion	30%	
Ewing's sarcoma (PNET)	t(11;22)(q24;q12) t(21;22)(q22;q12) t(2;22)(q33;q12) t(7;22)(p22;q12) t(17;22)(q12;q12) inv(22)(q12)(q12)	*EWS–FLI1* fusion *EWS–ERG* fusion *EWS–FEV* fusion *EWS–ETV1* fusion *EWS–E1AF* fusion *EWS–ZSG* fusion	>80% 5–10% <5% <5% <5% <5%	FLI1 can be detected by IHC but is not specific for Ewing's
Extraskeletal myxoid chondrosarcoma	t(9;22)(q22;q12) t(9;17)(q22;q11) t(9;15)(q22;q21)	*EWS–NR4A3* fusion *TAF2N–NR4A3* fusion *TCF12–NR4A3* fusion	>75% <10% <10%	
Fibromatosis (desmoid)	Trisomies of 8 and 20 Deletion of 5q	*APC* inactivation	30% 10%	
Fibromyxoid sarcoma, low grade	t(7;16)(q33;p11.2)	*FUS–BBF2H7* fusion	Unknown	
Fibrosarcoma, infantile	t(12;15)(p13;q26) Trisomies 8, 11, 17, 20	*ETV6–NTRK3* fusion	>75% >75%	The same translocation is seen in cellular mesoblastic nephroma
Gastrointestinal stromal tumor	Monosomies 14 and 22 Deletion of 1p	*KIT* or *PDGFRA* mutation	> 75% >25% >90%	CD117 (KIT) is detected by IHC and is useful for diagnosis. Gleevec[c] is effective against tumors with activating mutations in either gene
Germ cell tumors	Isochromosome 12p	*KIT* mutations	>80–90% 25–70%	Includes all histologic subtypes Seminomas
Giant cell tumor	Telomeric changes		>50%	

Table 7-33 Common cytogenetic and genetic changes in solid tumors of diagnostic or therapeutic significance—*cont'd*

TUMOR TYPE	CHARACTERISTIC CYTOGENETIC CHANGES	GENETIC CHANGES	FREQUENCY	COMMENTS
Giant cell tumor, diffuse type (PVNS)	Trisomies 5 and 7 t(1;2)		>25%	
Hepatoblastoma	Trisomies 2q and 20		>75%	
Hibernoma	11q13 rearrangement		>50%	
Inflammatory myofibroblastic tumor	2p23 rearrangement	*ALK* fusion with multiple partners	50%	ALK can be detected by IHC in one third of cases
Leiomyoma, Uterine	t(12;14)(q15;q24) deletion of 7q	*HMGA2* rearrangement	40%	Uterine leiomyosarcomas have more complex karyotypes
Lipoblastoma	8q12 rearrangement polysomy 8	*PLAG1* oncogene	>80%	
Lipoma Typical	12q15 rearrangement 6p21 rearrangement Deletion of 13q or 16q	*HMGA2* rearrangement *HMGA1* rearrangement	60%	
Spindle cell or pleomorphic Chondroid	t(11;16)(q13;p12-13)		>75%	
Liposarcoma Well-differentiated	Ring form of chrom 12q1,5/giant markers	*HMGA2, MDM2* amplification	>75%	
Myxoid/round cell	t(12;16)(q13;p11) t(12;22)(q13;q12)	*FUS–CHOP* fusion *EWS–CHOP* fusion	>75% <5%	
Pleomorphic	Complex		90%	
Lung adenocarcinomas that respond to gefitinib (most have features of bronchioloalveolar carcinoma)	Fewer changes than seen in carcinomas associated with smoking	*EGFR*—small deletions or amino acid substitutions	10–20% of all lung carcinomas	Mutations predict response to the tyrosine kinase inhibitor gefitinib (Iressa)[d] 40–80% of lung carcinomas show *EGFR* overexpression by IHC, but only carcinomas with specific mutations respond to gefitinib
Medulloblastoma	Isochromosome 17q		>25%	
Meningioma	Monosomy 22 1p deletion		90% 25%	
Mesothelioma	Deletion of 1p Deletion of 9p Deletion of 22q Deletions of 3p and 6q	? *BCL10* inactivation p15, p16, and p19 inactivation *NF2* inactivation	>50% >75% >50% >50%	Cytogenetic changes are less complex than those seen in carcinomas. Cytogenetic analysis of cytologic specimens (e.g., pleural fluid) can be of value if larger biopsies are not available
Mucoepidermoid carcinoma	t(11;19)(q21;p13)	*MECT1–MAML2* fusion	>50%	
Neuroblastoma	Hyperdiploid, no 1p deletion		40%	Good prognosis
	1p deletion Double minute chromosomes	N-*myc* amplification	40% >25%	Poor prognosis

Table 7-33 Common cytogenetic and genetic changes in solid tumors of diagnostic or therapeutic significance—*cont'd*

TUMOR TYPE	CHARACTERISTIC CYTOGENETIC CHANGES	GENETIC CHANGES	FREQUENCY	COMMENTS
Oligodendroglioma	Deletion of 1p36 and 19q13.3 9p21 deletion	 CDKN2A (p16) deletion	50%	Useful for diagnosis and to predict response to radiation and/or chemotherapy Occurs in some anaplastic oligodendrogliomas. Poor prognostic factor
Osteochondroma	Deletion of 8q	EXT1 inactivation	>25%	

Osteosarcoma
  Low grade
  High grade
	
	Ring chromosomes
	Complex
		
		RB and P53 inactivation
			
			>50%
			>80%	

Pheochromocytoma
  Sporadic (70%)
  Hereditary (30%)
		Losses on 1p
		Germline mutations in RET, VHL, NF1, SDHB, SDHD, MEN2A, MEN2B
			>80%
			>90% of hereditary cases
				Patients are more likely to be young (<50), have multiple tumors, and have a family history of pheochromocytoma, paraganglioma, or medullary carcinoma of the thyroid

Pleomorphic adenoma (salivary)	8q12 rearrangement 12q15 rearrangement	PLAG1 fusion genes HMGIC oncogenes	>50% <20%	

Renal tumors
  Clear cell carcinoma
  Papillary carcinoma: adult
 	
"Papillary-like" carcinoma: young adults
 	
Oncocytoma
 	
Chromophobe carcinoma
	
	Deletion of 3p
	Trisomies 3, 7, 12, 16, 17, and 20
	
	t(X;1)(p11.2;q21)
	t(X;1)(p11.2;p34)
	inv(X)(p11.2q12)
	t(X;17)(p11.2;q25.3)
	t(6;11)(p21.1;q12)
	
	−1, −X or −Y
	11q13 rearrangement
	Monosomies 1, 2, 3, 6, 10, 13, 17, and 21
		
		KIT mutations
		
		PRCC–TFE3 fusion
		TFE3–PSF fusion
		TFE3–NonO fusion
		RCC17(ASPL)–TFE3 fusion
		TFEB-Alpha fusion
			
			>90%
			>90%
			
			>90%
			
			>25%
			>25%
			>75%
				
				CD117 (c-kit) present by IHC in cytoplasm and is associated with activating mutations
				The majority of these carcinomas are associated with fusion proteins involving TFE3 or TFEB.
				The ASPL–TFE3 fusion is also present in alveolar soft part sarcoma
				
				CD117 (c-kit) is present by IHC on membranes, but activating mutations have not been detected

Retinoblastoma	13q14 deletion Isochromosome 6p	RB1 inactivation	>75% 25%	40% of cases are due to germline mutations in RB1
Rhabdoid tumor of the kidney and Atypical teratoid/rhabdoid tumor (AT/RT)	Normal karyotype Monosomy 22	hSNF5/INI1 (22q11.2) deletions and mutations hSNF5/INI1 deletions and mutations	>90%	Infants and children with both tumors have a germline mutation in INI1 (rhabdoid predisposition syndrome) Choroid plexus carcinomas are also associated with non-function of this gene (70%)

Table 7-33 Common cytogenetic and genetic changes in solid tumors of diagnostic or therapeutic significance—*cont'd*

TUMOR TYPE	CHARACTERISTIC CYTOGENETIC CHANGES	GENETIC CHANGES	FREQUENCY	COMMENTS
Rhabdomyosarcoma				
Alveolar	t(2;13)(q35;q14)	*PAX3–FKHR* fusion	>75%	Poor 4-year survival if metastatic (8%)
	t(1;13)(p36;q14), double minutes	*PAX7–FKHR* fusion	10–20%	Better 4-year survival if metastatic (75%)
Embryonal	Trisomies 2q, 8, and 20		>75%	
		LOH 11p15	>75%	
Schwannoma and perineurioma	Deletion of 22q	*NF2* inactivation	>80%	5% of cases of vestibular schwannomas are associated with neurofibromatosis type 2 (germline *NF2* mutations)
Synovial sarcoma				
Monophasic	t(X;18)(p11;q11)	*SYT–SSX1/SYT–SSX2* fusion	>90%	
Biphasic	t(X;18)(p11;q11)	*SYT–SS1* fusion	>90%	
Thyroid carcinoma				
Papillary	10q11 rearrangement	*RET* fusion oncogenes	>30%	
	1q21 rearrangement	*NTRK1* fusion oncogenes	>10%	
		BRAF oncogenes	30%	
Follicular	t(2;3)(q13;p25)	*PAX8–PPARG* fusion	>40%	
Medullary				
Sporadic (75%)		*RET* activating mutations	>90%	
Hereditary (25%)		Germline *RET, MEN2A,* or *MEN2B* mutations	>90%	Indication for screening for pheochromocytoma and screening family members
Wilms' tumor, pediatric	Deletion 11p13	*WT1* inactivation	25%	Germline mutations occur in several syndromes. WT1 mutations also occur in sporadic tumors
	Trisomy 12		40%	

^a Trastuzumab (Herceptin) is a monoclonal antibody directed against the HER-2/neu receptor. Patients are selected for treatment by testing carcinomas with IHC or FISH.

^b Cetuximab (C225, Erbitux ™) is a monoclonal antibody directed against the EGFR receptor. A test has been approved by the FDA for the determination of EGFR (DakoCyomation, EGFR PharmDX). This test is not used for lung carcinomas (see note "d" below).

^c Imatinib mesylate (STI571, Gleevec™, Glivec™) is a small molecule tyrosine kinase inhibitor that may be used for the treatment of tumors overexpressing tyrosine kinases:

> Bcr–Abl tyrosine kinase: CML, ALL (Ph+)
> KIT tyrosine kinase: GIST, systemic mastocytosis, some types of AML
> PDGFR kinase: CMML, chronic eosinophilic leukemia, rare cases of GIST.

The KIT protein (CD117) is encoded by the c-*KIT* proto-oncogene and is a transmembrane receptor protein with tyrosine kinase activity. Mutations may render KIT independent of its ligand, SCF (stem cell factor). Mutated proteins may or may not respond to therapy with imatinib. Wild-type KIT and KIT with mutations in the juxtamembrane domain (the intracellular segment between the transmembrane and tyrosine kinase domains) are found in GISTs and are sensitive to imatinib. Other tumor types are associated with mutations in the enzymatic domain and the altered protein is generally not sensitive to imatinib. Overexpression of the protein is detected by IHC.

^d Gefitinib (Iressa) is a tyrosine kinase inhibitor effective against a small subset of lung adenocarcinomas with specific activating mutations in EGFR. IHC for EGFR is not helpful for identifying carcinomas likely to respond to treatment.

For additional information on specific genes, see Online Mendelian Inheritance in Man (OMIM; www.ncbi.nlm.nih.gov).

Table 7-34 Common cytogenetic changes in lymphomas and leukemias

TUMOR TYPE	CYTOGENETIC CHANGES	MOLECULAR EVENTS	FREQUENCY	COMMENTS
Chronic leukemias and mastocytosis				
CML (Ph[1])	t(9;22)(q34;q11.2)	BCR–ABL fusion (usually p210, but also p190 and p230 fusion proteins)	90–95%	Philadelphia chromosome. Also present in 5% of children and 15–30% of adults with ALL and 2% of patients with AML Treated with the ABL tyrosine kinase inhibitor imatinib (Gleevec)[a]
	Other variants or cryptic translocations	BCR–ABL fusion (usually p210, but also p190 and p230 fusion proteins)	5–10%	
CML, accelerated phase or blast phase	Additional changes: extra Ph, +8, or i(17)(q10)		80%	May be myeloid (70%) or lymphoid (30%)
Chronic myelomonocytic leukemia with eosinophilia	t(5;12)(q33;p13)	ETV6 (also called TEL) –PDGRFbeta fusion	Rare	Excellent response to imatinib[a]
Chronic eosinophilic leukemia/hyper-eosinophilic syndrome	Cryptic del(4)(q12) – interstitial 800 kb deletion	FIP1L1–PDGFRalpha fusion	~50%	The fusion protein is an activated tyrosine kinase. Excellent response with the tyrosine kinase inhibitor imatinib[a]
	t(1;5)(q23;q33)	myomegalin–PDGFRbeta fusion protein	? Rare	May be more common in infants and women. Excellent response to imatinib[a]
Mastocytosis		c-KIT point mutations (Asp816Val)	100%	CD117 (c-kit) is detected by IHC in normal and abnormal mast cells. The most common mutations do not result in proteins sensitive to imatinib
	Cryptic del(4)(q12) – interstitial 800 kb deletion	FIP1L1–PDGFRalpha fusion	~60% of patients with eosinophilia	Found in mastocytosis with associated eosinophilia. These patients do not have the typical c-KIT mutation. Excellent response to treatment with imatinib[a]
Acute myeloid leukemia				
AML	Normal karyotype		20%	
		FLT3 (13q12) internal tandem duplications (ITD, 20%) or point mutations (7%)	20–30% of AML with normal karyotype	More common in monocytic AML (M5), less common in myeloblastic leukemia with maturation (M2) or erythroleukemia (M6). Less common in AML with cytogenetic changes (10%). Poor prognostic factor Results in an activated tyrosine kinase. Current trials are evaluating response to a kinase inhibitor, PKC412.
AML (M1, M2, or M4)	t(6;9)(p23;q34)	DEK–CAN fusion	1% of all AML	Poor prognosis
		FLT3 ITDs	90% of this AML type	

Table 7-34 Common cytogenetic changes in lymphomas and leukemias—*cont'd*

TUMOR TYPE	CYTOGENETIC CHANGES	MOLECULAR EVENTS	FREQUENCY	COMMENTS
Acute myeloid leukemia				
AML with t(8;21) (M2)	t(8;21)(q22;q22)	*AML1–ETO* fusion	5–12% of AML	30% of cases of AML with karyotypic abnormalities and maturation. Maturation in neutrophilic lineage. Usually younger patients, good prognosis
		c-*KIT* mutations	~50% of this AML type	Response to imatinib[a] untested
Acute promyelocytic leukemia (M3, M3v.)	t(15;17)(q22;q11-12) t(11;17)(q23;p21) t(5;17)(q34;q12) t(11;17)(p13;q21)	*PML–RARα* fusion *PLZF–RARα* fusion *NPM1-RARα* fusion *NUMA–RARα* fusion	5–8% of AML (95–100% of APML)	Abnormal promyelocytes predominate. Usually occurs in adults in mid-life. Treatment with all *trans*-retinoic acid acts to differentiate the cells. Favorable prognosis
		FLT3 ITDs	32% of APML	
AML with inv(16) or t(16;16)	inv (16)(p13)(q22) t(16;16)(p13;q22) del(16q) Other rare variants or cryptic translocations	*CBFbeta–MYH11* fusion	10–12% of AML (100% of M4EO)	Monocytic and granulocytic differentiation and abnormal eosinophils in the marrow. Usually younger patients. Favorable prognosis
		c-*KIT* mutations	~50% of this AML type	Response to imatinib[a] untested
AML with 11q23 abnormalities	11q23 abnormalities	*MLL* fusion with numerous different partners	5–6% of AML	Usually associated with monocytic features. Occurs in infants and in patients after therapy with topoisomerase II inhibitors. Intermediate prognosis
AML and MDS, therapy related	5q–/7q–/12p–/20q– t(9;11), t(11;19), t(6;11) Other less common changes			Occurs after alkylating agents and/or radiation, usually 5 to 6 years after treatment. Poor prognosis
		MLL balanced translocations		Occurs after DNA-topoisomerase II inhibitors, usually 3 years after treatment. Long-term prognosis unknown
B Cell				
Precursor B-lympho-blastic leukemia/ lymphoblastic lymphoma (ALL)	t(9;22)(q34;q11.2)	*BCR–ABL* fusion (usually p190 (esp. in children), but also p210 protein)	5% of childhood ALL 20–25% of adult ALL	Philadelphia chromosome Poor prognosis
	t with 11q23 t(12;21)(p13;q22)	*MLL* rearrangements *TEL–AML1* fusion	>50% of childhood ALL or hyperdiploid	Poor prognosis. Usually infants Good prognosis. This translocation is not detected by standard cytogenetics
	t(1;19)(q23;p13.3)	*PBX1–E2A* fusion	5–6%	Pre-B-ALL; most common translocation in childhood. Unfavorable but modified by therapy

Table 7-34 Common cytogenetic changes in lymphomas and leukemias—*cont'd*

TUMOR TYPE	CYTOGENETIC CHANGES	MOLECULAR EVENTS	FREQUENCY	COMMENTS
B Cell				
	Hypodiploid			Poor prognosis
	Hyperdiploid >50			Good prognosis (= DNA Index 1.16 to 1.6)
	t(5;14)(q31;q32)	IL3–IGH fusion		Poor prognosis
	t(8;14)(q24;q32)	MYC–IGH fusion		Good prognosis
	t(2;8)(p12;q24)	IGK–MYC fusion		Good prognosis
	t(8;22)(q24;q11)	MYC–IGL fusion		Good prognosis
	t(17;19)(q21;p13)	HLF–E2A fusion		Poor prognosis
	t(4;11)(q21;q23)	MLL–AF4 fusion		Poor prognosis
ALL, therapy related				Similar to therapy related AML
Small lymphocytic lymphoma/CLL	Trisomy 12		16%	Usually do not have I_gV_H mutations. Aggressive clinical course
		del(11q22-23)—ATR	18%	Poor prognosis Detected by FISH
		del(13q14) —DBS319	55%	Usually do have I_gV_H mutations Long-term survival Detected by FISH
		17p — p53	7%	Worse prognosis Detected by FISH
		I_gV_H not mutated	40–50%	Worse prognosis (<8 year median survival)
		I_gV_H (mutated, >2% difference in nucleotide sequence)	50–60%	Better prognosis (median survival >24 years)
Lymphoplasmacytic lymphoma/ Waldenström's macroglobulinemia	t(9;14)(p13;q32)	PAX-5–IGH fusion	50%	This rearrangement may be less common in cases associated with Waldenström's macroglobulinemia or if node-based
Mantle cell lymphoma	t(11;14)(q13;q32)	CCND1–IGH fusion ATM point mutations	>95%	Overexpression of cyclin D1 detected by IHC
Marginal zone lymphoma (MALT)	+3		60%	
	t(1;14)(p21;q32)	BCL-10–IGH fusion		
	t(11;18)(q21;q21)	API2–MALT1 fusion	25–50%	
	t(11;14)(q21;q32)	MALT1–IGH fusion		
Follicular lymphoma	t(14;18)(q32;q21)	IGH–BCL-2 fusion	70–95%	
	t(2;18)(p12;q21)	IGK–BCL-2 fusion	Rare	
Burkitt's lymphoma and Burkitt-like lymphoma	t(8;14)(q24;q32)	MYC–IGH fusion	85%	
	t(2;8)(p12;q24)	MYC–IGK fusion	Rare	
	t(8;22)(q24;q11)	MYC–IGL fusion	Rare	
Mediastinal (thymic) large B-cell lymphoma	9p+	REL amplification		
Diffuse large B-cell lymphoma	t(3q27;v)	BCL6 translocations with many partners	30%	BCL6 is detected by IHC in most cases, BCL2 in some cases
	t(14;18)(q32;q21)	BCL2–IGH fusion	20–30%	
Hairy cell leukemia				No consistent changes
Primary effusion lymphoma				No consistent changes

Table 7-34 Common cytogenetic changes in lymphomas and leukemias—*cont'd*

TUMOR TYPE	CYTOGENETIC CHANGES	MOLECULAR EVENTS	FREQUENCY	COMMENTS
B Cell				
Plasmacytoma/myeloma	t(11;14)(q13;q32) t(6;14)(p21;q32) t(4;14)(p16;q32) t(14;16)(q32;q23) Monosomy 13/13q–	*CCND1–IGH* fusion *CCND3–IGH* fusion *FGF23–IGH* fusion *IGH–MAF* fusion	 15–40%	Best prognosis Adverse prognosis Adverse prognosis
T Cell				
Precursor lymphoblastic leukemia/lymphoblastic lymphoma	Translocations involving *TCR* alpha, beta, delta, and gamma and partner genes *MYC*, *TAL1*, *RBTN1*, *RBTN2*, *HOX11*, and LCK del(1) t(1;14) t(5;14) del(9p)	 *Tal1* (small deletion) *Tal1–TCRdelta* fusion *HOX11L2–TCRdelta* fusion *CDKN2A* deletion	30% 30% 25% >30%	 Adolescents Adolescents Young children
T-cell prolymphocytic leukemia	inv(14)(q11)(q32) t(14;14)(q11;q32) t(7;14)(q35;q32.1) chrom 8 abnormalities	*TCRα/β–TCL1* & *TCL1b* fusion *TCRα/β–TCL1* & *TCL1b* fusion *TCRβ–TCL 1A* fusion	80% 10% 70–80%	
Adult T-cell lymphoma/leukemia				No consistent changes
Mycosis fungoides and Sézary syndrome				No consistent changes
Peripheral T-cell lymphoma, NOS				No consistent changes
Hepatosplenic T-cell lymphoma	i(7q)(q10)		100%	
Panniculitis-like T-cell lymphoma				No consistent changes
Angioimmunoblastic lymphoma	Trisomy 3, trisomy 5, + X			
Enteropathy-type T-cell lymphoma				No consistent changes.
Anaplastic large cell lymphoma (CD30+)	t(2;5)(p23;q35) 2p23 rearrangements	*NPM1–ALK* fusion protein (p80) *ALK* fusion with other partners	70–80%	ALK detected by IHC in nucleus, nucleolus, and cytoplasm ALK detected by IHC in cytoplasm

Table 7-34 Common cytogenetic changes in lymphomas and leukemias—*cont'd*

TUMOR TYPE	CYTOGENETIC CHANGES	MOLECULAR EVENTS	FREQUENCY	COMMENTS
T Cell				
Extranodal NK/T-cell lymphoma, nasal type				No consistent changes.
Blastic NK-cell lymphoma				No consistent changes.

[a] Imatinib mesylate (STI571, Gleevec™, Glivec™) is a small molecule tyrosine kinase inhibitor that may be used for the treatment of tumors overexpressing tyrosine kinases:

Bcr-Abl tyrosine kinase: CML, ALL (Ph+)
KIT tyrosine kinase: GIST, systemic mastocytosis, some types of AML
PDGFR kinase: CMML, chronic eosinophilic leukemia, rare cases of GIST

The KIT protein is encoded by the c-*KIT* proto-oncogene and is a transmembrane receptor protein with tyrosine kinase activity. Mutations may render KIT independent of its ligand, SCF (stem cell factor). Mutated proteins may or may not respond to therapy with imatinib. Wild-type KIT and KIT with mutations in the juxtamembrane domain (the intracellular segment between the transmembrane and tyrosine kinase domains) are found in GISTs and are sensitive to imatinib. Other tumor types are associated with mutations in the enzymatic domain and the altered protein is generally not sensitive to imatinib.
For additional information on specific genes, see Online Mendelian Inheritance in Man (OMIM; www.ncbi.nlm.nih.gov).

Tumors and diseases associated with germline mutations

The following features are suggestive of a hereditary susceptibility to cancer:

- Two or more close relatives on the same side of the family with cancer
- Evidence of autosomal dominant transmission
- Early development of cancer in the patient and relatives (in general, under 50 years of age)
- Multiple primary cancers
- Multiple types of cancers
- Unusual pathologic features of tumors (Table 7-35)
- A constellation of tumors suggestive of a specific syndrome (Table 7-36).

Pathologists can aid in the detection of hereditary carcinomas by being aware of the types and pathologic characteristics of carcinomas associated with these syndromes. Patients with germline mutations are important to identify in order to:

- Screen patients for other common tumors or other components of the disease
- Consider prophylactic surgery or preventive interventions
- Offer screening to family members at risk and genetic counseling.

Although the sporadic forms of cancers in general far outnumber cases associated with germline mutations, in some cases the appearance or site of a carcinoma is highly suggestive of a known syndrome and further investigation may be warranted.

Table 7-35 Pathologic features of tumors and diseases suggestive of a germline mutation

TYPE OF TUMOR	PERCENTAGE OF CASES RELATED TO KNOWN GERMLINE MUTATIONS	SYNDROMES/GENES INVOLVED	CLUES FOR THE PATHOLOGIST
Adrenocortical carcinoma in children	50–100%	Li–Fraumeni, Beckwith–Wiedemann, MEN1	Unusual occurrence in a child
Angiomyolipoma of kidney	20%	Tuberous sclerosis	Patients may be screened for other features of tuberous sclerosis
Basal cell carcinoma	Rare if solitary	Nevoid basal cell carcinoma syndrome	Risk of a mutation is increased if multiple or if tumor occurs at <30 years of age
Breast cancer, poorly differentiated, ER negative[a]	>25% if <35 years old, <10% if >35 years old	BRCA1	BRCA1 cancers are more likely to have "medullary" features, and be ER− PR− HER-2/neu−. BRCA1 mutation more likely if patient has a family history or has bilateral cancer
Breast cancer, male	4–14%	BRCA2	Cancers are of no specific type
Colorectal carcinoma, poorly differentiated, mucinous, or with prominent lympho-cytic infiltrate	~10–15% overall, ~80% if patient is <40	HNPCC	HNPCC carcinomas are more likely right-sided (two thirds), poorly differentiated ("medullary"), mucinous, signet ring, lymphocytic infiltrate. IHC for MSH2 and MLH1 can be used to detect many, but not all, cases, but MLH1 may also be absent in sporadic cases
GI neuroendocrine tumors: Somatostatinoma PPoma Non-functioning Gastrinoma Glucagonoma VIPoma Insulinoma Carcinoid	45% 18–44% 18–44% 20–25% 1–20% 6% 4–5% Rare	MEN1 mutations	MEN1 mutations are also found in 15–70% of sporadic neuroendocrine tumors
Hirschsprung's disease	20–40%	MEN2A (RET mutations in codons 609, 618, 620)	
Juvenile (hamar-tomatous) polyps	Rare if solitary	Juvenile polyposis syndrome (JPS)	Suspect JPS if there are >5 polyps, if present throughout the GI tract, or if there is a family history of juvenile polyps
Medullary carcinoma of the thyroid	25%	MEN2A, MEN2B, Familial medullary carcinoma (RET mutations)	May be multiple and associated with C-cell hyperplasia Cancers in occur in children in MEN2B and in young adults in MEN2A
Medulloblastoma	Rare (?)	Nevoid basal cell carcinoma syndrome	If <3 years of age or of desmoplastic type, risk of mutation is increased
Myxoma, cardiac	<5%	Carney complex	Increased likelihood if multiple, right sided, and/or recurrent and in young patients (<30)
Neurofibromas	~10% if solitary but > 90% if plexiform	Neurofibromatosis type 1	Increased risk if there are ≥2 neurofibromas or one plexiform neurofibroma

Table 7-35 Pathologic features of tumors and diseases suggestive of a germline mutation—*cont'd*

TYPE OF TUMOR	PERCENTAGE OF CASES RELATED TO KNOWN GERMLINE MUTATIONS	SYNDROMES/GENES INVOLVED	CLUES FOR THE PATHOLOGIST
Ovarian carcinoma	Rare	BRCA1, BRCA2	Increased risk if there is a history of breast cancer BRCA1-associated carcinomas are more likely to be serous in type
Pheochromocytoma	30% of all cases, 59% if patient is <18, 84% if bilateral	MEN2A, MEN2B, VHL, isolated familial pheochromocytoma	Multiple tumors, hyperplasia of the medulla
Primary pigmented nodular adreno-cortical disease	>90%	Carney complex	May present with Cushing's syndrome Most are associated with germline mutations, but patients may not have other manifestations of the Carney complex
Retinoblastoma	40% of all cases, 100% if bilateral or with a positive family history	RB mutations (13q14.1-q14.2)	
Rhabdomyoma of heart in infants	50%	Tuberous sclerosis	
Sarcoma, children	7–33%	Li–Fraumeni, basal cell nevus syndrome, neurofibromatosis type 1, pleuropulmonary blastoma syndrome	
Sebaceous carcinoma	~10% if ocular, 40% if above the chin, 80% if elsewhere	HNPCC	Increased likelihood if the tumor has cystic degeneration or features of keratoacanthoma Usually due to germline MSH2 mutations
Schwannoma, psammomatous melanotic	>50%	Carney complex	Higher likelihood if patient is young (<30 years) and/or multiple tumors present
Schwannoma, vestibular	5%	Neurofibromatosis type 2	Risk is increased if the patient is <30 or if there is bilateral involvement Sporadic cases almost all have somatic NF2 mutations
Sertoli cell tumor, large-cell calcifying	25–35%	Carney complex, Peutz–Jeghers	Most are bilateral and multifocal in young patients. Rarely malignant
Trichilemmoma, facial, multiple	~80%	PTEN	Sporadic tumors also have loss of PTEN, which can be shown by IHC.
Wilms' tumor	10–15%	Germline mutations in WT1 (11p13)	Nephrogenic rests are present and may be extensive 5–10% of cases associated with germline mutations are multicentric or bilateral Associated with WAGR syndrome (Wilms' tumor, aniridia, GU anomalies, mental retardation) and Denys–Drash syndrome

[a] See reference 17 for additional information relating pathologic characteristics to risk of a BRCA1 mutation.

Table 7-36 Hereditary syndromes associated with multiple tumors

SYNDROME	GERMLINE MUTATIONS	TUMORS (% OF PATIENTS DEVELOPING TUMOR)	COMMENTS
Beckwith–Wiedemann syndrome	11p15 abnormalities (loss of methylation, uniparental disomy, mutations in *CDKN1C*)	Wilms' tumor, neuroblastoma, hepatoblastoma, adrenocortical carcinoma, rhabdomyosarcoma	Macrosomia, macroglossia, visceromegaly, ear creases and pits, omphalocele, hypoglycemia
BRCA1 and 2	*BRCA1* (17q21), *BRCA2* (13q12.3)	Breast (85%), ovary (BRCA1 63%, BRCA2 27%), prostate carcinoma, others	BRCA1 breast cancers are more often poorly differentiated, have medullary features, are ER– PR– HER-2/neu–, and have p53 mutations. Ovarian carcinomas are generally serous (90%), high grade, and bilateral. BRCA2 cancers do not have specific pathologic features
Carney complex	Type 1 (CNC1): PRKAR1A (17q23-24) Type 2 (CNC2): locus at 2p16	Myxomas (cardiac, cutaneous, breast), primary pigmented nodular adrenocortical disease (25%), large-cell calcifying Sertoli cell tumors (>90% males), multiple thyroid nodules or carcinoma (75%), growth hormone producing pituitary adenoma (10%), psammomatous melanotic schwannoma (10%), breast duct adenomas, osteochondromyxoma of bone Pigmented skin lesions (lentigos, blue nevi (especially epithelioid blue nevus), cafe-au-lait spots)	
Carney triad	Unknown	Gastric gastrointestinal stromal tumor, pulmonary chondroma, extra-adrenal paraganglioma Also esophageal leiomyomas and adrenocortical tumors	Most patients are young and female. Only 22% have all three tumors. Most family members are not affected
Familial adenomatous polyposis (FAP; including Gardner syndrome and Turcot syndrome)	*APC* (5q21-22)	Colorectal carcinoma, upper GI carcinoma, desmoid, osteoma, thyroid, brain (one third to two thirds are medulloblastomas—Turcot syndrome)	
Familial medullary thyroid carcinoma	*RET* mutations in codons 10, 11, 13, 14 (10q11.2)	Medullary thyroid carcinoma	Cancers usually occur in adults
Hereditary diffuse gastric cancer syndrome	*CDH1* (e-cadherin) (16q22.1)	Signet ring cell carcinoma of the stomach (67% men, 83% women), lobular carcinoma of the breast (39% women)	50% of sporadic signet ring cell carcinomas have *CDH1* somatic mutations and all show loss of e-cadherin by IHC
Hereditary non-polyposis syndrome	Mismatch repair genes: *MSH2* (2p22-p21) (40%), *MLH1* (3p21.3) (40%), *MSH6* (2p16) (5–7%), *PMS2* (7p22) (rare)	Colon carcinoma (80%), endometrial carcinoma (20–60%), ovarian carcinoma (9–12%), stomach carcinoma (11–19%), hepatobiliary tumors (2–7%), transitional cell carcinoma (4–5%, esp. ureter and renal pelvis), small bowel tumors (1–4%), lymphoma (rare) Sebaceous skin tumors, adenomas, epitheliomas, carcinoma, keratoacanthomas (Muir–Torre, usually *MSH2*)	Colon carcinomas are more likely (overall, 66%) to be on the right side, poorly differentiated ("medullary"), mucinous, signet ring, or undifferentiated, with a prominent lymphocytic infiltrate IHC can be used to detect the absence of *MSH2* (usually

Table 7-36 Hereditary syndromes associated with multiple tumors—*cont'd*

SYNDROME	GERMLINE MUTATIONS	TUMORS (% OF PATIENTS DEVELOPING TUMOR)	COMMENTS
			due to germline mutations) and *MLH1* (can be due to germline mutations, epigenetic changes, or less commonly, somatic mutations) in many patients MSI testing is also used
Juvenile polyposis syndrome	*MADH4* (or *SMAD4*) (18q21.10) (15%) or *BMPR1A* (10q22.3) (25%)	Hamartomatous (juvenile) polyps, GI carcinomas	
Li–Fraumeni	p53 (17p13.1), rarely *CHEK2* (22q12.1)	Sarcomas, breast cancer, leukemia, osteosarcomas, brain tumors, adrenocortical carcinoma, others	
MEN1	*MEN1* (11q13)	Pituitary adenoma, pancreatic islet cell tumors, parathyroid adenomas, adrenocortical tumors, carcinoids, lipomas	*MEN1* mutations also occur in 15–70% of sporadic neuroendocrine tumors
MEN2A	*RET* exon 10 and 11 missense mutations (10q11.2)	Medullary thyroid carcinoma (95%), hyperplasia of the parathyroids (15–30%), pheochromo-cytoma (50%), ganglioneuromatosis of GI tract Subsets of patients have Hirschsprung's disease or cutaneous lichen amyloidosus	Specific mutations correlate with age at development of medullary thyroid carcinoma
MEN2B	*RET* missense mutation in exon 16 (10q11.2)	Medullary thyroid carcinoma (100%), pheochromocytoma (50%) Mucosal neuromas of lips and tongue	Marfanoid habitus, distinctive facies
Nevoid basal cell carcinoma syndrome (Gorlin syndrome)	*PTCH* (9q22.3)	Basal cell carcinomas (90%), odontogenic keratocysts (90%), cardiac or ovarian fibromas (20%), medulloblastoma in childhood (5%)	Macrocephaly, skeletal anomalies, palmar or plantar pits, calcification of falx (90%)
Neurofibromatosis type 1	*NF1* (17q11.2)	Neurofibromas (esp. plexiform) (100%), optic gliomas, adrenal ganglioneuromas, pheochromo-cytoma (0.1–6%), MPNST (10%), leukemia, ganglioneuromatosis of the GI tract	Café-au-lait macules (95%), iris hamartomas (Lisch nodules), axillary freckling
Neurofibromatosis type 2	*NF2* (22q12.2)	Bilateral vestibular schwannomas (100%, 40% have lobular pattern), schwannomas of other nerves, meningiomas (50%, often fibroblastic)	
Peutz–Jeghers (hamartomatous polyp) syndrome	*LKB1/STK11* (19p13.3)	Colon, breast, stomach, pancreas, small bowel, thyroid, lung, uterus, sex cord stromal tumors, calcifying Sertoli cell tumors Hamartomatous polyps of GI tract	Perioral pigmentation
Pheochromo-cytoma or paraganglioma, familial	*SDHB* (1p36.1-p35), *SDHD* (11q23) *SDHC* (1q21) (paraganglioma)	Pheochromocytoma, paraganglioma	Patients are more commonly young (<40), with multifocal adrenal tumors, or extra-adrenal disease *SDHD* is imprinted and only confers susceptibility after paternal transmission

Table 7-36 Hereditary syndromes associated with multiple tumors—*cont'd*

SYNDROME	GERMLINE MUTATIONS	TUMORS (% OF PATIENTS DEVELOPING TUMOR)	COMMENTS
PTEN hamartoma syndrome (including 80% of Cowden's syndrome, 50–60% of Bannayan–Riley–Ruvalcaba syndrome)	*PTEN* (10q23.31)	Breast cancer (25 to 50%), thyroid carcinoma (10%, esp. follicular), endometrial carcinoma (5–10%), hamartomatous polyps of GI tract Multiple facial trichilemmomas, acral keratosis, oral papillomatous lesions, mucosal lesions	Macrocephaly (megalencephaly, 97th percentile), Lhermitte–Duclos disease
Tuberous sclerosis	*TSC1* (9q34), *TSC2* (16p13.3)	Subependymal glial nodules (90%), cortical or subcortical tubers (70%), angiomyolipoma of kidney (70%), lymphangiomyomatosis of lung (1–6%), rhabdomyoma of heart (47–67%) Skin lesions (100%, including myomelanotic macules, multiple facial angiofibromas, shagreen patch, fibrous facial plaque, ungual fibroma)	Seizures (80%), developmental delay or retardation (50%)
Von Hippel–Lindau (VHL)	*VHL* (3p26-p25)	Hemangioblastomas (retinal, cerebellar, spinal cord) (80%), renal cell carcinoma (40%), renal cysts, pancreatic cysts, Pheochromocytoma, endolymphatic sac tumors (10%), epididymal cystadenomas	

For additional information on most syndromes, see http://www.genetests.org/ and Online Mendelian Inheritance in Man (OMIM; www.ncbi.nlm.nih.gov).

■ ANALYTICAL CYTOLOGY (FLOW CYTOMETRY)

Flow cytometers analyze populations of thousands of disaggregated cells as they pass by stationary detectors. Cell size and cytoplasmic granularity can be measured as well as DNA content and the presence or absence of immunohistochemical markers added to the cell suspension. Newer techniques can analyze three or more features simultaneously to divide cells into unique populations. DNA content can be used to determine the number of cells in S-phase (a measure of proliferation—S-phase fraction). Because cells are not visualized by this technique, it is important to be sure that only lesional tissue is submitted.

Indications for ploidy and S-phase analysis

- Hydatidiform moles: complete (diploid), partial (triploid).
- Some carcinomas: DNA ploidy and S-phase fraction have been reported to be of prognostic significance for some carcinomas (e.g., colon, breast, and prostate) but the analysis is not routinely performed at all institutions or used by all oncologists.

Indications for cell surface marker analysis

- Lymphomas.
- Leukemias.

Method for submitting tissue

Single cell suspensions are necessary for analysis. For fresh tissues, cells must be viable. Fresh tissue (approximately 0.3 to 0.5 cm³) is placed in a specimen container and kept moist with HBSS. Tissues can be held overnight in the refrigerator.

Formalin-fixed paraffin-embedded sections may also be used for DNA ploidy analysis by the Hedley method, although the results are not as satisfactory due to nuclear fragmentation.

Results

The results are usually incorporated into the final surgical pathology report.

■ CYTOLOGIC PREPARATIONS FROM SURGICAL SPECIMENS

Cytologic preparations of surgical specimens often provide additional information.

Intraoperative diagnosis. Touch preps or smears are especially valuable for:

- Infectious cases (to avoid contamination of the cryostat and aerosolization of infectious agents)
- Neuropathology cases, for diagnosis and for the performance of cytogenetic (FISH) analysis

- Tumors (for excellent cytologic detail, especially lymphomas and papillary carcinomas of the thyroid).

Special stains. Stains for microorganisms can be performed the same day on cytologic smears of specimens from critically ill patients. Do not submit air dried smears of infectious cases for staining as the unfixed material may constitute a hazard to laboratory personnel.

Fat is dissolved during routine processing, but can be demonstrated with fat stains on air dried slides.

Genetic studies (FISH). Nuclei are intact in touch preparations, unlike tissue sections in which the only partial nuclei are present. This feature makes touch preparations superior for techniques such as FISH and image analysis.

It is always a useful exercise to look at cytology preparations and the corresponding surgical specimen to learn the comparative morphology of these techniques.

■ SPECIMEN RADIOGRAPHY

Specimen radiographs are often preferred to patient radiographs:

- A permanent record of the radiograph can be kept with the case.
- A radiograph of the specimen may reveal more details of the underlying process (e.g., fewer structures may be present to complicate the appearance).
- A significant time interval may have elapsed between the patient radiograph and the surgical excision.
- The radiograph often indicates sites that are important to examine histologically (tumor invasion into a rib or microcalcifications in a breast biopsy).
- The specimen radiograph can confirm that the clinical lesion was removed.

Indications

- Tumors of bone and cartilage.
- Tumors invading into bone.
- Avascular necrosis.
- All bioprosthetic heart valves (to document the degree of calcification).
- Breast biopsies or mastectomies performed for mammographic lesions that cannot be located grossly. Paraffin blocks of breast tissue can be radiographed if microcalcifications were seen by specimen radiography but not in histologic sections and were not identified prior to processing.

Calcifications can dissolve in formalin over several days. If the demonstration of calcifications is important (e.g., mammographically detected calcifications) it is preferable to process the tissue within 1 to 2 days. If processing is to be delayed, the tissue can be stored in ethanol.

Method

Radiographic equipment is available in radiology departments and in some pathology departments. The specimen may be placed on a piece of wax paper (to keep the surfaces clean) lying on the film. Specimens can be radiographed after decalcification (not all calcium is removed) but best results are obtained on fresh undecalcified specimens. Lungs should not be inflated prior to radiography.

If the specimen is small, two exposures at different settings or at different angles may be useful. Lead sheets can be used to allow two exposures on one piece of film.

If the film is too dark (overexposed), the exposure is too high and a lower setting should be tried. If the film is too light (i.e., unexposed) the exposure is too low and a higher setting is indicated.

Special injection techniques with radiocontrast media are available for unusual specimens such as a recipient lung with pulmonary hypertension or vascular ectasia of the bowel.

Octreotide and sentinel nodes. Labeled compounds are sometimes used to localize certain types of tumors (generally neuroendocrine) or sentinel lymph nodes. The patient is injected with the isotope prior to surgery and the surgeon uses a handheld probe to identify the labeled tissue. The amount of radioactivity in the tissue is small; generally it does not pose a hazard to pathologists handling the tissue and does not need special disposal methods. However, each pathology department should consult with the radiation safety department to ensure appropriate handling of such tissues. In some cases, if a gross lesion is not present corresponding to the area of octreotide uptake, specimens can be imaged using a gamma camera.

Results

The radiographs are documented in the gross description and any information gained from the radiograph is incorporated into the surgical pathology report.

■ TISSUE FOR RESEARCH: TUMOR BANK

The pathology department is a unique resource for researchers who need human tissues. The pathologist plays a key role as patient advocate and diagnostician in order to provide appropriate human tissues for biologic research. Most hospitals have a policy that allows the release of tissue for research *if it would otherwise be discarded*. Therefore, tissue is never given away for research until all necessary tissue has been taken for diagnosis. Tissue from primary diagnostic breast biopsies and open lung biopsies without gross lesions should not be given away. It is in the best interest of the patient that a pathologist evaluates the specimen rather than have tissue given away by a nonpathologist who is not aware of what is needed for diagnosis.

Indications

By request of researchers who have obtained permission from the hospital Human Studies Committee.

Method

Adequate information must be provided by the clinician to allow the pathologist to determine how much of the tissue is needed for diagnostic purposes. Research laboratories should provide containers for the transport of specimens. The name of the laboratory, the type of tissue, and the amount of tissue allocated for research must be carefully documented. Tissue should never be given away if there is any question as to the need for the tissue for diagnostic purposes. In some cases it may be preferable (or possibly required) to withhold the name or other identifiers of the patient for medical confidentiality.

■ MICROBIOLOGIC CULTURE AND SMEARS

The investigation of infectious disease by culture is complementary to its investigation by histologic sections (Table 7-37).

Table 7-37 Identification of infectious diseases

CULTURE	HISTOLOGIC SECTIONS
Can be performed on aspirates, swabs, fluids, or tissues	Requires surgical excision of tissues
Cultures amplify the number of organisms present, allowing them to be recognized	Organisms may be rare, or not seen in tissue sections
The specific organism can be identified and tested for drug susceptibility	Categories of organisms can be recognized but specific identification may not be possible
Some organisms cannot be cultured	Many organisms can be identified that will not grow in culture or that require long culture times (e.g., *Mycobacterium tuberculosis*)
It may be difficult to exclude contamination for a positive culture	Morphologic evidence of an inflammatory response provides evidence for a clinical infection. The location of the infection may be of diagnostic importance (e.g., cellulitis versus necrotizing fasciitis or superficial colonization of devitalized tissue versus deep infections involving viable tissues)

Indications

- Suspected infectious processes.
- Suspected sarcoid to exclude an infectious process.

Method

Tissue is kept as sterile as possible. Suture removal kits are a convenient source of sterile scissors and forceps. Serially section the specimen to determine whether there are focal lesions. Place representative sections in a sterile specimen container. Label with the patient's name and unit number, patient's physician, type of specimen, collection date, and time of collection (required for JCAHO accreditation).

Three different types of culture are often requested (requiring three different requisition forms):

1. Routine culture. The usual request for routine specimens would be:

- Bacteria (only includes aerobic culture)
- Mycobacteria
- Fungal.

Other organisms require special culture techniques and must be specifically requested:

- Anaerobic bacteria
- *Salmonella*, *Shigella*, and *Campylobacter*
- *Nocardia*
- *Neisseria gonorrhoeae*
- *Brucella*
- *Legionella*
- *Francisella tularensis*
- *Helicobacter*.

2. Viral culture. CMV, varicella zoster, adenovirus, and herpes simplex are most commonly requested. Cultures for influenza A and B, Respiratory synctial virus, and parainfluenza require special techniques.

3. Mycoplasma. Usually requires special cultures. Occasionally, mycoplasma can be detected on anaerobic cultures, but this is not the optimal means for identifying this organism.

Results

The results are generally reported by the microbiology laboratory. It is helpful to correlate the results with the pathologic findings, when possible.

REFERENCES

1. Werner M, Chott A, Fabiano A, Battifora H. Effect of formalin fixation and processing on immunohistochemistry. Am J Surg Pathol 24:1016-1019, 2000.
2. Arber JM, Arber DA, Jenkins KA, Battifora H. Effect of decalcification and fixation in paraffin-section immunohistochemistry. Appl Immunohistochem 4:241-248, 1996.

3. DiVito KA, Charette LA, Rimm DL, Camp RL. Long-term preservation of antigenicity on tissue microarrays. Lab Invest 84:1071-1078, 2004.

4. Jacobs TW, Prioleau JE, Stillman IE, Schnitt SJ. Loss of tumor marker immunostaining intensity on stored paraffin slides of breast cancer. J Natl Cancer Inst 88:1054-1059, 1996.

5. Bertheau P, Cazals-Hatem D, Meignin V, et al. Variability of immunohistochemical reactivity on paraffin slides. J Clin Pathol 51:370-374, 1998.

6. van den Broek LJ, van de Vijver MJ. Assessment of problems in diagnostic and research immunohistochemistry associated with epitope instability in stored paraffin sections. Appl Immunohistochem Mol Morphol 8:316-321, 2000.

7. Battifora H. Assessment of antigen damage in immunohistochemistry, the vimentin internal control. Am J Clin Pathol 6:669-671, 1991.

8. Chu PG, Weiss LM. Keratin expression in human tissues and neoplasms. Histopathology 40:403-439, 2002.

9. Gyure KA, Morrison AC. Cytokeratin 7 and 20 expression in choroid plexus tumors: utility in differentiating these neoplasms from metastatic carcinomas. Mod Pathol 13:638-643, 2000.

10. Wang NP, Zee S, Zarbo RJ, Bacchi CE, Gown AM. Coordinate expression of cytokeratins 7 and 20 defines unique subsets of carcinomas. Appl Immunohistochem 3:99-107, 1995.

11. Mierau GW, Berry PJ, Malott RL, et al. Appraisal of the comparative utility of immunohistochemistry and electron microscopy in the diagnosis of childhood round cell tumors. Ultrastruct Pathol 20:507-517, 1996.

12. Varadhachary GR, Abbruzzese JL, Lenzi R. Diagnostic strategies for unknown primary cancer. Cancer 100:1776-1785, 2004.

13. Corson J. Pathology of mesothelioma. Thorac Surg Clin 14: 447-460, 2004.

14. Banks PM. Incorporation of immunostaining data in anatomic pathology reports. Am J Surg Pathol 16:808, 1992.

15. Electron microscopy of tumors. Semin Diagn Pathol 20: 2003. *The entire February 2003 issue is devoted to EM.*

16. Wittel VA, Goel A, Varshney GC, Batra SK. Mucin antibodies – new tools in diagnosis and therapy of cancer. Front Biosci 6: D 1296-310, 2001.

17. Lakhani SR, et al. The pathology of familial breast cancer: predictive value of immunohistochemical markers estrogen receptor, progesterone receptor, HER-2, and p53 in patients with mutations in BRCA1 and BRCA2. J Clin Oncol 20:2310-2318, 2002.

Safety precautions

8

A pathology department can be a dangerous place to work. Hazards include physical injury (scalpel cuts, needlestick injuries), infectious disease, radioactivity, and noxious chemical fumes. Although we all take risks when we work with specimens from patients, these risks can be minimized for both ourselves and our coworkers by following the procedures outlined below.

■ INFECTIOUS DISEASE: THE BAD NEWS

The incidence of infectious diseases, particularly those that are incurable or difficult to treat, is rising. In a study of patients undergoing major surgery in New York,[1] 5.2% were HCV positive, 1.4% HBV positive, and 1.6% HIV positive (or 6.7% with one or more of these viruses). Often, the presence of infection is unknown or is not reported to the pathology department. Healthcare workers are at risk for contracting these diseases when working with patients (Box 8-1). The risk is lower for pathology personnel, but exposure can occur by aerosolization of tissues, needlestick injury, scalpel wounds, and mucocutaneous exposure during the processing of pathology specimens.

Other infectious agents (e.g., other types of bacteria or fungi, *Pneumocystis carinii*, other viral agents) are also

---

Box 8-1

Diseases that have been transmitted to healthcare workers

- Hepatitis B, C, and A
- Tuberculosis (including strains resistant to multiple drugs)
- HIV
- Syphilis
- Creutzfeldt–Jakob disease
- *Coccidioides immitis* (the risk arises primarily from cultures of the fungus in microbiology laboratories); if this infection is suspected, all specimens must be labeled appropriately
- Parvovirus and *H. pylori* infection, cryptosporidiosis, scabies, pertussis

---

potential dangers, particularly to immunocompromised healthcare workers, but transmission is very rare and has not yet been reported.

■ INFECTIOUS DISEASE: THE GOOD NEWS

The actual incidence of transmission of infectious agents from *unfixed surgical specimens* to pathology department personnel is extremely low. There are only three reported cases, all involving conversion to positive tuberculin skin tests after use of an aerosolized gas coolant to freeze a tissue block during an intraoperative consultation.[2,3] However, transmission of other types of infectious disease is theoretically possible: transmission of HBV, HIV, and TB has occurred during the performance of autopsies.

The good news is that pathology personnel can take action to protect themselves by educating themselves about risks, taking physical precautions to protect themselves and others, avoiding the use of hollow-bore needles, and making sure they are vaccinated for HBV (Table 8-1). Personnel who are immunocompromised must be especially vigilant.

Hepatitis B virus[4,5]

The CDC estimated that 18,000 healthcare workers whose jobs entailed exposure to blood became infected with HBV each year prior to widespread vaccination. Of these, 200 to 300 died of complications of HBV infection. Prior to widespread vaccination, 25% to 30% of pathologists were positive for HBV, their exposure likely being due to the performance of autopsies. However, the incidence of HBV infection has sharply declined with vaccination. All pathology department workers who come into contact with tissue should be vaccinated. OSHA bloodborne standards require that employers offer the vaccine at no cost to all employees at risk. (http://www.osha.gov).

After a needlestick injury, the seroconversion rate is 30% from HBeAg-positive blood and <6% from HBeAg-negative blood in non-vaccinated individuals. Mucocutaneous exposure can also occur.

Table 8.1 Risk of exposure to common infectious agents

AGENT	PERCENTAGE OF HOSPITAL PATIENTS	RISK OF INFECTION AFTER PERCUTANEOUS INJURY[a]	RISK AFTER MUCOCUTANEOUS EXPOSURE	RISK OF ENVIRONMENTAL EXPOSURE	POSTEXPOSURE PROPHYLAXIS AVAILABLE
HIV	~0.2–14%	0.3%	0.09%	Possible, but very rare	Yes, effective
HCV	~2–5%	1.8%	Rare	Yes, but rapidly degrades	No, not shown to be effective
HBV	~2%	30%	Yes, probably high	Occurs, can be found in dried blood ~1 week	Yes, effective
TB	~10%	Yes, risk not quantified	Yes, risk not quantified	Yes	No, treatment initiated only if skin test converts

[a] Percutaneous injury: needlestick injury (majority) or other penetrating injury with a sharp object (e.g., scalpel, broken glass).

Postexposure prophylaxis with HBV hyperimmune globulin and vaccine is suggested for non-vaccinated individuals or vaccinated persons with low antibody titers. Treatment provides approximately 75% protection from infection if instituted within a week.

Hepatitis C virus[4-6]

The seroprevalence of HCV in healthcare workers has ranged from 0% to 1.7% in multiple studies. Occupational infections in pathology personnel have not been reported. Eighty percent to 90% of infections will become chronic with risk for the development of chronic hepatitis, cirrhosis (3% to 20% of patients), and hepatocellular carcinoma. HCV has also been linked to cryoglobulinemia and many other immune system related diseases.

The risk is approximately 1–8% for HCV transmission after a needlestick injury. The risk after skin or mucous membrane exposure is likely to be very low.

Postexposure treatment has not been shown to be effective. If there has been a potential exposure, the person should be monitored for infection in order to start treatment as early as possible.

Human immunodeficiency virus[5,7-10]

As of 2001, 57 healthcare workers had developed HIV infection following documented occupational exposure; an additional 138 workers were considered possible cases. Most exposures (88%) were percutaneous and involved hollow-bore needles, scalpels, and broken vials: 20% of exposures occurred during the disposal of sharp objects. Mucous membrane and skin exposure were responsible in about 10% of cases. The source in almost all cases was infected blood (86%). The risk is increased with the volume of blood, the depth of the injury, and the viral titer of the patient (with an increased risk with patients close to death).

A pathologist was infected by HIV after a scalpel wound to the hand during an autopsy.[11] Surgical specimens containing blood could also potentially transmit the virus, if an injury occurs. HIV can be cultured from cadavers hours to days after death.[12] The effect of fixation has not been studied but would presumably lower or eliminate risk.

> Approximately 0.3% of persons will seroconvert after a needlestick exposure to HIV, 0.1% after mucocutaneous exposure, and <0.1% after skin exposure.

Postexposure treatment with antiviral agents can decrease the risk of seroconversion by 81%. Treatment should be started as soon as possible, as it may be less effective after 2 to 3 days. Additional agents used in combination for prophylaxis may be more effective, as the source patients for occupational cases have a high prevalence of drug-resistant HIV.[13] There have been 21 cases of healthcare personnel becoming infected with HIV despite postexposure prophylaxis.

Tuberculosis

The risk of transmission of TB to autopsy personnel during the performance of necroscopies is well documented. TB can be transmitted not only as an aerosol but also percutaneously.[14] It must be kept in mind that many cases of TB are first diagnosed after death. Multiple individuals had conversion to a positive skin test after the autopsy of an infected person.[15] Exposure can be diminished by wearing special respiratory protection.

Healthcare workers also have a significant risk of contracting multiple-drug-resistant tuberculosis. Although healthcare workers have been infected by drug-resistant TB, no fatal case has yet been reported in the absence of an underlying immunodeficiency disorder.

There are no definitive studies on the survival of mycobacteria in fixed surgical specimens.[16,17] Formalin probably kills mycobacteria, but the time required for it to do so is unknown.

Special respiratory protective devices are recommended for personnel who may be exposed to tuberculosis.

If an exposed person does not develop a positive skin test, no treatment is necessary. Converters and persons who are immunocompromised should be treated.

Hospital workers are required to undergo yearly TB testing.

Severe acute respiratory syndrome[18]

Severe acute respiratory syndrome (SARS) was first identified in China in late 2002. It is caused by SARS-associated coronavirus (SARS-CoV) and spreads via respiratory droplets contacting the mucous membranes of a second person. Occupationally acquired cases have occurred among healthcare workers. The risk to surgical pathology personnel is likely to be low, as most patients will not undergo surgical procedures. However, autopsies may be performed.

There are no reported cases of SARS being transferred via the handling of pathology specimens. However, as there is little experience with this virus, all cases from patients with known or suspected SARS may best be handled as for cases of HBV. All tissue should be promptly fixed and the cryostat decontaminated if necessary.

Creutzfeldt–Jakob disease[19,20]

The only cases of infection in laboratory personnel from *fixed tissue* are due to Creutzfeldt–Jakob disease (CJD). As of 1995, 24 healthcare workers had developed CJD, including two histotechnologists and one pathologist. Infectious units are present in fixed and paraffin-embedded tissue for years. Any adult patient with a rapidly progressive dementia, myoclonus, and nonspecific neurologic findings should be considered as potentially having the disease.

All tissues from affected patients can potentially cause infection. The virus is not inactivated by standard formalin fixation or boiling water. Tissues should be fixed in formalin for 24 hours, then in 95% formic acid for one hour followed by formalin fixation for one day.

■ BIOLOGIC TERRORISM[21-27] (Table 8-2)

It is to be hoped that pathologists will not receive specimens from acts of biologic terrorism, but, should such an event occur, pathologists can aid in recognizing the disease and the likely method of infection. The first anthrax case in 2001 was suspected when typical organisms were seen on a Gram stain of CSF. The autopsy determined that the mode of exposure was inhalation and this finding helped direct investigators to search for possible sources of airborne spores.

In the event of an actual or threatened bioterrorist attack, local health and law enforcement agencies should

be contacted. Additional information can be found at www.bt.cdc.gov/emcontact/index.asp or the CDC Emergency Response Hotline 770-488-7100.

The CDC recommends saving tissue from autopsies (and other specimens) from possible victims of biologic terrorism:

- Fixed tissue: Histologic examination for patterns of tissue damage and special stains for identification of organisms. IHC and DFA assays are available at the CDC and most can be performed on fixed tissue.
- Blood, CSF, tissue samples or swabs for bacterial and viral culture. Mucosal swabs for cases of possible botulinum toxin inhalation.
- Serum for biologic and serologic assays.
- Frozen tissue for PCR.
- Fixed tissue (glutaraldehyde) for EM to identify viral particles.

The Laboratory Response Network

The Laboratory Response Network (LRN) is a partnership of local, state, and federal public health laboratories, and veterinary, food, and environmental laboratories, the CDC, the Food and Drug Administration, the Environmental Protection Agency, the US Army Medical Research Institute of Infectious Diseases, and other Department of Defense laboratories. The network functions to channel specimens from sentinel laboratories to advanced laboratories for confirmation and final identification of pathogens. Specimens from cases suspected to be related to biologic terrorism can be submitted to the state public health laboratory. Contact information for all state laboratories is included in the CDC guidebook listed in the resources. If the suspected agent is smallpox, the state laboratory should be notified as such specimens may be transported directly to the CDC.

Risks to pathology personnel

All of the infectious agents listed in Table 8-2 could potentially be transmitted to personnel during the performance of an autopsy or by handling fresh tissue, except for botulinum toxin. Smallpox, tularemia, and viral hemorrhagic fevers have been transmitted to persons performing autopsies. Biologic terrorism raises an additional risk of surface contamination by the agent (e.g., powders used to transmit anthrax or botulinum toxin). Because of the incubation period, it is likely victims will have changed clothes and bathed so that such contamination, in most cases, will likely be minimal. Standard universal safety precautions should be used in all cases and should be protective.

Cadavers of patients dying of *B. anthracis*, *Y. pestis*, or botulinum toxin are unlikely to pose a threat to non-autopsy personnel (e.g., funeral home workers). However, smallpox virus and hemorrhagic fever viruses could be

Table 8.2 Agents most likely to be used for biologic terrorism (category A agents)

AGENT MODE OF TRANSMISSION	CLINICAL SYNDROME	PATHOLOGIC FINDINGS	APPEARANCE OF ORGANISM/ AVAILABLE TESTS[a]	TREATMENT/PROPHYLAXIS
Smallpox virus (variola major) Inhalation: aerosols Direct contact with lesions or contaminated surfaces Person to person spread	Diffuse rash (including palms and soles): deep-seated, firm/hard, round well-circumscribed vesicles or pustules, all in same stage of development Hemorrhage into skin and GI tract	Early vesicles are multilocular (but coalesce in later stages), ballooning degeneration of epithelial cells (not multinucleated), eosinophilic intracytoplasmic viral inclusions (Guarnieri bodies)	Viral inclusions present in cytoplasm IHC EM: fluid from vesicles can be used to detect viral particles PCR: viral DNA	Vaccine available.[b] Routine vaccination in the US ended in 1972. Persons with remote vaccination probably have some, but not complete, immunity
Bacillus anthracis (anthrax) Direct contact with spores (skin or ingestion) Inhalation of spores No person to person spread	Cutaneous: eschar with hemorrhage, edema, necrosis, perivascular infiltrate, vasculitis Gastrointestinal: hemorrhagic enteritis, hemorrhagic lymphadenitis, mucosal ulcers with necrosis in the terminal ileum and cecum, peritonitis Inhalational: hemorrhagic mediastinitis, hemorrhagic lymphadenitis, hemorrhagic pleural effusion CNS: hemorrhagic meningitis	Skin: edema, focal necrosis, vasculitis, acute inflammation, ulceration Organisms only rarely seen by H&E Lymph nodes: hemorrhage, necrosis After antibiotic treatment, organisms may only be visible by silver stains and IHC	Gram, silver stains: large, broad (3 × 5 μm) encapsulated Gram-positive bacilli with flattened ends in short chains India ink: shows capsule in blood and CSF IHC: sensitive and specific DFA (but cannot be used on formalin-fixed tissue) PCR: formalin or fresh tissue	Vaccine available[b] Antibiotic prophylaxis available
Yersinia pestis (plague) Flea bites Inhalation: aerosols Person to person spread	Bubonic: acute lymphadenitis with surrounding edema (a bubo is a local painful swelling) Pneumonic: severe, hemorrhagic bronchopneumonia, often with fibrinous pleuritis, diffuse alveolar damage (ARDS), sepsis with DIC CNS: meningitis	Lung: Severe, confluent, hemorrhagic, necrotizing bronchopneumonia, often with fibrinous pleuritis Lymph nodes: Necrosis—preferred for histologic examination and culture	Gram, silver, Giemsa stains: short, silver, fat Gram-negative bacilli IHC DFA	Vaccine available (but does not protect against pneumonia)[b] Antibiotic prophylaxis available
Clostridium botulinum toxin (botulism) Ingestion or inhalation of preformed neurotoxin No person to person spread	CNS: hyperemia and microthrombosis of small vessels associated with symmetrical, descending pattern of weakness and paralysis of cranial nerves, limbs, and trunk	No specific findings for cases due to ingestion or inhalation of preformed toxin Swabs of mucosal surfaces or serum may be used for the botulinum toxin mouse bioassay Samples should be taken prior to the use of antitoxin	Gram-positive bacteria – however organisms unlikely to be present in a terror attack	Antitoxin available

Table 8.2 Agents most likely to be used for biologic terrorism (category A agents)—cont'd

AGENT MODE OF TRANSMISSION	CLINICAL SYNDROME	PATHOLOGIC FINDINGS	APPEARANCE OF ORGANISM/ AVAILABLE TESTS[a]	TREATMENT/PROPHYLAXIS
Francisella tularensis (tularemia) Tick bite Direct contact with infected fluids or tissues Ingestion of infected meat No person to person spread	Ulceroglandular: skin ulcer with associated suppurative lymphadenitis Glandular: suppurative necrotizing lymphadenitis without associated skin ulcer Oculoglandular: eyelid edema, acute conjunctivitis and edema, small conjunctival ulcers, regional lymphadenitis Pharyngeal: exudative pharyngitis or tonsillitis with ulceration, pharyngeal membrane formation, regional lymphadenitis Typhoidal: systemic involvement, DIC, focal necrosis of major organs Pneumonic: acute inflammation, diffuse alveolar damage	Ulcer with a nonspecific inflammatory infiltrate and a granulomatous reaction. In some cases, large necrotizing granulomas with giant cells may be present Lymph nodes: extensive necrosis, irregular microabscesses and multiple granulomas with caseous necrosis Lung: necrotizing pneumonia with abundant fibrin, acute inflammation	Small encapsulated Gram-negative coccobacilli—difficult to see with histochemical stains IHC DFA	Antibiotic prophylaxis available
Hemorrhagic fever viruses, including filoviruses (including Ebola and Marburg viruses) and arenaviruses (e.g., Lassa fever) Close personal contact with infected person, blood, tissue, or body fluids	Diffuse rash, massive hepatocellular necrosis, extensive necrosis in other major organs, diffuse alveolar damage	Massive hepatic necrosis with filamentous viral inclusions in hepatocytes, extensive necrosis of other organs	Viral inclusions in hepatocytes IHC EM: viral inclusions PCR	No specific treatment

ARDS, acute respiratory distress syndrome; DFA, direct fluorescent assay; DIC, disseminated intravascular coagulopathy; IHC, immunohistochemistry.
[a] IHC and DFA tests for each of these organisms are available at the CDC. Consult the CDC website to determine how to decide if a specimen is appropriate for testing and how to send such a sample: call the CDC at 404-639-3133 or fax the CDC at 404-639-3043 for more information.
[b] Vaccination is not currently recommended for individuals without a known exposure. Vaccination for smallpox may be considered for selected personnel who would be first responders for the examination of the remains or specimens from patients dying of smallpox.

transmitted and should only be handled with safety precautions. In general, such bodies should not be embalmed as this might impose increased risk.

Sending specimens to reference laboratories

Detailed instructions for the packaging and shipping of specimens to reference laboratories are available at the CDC website (www.cdc.gov). In general, such specimens must have three levels of containment and must be marked with an "Infectious Substance" label. The laboratory director of the state health department should be contacted before a specimen with a suspected biologic agent is shipped.

■ TRANSMISSION OF TUMORS

In general, malignant tumors do not pose a risk to any person other than the patient. However, malignancies can be transferred from a graft to an organ transplant recipient.[28]

There has been one case of a sarcoma transferred to the hand of a non-immunocompromised surgeon after a scalpel injury.[29] Thus, although the risk is extremely small, tumors (and all human tissue) must be handled with appropriate safety precautions.

■ GUIDELINES FOR PROCESSING SPECIMENS WITH KNOWN OR PROBABLE INFECTIOUS DISEASE

- **Specimens from patients with infections not posing a risk to immunocompetent individuals** (e.g., routine bacterial and fungal infections, opportunistic pathogens) can be processed as for other pathology specimens using universal precautions. Specimens from patients with infections (or suspected infections) posing a greater risk to pathology personnel (TB, HBV, HCV, HIV, CJD) must be handled with special precautions. All specimens must be fixed as soon as possible and stored in rigid leak-proof containers. *Gloves must always be worn when handling specimens.*
- **Fresh tissues** are potentially infective and all specimens are placed in fixative as soon as possible. Formalin effectively inactivates viruses (including HIV and HBV) and reduces the infectivity of mycobacteria. Procedures that could aerosolize an infectious agent (e.g., cutting a specimen with a bone saw) should not be performed. Tissue from a CJD patient requires special procedures for handling it safely (see "Creutzfeldt–Jakob disease," above).
- **Small specimens** (e.g., colon biopsies and open lung biopsies) are usually of immediate diagnostic importance

and can be processed as usual as long as the specimens are fixed in formalin for at least 4 to 6 hours.
- **Larger specimens**, if of no immediate diagnostic importance (e.g., a placenta from a normal delivery or a colon resection for trauma), can be sectioned thinly and placed in an adequate volume of fixative (1:10 specimen/formalin fixative ratio) for 72 hours before submitting for histologic processing. Placentas and products of conception must be fixed for 7 days before processing. If such a specimen is of diagnostic importance, small sections can be cut for blocks and fixed as above before processing.
- **Potentially infectious cases are not photographed in the fresh state.** If it is an especially interesting case, pictures may be taken after fixation if special precautions are used in order not to contaminate surfaces or the camera.
- **Frozen sections** on potentially infectious cases may be performed but should be avoided if cytologic preparations can be used or an intraoperative diagnosis is not necessary. Freezing does not inactivate infectious agents. If an infectious case is cut in a cryostat, the cryostat should be decontaminated. Pressurized sprays should not be used as this can aerosolize infectious agents. Air-dried slides should be considered potentially infectious and are not saved or submitted to the histology laboratory. Any smears submitted for special stains must be fixed in methanol.

Prevention of injuries and exposures

Prevention of injuries and exposures is the goal of all pathology personnel. Most injuries and exposure to blood and other body fluids can be prevented if the following guidelines are followed:

Gloves
- All fresh and fixed tissues must be handled with gloves. The use of two pairs of gloves is recommended as small tears in gloves are common. Metal mesh and Kevlar cloth type gloves are available and should be worn if puncture injuries are possible.
- Latex gloves protect against biohazards but not against fixatives. Nitrile gloves provide protection from fixatives. Some individuals (5% to 10%) have or develop allergic reactions (usually dermatitis but sometimes asthma or anaphylaxis) to latex antigens.
- Do not touch objects in general use (door handles, telephone, computer, etc.) with contaminated gloves. Hands must always be washed after handling specimens and after leaving a specimen handling area because gloves are not completely leak-proof.

Protective clothing
- Scrub suits or disposable jumpsuits are recommended if large, bloody specimens need to be processed.

- Aprons must be worn when handling many specimens (e.g., at a cutting bench) or handling large specimens.
- Protective clothing, including gloves, must be removed and disposed of properly before leaving the surgical cutting or OR consultation rooms.

Sharps

- Any person using a scalpel blade, razor blade, or syringe needle is responsible for disposing of it properly. Scalpel blades are removed from the handle with extreme caution after gross blood and tissue have been removed. OCT blocks are not removed from the chuck with a razor blade. Holding the stem for a few seconds will melt the OCT sufficiently for removal with a fingertip. Syringe needles are never recapped. All blades, needles, and disposable scissors must be discarded into impervious labeled sharps containers. Broken glass slides and coverslips must also be disposed of into designated containers.
- The most common site of an injury is the nondominant hand.
- Reusable but contaminated equipment should be decontaminated with bleach.

Tissue fixation

- All tissues are fixed as soon as possible. Unfixed specimens must be kept in leak-proof containers and stored in an appropriate biohazard refrigerator or freezer.
- Always dispose of all blood and tissue fragments before leaving a worksite. All tissues, or non-reusable material contaminated by any body fluid or tissue, must be disposed of in labeled hazardous waste containers (containers with red bags and biohazard symbols). Urine, blood, and feces may be disposed of directly into the municipal sewerage system.

Eye protection

- Areas contaminated after handling a known infectious case should be immediately cleaned with dilute bleach.
- Eye protection should be worn when cutting into large specimens. Cysts may feel deceptively solid when filled with fluid. Such fluid may be under pressure and can travel several feet when the cyst is opened (this has been documented by many pathologists!). Place the specimen near a sink on a surgical drape or blue barrier and make a small nick near the bottom in order to let fluid slowly drain out of the cyst.

Food

- Food or beverages must not be consumed, or brought into, the cutting room or the OR consultation room. Foods cannot be stored in refrigerators used to store specimens. Food or food containers (e.g., an empty coffee cup) cannot be disposed of into containers in these areas as this may be used as evidence that food consumption is occurring in these areas. Evidence of food consumption is monitored by OSHA and can be grounds for penalties or closure.

■ RECOMMENDATIONS FOR POSTEXPOSURE TREATMENT AND INCIDENT REPORTING

Unfortunately, accidents will occasionally occur. First aid is administered at the site. Bleeding injuries are allowed to bleed liberally. The site should be cleaned with soap and water. If there has been an eye or mucous membrane exposure, these sites are liberally flushed with water.

All exposures involving percutaneous inoculation or contact with an open wound, non-intact skin (e.g., chapped, abraded, weeping, or dermatitic), or mucous membranes by blood or tissue should be seen by a physician. The exposed person should record the name of the patient and the surgical specimen number and file an incident report.

The exposed individual should be informed of current recommendations for postexposure prophylaxis (HIV and HBV). The exposed individual should be counseled on the relative risks and benefits of this treatment, if available.

The blood of the source individual can only be tested for HIV after appropriate consent is obtained. The results of such a test may be made available to the exposed individual after he or she is made aware of applicable laws and regulations concerning disclosure of the identity and infectious status of a source individual and after signing a confidentiality statement.

■ RADIATION

Radioactive substances are widely used in the evaluation of patients and may be present in tissues submitted to pathology departments. In some cases patients have been injected with radioactive agents for the purpose of localizing and surgically removing a lesion (e.g., sentinel nodes, octreotide-positive lesions). Little published information is available about the incidence of such specimens and the risk to pathology personnel.[30] In general, patients are injected with small amounts (<5 millicuries) and typical half-lives are short. Specimens should have minimal residual radioactivity and can be generally handled and disposed of without special precautions. However, radiation safety personnel should be consulted for unusual cases or unusual isotopes.

REFERENCES AND RESOURCES

1. Montecalvo MA, Lee MS, DePalma H, et al. Seroprevalence of human immunodeficiency virus-1, hepatitis B virus, and hepatitis C virus in patients having major surgery. Infect Control Hosp Epidemiol 16:627-632, 1995.
2. Tuberculosis infection associated with tissue processing. MMWR 30:73-74, 1981.
3. Duray PH, Flannery B, Brown S. Tuberculosis infection from preparation of frozen sections. N Engl J Med 305:167, 1981.

4. CDC Hepatitis information line: 888-443-7243 (www.cdc.gov/hepatitis).

5. Updated US Public Health Service Guidelines for the Management of Occupational Exposures to HBV, HCV, and HIV and Recommendations for Postexposure Prophylaxis (June 29, 2001): http://www.cdc.gov/mmwr/preview/mmwrhtml/rr5011a1.htm

6. NIH Consensus statement on management of Hepatitis C: 2002: htttp://consensus.nih.gov

7. Do AN, Ciesielski CA, Metler RP, Hammett TA, Li J, Fleming PL. Occupationally acquired human immunodeficiency virus (HIV) infection: national case surveillance data during 20 years of the HIV epidemic in the United States. Infect Control Hosp Epidemiol 24:86-96, 2003.

8. Gerberding JL. Occupational exposure to HIV in health care settings. N Engl J Med 348:826-833, 2003.

9. National Clinician's Post-Exposure Prophylaxis Hotline (PEPline). University of California, San Francisco, San Francisco General Hospital: 888-448-4911 (http://www.ucsf.edu/hivcntr).

10. Needlestick! (an on-line decision-making support for clinicians). Emergency Medicine Center, UCLA School of Medicine: http://www.needlestick.mednet.ucla.edu

11. Johnson MD, et al. Autopsy risk and acquisition of human immunodeficiency virus infection. Arch Pathol Med 121:64-66, 1997.

12. Nyberg M, et al. Isolation of human immunodeficiency virus (HIV) at autopsy one to six days postmortem. Am J Clin Pathol 94:422-425, 1990.

13. Beltrami EM, Cheingsong R, Heneine WM, et al. Occupational HIV Exposure Study Group. Infect Control Hosp Epidemiol 24:724-730, 2003.

14. Goette DK, Jacobson KW, Doty RD. Primary inoculation tuberculosis of the skin. Prosector's paronychia. Arch Dermatol 114:567-569, 1978.

15. Templeton GL, Illing LA, Young L, Cave MD, Stead WW, Bates JH. The risk for transmission of *Mycobacterium tuberculosis* at the bedside and during autopsy. Ann Intern Med 122:922-925, 1995.

16. Anhalt JP, Witebsky FG. CAP Today, Illinois, American College of Pathologist, 75-76, 1996.

17. Kappel TJ, Reinartz JJ, Schmid JL, Holter JJ, Azar MM. The viability of Mycobacterium tuberculosis in formalin-fixed pulmonary autopsy tissue: review of the literature and brief report. Hum Pathol 27:1361-1364, 1996.

18. National Institute for Occupational Safety and Health: http:www.cdc.gov/niosh/topics/SARS.

19. Brumbeck RA. Routine use of phenolized formalin on autopsy brain tissue. N Engl J Med 319:654, 1988.

20. Brown P, Wolff A Gajdusek DC. A simple and effective method for inactivating virus activity in formalin-fixed tissue samples from patients with Creutzfeldt–Jakob disease. Neurology 40:887-890, 1990.

21. Burgess TH, Steele KE, Schoneboom BA, Grieder FB. Clinicopathologic features of viral agents of potential use by bioterrorists. Clin Lab Med 21:475-493, 2001.

22. Caya JG, Agni R, Miller JE. *Clostridium botulinum* and the clinical laboratorian. A detailed review of botulism, including biologic warfare ramifications of botulinum toxin. Arch Pathol Lab Med 128:653-662, 2004.

23. Guarner J, Jernigan JA, Shieh WJ, et al and the Inhalation Anthrax Working Group. Pathology and pathogenesis of bioterrorism-related inhalational anthrax. Am J Pathol 163:701-709, 2003.

24. Medical examiners, coroners, and biologic terrorism. A guidebook for surveillance and case management. Morbidity and Mortality Weekly Report, supplement vol. 53, No. RR-8, 2004.

25. Robinson-Dunn B. The microbiology laboratory's role in response to bioterrorism. Arch Pathol Lab Med 126:2910294, 2002.

26. Rollins SE, Rollins SM, Ryan ET. *Yersinia pestis* and the plague. Am J Clin Pathol 119 Suppl:S78-85, 2003.

27. Shieh Wun-Ju, Guarner J, Paddock C, et al and the Anthrax Bioterrorism Investigation Team. The critical role of pathology in the investigation of bioterrorism-related cutaneous anthrax. Am J Pathol 163:1901-1910, 2003.

28. Loh E, Couch FJ, Hendricksen C, et al. Development of donor-derived prostate cancer in a recipient following orthotopic heart transplantation. JAMA 277:133-137, 1997.

29. Gärtner H-V, Seidl C, Luckenbach C, et al. Genetic analysis of a sarcoma accidentally transplanted from a patient to a surgeon. N Engl J Med 335:1494-1496, 1996.

30. Warren S. Safe handling of tissue containing radioactive substances. Ann Clin Lab Sci 6:207-208, 1976.

Microscopy and photography

9

A pathologist without a microscope is like a surgeon without a scalpel or a dermatologist without steroid cream: these tools are essential to our practice of medicine. Although it is not necessary to have an advanced degree in optics, it is important to understand the basics of microscope use, special techniques useful to the pathologist, and the optical properties of biologic and synthetic materials present in clinical specimens. These topics are covered in the sections below.

■ OPTIMAL OPTICS

Definitions

- *Field diaphragm.* Source of light at the base of the microscope. Adjusted by moving the circular ring around it.
- *Substage condenser.* Located just below the stage. It can be moved up and down and centered with two screws.
- *Aperture iris diaphragm.* Located in the substage condenser. Adjusted by using a rotating ring on the front of the condenser.

Optimal image formation occurs when the image is in focus and the illumination is appropriately adjusted. First, the eyepieces should be adjusted for width (by sliding them back and forth) in order to form a single image. Secondly, each eye is closed in turn individually to adjust the focus of each eyepiece. Many people have subtle differences between their two eyes. Finally, the illumination is adjusted to ensure that the light is bright, evenly dispersed, and glare free, and that good image contrast is achieved. This procedure is termed "Koehler illumination" after the person who first determined the optimal settings.

The microscope is now optimally adjusted for the objective. Other objectives will require readjustment, and in practical terms a compromise position is usually used that is adequate for all of the objectives. A reasonable solution is to center the field diaphragm for a 40× objective and maintain its opening for a 10× field. The substage condenser should be slightly below the level where dust is brought into focus under 10×. As objectives

Adjusting a microscope for Koehler illumination

1. Open the aperture diaphragm and the field diaphragm completely. Using a 20× objective, focus on a slide on the stage.
2. Close the field diaphragm almost completely. Raise the condenser until the edges of the diaphragm are sharply focused (the condenser is usually at about its highest position).
3. Use the centering screws on the substage condenser to center the image of the field diaphragm. Slowly open the field diaphragm until it just disappears from view.
4. Remove one eyepiece objective and look into the tube. Open and close the aperture diaphragm until only 66% to 77% of the back lens is illuminated (see Fig. 9-1). This prevents unnecessary light from entering and creating glare.

are changed, only the aperture diaphragm need be changed to optimize contrast.

If the light intensity needs to be adjusted, it is accomplished by using the transformer, not by changing the position of the condenser or diaphragm.

Contrast can be increased by closing the aperture diaphragm below 60% or by lowering the substage condenser. However, resolution and sharpness are reduced. This maneuver may be useful if looking for refractile material (see "Optical properties," below).

■ OIL IMMERSION MICROSCOPY

Oil immersion lenses (usually 100×) can achieve higher magnifications than dry lenses. Because the refractive index of oil is higher than that of air, light rays coming from the slide are bent to a greater degree and thus an oil objective can capture more of these light rays, which results in greater resolution.

There are two major uses in surgical pathology for oil immersion magnification:

1. Hematologic specimens (due to the generally small size of the cells and the importance of subtle nuclear and cytoplasmic features for characterization)

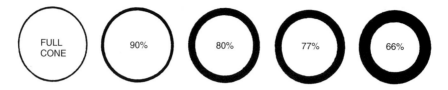

Figure 9-1 Aperture size.

2. Small micro-organisms (e.g., acid-fast bacilli or microsporidia).

There is virtually no other use for oil immersion lenses. The use of oil should be avoided outside of the applications cited above due to the frequent contamination of the microscope and other objectives with oil if great care is not used.

Only immersion oil designed for microscopic use should be employed. Lint-free tissues or lens paper should always be available to wipe away any excess oil before it drips into the microscope or onto other surfaces.

Using an oil immersion lens

1. Focus the microscope using the highest magnification available with a dry objective. It is helpful to identify and mark the area(s) of the slide to be examined under oil with ink to avoid the need to scan the slide after oil is applied.
2. Swing this objective away (in the direction to bring the oil objective into place) and place a small amount of oil on the slide.
3. Swing the oil objective into place, making sure that the space between the objective and the slide is filled with oil. The slide may now be observed.
4. After viewing, again swing the oil objective partially away from the slide.
5. Immediately wipe the objective with lens paper to prevent oil from dripping onto the microscope.
6. Remove the slide and wipe off excess oil with lens paper. The slide may then be cleaned with a small amount of xylene. Peripheral blood smears are often viewed under oil without using a coverslip. The oil can be wiped directly off the slide.

Do not attempt to view a slide with a high-power dry objective while there is oil on the slide! If it is necessary to scan a slide, place a 4× objective adjacent to the oil objective. One can safely alternate between these two objectives without contaminating the 4× objective with oil. It is very difficult to clean oil off a dry objective (see "Cleaning and care of the microscope and glass slides" on page 188).

■ OPTICAL PROPERTIES

The optical properties of microscopic objects reveal clues about their structure and identity. Table 9-1 lists the most common findings for noncellular materials. However, materials can be altered by in vivo responses, fixation conditions, and staining. Energy dispersive x-ray analysis (EDAX), as well as other methods, can be used to identify small deposits of elements in tissue specimens. Other types of spectroscopy can also be used.

"Refractile" objects

Refractile objects have a refractive index different from that of normal tissue. Refractility can be highlighted by increasing the contrast (i.e., by lowering the condenser or closing the aperture diaphragm). Refractile objects look brighter and shinier than tissues. This material is usually foreign (e.g., suture material) but can be endogenous. "Doubly refractile" is sometimes used to describe objects that are polarizable.

"Polarizable" objects

Polarized light is light oriented in one specific plane; it is produced by using two crossed polarizing filters. Most tissues are isotropic and do not change the quality of light passing through them. They appear dark under polarized light as very little light passes through the filters in any given plane.

"Polarizable," "birefringent," and "anisotropic" are terms used to describe substances that change the direction and speed of the light passing through them. Polarized light passing through such an object is deviated in a particular plane or planes and can pass through a second polarizing filter at an angle to the first. A "polarizable" object appears bright in comparison to the surrounding dark non-polarizable tissue. Some substances can reflect light at two different wavelengths (e.g., the "dichroic birefringence" of amyloid). Many of these polarizable substances have regular repeating structures (e.g., crystalline) and may be biologic (e.g., amyloid or collagen) or synthetic (e.g., polyethylene).

Polarizing objects

Some microscopes have built-in high-quality polarizers. Polarizing material may also be purchased as sheets and has the advantage of being transportable. It is available from Edmund Scientific Company (101 East Gloucester Pike, Barrington, NJ 08007-1380, (609) 573-6879; TECHSUP@EDSCI.COM or www.edsci.com). However,

Table 9–1 Optical properties of commonly seen noncellular material[1–7]

Endogenous material

TYPE	POLARIZABLE	REFRACTILE	LOCATIONS USUALLY SEEN	APPEARANCE/STAINS	COMMENTS
Amyloid	Yes	Yes/no	Bone marrow (multiple myeloma), medullary carcinoma of the thyroid, periarticular tissue in dialysis patients, many other sites	Acellular homogeneous pink material, sometimes with giant cells. Congo red positive: orange/red without polarization and apple green with polarization	Immunoperoxidase studies can be used to identify specific types of amyloid: Multiple myeloma: lambda and kappa chains Medullary carcinoma of the thyroid: calcitonin Dialysis-related amyloidosis: β_2-microglobulin EM can also be used to recognize amyloid
Bile	No	No	Liver: hepatocytes or intracanicular	Dark green-brown globules (intra- or extracellular). PAS positive	May be helpful for recognition of HCC
Bone and collagen	Yes	No	Joints and connective tissue	Normal bone: polarization shows regular osteoid seams (not seen in woven bone) Type I collagen is polarizable. Type III collagen (reticulin) is not polarizable	Bone and collagen overstained with Congo red will also be apple green after polarization. The background must not show staining Trichrome stains and reticulin stains can be used to identify collagen Nodular sclerosing Hodgkin's disease is associated with polarizable collagen
Calcium oxalate	Yes	Yes	Apocrine cysts of the breast, benign thyroid follicles, giant cells in sarcoidosis	Flat rhomboid (sometimes needle-shaped) colorless or pale yellow crystals. Can be difficult to see without polarization	Can be the source of mammographic calcifications in breast biopsies Also present in congenital hyperoxaluria
Calcium phosphate	No	No	Benign and malignant breast lesions, areas of chronic inflammation or necrosis, deposition on collagen (e.g., heart valves), pulmonary blue bodies	Purple granular material. Calcium stain positive	Most common source of mammographic calcifications
Calcium pyrophosphate dihydrate crystals ("pseudogout" or chondrocalcinosis)-	Yes	Yes	Large joints in periarticular tissues (uncommon in small joints of foot or hand)	Blue to purple short rhomboid crystals (but may be needle-shaped)	The crystals are water soluble and require anaqueous processing for best demonstration

Table 9–1 Optical properties of commonly seen noncellular material[1–7] —cont'd

TYPE	POLARIZABLE	REFRACTILE	LOCATIONS USUALLY SEEN	APPEARANCE/STAINS	COMMENTS
Charcot–Leyden crystals	No	Yes	Sites of eosinophil accumulation (e.g., chronic sinusitis, parasitic infections, asthma)	Bright-red, needle-like crystals	
Corpora amylacea	No	No	Prostate, brain, lung	Extracellular laminated light pink spherical structures	Incidence increases with age
Gamna–Gandy nodules	No	Yes/no	Spleen, lymph nodes, thymus gland, thyroid, cardiac myxomas	Granulomas consisting of hemosiderin, calcium, foreign body giant cells, and ovoid or bamboo-shaped structures	"Siderotic granulomas" found in sites of prior hemorrhage. Can mimic fungal mycelia or parasite eggs
Hamazaki–Wesenberg bodies	No	Yes	Areas of prior hemorrhage, lymph nodes (sinusoids)	Small round to ovoid brown bodies that may appear to be budding	Can mimic pigmented fungal forms or bacteria[8]
Hemosiderin	No	Yes	Any area of hemorrhage. Liver in hemochromatosis and hemosiderosis	Coarse granular brown intra and extracellular granules. Iron stain positive	A complex of iron and ferritin. Useful in distinguishing prior bleeding from intraoperative bleeding
Liesegang rings	No	No	Any area of old hemorrhage	Round extracellular concentric laminated or fibrillated concretions of precipitated proteins	May be mistaken for the giant kidney worm or fungal organisms[9]
Lipids	No/Yes	No	Polarizable lipids may be present in xanthomas, histiocytosis X, and other dermatopathologic entities, and fat necrosis secondary to pancreatitis. Cholesterol crystals are often seen as empty clefts in areas of cell injury	Needle-shaped clear crystals of varying size, plate-like structures, or intracellular rounded structures. Oil red O positive. Sudan black positive	Must have special processing or frozen sections to avoid loss during processing. Also present in metabolic storage diseases such as Gaucher's, Niemann–Pick's, and Wolman's. Fat necrosis due to pancreatitis.[10]
Lipofuscin (oxidized lipid precursors)	No	No	Sites of atrophy or chronic injury	Fine yellow-brown granules to coarse granules resembling hemosiderin. PAS positive	Ochrocytes are histiocytes containing lipofuscin
Malaria pigment (haemozoin, hematin)	Yes	No	Macrophages and erythrocytes	Brown to black granules inside macrophages	Present in malaria and schistosomal infections or severe hemolytic anemia. Formalin pigment can resemble malaria pigment

Table 9–1 Optical properties of commonly seen noncellular material[1–7] —cont'd

TYPE	POLARIZABLE	REFRACTILE	LOCATIONS USUALLY SEEN	APPEARANCE/STAINS	COMMENTS
Melanin	No	No	Normal melanocytes in basal epithelium, pigmented malignant melanomas	Fine brown or black granules but can sometimes resemble hemosiderin. Fontana Masson positive	
Michaelis–Gutmann body macrophages	No	No	Malakoplakia	Concentric targetoid bodies ("owl-eye"), intra- and extracellular. Iron stain positive, Von Kossa positive, PAS positive	These bodies may form due to defective phagocytosis of bacteria—most patients have a chronic coliform infection
Prostatic crystalloids	No	Yes	Prostate carcinomas	Bright eosinophilic angulated crystals in lumens of adenocarcinomas	Always associated with cancer—if present on a core needle biopsy, additional levels should be examined. Similar crystals are rarely seen in DCIS of the breast
Psammoma body	No	No	Papillary carcinoma of the thyroid, ovarian carcinoma, breast, others	Laminated concentric rings of calcium phosphate	Very specific in the thyroid for papillary carcinoma
Reinke crystals	No	Yes	Leydig cells of the testis, hilus cells of ovary, and their tumors	Rod-shaped eosinophilic crystals. Masson's trichrome positive (magenta)	
Schaumann bodies	No	No	Lymph nodes in sarcoidosis	Concentric basophilic rings	The other two types of inclusions in sarcoidosis are calcium oxalate and asteroid bodies (spider-shaped inclusions). These findings are not specific for sarcoid
Spironolactone bodies	No	No	Adrenal adenomas associated with Conn's syndrome	Concentric laminated eosinophilic inclusions (2 to 12 μm) in cytoplasm. PAS positive	Found in tumors in patients with Conn's syndrome treated with spironolactone. IHC can identify aldosterone in the bodies
Uric acid crystals (gout)	Yes	Yes	Periarticular tissues around joints, other areas of connective tissue	Long needle-shaped crystals (sheaves of wheat) are characteristic but may be fractured and appear to be smaller crystals	Requires anaqueous processing for preservation. In routine H&E sections only needle-shaped holes may be seen where the crystals are dissolved. The crystals may be seen in routinely fixed tissue if the tissue is unstained

Iatrogenic material

TYPE	POLARIZABLE	REFRACTILE	LOCATIONS USUALLY SEEN	APPEARANCE/STAINS	COMMENTS
Barium sulfate	No/Yes	Yes	In GI tract after radiologic examination, in peritoneum after perforation, within bone cement	Golden refractile granular material. May be intra- or extracellular	Rarely incites an inflammatory reaction

Table 9–1 Optical properties of commonly seen noncellular material[1-7] —cont'd

Iatrogenic material cont'd

TYPE	POLARIZABLE	REFRACTILE	LOCATIONS USUALLY SEEN	APPEARANCE/STAINS	COMMENTS
Cotton fibers	Yes	Yes	Around surgical sites	Hollow discoid fibers, present intra- or extracellularly	
Cornstarch	Yes	No	In surgical sites	3 to 20 μm spheres. Maltese cross appearance after polarization. PAS positive, MSS positive	Used to lubricate surgical gloves. However, cornstarch may be avoided as it can incite a granulomatous response
Formalin pigment	No	Yes	Most commonly seen in bloody tissues	Brown or black finely granular extracellular deposits	Due to a reaction between formic acid and heme during fixation. Can be avoided by using buffered formalin. Can be mistaken for malaria pigment
Gelfoam	No/Yes	No/Yes	Within vascular spaces of hemangiomas or other vascular lesions, sometimes used to mark breast core needle biopsy sites	Irregular fenestrated bluish or clear material	See reference 11
Gold	Yes	No	Skin, lymph nodes, organs of patients treated with gold for RA	Small intracellular black particles in histiocytes	Gold in intramammary lymph nodes can mimic mammographic calcifications. See also reference 12
Graft material: Gore-Tex or Dacron	Yes	Yes	Grafts	Numerous uniform round filaments with small black granules	
India ink (tattoo pigment)	No	No	Injected into the site of biopsied colonic polyps	Black granular pigment in stroma or within histiocytes	May be useful to document the site of a previously biopsied polyp that has been completely removed
Melanosis coli	No	No	Lamina propria of the colon	Fine brown to black granules in macrophages. PAS positive, silver stain positive	Associated with anthracene-derived bowel cathartics. Can cause grossly pigmented colonic mucosa
Mercuric chloride	Yes/No	No	Tissues fixed in mercury-containing fixatives	Dark brown granular extracellular deposits throughout the tissues	Should be removed by proper tissue processing
Metal	No	No	Tissue around prosthetic joints	Small black irregular angulated or needle-shaped fragments that may be intra- or extracellular	
Minocycline	No	No	Thyroid, atheromatous plaques, substantia nigra	Black granular pigment	Found in patients treated with minocycline

Table 9–1 Optical properties of commonly seen noncellular material[1-7] —cont'd

Iatrogenic material cont'd

TYPE	POLARIZABLE	REFRACTILE	LOCATIONS USUALLY SEEN	APPEARANCE/STAINS	COMMENTS
Myo--spherulosis	No	No	Nasal cavity and paranasal sinuses	Sac-like structures with outer lipid surrounding endobodies (red blood cells)	Due to packing with a petroleum-based ointment Can be mistaken for protothecosis or fungi
Polyethylene	Yes	Yes	Tissue around prosthetic joints	Large fragments, filaments, shards, or small intracellular fragments. Often with a giant cell reaction. Oil red O positive	
Poly-methyl-methacrylate (bone cement)	No	No	Tissue around prosthetic joints	Round to oval holes surrounded by a giant cell reaction	Dissolves in xylene. Barium sulfate may be present within the bone cement
Silicone	No	Yes	In tissue around implants, rarely in draining lymph nodes	Silicone may be removed during processing and appear as empty holes with residual refractile material around the edge	Intracellular silicone appears like multiple vacuoles in histiocytes that can be mistaken for lipoblasts Other organic oils can have the same appearance
Sodium poly-styrene sulfonate (Kayexalate)	No	Yes	Gastrointestinal tract	Irregular eosinophilic crystals present in the lumen or within ulcers. PAS positive and AFB positive	See reference 13
Sutures Surgical gut	Yes	No	Prior biopsy sites (often seen in breast)	Ovoid deeply eosinophilic monofilament often surrounded by a chronic inflammatory response and giant cells	Nuclei may be spindle-shaped (due to sterilization by cautery) and the suture may develop jagged edges during resorption. Gut sutures may be mistaken for metaplastic bone
Other sutures	Yes	Yes	Surgical sites	May be monofilament or polyfilament. Often colorless	Absorbable sutures may be surrounded by chronic inflammation
Talc	Yes	Yes	Pleura after talc pleurodesis, granulomas in intravenous drug abusers	Irregular clear to yellow crystalline material	
Thorotrast	No	No	Liver and spleen	Coarse light brown or gray granules in histiocytes or stroma—similar to the appearance of hemosiderin	This radiocontrast agent is no longer used as it is associated with cirrhosis, HCC, bile duct carcinoma, and angiosarcomas of the liver and spleen. It has a half-life of 400 years

Table 9–1 Optical properties of commonly seen noncellular material[1-7] —cont'd

Environmental material

TYPE	POLARIZABLE	REFRACTILE	LOCATIONS USUALLY SEEN	APPEARANCE/STAINS	COMMENTS
Anthracotic pigment (carbon)	No	No	Lymph nodes of the respiratory tract	Black granular deposits in macrophages	
Asbestos fibers	No/Yes	No	Lung	Thin fibers encrusted with beaded protein and iron (ferruginous bodies)	Specific identification requires spectroscopic analysis. Similar bodies can be seen with aluminum silicate, fiberglass, or lung elastin. Quantification and identification of fibers can be performed by energy dispersive x-ray analysis
Insects (flies and ticks)	Yes	Yes	Skin and subcutaneous tissue	Variable	
Silica	Yes	No	Lymph nodes of the respiratory tract, silicotic nodules	Minute polarizable material in histiocytes and fibrotic nodules	May be seen in workers exposed to silica. Lung disease is often complicated by superimposed infections
Plant material	Yes	Yes	Colonic rupture, lung (if aspirated)	Cell walls are readily identifiable by polarization	Can be useful to document colonic rupture

polarizing material varies greatly in quality. Tissues (especially those with suspected amyloid) should be

Definitions

- *Polarizer.* The polarizing disk below the condenser.
- *Analyzer.* The polarizing disk above the specimen (laid on top of the slide or built into microscope above the objectives).

observed using the higher quality built-in polarizers before it is determined that polarizable material is not present.

When the polarizer and the analyzer are at ninety degrees to each other, no light can pass through and the field is dark. As the angle between the filters is changed by rotating the polarizer, substances that preferentially reflect light in a specific direction (i.e., polarizable materials) allow light to pass through the analyzer and will appear bright.

The determination of "positive" and "negative" birefringence requires the use of a compensating first order red filter under polarized light and can be used to distinguish uric acid crystals from CPPD crystals. However, this determination is best performed on crystals in solution and cannot be reliably performed on fixed tissue.

Substances may be neither refractile nor polarizable (most tissues and cells), refractile but not polarizable (e.g., hemosiderin), polarizable but not (or poorly) refractile (e.g., amyloid), or both refractile and polarizable (e.g., suture material).

■ MEASURING WITH THE MICROSCOPE

In some instances it is necessary to accurately measure microscopic sizes. For example:

- Depth of invasion of malignant melanomas
- Depth of invasion of cervical carcinomas
- Fuhrman nuclear grading
- Standardization of microscopic field size for counting mitoses (especially in breast carcinoma grading).

Different methods are available depending upon the need for accuracy, the size of the object to be measured, and the equipment available.

Method	Approximate accuracy
Estimation from known field diameters	1–2 mm

Direct measurement on the slide	1–2 mm
Vernier scale on a movable stage	0.1 mm
Ocular reticle (graticule)	0.01 mm (10 mm)

Estimation from known field diameters

The field diameters on a microscope can be used to rapidly gauge the size of an object. The field diameter must also be known in order to use some types of grading systems as the number of mitoses scored must be standardized to a given area.

The size of a microscope field is affected by:

- The brand of the microscope
- The eyepiece magnification and the objective magnification
- The distance between the eyepiece and the objective (the distance may be lengthened by additional heads added to the microscope and built-in polarizing lenses).

For example, in our department the diameters of 40× fields varied from 0.39 to 0.52 mm and were significantly smaller than the 0.59 mm diameter used in a published system for breast cancer grading.[14] The number of mitoses per 10 high-power fields required for a score of 3 in this system is >20, based on a diameter of 0.59 mm. However, in our department, the number ranged from >8 to >16 mitoses per 10 high-power fields depending on the microscope used.

The size of a microscope field can be determined by:

- Carefully marking two edges of the field on a glass slide and measuring with a ruler.
- Using the Vernier scale (see below). The edge of a coverslip is a convenient landmark that can be moved across the field.
- Using a stage micrometer to measure a high-power field directly (most micrometers are too small to measure the other fields). The size of the other fields can be calculated with the following formula:

$$\text{Eyepiece magnification} \times \text{objective magnification} \times \text{field diameter} = \text{a constant}$$

Once the field sizes are known (and conveniently posted on the microscope) the size of objects can be estimated by determining the relative size to the microscopic fields (typically ranging between 0.05 and 1 cm). If grading systems using the number of mitoses per HPF are employed, it is also useful to make a table of equivalent mitotic counts per area for the microscope.

Comparison can also be made to cells with relatively constant sizes:

A lobe of a neutrophil nucleus	2 μm
Nucleus of a small lymphocyte	5–6 μm
A red blood cell	7 μm
A histiocyte nucleus	10 μm

Direct measurement on slides

Direct measurement is the most convenient method for objects measuring several millimeters in size. The borders to be measured are carefully marked by ink and an accurate ruler used to make a direct measurement. Small breast carcinomas can often be measured using this method as the gross measurements may underestimate or overestimate the extent of the invasive carcinoma.

Some coverslip films are permanently marked by ink. Marking on such slides should be minimized.

Vernier scale

The Vernier scale is found on the edge of most microscope stages and is used to measure the movement of the stage. Because the movement of the stage is measured directly, the eyepiece and objective magnifications are irrelevant to the measurement.

Definitions

- *Rule scale.* Located on the stage and divided into millimeters.
- *Vernier scale.* Adjacent to the rule scale but fixed in position. It is divided into 10 divisions, each measuring 0.9 mm.

There are usually two sets of scales corresponding to X and Y axes.

Measuring with the Vernier scale

1. The first reading is taken as the number of millimeters on the rule scale immediately before the "0" on the Vernier scale.
2. The decimal place is read off the Vernier scale and is the number at which there is perfect alignment between the two scales.
3. To measure an object, a reading is taken with the object at the edge of the field of view. The stage is then moved over the length of the object and a second reading is taken. The first number is subtracted from the second number to determine the distance the stage has moved.

The use of the Vernier scale is clearly described and illustrated by Warren et al.[15] Its use in measuring objects not aligned in the X and Y axis is described by Clark and Kung.[16] This method can be more reproducible than other measuring techniques.[17]

Ocular reticle

The most precise measurements may be made using a scale mounted in an eyepiece objective that has been calibrated. The disadvantage of this method compared to other methods is that two special pieces of equipment are required:

- **Reticle.** A reticle (graticule) has either a line scale or grid inscribed on the surface of a disc (either glass or plastic). It is used in conjunction with a focusing objective. The scale distances are arbitrary and must be calibrated for each microscope.
- **Stage micrometer.** This is a glass slide with a very accurate scale of known size etched into its surface. Typically the scale is 1 mm in length divided into 100 equal divisions (1 mm = 1000 μm, thus each division equals 10 μm).

Reticles cost from $30 to $90, focusing eyepieces from $70 to $130, and stage micrometers from $100 to $200. After a reticle is calibrated for a microscope, the stage micrometer is no longer needed. Most measurements (with the exception of the thickness of melanomas) can be made using the diameter of microscopic fields. Therefore, one reticle and stage micrometer can suffice for an entire department.

Reticles and stage micrometers are available from Edmund Scientific Company (101 East Gloucester Pike, Barrington, NJ 08007-1380, (609) 573-6879; TECHSUP@EDSCI.COM or www.edsci.com).

Calibrating a reticle and measuring objects

1. The measuring reticle is placed in one eyepiece in the microscope. If possible, it is most convenient to have a focusing objective with the reticle permanently installed.
2. The stage micrometer is viewed through the objective. The distance between the lines on the reticle is measured.
3. This is repeated for all the objectives on the microscope.
4. A table giving the calibration of the markings on the reticle is made and kept with each microscope. It is also useful to include the diameter of each microscope field.

Measuring microscopic objects using a reticle

1. The measuring reticle is placed in one eyepiece in the microscope.
2. The calibration line is placed over the object or distance to be measured.
3. The object or distance is measured by determining the number of units spanned on the calibration line. This number can then be converted to μm or millimeters using the table prepared for the microscope.

■ CLEANING AND CARE OF THE MICROSCOPE AND GLASS SLIDES

The microscope

The best method of keeping a microscope clean is to prevent it from getting dirty by covering it when it is not in use and avoiding the use of immersion oil. However, inevitably microscopes do gather dust or oil on the objectives. Only lens paper should be used to touch the objectives. Other types of paper may be too coarse or may be dusty and will scratch the lens. Fingers contain oils that may damage the coatings. If wiping the objective does not remove the dirt, a small amount of xylene or other cleaning solution applied to a piece of lens paper may be used. Do not place cleaning solution directly onto the objective as it may seep inside of the objective. Xylene should be wiped away immediately as it will damage the adhesives used to construct the objective. Do not use alcohol, as this substance will damage the objective.

Glass slides

The day a microscope slide is made, the mounting medium will still be wet. It takes 6 to 7 days to dry and may not be completely dry for 1 to 2 months. Therefore, special care must be taken when cleaning the coverslip as it is easily moved, which may damage the underlying tissue. The corner of the coverslip should be held with the tip of the finger to prevent dislodging it. For the same reason, slides should not be filed until the following day. An adhesive footplate on the end opposite the label can help prevent slides from sticking together.

Microscope slides often become soiled due to handling. Smears and oil can be cleaned using a small amount of xylene on a lint-free tissue. Excess dried mounting medium can be gently scraped off on the side of the microscope stage. Peripheral blood smears often do not have a coverslip. Oil can be gently wiped off the surface.

Sometimes slides will be received with air bubbles caught under the coverslip. As a temporary measure, before the mounting medium has dried, a small amount of xylene can be introduced under the coverslip to allow viewing of the tissue. However, these slides should be re-coverslipped to avoid permanent damage to the tissue by drying.

If one wishes to note findings on a glass slide it is convenient to write them on a small adhesive footplate on the opposite end of the slide from the label. These footplates are easily replaced, unlike the surgical number label, and also serve to protect the slide when filed.

If a slide cannot be focused, it may be upside down on the stage. Rarely, a coverslip has been placed on the wrong side or two coverslips may be present.

■ PHOTOGRAPHY

One of the most important roles of a pathologist is as an educator. Most doctors, including surgeons, never have the opportunity to see directly the disease processes that they diagnose and treat. Photography is an excellent means to convey to clinicians the pathology of disease. For example, the stellate appearance of a mass on a mammogram or the irregular feel of a breast mass on physical examination can be correlated with the irregular margins of a breast carcinoma in a gross specimen. The underlying histologic finding of infiltration of fibroadipose tissue by the carcinoma can then be appreciated.

Photomicroscopy

Photomicrographs are invaluable additions to teaching conferences and publications. Most photographs are now taken with a digital camera and then manipulated in Photoshop.

Slide selection. The tissue should be well cut and stained without wrinkles or bubbles. Any ink present on the coverslip should be removed. The slide and coverslip should be wiped clean of dust and oils before photography.

Magnification. For the novice, it is often tempting to take photographs of the same image at each available magnification. However, the maximum amount of information is usually obtained with one lower power picture to show the general location and architecture of the tissue and one higher power picture to show the specific important pathologic features. If you find yourself repeatedly saying at conference "And here is another picture of X," then you are taking too many photographs. Each image should reveal a different feature of the tumor or pathologic process.

Multiple panel photographs. For non-pathologists, it is easier to appreciate the differences between two processes rather than the important features of a single pathologic entity. Double or multi-panel images are very useful for illustrating important points. Examples include showing mucinous versus serous epithelium, immunoperoxidase for B cells versus immunoperoxidase for T cells, a benign lobule versus one involved by LCIS, or normal skin versus psoriasis.

Adding text to photographs. Simple additions (e.g., letters indicating the type of immunoperoxidase stain represented), text, arrows, or graphics can greatly enhance the information provided by the microscopic image.

Modifications of digital images. Images can be markedly improved with a few of the tools available in imaging processing programs:

- Focus ("unsharp mask"), but overuse will lead to pixillated pictures.
- Color: background color can be corrected to white.
- Cropping: use to remove unnecessary peripheral areas.
- Rips in the tissue, uneven staining, ink spots, and other distracting marks: remove or copy over using erasing and cloning tools.

Photography of gross specimens

Specimens for which photography may be helpful
• Surgical resections of tumors • Colon resections for inflammatory bowel disease • Artificial heart valves and intact native valves • Transplant lungs, kidneys, and hearts • Possible medicolegal cases (e.g., amputations due to trauma, explanted permanent silicone implants, and bullets) • Pertinent negative specimens (e.g., a resection for a tumor if the tumor was not present on pathologic examination) • Unusual specimens or specimens with examples of classic pathology (e.g., a classic porcelain gallbladder, Paget's disease of the nipple, rare grossly evident prostatic carcinomas).

Preparing the specimen

Most specimens are best photographed prior to fixation. Blood, bile, and fecal material should be gently rinsed off the specimen using saline. Immersion in 80% ethanol for 15 to 30 minutes will restore some of the original color to the specimen.

Some specimens are better demonstrated after fixation in an inflated state, such as lung, bladder, or colon resections for diverticulosis.

Dissection

Most pathologic lesions are best demonstrated after partial dissection of the specimen. Think about how best to demonstrate the lesion before starting dissection; however, do not alter the specimen in a way that will impair the final diagnosis. Cross-sections of tumors offer much more information about tumor appearance and relationships with normal structures. Examples include:

- **Colon carcinoma.** A cross-section can reveal residual villous adenoma at the edge of the tumor as well as tumor invasion into and through the muscularis propria.
- **Whipple specimen.** A photograph of a section taken through the plane of the common bile duct, the pancreatic duct, and the ampulla of Vater will reveal the appearance of the tumor and its relationship (obstruction, invasion, dilation) to these structures.

Photographing under saline

Saline supports delicate tissues and can be very helpful in bringing out fine textures. Sections of lungs (e.g., severe emphysema) or papillary structures (e.g., villous adenomas, PVNS, placental villi) can be demonstrated best under saline. Transillumination through saline on a light box often gives the best demonstration of a delicate floating structure.

Probes and arrows

In some cases the informational value of a picture is enhanced if certain features are emphasized. For example, a Whipple resection may be photographed with a probe in the ampulla of Vater to demonstrate the relationship of the tumor to the ampulla, or a probe can be used to indicate the site of a colon perforation. Small arrows may be cut out of white cardboard and used to indicate subtle features. Some specimens may need to be propped open (e.g., laryngectomies) to show the important lesions. The handle of a Q-tip (with the tip cut off) can be used. Avoid including hands in the picture. If something needs to be held, grasp it with a hemostat.

Composition of the photograph
Label

A label with the surgical pathology number and a ruler are always included.

Place the ruler/label in an anatomically appropriate orientation (e.g., with the upper pole of the kidney at the upper part of the photograph) so that it will be legible when the picture is displayed.

Orient the ruler/label with the edge of the photograph. Do not place ruler/labels diagonally as they will be more difficult to read and crop if necessary. The ruler should be closer to the specimen than the label in order to be able to crop the label but leave the ruler if the photograph is used for publication.

Do not allow the ruler/label to touch or overlap the specimen. If the specimen will fill the entire field, take one lower magnification picture first to include the ruler/label, or take one picture with the label over the specimen first, and then remove it to take the remaining photographs.

Always keep the label clean. It is generally best to prepare the label first, before handling the specimen, or to change gloves before making the label. The label can be attached to a clean glass microscope slide in order to handle it without soiling it.

The ruler/label and the lesion of interest should be in the same plane of focus. Use blocks or specimen cassettes to elevate the ruler/label to the appropriate height.

Specimen placement

Most specimens photograph well on a dark background. For some specimens that are very dark (e.g., a metastatic melanoma or a thyroid after minocycline therapy), it may be more appropriate to select a light-colored background (e.g., a clean blue pad or drape).

Place the specimen in an anatomically reasonable position if possible. Avoid confusing ways of showing specimens. For example, if a kidney has been bivalved, photograph only half of the specimen. Orient the specimen so that it will fill the frame of the photograph.

Use as high a magnification as possible without leaving out important features of the specimen. It is often useful to take both a low-magnification and a high-magnification view. For example, clinicians might better understand a Whipple specimen if the photograph includes the stomach, duodenum, and pancreas. A second close-up photograph could be taken showing the relationship of the tumor to the ampulla.

REFERENCES

1. Donath K, Laa BM, Gunzl H-J. The histopathology of different foreign-body reactions in oral soft tissue and bone tissue. Virchows Arch A Pathol Anat 420:131-137, 1992.
2. Fechner RE, Nichols GE. Iatrogenic lesions. In: Silverberg SG, DeLellis RA, Frable WJ (eds) Principles and Practice of Surgical Pathology and Cytopathology, 3rd edn, Ch. 22. New York Churchill Livingstone, 1997.
3. Forest M, Tomeno B, Vanel D. Pathology of bone and joints after surgery. In: Forest M (ed) Orthopedic Surgical Pathology. Edinburg Churchill Livingstone, 1998:739-756.
4. Johnson FB. Crystals in pathologic specimens. In: Sommers SC (ed.) Pathology Annual. New York, Appleton-Century-Crofts, 1972:321-348.
5. Walley VM, Stinson WA, Upton RT, Santerre JP, Mussivand T, Masters RG, Ghadially FN. Foreign materials found in the cardiovascular system after instrumentation or surgery (including a guide to their light microscopic identification). Cardiovasc Pathol 2:157-185, 1993.
6. Wallington EA. Artifacts in tissue sections. Med Lab Sci 36:3-61, 1979.
7. Yeh I-T, Brooks JSJ, Pietra GG. Atlas of microscopic artifacts and foreign materials, Baltimore, Williams & Wilkins, 1997.
8. Ro JY, et al. Yellow-brown (Hamazaki-Wesenberg) bodies mimicking fungal yeasts. Arch Pathol Lab Med 111:555-559, 1987.
9. Tuur SM, et al. Liesegang rings in tissue. Am J Surg Pathol 11:598-605, 1987.
10. Keen CE, Buk SJA, Brady K, Levison DA. Fat necrosis presenting as obscure abdominal mass: Birefringent

saponified fatty acid crystalloids as a clue to diagnosis. J Clin Pathol 47:1028-1031, 1994.

11. Kepes JJ, Yarde WL. Visualization of injected embolic material (polyvinyl alcohol) in paraffin sections with Verhoeff-Van Gieson elastica stain. Am J Surg Pathol 19:709-711, 1995.

12. Al-Talib RK, Wright DH, Theaker JM. Orange-red birefringence of gold particles in paraffin wax embedded sections: an aid to the diagnosis of chrysiasis. Histopathology 24:176-178, 1994.

13. Rashid A, Hamilton SR. Necrosis of the gastrointestinal tract in uremic patients as a result of sodium polystyrene sulfonate (Kayexalate) in sorbitol. Am J Surg Pathol 21:60-69, 1997.

14. Elston E, Ellis IO. Pathologic prognostic factors in breast cancer. Histopathology 19:403, 1991.

15. Warren BI, Davies JD. Pierre Vernier's invention: a neglected tool of our trade. Histopathology 18:361-362, 1991.

16. Clark SP, Kung ITM. Measurement of Breslow depth [letter]. J Pathol 165:269-270, 1991.

17. Calder CJ, Campbell AP, Plastow SR. Measurement techniques for melanoma: a statistical comparison. J Clin Pathol 43:922-923, 1990.

Approaching perfection: avoiding errors in surgical pathology

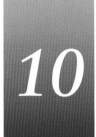

Start out with the conviction that absolute truth is hard to reach in matters relating to our fellow creatures, healthy or diseased, that slips in observation are inevitable even with the best-trained faculties, that errors in judgment must occur in the practice of an art which consists largely in balancing probabilities.

SIR WILLIAM OSLER[1]

Show me a pathologist who has never made a mistake, and I'll show you a liar or someone who has never looked down the end of a microscope.

A RESPECTED PROFESSOR OF PATHOLOGY
(QUOTED IN REFERENCE 2)

The standard of care is not perfection.

A MALPRACTICE DEFENSE ATTORNEY

When error is mentioned in medicine, the immediate presumption is that a physician failed to provide good care due to either negligence or ignorance. The thought of being responsible for such an error strikes dread into the heart of all pathologists. However, within the broad spectrum of possible medical errors, errors due to negligence or ignorance are rare. Other types of errors are much more common and most of these can be minimized by understanding how they occur and designing systems to detect and prevent them.[3–9]

The Institute of Medicine issued a report on medical error and patient safety on November 29, 1999.[3] The report stated that the current error rate was unacceptable and mandated a 50% reduction by 2004. Some changes have taken place at the regulatory and governmental level, but the most important steps will occur at the institutional and individual practitioner level.

Dr. Ronald Sirota has described the "culture of safety" that creates an environment that prioritizes patient safety and error reduction (Table 10.1).

■ SOURCES OF ERROR

Errors can occur before specimens arrive in the pathology department, during pathologic evaluation, or after the report leaves the pathology department (Box 10-1).

Pre-pathology errors

Both the CAP and the JCAHO have issued guidelines for the submission of specimens for pathologic examination. A Q-probes study revealed that 6% of specimens failed to meet these standards.[10] Errors constituted the following:

Discrepant or missing information	77.0%
Specimen not appropriately identified	9.6%
Specimen handling	3.6%

Table 10-1 The culture of safety[3-9]	
A TYPICAL MEDICAL SYSTEM	A BETTER MEDICAL SYSTEM
Patient safety and error reduction are important, but may not be given as much attention as other organizational goals	Patient safety and error reduction are top organizational priorities
Assumes that the system is perfect and that pathologists never make mistakes	Assumes that mistakes are inevitable
Systems (e.g., procedures, computer programs) are not designed to prevent and detect errors	Systems are designed to prevent and detect all types of error
All errors are considered to be the result of individual incompetence	Recognizes that there are many types of error. Only a small number are due to incompetence. Most are due to system failures
Creates strong incentives to not find errors or to conceal them	Creates strong incentives to find and correct errors. Errors are openly reported and discussed
Error detection results in shame and derision	Uses each error as an opportunity to improve the system and to educate others in error prevention

Box 10-1 Sources of error

Pre-pathology errors

- Failure to provide appropriate patient and specimen identification
- Failure to provide relevant clinical history
- Failure to provide tissue in a timely and appropriate manner to perform necessary pathology examination
- Failure to transport the specimen to the pathology laboratory

Pathology errors

- Loss of specimen
- Errors in accessioning specimens
- Errors in gross sampling of tissue
- Failure to preserve tissue in appropriate fixatives or for special studies necessary for diagnosis
- Failure to make the correct diagnosis or significant omissions to the pathology report
- Failure to provide a completed pathology report without typographical errors
- Billing errors—usually due to failure to document billable procedures in the report

Post-pathology errors

- Failure of the pathology report to be available to treating clinicians
- Failure of the clinician to understand the report
- Failure to inform clinicians directly of significant changes in diagnosis in addenda

Pathology errors

Specimen identification

Specimens must be correctly identified by the clinician submitting the specimen. This identification should be confirmed by the following:

1. The tissue must correspond to the site biopsied. If it does not, identify the problem as clinician error (e.g., endometrial curettings are actually colonic mucosa) or pathology error (mixed-up specimens or extraneous tissue).
2. Correlate the pathologic findings with the clinical setting. If they are discordant, consider the possibility of a misidentified specimen.

Clinicians often provide information that aids in detecting such errors. If a clinician questions a diagnosis, the possibility of an error should be addressed. In rare cases, it may be appropriate to identify the specimen by tissue typing.

Gross examination

Advances in disease detection have resulted in the removal of increasingly smaller tumors or in situ disease that may be difficult to find on gross examination.

Small specimens that are completely examined microscopically rarely present a problem; however, large resections, particularly after preoperative therapy, can pose problems. A recent study investigated the incidence of errors in breast pathology.[11] The investigators found that failure to adequately examine specimens grossly was responsible for major discrepancies in 5% of cases and minor discrepancies in 6% of cases, including missed cancers, missed metastatic carcinoma to lymph nodes, and undetected skin invasion. The majority (83%) of the major discrepancies occurred in mastectomy specimens. In contrast, review of the original glass slides revealed major discrepancies in only 1.5% of cases and minor discrepancies in 6%. Errors due to suboptimal gross examination may be reduced by the following procedures:

1. Provide increased supervision for first year residents or new pathology assistants for large complicated specimens. Most major discrepancies occurred when the prosector had limited experience.
2. Utilize additional techniques to find lesions when necessary. For example, specimen radiography may be necessary to localize small mammographic lesions in mastectomies when the diagnosis was made by needle biopsy.
3. Reexamine specimens grossly after microscopic evaluation if the following occurs:
   - Prior diagnostic findings are not confirmed (e.g., FNA was suspicious for papillary carcinoma but no carcinoma was found in the thyroid on initial sampling)
   - Fewer lymph nodes than expected are found
   - Prior biopsy or tumor site is not identified
   - Radiologic findings are not found—radiographic reexamination of the specimen can be helpful.

Microscopic examination

The major reasons for errors in the microscopic examination of specimens include the following:

Failure to see an area of a slide or an entire slide:
- Slides may be scanned on low power first to identify all tissue fragments.
- If there are many fragments on the slide, it can be helpful to mark a line around all the fragments (to facilitate screening the entire circled area) or to make a line interconnecting all the fragments (e.g., multiple lymph node sections).

Avoid distractions during sign-out. Some pathologists mark each slide as it is examined or reverse examined slides in the tray.

Failure to recognize a diagnostic entity. This is what most pathologists think of as an "error" although it constitutes only a small portion of the total number of errors possible. Pathologists do need to establish an adequate knowledge base and to know their limitations.

One should resist the temptation to make a rare diagnosis with which one has little familiarity and to have a low threshold to always be ready to seek consultation with colleagues or acknowledged experts.

This type of error is rare, occurring in less than 1% of cases.

Diagnostically difficult cases. Although there will be little variation in the diagnosis of some lesions (e.g., invasive colon carcinoma), other lesions can be very difficult to classify. Differences in opinion for such lesions do not, in general, constitute an error on the part of a pathologist who may disagree with another pathologist. Unfortunately, it is often difficult for non-pathologists to understand that there can be a differential diagnosis for pathologic lesions. In such cases it may be beneficial to obtain and document opinions from more than one pathologist in the final report.

Pathology reporting

Typographical errors. These are probably the most common type of error. Pathologists must be vigilant in detecting such errors, as they can sometimes change a final diagnosis. Computer systems with spell checkers can be helpful, but will not find many errors in meaning. Synoptic reports aid in typing reports and reducing spelling errors, but are difficult to proofread.

Errors of omission. Failure to provide information required for the treatment of patients can adversely affect patient care. To some extent, this is dependent on the information desired by the clinicians in each institution.

There are published recommendations for cancer reporting from the Association of Directors of Surgical Pathology (ADASP; www.panix.com/~adasp/) and the College of American Pathologists (CAP; www.cap.org). CAP protocols can also be purchased in a loose-leaf binder.[12] As of January 1, 2004, the American College of Surgeons Commission on Cancer (ACS CoC) requires the reporting of all scientifically validated or regularly used data elements of the CAP checklists in reports of cancer-directed surgical resection specimens (not including cytologic specimens, diagnostic biopsies, and palliative resection specimens) from CoC-approved cancer centers. The ACS does not require the actual use of the CAP checklists or any other specific format.

Post-pathology errors

Post-pathology errors consist of failure of the pathology information provided in a report to reach the relevant clinicians.

Unexpected diagnosis.
A clinician may not see a pathology report on a routine specimen until the patient is next seen for follow-up. If this appointment is delayed or does not occur, an important unexpected diagnosis may be overlooked. Examples include finding carcinoma in a hernia sac, endocarditis in a heart valve, and multiple myeloma in bone marrow from a joint replacement. In such cases, it is advisable to contact the clinician directly as well as to send the final report.

Amended diagnosis. Addenda can be easily lost or overlooked unless the original report specifically states that an addendum will be added. If important information needs to be added to a report at a later date, it is advisable to contact the clinician directly. These problems can be minimized as follows:

1. Avoid putting important information in an addendum. If additional important diagnostic tests are being performed or consultation is sought, then it may be preferable to hold the report until all information is available to render a final diagnosis.
2. The original report can state that an addendum will be added if it is known that additional information will be available later.
3. An amended report should be identified on the first page of the report. If the addendum is added to the end of the report, the clinician may not realize that additional information has been added.

Failure of the clinician to understand the diagnosis.
A recent study showed that surgeons misunderstood pathology reports 30% of the time.[13] Although the presence or absence of carcinoma was well understood, problems arose when surgeons had to interpret histologic descriptions. Such problems can be minimized as follows:

1. Provide specific, well understood, diagnostic terms whenever possible.
2. Standardize terminology within a department. Sign-out checklists can help in providing all the important information in a format familiar to clinicians.
3. Provide additional explanatory information if possible in the report (e.g., information on grading or classification systems).
4. Provide AJCC classifications for malignant tumors when possible.
5. Avoid providing misleading information. For example, clinicians may not understand that a specimen heading is not a diagnosis. If a specimen has been labeled "Left thigh sarcoma" but the lesion is not a sarcoma, it is advisable not to include the word "sarcoma" in the heading for the final diagnosis. The specimen heading can be documented in the gross description for medicolegal purposes.
6. Include important information from the gross examination in the final diagnosis. For example, the final determination of tumor size should be based on a final assessment of both the gross and microscopic appearance and should be recorded in the final diagnosis.

Similarly, the gross description should be edited after the microscopic examination to remove misleading information. For example, if the gross description states that a lymph node is grossly involved by tumor, but this later turns out to be false, this could potentially lead to confusion or the presumption that the pathologist has made an error.

7. Prioritize important information. The most important diagnosis should be stated first. A malignant diagnosis may be overlooked if placed within a paragraph describing benign findings.

Ten ways to avoid personal errors

1. Avoid signing out when tired, stressed, or ill. Have a low threshold for setting aside difficult, unusual, or clinically important cases (e.g., a diagnostic biopsy prior to a major resection). Reflecting on a case a few hours later or the next day can provide important insights.
   A rapid incorrect diagnosis is never better than a delayed correct diagnosis.

2. Know your limitations and always be ready to seek consultation with colleagues or acknowledged experts.

3. Require that all cases are logically consistent. If a case does not make sense to you (e.g., a surgeon has resected a completely normal length of bowel) there is likely missing clinical history (e.g., a subtle lesion has been missed during gross examination or the surgeon resected the wrong length of bowel).

4. Accept the fact that some lesions defy diagnostic certainty. A number of studies have shown that some lesions cannot be consistently classified, even by a panel of experts under ideal conditions. For such cases, a consensus opinion from a group of pathologists or an "expert" opinion may be helpful.

5. Establish error reduction systems and make sure coworkers are aware of the reason for the system. Explain the importance of "redundant" systems to those using them (see below).

6. Simplify tasks as much as possible for routine specimens, using:
   - Written procedures
   - Checklists
   - Synoptic reporting.
   Save creativity for the rare unusual case.

7. Be responsive when a clinician questions a pathology report, as this is an effective method of detecting and rectifying errors.

8. Demand sufficient clinical information when appropriate. On the other hand, remain appropriately skeptical of the information you do receive, as it may be incorrect or incomplete.

Clinical information is both our best friend and our worst enemy.

RONALD SIROTA, MD

9. Be aware of common pitfalls that other pathologists have fallen into, in order to avoid them yourself (see "Frequent diagnostic pitfalls," below).

10. Be appropriately grateful when someone discovers one of your errors, especially if patient harm has been avoided. Refrain from gloating over or reviling colleagues when you discover they have made a mistake.

■ REDUNDANT SYSTEMS

Redundancy, or requiring that more than one person perform the same task, can be an effective means of reducing error. For example, one person makes up cassettes with the appropriate specimen number and a second person checks the number on the cassette before using it for a specimen, or there may be a departmental requirement that some pathologic diagnoses are reviewed by two pathologists.

If each person makes one mistake out of 100 specimens, then the chance that two people will make the mistake on the same specimen is only one in 10,000.

However, it is human nature to minimize the amount of work one needs to do. If someone knows that another person is also performing the task, he or she is often less vigilant about performing it. Therefore, the error rate can increase for both people. The overall error rate may not only fail to be decreased, but may actually increase in a redundant system.

When redundant systems are in place, everyone must be aware of how the system works and why they must not rely on someone else to check for mistakes. Each person must take responsibility for any error made rather than blaming a single person. Almost every error is due to more than one person making multiple errors.

■ FREQUENT DIAGNOSTIC PITFALLS

There are some diagnostic situations that frequently pose problems for pathologists. Knowledge of these errors can help avoid them.

Dermatopathology specimens

Misdiagnosis of melanoma is the most common claim filed against pathologists in surgical pathology.

- **Making a diagnosis of melanoma (or failing to make the diagnosis) on an inappropriate small or shave biopsy.** Clinicians should be educated about appropriate biopsies of pigmented lesions.

- Melanomas versus Spitz nevi.
- **Failure to recognize desmoplastic melanoma.** This diagnosis may be difficult as this type of melanoma may not be immunoreactive for typical melanoma markers.
- **Metastatic melanoma versus a primary sarcoma or carcinoma.** Markers for melanoma are helpful.
- **Metastatic melanoma to a lymph node versus lymphoma.** This differential diagnosis is easily resolved with immunohistochemical markers.

Breast specimens

Breast specimens are the second most common source of malpractice claims.

- **Sclerosing adenosis versus invasive carcinoma.** This differential is made more difficult when the sclerosing adenosis is involved by apocrine metaplasia, LCIS, or DCIS. Smooth muscle α-actin or P63 will show myoepithelial cells in sclerosing adenosis. This is a frequent difficult diagnosis in needle biopsies.
- **Metastatic lobular carcinoma.** The cells can be quite small and infiltrate in a diffuse pattern without a stromal response. A high index of suspicion and keratin studies may be necessary for diagnosis.
- **Low-grade DCIS versus hyperplasia.** Some of these lesions defy accurate classification. Micropapillary DCIS is often overlooked. Suspect carcinoma when cells of a similar appearance are seen in multiple ductal spaces.
- **Freezing artifact in small lesions.** Small lesions should never be frozen in entirety. In general, frozen section should be avoided for any lesion less than 1 cm in size or if the pathologist thinks diagnosis would be compromised by freezing the lesion.

Pulmonary specimens

- **Crushed blue cells.** Transbronchial biopsies may contain crushed blue cells. The diagnosis of small cell carcinoma may be made without considering the possibility of carcinoid tumor or lymphocytes. If it is small cell carcinoma, mitoses or tumor necrosis should be present. Immunoperoxidase studies can be used to distinguish lymphocytes from small cell carcinoma.
- **Desmoplastic mesothelioma versus reactive pleuritis.** This can be a difficult differential diagnosis, particularly when the biopsy is small or the tumor is paucicellular. Repeat biopsies may be necessary. Cytogenetics on pleural fluid can be helpful if abnormal.

Genitourinary specimens

- **Atrophy versus prostate carcinoma.** IHC for basal cells can be helpful (see Chapter 7).
- **Basal cell hyperplasia versus PIN.** IHC for basal cells can be helpful (see Chapter 7).
- **Urothelial carcinoma in prostatic ducts versus PIN.** IHC can be helpful (see Chapter 7).

- **Seminal vesicle versus prostate carcinoma.** The seminal vesicle can contain enlarged "monster cells." However, surrounding cells will appear normal in appearance. The seminal vesicle has a characteristic papillary appearance and often has a golden yellow cytoplasmic pigment. The cells of the seminal vesicle are PSA negative.
- **Metastatic renal cell carcinoma.** The cells can often be quite bland and mistaken for histiocytes. Metastases can occur decades after the original diagnosis and can occur in unusual sites (e.g., the eyelid).

Gastrointestinal specimens

There are two types of pathologists. Those that have missed signet ring cell carcinoma and those that will someday miss signet ring cell carcinoma.

ANONYMOUS PATHOLOGIST

- **Signet ring cell carcinoma.** The cells can be very bland and infiltrate in the lamina propria without disrupting the surrounding architecture. A high index of suspicion is necessary for all gastric biopsies. Mucin stains or IHC studies for keratin can be helpful. In women, metastatic lobular carcinoma of the breast should also be considered.
- **Pancreatic carcinoma versus pancreatitis.** This is a difficult diagnosis on small specimens and on frozen section. Specific criteria for diagnosis have been published and are helpful in these situations (see page 60).
- **Carcinoma or pseudoinvasion in polyps.** Glands can become entrapped in the stalk of a polyp and can be difficult to distinguish from invasion. Invasive carcinoma in a polyp should be considered as a possibility in small biopsies, particularly from the rectum. Inappropriate surgery may be avoided by good communication between the pathologist, the endoscopist, and the surgeon.

Soft tissue specimens

- **Mistaking metastatic melanoma or carcinoma for sarcoma.** A good clinical history and immunoperoxidase studies are often necessary for appropriate diagnosis.
- **Nodular fasciitis.** These lesions can have markedly atypical cells and look very alarming. A good clinical history (a rapidly growing mass, usually in a young adult) and a familiarity with this entity are helpful.
- **Diffuse-type giant cell tumor** (previously known as pigmented villonodular synovitis) can be mistaken for a sarcoma, particularly if extra-articular.
- **Failure to recognize monophasic synovial sarcoma.**
- **Papillary endothelial hyperplasia (Masson's lesion) versus angiosarcoma.** Organizing thrombi can closely mimic an angiosarcoma. There is often a history of prior trauma and the lesion may be within a vessel or have a well-circumscribed border. There is no endothelial multilayering.

Gynecologic specimens

- **Metastatic carcinoma versus primary ovarian carcinoma.** IHC studies can be helpful (see Chapter 7).

Neuropathology

- **Pituitary adenoma versus multiple myeloma.** On smears, plasma cells can closely resemble the cells of an adenoma. See Folkerth[14] for tables of differential diagnoses of similar appearing lesions.

Hematopathology specimens

- **Lymphoma only partially involving a lymph node.** This type of missed diagnosis usually occurs in lymph nodes taken out as part of a larger resection.
- **Failure to diagnosis lymphoma in extranodal locations** (e.g., skin, nasal cavity, mediastinum, stomach).
- **Anaplastic lymphomas.** These lymphomas can partially involve a lymph node and can closely mimic a metastatic carcinoma. They are occasionally EMA positive and LCA negative. However, keratins are virtually always negative.

Head and neck pathology

- **Squamous cell carcinoma versus radiation changes.** This can be particularly difficult when the radiation changes involve small glands or ducts.
- **Follicular variant of papillary carcinoma.** Nuclear features of papillary carcinoma are present, but may be focal.
- **Pseudoepitheliomatous hyperplasia over a granular cell tumor mistaken for squamous cell carcinoma.**
- **Necrotizing sialometaplasia versus squamous cell carcinoma.**
- **Metastatic squamous cell carcinoma to a cervical lymph node versus a branchial cleft cyst.**

Bone specimens

- **Routine rib specimens.** The most common missed diagnoses are multiple myeloma and chronic lymphocytic leukemia. However, the latter diagnosis is usually known to the clinicians because of the patient's peripheral blood count. In rare cases, unsuspected cases of multiple myeloma may be detected in incidental specimens.

■ WHAT TO DO WHEN AN ERROR IS DETECTED

If an error is detected, the report must be corrected and the clinicians notified.

An original report that has been issued should not be altered or deleted, as this report is part of the patient's medical record. Minor errors can be corrected in an addendum. If a major error has occurred then it may be advisable to add a heading over the original diagnosis stating that a change in diagnosis has been made and directing the reader to the corrected diagnosis.

The circumstances and procedures leading to the error should be reviewed to determine how the error occurred and whether the system can be improved. In general, it is found that at least two people have made an error before an incorrect pathology report is released: for example, one person makes an error, but a second person fails to detect it. These occurrences should be viewed as excellent opportunities to discover ways to improve procedures and to educate pathology personnel on the importance of following the procedures in place to prevent errors.

REFERENCES

1. Stone MJ. The wisdom of Sir William Osler. Am J Cardiol 75:269-276, 1995.
2. Wolber R, Chercover D. [letter to the editor] Am J Surg Pathol 27:1020-1024, 2003.
3. Sirota RL. The Institute of Medicine's Report on Medical Error. Implications for pathology. Arch Pathol Lab Med 124:1674-1678, 2000.
4. Foucar E. Error in anatomic pathology. Am J Clin Pathol 116 Suppl:S34-46, 2001.
5. Foucar E. Error identification. A surgical pathology dilemma. Am J Surg Pathol 22:1-5, 1998.
6. Foucar E. Do pathologists play dice? Uncertainty and early histopathological diagnosis of common malignancies. Histopathol 31:495-502, 1997.
7. Goldstein NS. Diagnostic errors in surgical pathology. Clin Lab Med 19:743-756, 1999.
8. Renshaw AA. Measuring and reporting errors in surgical pathology. Lessons from gynecologic cytology. Am J Clin Pathol 115:338-341, 2001.
9. Troxel DB. Error in surgical pathology. Am J Surg Pathol 28:1092-1095, 2004. *There are also many other excellent articles by Dr. Troxel analyzing errors revealed by malpractice claims.*
10. Nakhleh RE, Zarbo RJ. Surgical pathology specimen identification and accessioning. A College of American Pathologists Q-Probes study of 1,004,115 cases from 417 institutions. Arch Pathol Lab Med 120:227-233, 1996.
11. Wiley EL, Keh P. Diagnostic discrepancies in breast specimens subjected to gross reexamination. Am J Surg Pathol 23:876-879, 1999.
12. College of American Pathologists. Reporting on Cancer Specimens. Case summaries and background documentation. A publication of the CAP cancer committee. Illinois, College of American Pathologists, 2004.
13. Powsner SM, Costa J, Homer RJ. Clinicians are from Mars and pathologists are from Venus. Arch Pathol Lab Med 124:1040-1046, 2000.
14. Folkerth RD. Smears and frozen sections in the intraoperative diagnosis of CNS lesions. Neurosurg Clin N Am 5:1-8, 1994.

Part 2

INTRODUCTION TO PART TWO

Part Two is a guide to the gross description, dissection, and processing of commonly received pathology specimens. The following protocols have been found useful for most specimens. However, the optimal procedure will vary according to specific issues associated with individual cases, institutional practices, and personal preferences of pathologists and clinicians.

Format of Part Two

Each section starts with a brief description of typical specimens and the commonly diagnosed disease processes.

"Relevant clinical history" lists the most important clinical information specific for the organ site that should be provided to the pathologist in order to enable full evaluation of the specimen. A clinical history is required by JCAHO when a specimen is accepted for examination by pathologists (see also Part One, "Request for pathologic examination" page 1). Important history for all specimens includes:

- The purpose of the procedure
- The organs/tissues resected
- Prior malignancies (type, location, stage)
- Prior treatment (radiation, chemotherapy, drugs that can alter the histologic appearance of tissues or increase susceptibility to infection)
- Immune system status (conditions that could result in immunocompromise)
- Current or recent pregnancy
- Unusual features of the clinical presentation
- Unusual features of the gross appearance at surgery.

"Processing the specimen" outlines the step by step description, dissection, and sampling of specimens in order to document all diagnostic and prognostic features.

"Special studies" lists tests beyond those applied to formalin-fixed tissue that might be helpful for some types of specimens.

"Gross differential diagnosis" describes the appearances of the most common tumors and disease processes. Illustrations are provided for the most common tumors and lesions.

"Microscopic sections" lists the types of tissue to be submitted and guidelines for the number of cassettes to submit.

"Sample dictations" are provided as examples of gross descriptions for common specimens.

"Pathologic prognostic/diagnostic features sign-out checklist" gives the major features of tumors that are used for diagnosis, prognosis, staging, correlation with clinical and radiologic findings, and treatment decision making. These lists are a guide to information that should be included in the final pathology report. The lists incorporate the published recommendations of the Association of Directors of Anatomic and Surgical Pathology (ADASP; see www.panix.com/~adasp/) and the College of American Pathologists (CAP) (their protocols can be purchased in a loose-leaf binder, *Reporting on Cancer Specimens, Case summaries and background documentation, A publication of the CAP cancer committee, 2004*, or are available on their website at www.cap.org), as well as other groups, when available. As of January 1, 2004, the American College of Surgeons Commission on Cancer (ACS CoC) requires the reporting of all scientifically validated or regularly used data elements of the checklists in reports of cancer-directed surgical resection specimens (not including cytologic specimens, diagnostic biopsies, and palliative resection specimens) from CoC-approved cancer centers. These items are followed by an asterisk in the checklists provided in this manual. The ACS does not require the actual use of the CAP checklists or any other specific format.

"AJCC classifications" are provided from the *AJCC Cancer Staging Manual*, Sixth Edition, 2002, when available. The Sixth Edition should be used to classify tumors diagnosed after January 1, 2003. Other classification systems used for staging are also provided.

The AJCC classification pertains to characteristics of a single tumor as determined at presentation, prior to treatment. The classification system uses suffixes and prefixes to indicate other situations:

M: indicates the presence of multiple tumors in a single site, e.g., T2 (m) N1 MX.

Y: indicates the classification of a tumor during or following therapy, e.g., ypT1 N0 MX.

R: indicates a recurrent tumor after a disease-free interval.

A: indicates the classification at autopsy.

"Grading systems" are provided for some specimens. Not all are universally accepted or used. Alternative grading systems are provided for some types of tumors.

Other types of information useful for the preparation of the final surgical pathology report are provided (e.g., Rosen criteria for lymphovascular invasion for breast cancer, evaluation of salivary gland biopsies for Sjögren's syndrome, endometrial dating).

Adrenal gland

11

Adrenal glands may be resected en bloc as part of a radical nephrectomy, to remove a clinically evident tumor (usually a functional cortical adenoma or a pheochromocytoma), or to investigate an incidental mass seen on CT scan (usually adenomas, rarely carcinomas). Cortical carcinomas, primary or secondary hyperplasia, and other benign lesions (e.g., myelolipomas, ganglioneuromas) are less common. Biopsies are usually fine needle aspirations to confirm the diagnosis of metastatic carcinoma.

Relevant clinical history (in addition to age and gender) See Table 11-1.

Processing the specimen

1. If a mass is present, or if the surrounding soft tissue is abnormal (e.g., grossly involved by tumor), ink the outer surface.
2. Serially section through the specimen at 2–3-mm intervals. If no mass is present and significant amounts of peri-adrenal soft tissue are present, the soft tissue is dissected away and the exact weight and size of the gland measured. Weight is an important feature in assessing hyperplastic glands as well as tumors.

Table 11-1 Relevant clinical history (in addition to age and gender)

HISTORY RELEVANT TO ALL SPECIMENS	HISTORY RELEVANT TO ADRENAL SPECIMENS
Organ/tissue resected or biopsied	Clinical symptoms of functional tumors:
Purpose of the procedure	Adrenocortical tumors
Gross appearance of the organ/tissue/lesion sampled	Cushing syndrome—increased cortisol (central obesity, striae, hypertension)
Any unusual features of the clinical presentation	Conn's syndrome—increased aldosterone (hypokalemia, hypertension)
Any unusual features of the gross appearance	Hypoglycemia
Prior surgery/biopsies—results	Combined excess syndromes
Prior malignancy	Pheochromocytomas/paragangliomas—elevated catecholamine levels (episodic hypertension, rare Cushing syndrome)
Prior treatment (radiation therapy, chemotherapy, drug use that can change the histologic appearance of tissues)	
Compromised immune system	Radiologic findings (e.g., incidental mass or found on studies for nonspecific symptoms of weight loss or malaise)
	Family or personal history of other endocrine tumors (see "Hereditary Tumor Syndromes")

Normal glands weigh from 4 to 6 g.

If a mass is present, and only a small amount of peri-adrenal soft tissue is present, the entire specimen may be weighed. If large amounts of soft tissue are present, take sections demonstrating margins and possible soft tissue invasion. Noninvolved soft tissue may then be removed before weighing.

3. Describe any lesion present including size, capsule (benign lesions are usually well encapsulated, malignant lesions may lack a capsule or invade into soft tissue), color (similar to normal cortex versus brown, yellow/white, or red/brown), and relationship to normal adrenal gland (adenomas and carcinomas arise from the cortex, pheochromocytomas arise from the medulla).

4. Describe the nonlesional portion of the gland (color: golden yellow cortex, inner band of reddish zona reticularis, with a central pearly gray medulla), average thickness of gland (normal is 0.7 cm), presence or absence of nodularity.

5. Carefully section through any adjacent soft tissue to search for additional tumor nodules or lymph nodes.

Special studies

Cytogenetics

Many adrenal tumors are associated with germline mutations (e.g., 50% to 100% of adrenocortical carcinomas in children are associated with Li–Fraumeni syndrome and 30% of pheochromocytomas are associated with MEN, as well as other syndromes) (see "Hereditary Tumor Syndromes" Table 7-36). Cytogenetic changes in sporadic cortical tumors have been associated with clinical behavior and may be helpful for their evaluation (see "Cytogenetics of Solid Tumors" Table 7-33). Cytogenetic studies are also important for pediatric adrenal tumors (see below).

Chromaffin reaction

Ninety percent of pheochromocytomas can be diagnosed grossly by a positive chromaffin reaction. Fresh tumor tissue placed in chromate solutions turns a mahogany brown or black. Zenker's fixative can be used, but is not as sensitive as it also contains acetic acid. A solution of potassium dichromate without acetic acid is preferable. Potassium iodide, 10% (which turns the tumors purple or magenta) may be used but may be less sensitive than potassium dichromate.

Pediatric adrenal tumors

Adrenal tumors in children are more likely to be neuroblastomas, ganglioneuroblastomas, and ganglioneuromas, although cortical tumors and pheochromocytomas also occur. As treatment decisions are based on biologic and morphologic variables, the pathologist plays a crucial role in managing the tissue allocation of neuroblastoma cases. In general, tumor tissue should be placed in sterile culture medium for cytogenetic studies, snap frozen in liquid nitrogen for molecular biology studies, saved as air-dried touch preparations for in situ hybridization (e.g., FISH), and possibly for EM.[1]

Gross differential diagnosis

Normal glands (Fig. 11-1A). A normal gland is a flat ovoid structures with a reticulated surface. On cross-section the cortex is a distinctive bright canary yellow color. Lesions of this color at other sites often correspond to adrenal rests. There is a narrow inner reddish brown band that corresponds to the zona reticularis. The medulla has a more homogeneous appearance and is a pearly gray color.

Hyperplastic glands (Fig. 11-1B). Hyperplastic glands show either diffuse (usually secondary hyperplasia due to increased ACTH) or nodular enlargement (usually primary hyperplasia) and commonly weigh more than 6 g. Multiple nodules may be present that are rarely encapsulated. There may be a dominant nodule but the entire cortex should be increased in size.

Adenomas (Fig. 11-1C). Adenomas are usually solitary and relatively small (less than 5 cm or 50 g) and arise from the cortex. Most have a homogeneous bright yellow parenchyma (like cortex) with a well-circumscribed border. Larger lesions may have areas of necrosis or hemorrhage. Rarely adenomas appear dark or black due to the presence of a pigment thought to be either lipofuscin or neuromelanin. These dark adenomas are usually nonfunctioning.

- *Cushing's syndrome*: Bright yellow and of moderate size. These adenomas cause suppression of ACTH by autonomously producing cortisol, and thus cause atrophy of the surrounding normal adrenal (as well as the contralateral gland). The cortex should measure less than 0.2 cm in thickness and there may be fibrous thickening of the capsule.
- *Conn's syndrome*: Often smaller (<2 cm) and paler in color than those associated with Cushing's syndrome. The normal gland is not suppressed and should be normal in size.
- *Adenomas associated with virilization or feminization*: Often large (>1000 g) and tan/white to brown.
- *"Incidentalomas"*: Adenomas found incidentally due to radiologic imaging of the adrenal glands for another reason. These lesions are usually nonfunctioning and may be present in 0.6% to 1.3% of patients. Less than 1% of these lesions will be adrenal carcinomas. Large lesions or lesions showing growth over time are usually resected.

Adrenal carcinomas. Carcinomas are usually much larger (i.e., over 100 g and 10 to 20 cm) but can be small. The tumors may be bright yellow but often have a variegated appearance with areas of necrosis and hemorrhage. A capsule may be present but is often invaded by tumor with extension into adjacent tissues. Vascular invasion is common and thrombosis or tumor embolism may be present. Half are functional and may cause atrophy of the surrounding cortex.

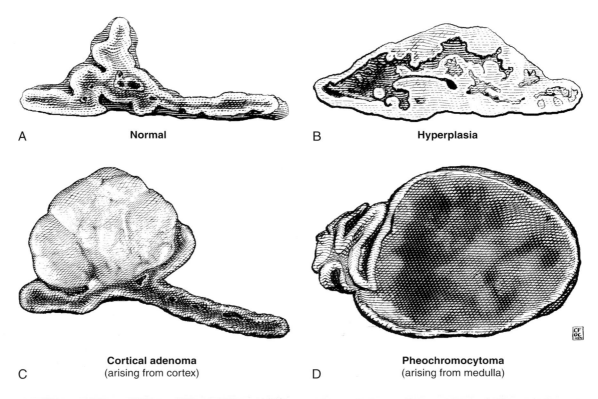

A   **Normal**   B   **Hyperplasia**

C   **Cortical adenoma** (arising from cortex)   D   **Pheochromocytoma** (arising from medulla)

Figure 11-1 Gross pathology of adrenal tumors.

Pheochromocytomas (Fig. 11-1D). These are yellow/white to red/brown and arise from the medulla. Small tumors tend to be unencapsulated whereas larger tumors usually have a capsule. Larger or malignant tumors may have areas of necrosis, hemorrhage, and cystic degeneration. Most are 5 to 8 cm in size and weigh 70 to 100 g. The surrounding cortex may be compressed.

The pheochromocytoma 10% rule
10% bilateral, 10% extraadrenal, 10% in children, 10% malignant

Pheochromocytomas associated with hereditary syndromes (approximately 30% of the total), are associated with medullary hyperplasia in the adjacent gland, and multiple nodules may be present. Adrenal medullary hyperplasia is usually associated with MEN IIa and IIb syndromes and consists of diffuse or nodular expansion of the medulla of both adrenal glands. A nodule measuring more than 1 cm is classified as a pheochromocytoma.

Neuroblastomas. These are the most common adrenal tumors in children. The tumors are soft and hemorrhagic and may be cystic. Necrosis may be present and may invade surrounding tissues. Ganglioneuroblastomas and ganglioneuromas are firmer, white to tan, and often have areas with calcification. Focal areas typical of neuroblastoma should be sought and sampled in such tumors.

Metastatic tumors. These are usually firm and white and appear to invade or destroy the adjacent adrenal. Multiple nodules may be present. Adrenal glands with metastasis from a distant site (usually lung, breast, or melanoma) would be an unusual surgical specimen as the diagnosis can often be made by FNA. However, if the adrenal gland is removed during a radical nephrectomy, the gland may harbor metastatic renal cell carcinoma (see Tables, 7–18. Adrenal and Renal Tumors").

Myelolipomas. A soft, fleshy, circumscribed mass that resembles adipose tissue with focal red or fibrous areas. The mass compresses the adjacent gland. Approximately 20% are associated with tuberous sclerosis.

Benign cysts. These are usually unilocular and small and are filled with serous or serosanguinous fluid. Hemorrhagic cysts may be filled with clotted blood. Most probably arise from blood vessels or lymphatics.

All other lesions not corresponding to the above descriptions may be highly interesting benign or malignant lesions (e.g., primary lymphomas of the adrenal, ganglioneuromas). Such lesions should be carefully documented, and tissue may be taken for special studies (e.g., frozen tissue, EM, cytogenetics).

Microscopic sections

Lesions
Small lesion (i.e., <2 cm): entire lesion including the capsule and relationship to adjacent adrenal gland. Large lesion (i.e., >2 cm): Three cassettes plus an additional cassette for each 1 cm of greatest dimension. Include the capsule and sample all areas that have different gross features (e.g., unusual color, necrosis, hemorrhage). Include relationship to the adjacent gland.

Normal gland
If no gross lesion is present, and was not suspected clinically, submit one representative section of the gland. If lesions are present, submit two sections of the junction of the nonlesional gland and the lesion.

Margins
If the tumor is infiltrating into soft tissue, submit perpendicular margins.

Lymph nodes
Serial section and submit (see Chapter 27).

Sample dictation

Received fresh, labeled with the patient's name and unit number and "right adrenal" is an adrenalectomy specimen (10 × 4 × 2 cm) completely surrounded by yellow/white unremarkable adipose tissue varying in thickness from 0.5 to 2.0 cm. There is a 20-g 3 × 3 × 2 cm ovoid well-circumscribed bright yellow tumor mass arising from the cortex of the adrenal, which is firm and lacks necrosis or hemorrhage. The tumor appears to compress the adjacent cortex, which is homogeneous and atrophic in appearance and measures 0.2 cm in thickness. The gray medulla is a narrow band and unremarkable. A single small (0.3 cm) lymph node is found in the adjacent soft tissue.

Cassette #1–4: Tumor including soft tissue margins, 4 frags, ESS.
Cassette #5: Remainder of tumor (ESS) and adjacent normal adrenal, 1 frag, RSS.
Cassette #6: Representative normal adrenal, 1 frag, RSS.
Cassette #7: Lymph node, 1 frag, ESS.

Pathologic prognostic/diagnostic features sign-out checklist for adrenal tumors

Specimen type*
Subtotal adrenalectomy, total adrenalectomy, biopsy (note if laparoscopic).

Laterality*
Right, left.

Tumor size*
Greatest dimension (optional: other dimensions). Most cortical tumors over 5 cm will be malignant.

Tumor weight*
In grams. Most benign cortical tumors weigh less than 50 g and most malignant tumors weigh more than 100 g.

Histologic type*
Cortical adenoma, cortical carcinoma, pheochromocytoma, neuroblastoma, ganglioneuroblastoma, ganglioneuroma, myelolipoma, other rare types. The WHO classification is recommended.

It is not always possible to determine whether a cortical or medullary tumor is benign or malignant in the absence of distant metastases. However, histologic features can be used to divide tumors into low- and high-risk groups (Boxes 11-1 to 11-3 and Table 11-2).

The Shimada classification system is used for pediatric neuroblastic tumors (Fig. 11-2).

Extent of invasion*
Confined to gland, extraglandular extension, involvement of other organs.
If present, specify if focal or over a broad front.

Regional lymph node metastasis*
Absent, present (number of nodes involved, number of nodes examined).

Distant metastasis*
Absent, present.

Margins*
Uninvolved, involved (specify site, extent of involvement)

Venous (large vessel) invasion
Absent, present.

Lymphovascular invasion
Present or absent

Fuhrman nuclear grade
For carcinomas (see under renal carcinomas for criteria)

Necrosis and hemorrhage
Present or absent, focal or extensive. Unusual in benign lesions. Lesions with zonal necrosis are more likely to be malignant.

Mitotic rate
Number of mitoses per 10 HPFs. For adrenocortical carcinomas, >20 mitoses per 10 HPFs is associated with a shorter disease-free survival (14 months) as compared to <20 mitoses (58 months). A mitosis-karyorrhexis index is used for neuroblastic tumors.

Nonlesional adrenal
Normal, atrophic, hyperplastic (cortex versus medulla).

This checklist incorporates information from the ADASP (see www.panix.com/~adasp/) and the CAP Cancer Committee protocols for reporting on cancer specimens (see www.cap.org/). The asterisked elements are considered to be scientifically validated or regularly used data elements that must be present in reports of cancer-directed surgical resection specimens from ACS CoC-approved cancer programs. The specific details of reporting the elements may vary among institutions.

Box 11-1

Weiss criteria for malignancy for cortical lesions in adults (>20 years of age)[2,3]

Fewer than 10% of cortical tumors behave in a malignant fashion. No single feature or group of features is able to separate benign from malignant lesions. However, the following criteria can be used to classify cortical lesions into high- and low-risk lesions:

1. Moderate to marked cellular pleomorphism, nuclear atypia (criteria of Fuhrman—see Table 20-4)
2. Mitotic rate >5 per 50 HPF
3. Atypical mitotic figures
4. Eosinophilic tumor cell cytoplasm (75% of tumor cells)
5. Diffuse architecture (33% of tumor)
6. Necrosis
7. Venous invasion (smooth muscle in wall)
8. Sinusoidal invasion (no smooth muscle in wall)
9. Capsular invasion (into or through capsule, with stromal reaction)

Criteria 2, 3, and 7 were seen only in malignant tumors. Ninety-five percent of malignant tumors had three or more of these criteria, whereas all benign lesions had two or fewer.

Box 11-2

Criteria for malignant clinical behavior for cortical lesions in children (<20 years of age)[4]

1. Tumor weight >400 g
2. Tumor size >10.5 cm
3. Extension into peri-adrenal soft tissue and/or adjacent organs
4. Invasion into vena cava
5. Venous invasion
6. Capsular invasion
7. Presence of tumor necrosis
8. >15 mitoses per 20 HPF (400×)
9. Presence of atypical mitotic figures

Some tumors that would be classified as malignant if the criteria for tumors in adults were used behave in a benign fashion in children.
0–2 criteria: benign long-term clinical outcome
3 criteria: indeterminate for malignancy (17% are malignant)
>3 criteria: poor clinical outcome (64% are malignant)

Box 11-3

Features associated with malignancy in pheochromocytomas[5]

Five to 15% of pheochromocytomas behave in a clinically malignant fashion, but it is impossible to predict this group based on any histologic feature. Even tumors with capsular invasion, vascular invasion, and invasion into adjacent soft tissue may be surgically curable. The following features are associated with a greater risk of malignant behavior:

- Male sex
- Large tumor size
- Coarse nodularity
- Tumor necrosis
- Predominantly small tumor cell size
- Absence of cytoplasmic hyaline globules
- Absence of neuropeptides and/or S100-positive sustentacular cells by IHC

Table 11-2 Staging system for adrenal cortical carcinomas[6]

T1	Tumor ≤5 cm, confined to gland
T2	Tumor >5 cm, confined to gland
T3	Tumor any size, locally invading out of the gland, but not involving adjacent organs
T4	Tumor any size, locally invading into adjacent organs
N0	No positive regional lymph nodes
N1	Positive regional lymph nodes
M0	No distant metastases
M1	Distant metastases

The AJCC does not have a staging system for adrenal carcinomas.

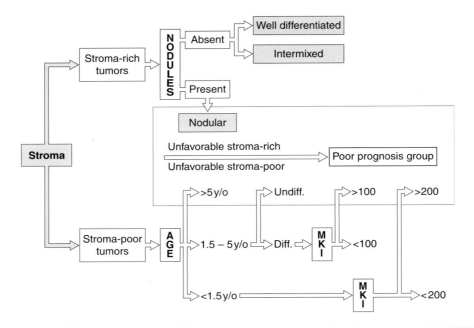

Figure 11-2 The age-linked Shimada classification of childhood neuroblastoma and ganglioneuroblastoma. The Shimada classification uses specific morphologic features (i.e., stroma, differentiation, mitosis-karyorrhexis index (MKI) nodularity, and calcification), age, stage, and nMYC status to evaluate pediatric neuroblastic tumors. The character of the stroma is important for prognosis. Unfavorable stroma-rich and stroma-poor categories are seen. (Reproduced with permission from Shimada H, Chatten J, Newton WA Jr et al. J Natl Cancer Institute 73:405-416, 1984.)

REFERENCES

1. Shimada H, Ambros IM, Dehner LP, Hata J, Joshi VV, Roald B. Terminology and morphologic criteria of neuroblastic tumors: recommendations by the International Neuroblastoma Pathology Committee. Cancer 86:349-365, 1999.

2. Weiss LM, Medeiros LJ, Vickery AL. Pathologic features of prognostic significance in adrenal cortical carcinoma. Am J Surg Pathol 13:202-206, 1989.

3. Medeiros LJ, Weiss LM. New developments in the pathologic diagnosis of adrenal cortical neoplasms. Am J Clin Pathol 97:73-83, 1992.

4. Wieneke JA, Thompson LDR, Heffess CS. Adrenal cortical neoplasms in the pediatric population: A clinicopathologic and immunophenotype analysis of 83 patients. Am J Surg Pathol 27:867-881, 2003.

5. Medeiros LJ, Weiss LM. Adrenal gland: Tumors and tumor-like lesions. In: Weidner N (ed.) The Difficult Diagnosis in Surgical Pathology. 377-407, Elsevier, St Louis 1996.

6. Henley DJ, et al. Adrenal cortical carcinoma—a continuing challenge. Surgery 94:926-931, 1983.

7. Shimada H, Ambros IM, Dehner LP, et al. The International Neuroblastoma Pathology Classification (the Shimada System). Cancer 86:364-372, 1999.

8. Shimada H, Chatten J, Newton WA Jr, et al. J Natl Cancer Inst 73:405-416, 1984.

Amputations and large resections

12

The most common reasons for amputations are peripheral vascular disease, trauma, and, occasionally, tumors.

Some amputation specimens may be requested by the patient (some religions require burial of the limb).

Relevant clinical history (in addition to age and gender)

See Table 12-1.

■ GENERAL GROSS DESCRIPTION

The description of all amputations includes the following:

Structures present:
- Left lower leg below the knee amputation, right foot, left index finger, etc.
- Dimensions of each structure (e.g., upper leg, lower leg, foot) including length and maximum circumference of limbs.

Type of procedure. Disarticulation (cartilage-covered joint surface present) versus amputation (exposed bone surface present).

Type of resection margin. For example, disarticulated femoral head, amputation of the third metacarpal, diaphysis of femur, 10 cm from distal surface of medial femoral condyle.

Table 12-1 Relevant clinical history

HISTORY RELEVANT TO ALL SPECIMENS	HISTORY RELEVANT TO AMPUTATION SPECIMENS
Organ/tissue resected or biopsied	Joint disease (e.g., gout or rheumatoid arthritis)
Purpose of the procedure	Reason for the amputation (e.g., vascular disease associated with diabetes, avascular necrosis, malignancy, pathologic fracture, traumatic amputation)
Gross appearance of the organ/tissue/lesion sampled	
Any unusual features of the clinical presentation	Prior malignancy (e.g., primary bone tumor, metastases to bone, or tumors such as lymphoma that involve bone marrow)
Any unusual features of the gross appearance	
Prior surgery/biopsies—results	Prior treatment (e.g., vascular grafts, treatment of malignant tumors)
Prior malignancy	
Prior treatment (radiation therapy, chemotherapy, drug use that can change the histologic appearance of tissues)	Radiologic findings (e.g., incidental mass or found on studies for nonspecific symptoms of weight loss or malaise)
Compromised immune system	

Smooth (surgical) or irregular (traumatic) resection margin.

Soft tissue at resection margin. Condition (e.g. grossly viable versus necrotic or ulcerated). Distance of skin and soft tissue from bony resection margin.

Skin. Color, lesions (ulcers, areas of discoloration, bruising, gangrene) or identifying marks (e.g., scars, tattoos).

Lesions. Bone fractures, blood vessels (atherosclerosis, thrombosis), osteomyelitis, tumor (if present), previous amputation sites.

Prior surgical procedures Amputations, vacular grafts, etc.

Decalcification. Decalcification must be documented as this procedure can alter the histologic appearance and immunogenicity of tissues and is required for appropriate billing.

■ TRAUMATIC AMPUTATIONS

Traumatic amputations may involve litigation, in which case the pathologic examination may become legal evidence. It is helpful to photograph such specimens for documentation. Process as described below for amputations for vascular insufficiency. The presence and extent of any peripheral vascular disease may be of clinical value.

■ DIGITS—NON-TUMOR

Fingers and toes are usually removed because of vascular insufficiency (toes) or trauma (usually fingers).

Processing the specimen

1. Describe, including the features listed in "General gross description", above.
2. Submit one section of soft tissue margin and an additional section of any skin lesion.
3. Fix the entire specimen overnight.
4. Decalcify the following day.
5. When the bone is sufficiently decalcified, take one section of bone at the resection margin and one additional section of bone if there is a question of osteomyelitis (e.g., bone below a deep ulcer bed).

Microscopic sections

Skin and soft tissue
One section of margin and additional section(s) to evaluate any skin lesions.

Bone
One section of the resection margin. Additional section(s) of bone beneath deep ulcers if there is a question of osteomyelitis.

Sample dictation

Received fresh, labeled with the patient's name and unit number and "toes," are two digits amputated through the first metatarsal bone with a smooth resection margin and measuring $2 \times 2 \times 1.5$ cm and $1.5 \times 1.5 \times 1$ cm. The larger digit has a deep ulcer on the plantar surface (1×1 cm) that grossly appears to extend to the underlying bone. The skin of the smaller digit has a purple/black color, but no ulceration is present. The nails are unremarkable. The resection margins consist of unremarkable bone and soft tissue. The bone is fixed and decalcified prior to submission.

Cassette #1: Larger digit, ulcer, 1 frag, RSS.
Cassette #2: Larger digit, skin at margin, 1 frag, RSS.
Cassette #3: Larger digit, bone below ulcer, 1 frag, RSS.
Cassette #4: Larger digit, bone at margin, 1 frag, RSS.
Cassette #5: Smaller digit, representative skin and soft tissue at tip, 1 frag, RSS.
Cassette #6: Smaller digit, skin at margin, 1 frag, RSS.
Cassette #7: Smaller digit, bone at margin, 1 frag, RSS.

■ LOWER EXTREMITY—NON-TUMOR

Vascular insufficiency

Vascular insufficiency is the most common reason for amputations. Often there will be prior amputations (e.g., several toes) and skin lesions (ulcers or frank gangrene). To document the disease process, dissect and examine the vessels of the leg.

Dissection of the vessels of the lower extremity (Fig. 12-1)

1. Make a skin incision that starts just behind the medial malleolus and extends proximally in an oblique manner to reach the posterior aspect of the leg and thence straight upwards to the line of resection.
2. Identify the posterior tibial neurovascular bundle behind the medial malleolus. Sever the distal ends and proceed to strip the vessels upwards, dissecting the muscle and subcutaneous tissue away from the vessels. Stop when the junction of the posterior tibial and the popliteal arteries is reached at the interosseous membrane between the tibia and fibula.
3. Return to the ankle region and extend the original incision distally and then laterally to traverse the dorsum of the foot just distal to the ankle. Reflect the skin flap to expose the anterior compartment of the leg.
4. Identify the anterior tibial neurovascular bundle at the ankle (the anterior tibial artery becomes the dorsalis pedis artery and traverses the dorsum of the foot at this site). Sever the distal ends and reflect proximally as for the posterior tibial. When the interosseous membrane is reached, dissect bluntly around the vessel to free it. Then return to the posterior aspect of the leg and pull the anterior tibial vessels through the interosseous membrane.
5. Complete the removal of the vessels by continuing the reflection of the popliteal artery to the lines of resection.

Usually the vessels are densely calcified and will require decalcification before cutting.

Processing the specimen

1. Record the measurements and features described in "General gross description", above.
2. Dissect out the anterior and posterior vessels and any grafts if present (see above). If vein grafts are present, describe their anatomic relationships to other vessels, the status of the anastomosis (intact, patent, obstructed) and the presence or absence of thrombi.
3. Take skin and soft tissue sections from the margin and from any lesions present. Take a cross-section of the soft tissue of one of the grossly normal toes to look for small vessel disease. Bone sections need not be taken if there is no gross lesion. If there is a suspicion of bone involvement (osteomyelitis), that section of bone is resected with the bone saw for fixation and decalcification.

    The metatarsophalangeal joint of the great toe is dissected open and examined for evidence of joint disease (see Chapter 14, "Synovium," for gross differential diagnosis of joint disease).

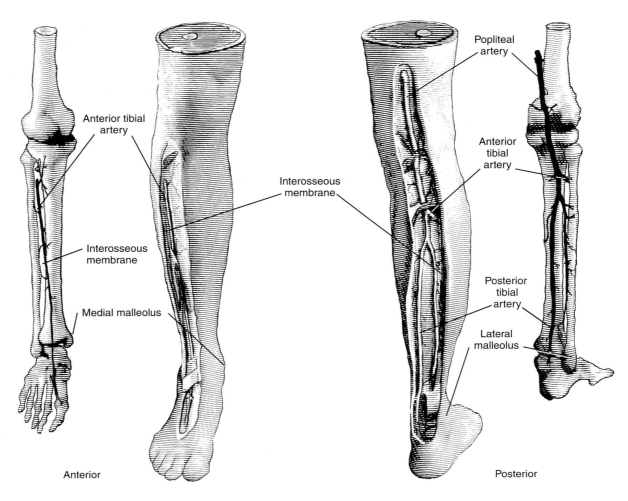

Anterior tibial artery

Interosseous membrane

Medial malleolus

Interosseous membrane

Popliteal artery

Anterior tibial artery

Posterior tibial artery

Lateral malleolus

Anterior

Posterior

A

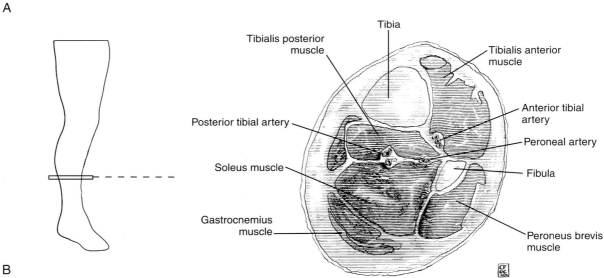

B

Tibia

Tibialis posterior muscle

Tibialis anterior muscle

Posterior tibial artery

Anterior tibial artery

Soleus muscle

Peroneal artery

Fibula

Gastrocnemius muscle

Peroneus brevis muscle

Figure 12-1 Dissection of the lower extremity.

The marrow can be removed from the cut section of the bone and prepared as for a rib marrow squeeze if there is a clinical suspicion of disease involving the marrow.

4. Fix the tissue sections and blood vessels in small formalin containers with appropriate labels (e.g., "anterior vessels and margin," "posterior vessels and skin lesion"). The remainder of the specimen is kept unfixed but refrigerated.

5. The following day the soft tissue is submitted for processing: one cassette of margin, cassette(s) of lesion(s), cassette of soft tissue of toe. The vessels are decalcified.

6. The following day the vessels and grafts are serially sectioned. Record the location and extent of occlusions (calcified plaque, thrombosis). Submit multiple cross-sections in two separate cassettes from the anterior and from the posterior vessels of the areas of greatest occlusion. If a graft is present, submit areas of obstruction and the vein–artery anastomotic site.

Microscopic sections

Skin and soft tissue
One section of margin and additional section(s) to evaluate any skin lesions.

Cross-section of toe
One cross-section (to evaluate small vessel disease).

Bone
Only submit section(s) of bone if there is a question of osteomyelitis or if bony lesions are present. The margin need not be submitted.

Vessels and grafts
Submit one cassette each of anterior and posterior vessels showing area(s) of greatest occlusion. Submit area of greatest occlusion of grafts and the vein–artery anastomotic site.

Bone marrow
Only submit if there is a clinical suspicion of disease affecting the bone marrow.

Joint
Only submit if there is clinical suspicion or gross evidence of disease affecting the joints (e.g., gout).

Sample dictation

Received fresh, labeled with the patient's name and unit number and "leg," is a right lower extremity amputated through the tibia and fibula with a smooth resection margin (length of leg 37 cm; circumference of calf 40 cm; foot 26 × 9 cm). The fourth and fifth digits have been previously amputated. The skin is diffusely mottled purple and red. There are ulcerations present on the lateral aspect of the foot (3 × 1 cm) and on the plantar surface of the great toe (1 × 1 cm). The anterior vessels are diffusely calcified with luminal obstructions of up to 80%. The posterior vessels are diffusely calcified with luminal obstructions of up to 50%. The metatarsophalangeal joint of the great toe consists of smooth glistening white cartilage and is grossly unremarkable. The bone and soft tissue at the resection margin are unremarkable. A cross-section of the third digit is fixed and decalcified prior to submission.

Cassette #1: Skin, ulcers, 2 frags, RSS.
Cassette #2: Skin and soft tissue at margin, 1 frag, RSS.
Cassette #3: Cross-section of third digit, 1 frag, RSS.
Cassette #4: Anterior vessels, 1 frag, RSS.
Cassette #5: Posterior vessels, 1 frag, RSS.

■ AMPUTATIONS OR LARGE RESECTIONS FOR TUMOR

Large tumor resections are unusual and usually involve either tumors of bone or cartilage, or soft tissue tumors involving major neurovascular bundles[1-4]. See Chapter 14, "Bone resections for tumors" and Chapter 32 respectively for additional information on these specimens.

If bone is present, radiographs of the specimen are helpful to document the bony structures and to identify areas of destruction of normal bone or abnormal bone formation for sampling. Tumors involving bone may require sectioning (either longitudinal or cross sections) with an electric handsaw or a band saw. If the distal limb is not involved, separating this part of the specimen may simplify dissection and fixation.

Diagrams are often useful to document complex specimens and can be used to designate the location of tissue blocks. Polaroid photographs and photocopies have also been used for this purpose.[5]

Describe the specimen as outlined in "General gross description", above. Identify the muscles, nerves, and arteries present at the margin of the specimen and the sites of any prior biopsies. The best way to process the specimen will depend on the type and location of the tumor. Tumors involving nerve bundles may be best demonstrated by partial dissection of nerve trunks.

Describe the tumor including size, appearance (color, necrosis, bone formation, cartilage formation), location (tissue compartment), relationship to surrounding structures (bone, vessels, nerves, muscle), center of tumor (epiphysis, metaphysis, diaphysis, intramedullary, periosteal), erosion of cortex, extension into soft tissue (compression or true invasion), extension through epiphyseal plate, extension into or across joint space, vascular involvement, skip metastases, and distance from each margin.

After all soft tissue sections have been removed, tumors involving bone can be decalcified after fixation. Overdecalcification, which results in loss of histologic detail, should be avoided by periodically checking the specimen to minimize exposure. Bone dust may create histologic artifacts (i.e., bone fragments within the marrow space). To avoid this, small sections of bone should be decalcified, the decalcified tissue thinly sectioned with a scalpel, and the tissue sections embedded so that the surface away from that cut by the saw is used to prepare tissue for slides.

All margins, usually perpendicular, must be evaluated including soft tissue, blood vessels, nerves, and bone. Bone margins can be removed with a bone saw and decalcified separately.

Special studies

Untreated tumors

Most amputations are performed for sarcomas, bone tumors, or other unusual tumors. It is often helpful to save tumor for rapid formalin fixation, electron microscopy, snap freezing, and cytogenetics.

Treated tumors

If the tumor has been previously diagnosed and special studies performed, and the patient has received preoperative chemotherapy and/or radiation therapy, the tumor may be largely necrotic and additional studies may not be possible. However, a complete cross-section of the tumor (using multiple cassettes with locations indicated on a diagram) may be helpful to evaluate the extent of necrosis in response to treatment (see Chapter 14).

Microscopic sections

Tumor

At least one section per cm including areas of intratumoral heterogeneity, relationship to adjacent normal structures, and relationship to margins. A diagram with a section code is usually needed.

Margins

All margins, including soft tissue and bone, are sampled using perpendicular sections.

Normal structures

Representative sections of normal structures (e.g., blood vessels, major nerve bundles).

Lymph nodes

Submit all lymph nodes found (see Chapter 27).

REFERENCES

1. Barnes L, Johnson JT. Pathologic and clinical consideration in the evaluation of major head and neck specimens resected for cancer, Part 1. Pathol Annu 21(Part 1):173-250, 1986.

2. Barnes L, Johnson JT. Pathologic and clinical consideration in the evaluation of major head and neck specimens resected for cancer, Part 2. Pathol Annu 21(Part 2):83-110, 1986.

3. Weatherby RP, Krishnan KU. Practical aspects of handling orthopedic specimens in the surgical pathology laboratory. Pathol Annu 17(Part 2):1-31, 1982.

4. Patterson K. The pathologic handling of skeletal tumors. Am J Clin Pathol 109 (Suppl 1):S53-S66, 1998.

5. Olson DR. Specimen photocopying for surgical pathology reports. Am J Clin Pathol 70:94-95, 1978.

Biopsies, small

13

Small biopsies are minute tissue fragments taken either by pinching and tearing tissue (e.g., endomyocardium, gastrointestinal tract, bladder, synovium, larynx, or lung) or with a core needle biopsy (e.g., liver, kidney, bone marrow, prostate, and breast) for a wide variety of reasons (e.g., malignancy, infection, inflammatory diseases, radiologic lesions, transplant rejection). The anatomic site of the tissue is usually unidentifiable.

Relevant clinical history (in addition to age and gender)

See Table 13-1.

Biopsies of the small bowel, breast, heart, liver, bladder, lung (transbronchial), colon, synovium, brain, stomach, temporal artery, bone marrow, kidney, and skin have additional processing protocols, described in the respective chapters.

Table 13-1 Relevant clinical history (in addition to age and gender)

HISTORY RELEVANT TO ALL SPECIMENS	HISTORY RELEVANT TO SMALL BIOPSIES
Organ/tissue resected or biopsied	Type of biopsy (e.g., needle, forceps, wedge, curettage, punch)
Purpose of the procedure	
Gross appearance of the organ/tissue/lesion sampled	Number of biopsies or fragments
Any unusual features of the clinical presentation	Appearance of the clinical lesion
Any unusual features of the gross appearance	
Prior surgery/biopsies—results	
Prior malignancy	
Prior treatment (radiation therapy, chemotherapy, drug use that can change the histologic appearance of tissues)	
Compromised immune system	

Processing the specimen

1. Record:
- Number of fragments. If many, give an estimate, not "many" or "numerous".
- Aggregate dimensions.
- Greatest dimension of largest fragment. If there are only a few fragments (e.g., two to three), the dimensions of each one may be given.

   At sign-out it is important to correlate the number of fragments on the slide with the number of tissue fragments received to ensure that all tissue fragments are represented microscopically.

Check the sides and lid of the container for small fragments that may have stuck there. Every piece of tissue is important because sometimes a diagnosis can be made on only a few cells!

On the other hand, small specimens are particularly susceptible to cross contamination from other specimens. The work area must be kept fastidiously clean and all dissecting tools cleaned between cases.

Specimens may be submitted on gauze: this can introduce artifacts into tissues that look like perpendicular empty hatchmarks under the microscope and correspond to the weave of the cloth.

2.   Record the shape of the fragments: needle cores or small irregular fragments.

3.   Record the color and consistency of the fragments:
- White, firm—usual appearance of tissue
- Yellow, soft—adipose tissue, may fragment and not be seen well on slides
- Red, friable—usually blood clot, may not survive processing
- Brown, hard—may be foreign matter (e.g., seeds) sometimes present in colon biopsies.
  These features can be used to distinguish tissue fragments from non-tissue material to correlate with the number of fragments on the final slides.

4.   Small biopsy specimens should not be cut or inked. If the specimen is large enough to orient (e.g., colon polyps, skin, or temporal arteries), see the specific chapter concerning this type of biopsy.

5.   All small biopsies must be supported within the cassette to prevent tissue loss during processing. All fragments are submitted.

- **Lens paper** can be used for very small specimens and avoids introducing artifacts. Place the specimen in the center of a square of lens paper moistened in formalin. Fold carefully (four folds and crease). Overfolded specimens may be difficult to unfold for tissue embedding; underfolding may result in unfolding during processing with loss of the specimen. Needle biopsies may become clumped and difficult to embed in a single plane when wrapped in paper. Clumping can be minimized by wrapping the needle biopsies on a flat surface and placing a sponge in the same cassette to hold the specimen flat. Lens paper can also be used for cell blocks.
- **Nylon specimen bags** can be used in the same manner as lens paper. Make sure the fragments are near the bottom of the bag. Fold twice and place in a cassette. Specimen bags can also be used for cell blocks. The cell suspension can be poured through a nylon bag. The filtered formalin should be collected in a clean specimen cup in order to retrieve specimens in case of spillage.
- **Sponges** hold the tissue flat and aid in embedding the tissue in the same plane. However, sponges can create artifacts within the tissue (i.e., angulated "holes" within the tissue). They cannot be used for cell blocks. Wrapping the tissue in paper before placing between sponges may minimize tissue distortion.

6.   Most types of biopsies have standard numbers of levels and special stains (see Chapter 3).

Sample dictations

Example 1

Received in formalin, labeled with the patient's name, unit number, and "heart biopsies," are five fragments of soft tissue, each measuring approximately 0.4 × 0.3 × 0.3 cm. Three of the fragments are brown, one is white, and one is friable and red/brown.

Cassette #1: five frags, ESS.

Example 2
Received in formalin, labeled with the patient's name, unit number, and "PNBX left," are three white/tan needle biopsies measuring 0.1 cm in diameter and 0.7, 0.5, and 0.3 cm in length.

Cassette #1: three frags, ESS.

Example 3
The specimen consists of three parts, all received in formalin, labeled with the patient's name and unit number.
The first part is labeled "Transverse" and consists of a single fragment of tan soft tissue (0.4 × 0.4 × 0.4 cm).

Cassette #1: one frag, ESS.

The second part is labeled "Sigmoid" and consists of two fragments of white/tan soft tissue, each approximately 0.3 × 0.3 × 0.3 cm.

Cassette #2: two frags, ESS.

The third part is labeled "Rectum" and consists of three fragments of white/tan soft tissue, each approximately 0.4 × 0.3 × 0.2 cm, and one fragment of friable tan/brown material measuring 0.2 × 0.2 × 0.2 cm.

Cassette #3: four frags, ESS.

Example 4
Received in formalin, labeled with the patient's name, unit number, and "Bladder tumor," are approximately 20 fragments of soft tan/white tissue with a micropapillary architecture, measuring in aggregate 0.7 × 0.7 × 0.3 cm, the largest fragment measuring 0.4 × 0.4 × 0.4 cm.

Cassette #1: mult frags, ESS.

Bone and joints

14

Bones are common surgical specimens that may be submitted after reconstructive or joint replacement surgery, as part of a larger soft tissue resection, to diagnose metabolic bone disease, or after resection of tumors primary to bone.

Relevant clinical history (in addition to age and gender)

See Table 14-1.

Table 14-1 Relevant clinical history (in addition to age and gender)	
HISTORY RELEVANT TO ALL SPECIMENS	HISTORY RELEVANT TO BONES AND JOINTS
Organ/tissue resected or biopsied	Reason for the procedure (e.g., degenerative joint disease, failed joint replacement, fracture, infection, malignancy, osteonecrosis, evaluation of metabolic bone disease)
Purpose of the procedure	Joint disease (e.g., gout, rheumatoid arthritis)
Gross appearance of the organ/tissue/lesion sampled	
Any unusual features of the clinical presentation	
Any unusual features of the gross appearance	
Prior surgery/biopsies—results	
Prior malignancy	
Prior treatment (radiation therapy, chemotherapy, drug use that can change the histologic appearance of tissues)	
Compromised immune system	

■ TOTAL JOINT ARTHROPLASTY (HIPS AND KNEES)

Bone, cartilage, and adjacent soft tissues are removed during artificial joint replacements, usually for cases of degenerative joint disease but also for rheumatoid arthritis, osteonecrosis, traumatic fractures, and pathologic fractures. Specimens are submitted for documentation and to exclude clinically unsuspected diseases (e.g., hemochromatosis, rheumatoid arthritis, gout, and rarely tumors such as metastatic prostate carcinoma or multiple myeloma).

The value of histologic examination of "routine" arthroplasty specimens has been questioned.[1,2] For a full discussion of this issue, see "Gross Examination, Chapter 21" It is unusual to find unsuspected inflammatory synovitis (4 in 1000 cases) or malignancy (1 in 1000 cases). A decision to not examine well-defined "routine" specimens (therapeutic procedures in patients without a history of malignancy, infection, or immunocompromise, and with normal gross findings) should be made jointly between pathologists and clinicians, in accordance with JCAHO standards, be part of a written hospital or laboratory policy.

Processing the specimen

1. Describe the number of fragments of bone (estimate if many), size in aggregate, range of sizes. Describe any recognizable portions of bone: femoral head (see "Specimens with intact femoral heads", page 224), tibial plateau, and femoral condyles.

2. Describe the articular surface including color (usually white, black if ochronosis, brown/green if hemochromatosis), crystalline deposits (both gout and chondrocalcinosis will produce chalky white deposits), erosions or pits, or eburnation (bone which is markedly thickened and smooth like ivory, due to complete loss of the overlying cartilage—do not mistake eburnated bone for cartilage!). Describe subchondral cysts or osteophytes if present.

3. Describe the number of fragments of soft tissue (estimate if many), size in aggregate, range of sizes.

4. Describe the color and consistency of the soft tissue:
- Normal: white/tan, delicate, villous.
- Hemochromatosis: brown/green.
- β_2-microglobulin amyloidosis: tan/yellow, firm, and homogeneous.
- Giant cell tumor, diffuse type (pigmented villonodular synovitis or PVNS): red/brown and shaggy (delicate villi with small nodules may be appreciated if the tissue is floated in saline). Necrotic foci may appear yellow due to the presence of histiocytes.
- Gout or chondrocalcinosis: chalky white crystalline material.

     See "Synovium, page 234" for a more complete description and special processing of unusual specimens.

5. The bone is separated from the soft tissue. Submit one section of soft tissue, including synovium if possible. Normal synovium looks like a thin delicate membrane. Fix the bone overnight in formalin and decalcify the following day. All decalcification procedures must be documented in the gross description.

6. Serially section through the decalcified bone to find the best areas for diagnostic study. One fragment of bone should include the junction of normal and abnormal cartilage and the other fragment should be from the periphery to include exostosis and/or pannus. The sections should be approximately 2×1 cm in size with the short axis perpendicular to the cartilage surface including 5 to 10 mm of subchondral bone.

     If osteonecrosis is suspected, the entire specimen must be serially sectioned to look for the characteristic gross findings (see below). Submit sections to document the interface of normal and abnormal bone. Radiography of the specimen may be helpful to identify the area of necrotic bone.

Special studies

Crystal disease

Chalky white deposits in soft tissue may be urate crystals (in gout) or calcium pyrophosphate dihydrate crystals (in calcium pyrophosphate dihydrate deposition disease [CPPD], also known as pseudogout and chondrocalcinosis). Tissue must be saved in absolute (100%) alcohol because these crystals are soluble in aqueous solutions. The tissue must be hand processed and stained with an anaqueous Wright stain. Crystals can also be visualized in unstained sections. See also Chapter 9 for a description of polarization.

Crystals sometimes survive routine processing in aqueous solutions but are lost in the final staining steps. Look for preserved crystals in tissue folds if present. An unstained slide may also be requested and examined under polarized light after deparaffinizing.

Crystals can also be examined directly by smearing the unfixed crystals on a slide or suspending in absolute alcohol as necessary (remember that they will dissolve in water). If the crystals are viewed using a compensating first order red filter under polarized light, uric acid can usually be distinguished from CPPD crystals. The crystals are aligned parallel to the line on the compensating filter. If such a microscope is not available in the pathology department, most rheumatologists will have one available for examination of synovial fluids. Crystals will polarize in properly fixed and stained histologic sections, but positive and negative birefringence cannot be reliably performed on fixed tissue.

Uric acid	Needle shaped
	Strong negative birefringence, bright yellow
CPPD crystals	Rhomboid
	Weakly positive birefringence, less bright and blue

Calcium oxalate crystals can be seen in bone, articular cartilage, and bone marrow in patients with primary (familial) oxalosis or secondary oxalosis (usually resulting from chronic renal failure). The crystals are needle shaped, refractile, and are arranged in radial clusters. The crystals are polarizable. They can dissolve in formalin, but only after several days. The type of crystal can be identified by chemical analysis, x-ray diffraction, or electron diffraction.

Metastasis

Determine from the clinical history if there is a known primary. If not, additional studies may be warranted (e.g., snap freezing, EM, immunohistochemistry). Remove as much soft tissue as possible to avoid exposing potential tumor to decalcification.

Gross differential diagnosis

Degenerative joint disease. The cartilage surface shows fibrillation and loss over the center of the femoral head or over the tibial plateau. The exposed bone becomes thickened and smoothly polished ("eburnated" or "like ivory") and can be mistaken for a cartilage surface. Fractures through articular bone result in subchondral cysts and collapse of the bone. The femoral head is often flattened and misshapen. Osteophytes commonly form around the edge of the articular surface. The soft tissue is relatively unaffected and may be fibrotic.

Rheumatoid arthritis. Patients usually undergo arthroplasty after significant secondary degenerative changes have occurred. Thus, most show the changes of degenerative joint disease, and features of rheumatoid arthritis may be subtle or absent. Findings characteristic of rheumatoid arthritis are an edematous hyperplastic synovium with growth over the cartilage surface to form a pannus.

Gout or CPPD. Chalky white crystalline deposits are present in soft tissue and cartilage, and sometimes erode bone. The synovium becomes fibrotic, thickened, and hyperplastic and forms a pannus overlying cartilage. It is usually not possible to distinguish gout from chondrocalcinosis grossly in mid-sized joints, in which both are common. However, CPPD crystals may preferentially be found within the cartilage and uric acid crystals in periarticular soft tissue. Gout is much more common in small joints of the foot and hand. Neither commonly affects the hip. Joint replacement is usually performed after significant secondary degenerative changes have occurred (see above). Crystals should be saved in alcohol (see "Special studies").

Osteonecrosis (aseptic necrosis, avascular necrosis). Osteonecrosis of bone is a common cause of joint disease (approximately 10% of joint replacements) and is often bilateral. Patients are younger than the typical patient with degenerative joint disease (55 versus 67 years) and often have predisposing conditions such as steroid use, sickle cell disease, or alcoholism. The pathogenesis is poorly understood but is thought to result from ischemic infarction of subchondral bone.

There is a characteristic wedge-shaped area of pale yellow necrotic bone below the cartilage surface. A band of hyperemia is often present below this area. Usually the overlying cartilage has separated away from the bone. The infarcted bone may collapse with distortion of the cartilage and resultant degenerative changes. Radiographs of bone slices can be helpful to look for areas of abnormal mineralization.

Metastatic disease. A joint replacement is sometimes performed to repair a known or suspected pathologic fracture, generally within the femur. The metastatic tumor may be subtle and only apparent after histologic examination of numerous sections. The bone destruction observed radiologically is usually produced by soluble factors produced by the tumor cells and not replacement of bone marrow by tumor per se. Therefore, in such cases histologic sampling of the fracture site is necessary to evaluate the presence of tumor. If a pathologic fracture is strongly suspected clinically or grossly, and the primary site is unknown, consider taking tissue for special studies (e.g., snap freezing, EM).

Microscopic sections

Soft tissue
One section including any grossly recognizable synovium.
If a metastatic deposit is suspected, submit as much soft material from the possible tumor/fracture site as possible that will not need decalcification.

Bone
One section including the junction of normal and abnormal cartilage and one from the periphery.
If osteonecrosis is known or suspected, submit one to two sections of necrotic bone including interface with normal bone and the area below the detached cartilage.

Crystals
If crystals are present, submit one section fixed in absolute alcohol for special anaqueous processing. Order 1 H&E, 1 anaqueous Wright stain, and one unstained slide.

Sample dictation

Received fresh, labeled with the patient's name and unit number and "left total knee" are multiple fragments of bone (in aggregate 5 × 5 × 3 cm, largest 2 × 1 × 1 cm) and soft tissue (4 × 3 × 2 cm, largest 3.5 × 2 × 1 cm). The bone fragments include recognizable portions of the tibial plateau and femoral condyles. The articular surface is markedly roughened with areas of cartilage loss and eburnation of the bony surface. The soft tissue is tan/pink and includes fragments of meniscus. The bone is fixed and decalcified.

Cassettes #1: bone with articular surface, 4 frags, RSS.
Cassette #2: soft tissue, 3 frags, RSS.

Specimens with intact femoral heads

Processing the specimen

1. The femoral head is cut into thirds, parallel to the long axis, with the bone saw. The central section must be thin, approximately 0.5 cm in width.
2. Describe the femoral head including dimensions, shape (flattened, round), cartilage surface (smooth and glistening, erosions, pits, eburnation of bone surface, fibrillation of cartilage, pannus formation), detachment of cartilage (as in osteonecrosis), presence of exostoses. Describe the quality of the bone (osteoporotic, sclerotic, pale as in osteonecrosis) and subchondral cysts.
3. Describe the resection margin including surface (flat and smooth if surgical, jagged and with medullary hemorrhage if fracture), quality of adjacent bone (soft may indicate a metastasis, osteoporotic, sclerotic). If the fracture site is grossly or clinically suspicious for

a pathologic fracture, save as much soft tissue from this site as possible in a cassette without bone (to avoid tissue alterations associated with decalcification) and consider taking tissue for special studies (see above).

4. Describe soft tissue (see description above) and submit one cassette including synovium if possible.

5. Fix the femoral head in formalin overnight and decalcify the following day.

Microscopic sections

Soft tissue
One section including any grossly recognizable synovium.

Bone
One section including the junction of normal and abnormal cartilage and one from the periphery.

Fracture site
Two representative sections in one cassette from the fracture site. If sufficient soft tissue (i.e., possible tumor) is present, submit an additional cassette of nondecalcified tissue.

Sample dictation: hip replacement for degenerative joint disease

Received fresh labeled with the patient's name and unit number and "left hip" is a 5 × 5 × 4 cm flattened femoral head and attached neck with a smooth resection margin. The articular surface is covered by irregularly surfaced cartilage with areas of cartilage loss and eburnation of the underlying bone. Multiple peripheral osteophytes are present. The bone is fixed and then decalcified. Also received are multiple fragments of pink/tan fibrous tissue measuring in aggregate 3 × 3 × 2 cm.

Cassette #1: Joint surface, 4 frags, RSS.
Cassette #2: Soft tissue, 3 frags, RSS.

Sample dictation: hip replacement after fracture

Received fresh labeled with the patient's name and unit number and "right hip" is a 5 × 5 × 3 cm round femoral head with a smooth white cartilage surface. The femoral neck resection margin is irregular and hemorrhagic. There are multiple smaller fragments of irregular bone measuring in aggregate 3 × 3 × 1 cm. There are no areas of soft tissue within the bone. The bone trabeculae are markedly thinned. The bone is fixed and then decalcified. Also received are multiple fragments of pink/tan fibrous tissue measuring in aggregate 3 × 3 × 2 cm.

Cassette #1: Fracture site, 2 frags, RSS.
Cassette #2: Joint surface, 2 frags, RSS.
Cassette #3: Soft tissue, 3 frags, RSS.

Sample dictation: hip replacement for avascular necrosis

Received fresh labeled with the patient's name and unit number and "right hip" is a 4.5 × 4 × 4 cm deformed flattened femoral head with a smooth resection margin. There is a wedge-shaped area of pale yellow bone immediately beneath the cartilage surface measuring 2 × 2 × 1 cm with a red/brown border. The overlying cartilage is intact but has pulled away from this area leaving a gap. The sliced section is radiographed. The bone is fixed and then decalcified. The remainder of the cartilage surface is smooth and unremarkable. Also received are multiple fragments of pink/tan fibrous tissue measuring in aggregate 3 × 2 × 2 cm.

Cassettes #1–2: Area of probable necrosis, 4 frags, RSS.
Cassette #3: Joint surface, 2 frags, RSS.
Cassette #4: Soft tissue, 3 frags, RSS.

■ REVISION TOTAL JOINT ARTHROPLASTY

Approximately 5% of prosthetic joints fail, either from mechanical loosening or due to infection. It may be difficult to distinguish clinically between these two possibilities as the presentation may be similar and false positive and negative culture results are possible. Prosthetic joints that have failed mechanically may be removed and replaced in the same procedure. If infection is present, drainage or removal of the prosthesis may be indicated and replacement may be delayed until after treatment. The most common acute pathogens are *S. epidermidis* and *S. aureus*; Gram-negative bacilli are more common in later infections. A frozen-section evaluation of periarticular soft tissue may be requested if infection is suspected (see Chapter 6).

Processing the specimen

1. The specimen usually consists of small fragments of unidentifiable bone, fibrous soft tissue, and often fragments of bone cement. Bone cement is usually light brown, homogeneous in appearance, and hard, and may be difficult to distinguish from bone. The soft tissue may be gray or black due to metallic debris.
2. Describe the number of fragments of bone (estimate if many), size in aggregate, range of sizes. Bone may not be present.
3. Describe the number of fragments of soft tissue (estimate if many), size in aggregate, range of sizes, color, presence of necrosis. If infection is suspected clinically or by gross examination, and cultures have not yet been sent, send tissue for bacterial culture.
4. The explanted prosthesis is described including number of parts, hip or joint prosthesis, identification markings (e.g., serial numbers, brand names), and the presence of any marked abnormalities (e.g., broken metal components, erosions, ridges, or pits in the articular surfaces).
5. The bone is separated from the soft tissue. Submit one section of soft tissue including synovium if possible. Fix the bone overnight in formalin and decalcify the following day. All decalcification procedures must be documented in the gross description.

Gross differential diagnosis

Detritic synovitis. Occasionally there is an exuberant papillary proliferation of synovium with hemosiderin deposition in response to foreign material that grossly mimics pigmented villonodular synovitis (giant cell tumor, diffuse type). However, unlike PVNS, there will be a history of an artificial joint, foreign material is present, and the process usually is superficial and does not extend deeply into soft tissue.

Foreign material from implants. Numerous types of foreign material derived from the implant can be found around failed prostheses and include bone cement (with barium to make the material radio-opaque), metal fragments, polyethylene, methylmethacrylate, silicone, and ceramic (see Chapter 9, Table 9–1). The tissue may be black due to deposits of oxidized metal.

Infection. The soft tissue from infected joints may be necrotic and purulent. Cultures should be sent either by the surgeon or the pathologist. Some infections may not be apparent grossly.

Microscopic sections

Soft tissue
One section including any grossly recognizable synovium.

Bone
One section.

Received fresh, labeled with the patient's name and unit number and "left hip" are multiple fragments of soft tissue and bone. There are five bone fragments, measuring in aggregate $3 \times 2 \times 2$ cm. No articular surfaces are present. The bone is fixed and decalcified prior to submission. There are approximately 20 fragments of tan/white fibrous soft tissue without recognizable synovium.

Also received is a joint prosthesis consisting of an acetabular component consisting of a white prosthetic socket ($6 \times 6 \times 4$ cm) inscribed with "ABDC" and femoral component consisting of a metallic ball attached to a stem ($15 \times 3 \times 2$ cm). A fragment of brown bone cement with a smooth outer surface is also present ($4 \times 2 \times 2$ cm).

Cassette #1: Bone, 4 frags, RSS.
Cassette #2: Soft tissue, 3 frags, RSS.

■ CORE BIOPSY FOR ASEPTIC (AVASCULAR) NECROSIS

Cores of bone may be submitted from patients with clinical and radiologic osteonecrosis. These cores are taken through the femoral head and into the area of necrosis in order to promote revascularization ("decompression") and are generally used for treatment and not diagnosis. There should be an area of osteonecrosis at one edge of the biopsy. These core biopsies are fixed in formalin and then gently decalcified. If the specimen will not fit in a cassette in entirety, section the specimen longitudinally.

■ BIOPSY, METABOLIC BONE DISEASE

Needle or core bone biopsies are sometimes submitted from patients with metabolic bone disease (osteomalacia, osteoporosis, hyperparathyroidism, effects of long-term hemodialysis, etc.) with a request for metabolic bone studies.

The evaluation of metabolic disease requires sectioning of nondecalcified bone, special stains, and morphometry. These techniques are generally performed by a specialty laboratory. The specialty laboratory will provide instructions for the fixation and transportation of these specimens.

■ CURETTINGS AND NEEDLE BIOPSIES, BONE TUMORS

Biopsies of bone lesions are occasionally performed for both benign and malignant lesions. See Chapter 6 for a description of how bone biopsies are processed in the frozen section room. See Chapter 12 and below for larger specimens.

Processing the specimen

1. Determine the type of specimen: needle biopsy or curettings. Grossly examine for the presence of bone and soft tissue. Most cases have at least small foci of soft, non-calcified, non-necrotic tissue that can be taken for special studies. However, if a definitive diagnosis of lesional tissue has not been made intraoperatively, most of the tissue should be reserved for routine sections and tissue should not be taken for studies that will preclude examination of the tissue (e.g., cytogenetics). The clinical and radiologic differential diagnosis is helpful in guiding apportionment of tissue.
2. Fix the specimen in formalin for 2 to 4 hours depending on size.
3. After fixation, the bone is gently decalcified for 4 to 12 hours. In unusual cases including larger pieces of bone, it may be necessary to fix overnight, decalcify during the day (with

periodic checks to see if the bone is soft), wash, fix again overnight, and decalcify again (up to four daily cycles) for optimal specimen preparation.

Special studies

Most of these tumors are unusual and warrant special studies. After lesional tissue has been taken for formalin fixation, additional tissue can be taken for snap freezing, EM, and/or Zenker's fixation, which decalcifies while preserving cytologic detail.

Cytogenetics. If definite lesional tissue is present then tissue can be submitted for cytogenetics. For example, Ewing's/PNET tumors have a characteristic t(11;22) and extraskeletal myxoid chondrosarcoma has a characteristic t(9;22) (see Chapter 7, Table 7–33, page 152). If no definitive lesional tissue is present, then all tissue should be examined histologically.

Gross differential diagnosis

In general, gross examination of these small fragmented specimens is not helpful.

Microscopic sections

Tumor
Entire specimen up to 10 cassettes. If little tissue is available (e.g., only one cassette is submitted), three levels are ordered.

Sample dictation

Received fresh, labeled with the patient's name and unit number and "femur lesion" are multiple irregular fragments of tan/brown tissue with minute areas of irregular bone, measuring in aggregate 1 × 1 × 0.5 cm (the largest fragment measuring 0.4 cm in size). Frozen-section examination is performed on a representative section. Tissue is apportioned for snap freezing, electron microscopy, and cytogenetics. The remainder of the tissue is fixed in Zenker's fixative or fixed in formalin and then decalcified.

Cassette #1: Frozen-section remnant, 1 frag, ESS.
Cassette #2: Tissue fixed in Zenker's, 3 frags, ESS.
Cassettes #3–9: Remainder of specimen in formalin and decalcified, mult frags, ESS.

■ BONE RESECTIONS FOR TUMORS

Bone resections may be performed for either benign (enchondromas, osteochondromas, osteoid osteomas, bone cysts, fibrous dysplasia, giant cell tumors) or malignant (most chondrosarcomas, some osteosarcomas) lesions.[3–5] The radiologic features of bone lesions are very helpful, and sometimes necessary, to distinguish benign from malignant tumors.

Processing the specimen

1. Determine the type of specimen (e.g., above-knee amputation, hip disarticulation). See Chapter 12 for additional information.

   Give the dimensions of each structure present, including length and maximum circumference of limbs.
2. Radiograph the intact specimen. The radiograph provides diagnostic information and is helpful to guide the specimen dissection.

3. Incise the soft tissue in a plane that will demonstrate the greatest extent of the tumor. A band saw can be used to bisect the specimen. Gently brush away bone dust under running water and photograph the specimen. It is useful at this point to make a diagram of the specimen to indicate where sections will be taken. For large specimens, an additional 0.5 cm parallel cut through bone should be made to produce a relatively thin cut section of the tumor. This section is also photographed if it yields additional information.

4. Describe the tumor including size, appearance (color, percentage of necrosis, bone formation, cartilage formation), location (tissue compartment), relationship to surrounding structures (bone, vessels, nerves, muscle), center of tumor (epiphysis, metaphysis, diaphysis, intramedullary, periosteal), erosion of cortex, extension into soft tissue (compression or true invasion), extension through epiphyseal plate, extension into or across joint space, vascular involvement, skip metastases, distance from each margin.

5. Take soft tissue sections of margins, representative structures (e.g., vessels and nerves), and any areas of noncalcified tumor showing relationships to soft tissues. Tumor can be taken for special studies if not previously performed. Carefully search for lymph nodes and submit.

6. Fix the entire specimen in formalin. After overnight fixation, gently decalcify the sections with bone. The specimen must be checked every few hours in order to avoid overdecalcification, which will adversely affect histologic examination.

7. Sections are taken to show the tumor, relationship to adjacent normal bone, invasion of contiguous structures (e.g., cortex, soft tissue, joint space), and margins. The location of sections taken is indicated on a diagram of the specimen. All areas of different radiologic appearance are sampled and correlated with the radiograph. For osteosarcomas, the extent of post-therapy tumor necrosis is important to determine. An entire cross-section of these tumors is mapped out and submitted for histologic examination.

Bone dust can create artifacts that may be difficult to interpret. Orient the sections so that the portion cut by the histology laboratory will be opposite the side cut by the saw (e.g., ink one side and indicate the appropriate side to be sectioned).

Special studies

Many of these tumors will have been pretreated with radiation, chemotherapy, or both and will be predominantly necrotic. Special studies in general are not performed on such tumors.

Cases with untreated tumors should have tissue sent for special studies. Refer to the sections on biopsies above.

Gross differential diagnosis (Fig. 14-1)

Ewing's sarcoma/PNET. These tumors are generally treated with radiation and chemotherapy and not resected. Therefore, they will usually be diagnosed in biopsy specimens (see sections on biopsies above). Grossly the tumors are grayish white with indistinct borders and may have hemorrhage, cystic degeneration, and necrosis. The adjacent bone is usually destroyed.

Osteoid osteoma. The lesion is usually present in the cortex of a long bone and is less than 2 cm in size. Grossly it may look like a bright red or pink nodule. Radiographs of the specimen can be helpful to demonstrate the characteristic central lucent zone with a rim of surrounding dense bone.

Fibrous dysplasia. There is fusiform expansion of the bone with thinning of the cortex and replacement of the bone by firm white/gray gritty tissue. Cysts and cartilage may be present in the lesion. There may be a fracture site through the lesion.

Aneurysmal bone cyst. This is a multiloculated cystic lesion with cysts lined by soft brown fibrous tissue. The cysts may contain blood clots. The telangiectatic variant of osteosarcoma

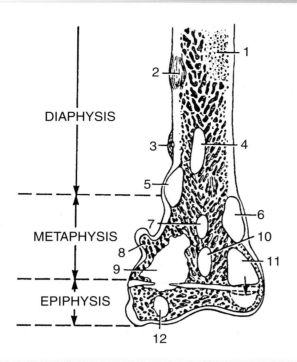

DIAPHYSIS

METAPHYSIS

EPIPHYSIS

1. Ewing's sarcoma, lymphoma, myeloma
2. Osseofibrous dysplasia, adamantinoma
3. Osteroid osteoma
4. Fibrous dysplasia
5. Chondromyxoid fibroma
6. Nonossifying fibroma
7. Bone cyst, osteoblastoma
8. Osteochondroma
9. Osteosarcoma
10. Enchondroma, chondrosarcoma
11. Giant cell tumor
12. Chondroblastoma

Figure 14-1 Most frequent locations of common osseous lesions. (From Fechner RE, Mills SE. AFIP Atlas of Tumor Pathology. Tumors of the Bones and Joints, 3rd series, fascicle 8. Washington, D.C., Armed Forces Institute of Pathology, 1993.)

can mimic an aneurysmal bone cyst radiologically and clinically. Extensive sampling may be necessary to exclude this diagnosis.

Osteochondroma. This is a mushroom-shaped subperiosteal projection or exostosis from the bone surface, usually juxta-articular. The bone merges with cortical bone and the medullary cavities are in continuity. The bone is covered by a thick cartilage cap.

Osteosarcoma. Osteosarcoma is a destructive bone-forming tumor that often invades through the cortex and may invade into adjacent soft tissue. Lytic areas may be present. The tumor replaces the normal marrow space with firm tissue. Bone and/or cartilage may be present within the tumor mass.

Chondrosarcoma. This usually appears as a lobulated grayish white or blue tumor mass that often is calcified. The tumor may invade into or through normal bone. Areas of necrosis may be present.

Enchondroma. Enchondroma is an intramedullary cartilaginous neoplasm consisting of multiple lobules of cartilage within bone.

Giant cell tumor. A well-defined lesion within the marrow space that consists of homogeneous tan/pink tissue. Hemorrhage and necrosis may be present.

Tumors after treatment. Treated tumors may be predominantly necrotic or be replaced by dense fibrous tissue. It may be difficult to find diagnostic areas.

Microscopic sections

Tumor
At least 1 section per cm showing relationship to cortex, medulla, adjacent joint, and soft tissue. Tumors that have been previously treated are blocked out in a complete cross-section in order to evaluate the extent of necrosis.

Margins
Usually will include both soft tissue and bone.

Normal structures
Representative sections of all normal structures (e.g., major vessels, major nerve trunks).

Lymph nodes
Submit all lymph nodes found (see Chapter 27).

Sample dictation

Received fresh, labeled with the patient's name, unit number, and "left distal femur" is an above-the-knee amputation with disarticulation of the knee (12 × 9 × 7 cm). The distal femur is 12 cm in length and surrounded by skeletal muscle. Centered within the metaphysis is a tan/yellow tumor (7.8 × 7 × 7 cm) that occupies the majority of the medullary cavity. The tumor appears to be entirely viable without gross areas of necrosis or hemorrhage. The tumor invades through the cortex medially, laterally, anteriorly, and posteriorly, and extends into soft tissue medially to form a soft tissue mass (2 × 1.8 × 0.4 cm). The tumor does not grossly involve the joint space. The tumor is located 3.5 cm from the proximal surgical resection margin, 0.4 cm from the posterior and lateral margins, and 0.1 cm from the anterior and medial margins. The tumor is 1 cm from the distal resection margin, which consists of the grossly unremarkable cartilage surface of the distal femur. There is an attached skin ellipse over the anterior/medial portion of the specimen, measuring 9.3 × 1.1 cm, with a centrally located well-healed surgical scar measuring 7.5 cm. There is a hemorrhagic biopsy cavity (1 × 1 × 0.6 cm) located 4.5 cm deep to the skin surface and adjacent to the tumor. The femoral artery and accompanying nerves and vein are not present. The specimen is radiographed. A diagram is prepared with the location of sections marked. Sections containing bone are fixed and decalcified prior to submission.

Cassette #1–15: Complete cross-section of tumor including relationship to cortex, submitted from proximal to distal, 15 frags, RSS.
Cassette #16: Tumor and medial margin including soft tissue extension, 1 frag, RSS.
Cassette #17: Tumor and lateral margin, 1 frag, RSS.
Cassette #18: Tumor and posterior margin, 1 frag, RSS.
Cassette #19: Tumor and anterior margin, 1 frag, RSS.
Cassette #20: Bone at proximal margin, 1 frag, RSS.
Cassette #21: Bone and cartilage at distal margin, 1 frag, RSS.
Cassette #22: Soft tissue at proximal margin, 1 frag, RSS.
Cassette #23: Soft tissue at proximal margin, 1 frag, RSS.
Cassette #24: Skin with scar, 1 frag, RSS.
Cassette #25: Biopsy site, 1 frag, RSS.

Pathologic prognostic/diagnostic features sign-out checklist for bone tumors

Histologic type
The most important feature. Usually the diagnosis will have been established prior to definitive resection.

Tumor grade
Used for some tumor types (Tables 14-2, 14-3).
All osteosarcomas are regarded as high grade with the exception of well-differentiated intramedullary (central) and paraosteal variants. Paraosteal osteosarcoma may show foci of (high-grade) dedifferentiation.

Location of tumor
Bones involved and site:

Epiphysis (articular cartilage to epiphyseal plate)
Metaphysis (epiphyseal plate to diaphysis)
Diaphysis (end of proximal metaphysis to beginning of distal metaphysis)
Medulla
Cortex
Periosteum

Size
Three dimensions

Invasion of adjacent structures
Confined to surface, confined to cortex, extends through cortex, extends into soft tissue, satellite (skip) lesions are present, tumor crosses the joint space.

Lymphatic or vascular invasion
Present or absent (present in 3% to 13% of osseous sarcomas).

Margins
Involvement of bone, soft tissue, marrow, and distance of tumor from margin
Neurovascular bundle at the margin: involved or not involved

Cystic change
Identified, not identified

Necrosis
Not identified, <25%, 26 to 75%, >76%

Hemorrhage
Identified, not identified

Response to therapy
Proportion of tumor viable or necrotic (Table 14-4).
This checklist incorporates recommendations of the ADASP (see www.panix.com/~adasp/).

Table 14-2 AJCC (6th edition) classification for bone tumors

Grade	GX	Grade cannot be assessed
	G1	Well differentiated—low grade
	G2	Moderately differentiated—low grade
	G3	Poorly differentiated—high grade
	G4	Undifferentiated—high grade
	Note: Ewing's sarcoma is classified as G4	
Tumor	TX	Primary tumor cannot be assessed
	T0	No evidence of primary tumor
	T1	Tumor 8 cm or less in greatest dimension
	T2	Tumor more than 8 cm in greatest dimension
	T3	Discontinuous tumors in the primary bone site
Regional lymph nodes	NX	Regional lymph nodes cannot be assessed
	N0	No regional node metastasis
	N1	Regional node metastasis
	Note: Lymph node involvement is rare. Tumors with no clinical involvement of lymph nodes can be classified as N0	
Distant metastasis	MX	Distant metastasis cannot be assessed
	M0	No distant metastasis
	M1	Distant metastasis
	M1a	Lung
	M1b	Other distant sites

This system is used for all primary malignant tumors of bone except lymphoma and multiple myeloma.

Table 14-3 Enneking staging for osteosarcomas[3]

STAGE	GRADE	SITE
IA	Low	One compartment
IB	Low	Two compartments
IIA	High	One compartment
IIB	High	Two compartments
III	Low or high	Distant metastases

■ INCIDENTAL RIBS

Portions of ribs are often removed to perform thoracotomies or nephrectomies. The rib is usually 2 to 5 cm long and is rarely of diagnostic importance. The most important missed histologic diagnosis on incidental ribs is multiple myeloma. The patients often survive for long periods of time, may have procedures performed that are not related to the disease (unlike, for example, acute leukemia), and the disease may not have been diagnosed clinically. Plasma cell dyscrasias can be diagnosed even on suboptimally fixed and decalcified tissue. Involvement by chronic lymphocytic leukemia is also occasionally found, but is usually clinically evident due to a high peripheral white blood count.

Specimen processing

Ribs resected from patients without malignant disease and without other clinical indication for examination (e.g., a known hematologic disorder) do not necessarily require histologic examination. There are two methods for examining all other specimens.

Decalcification method

The decalcification method should be used for all patients with a history of lymphoma or other hematologic disorder (treat as a diagnostic bone marrow biopsy, see Chapter 27), malignancies that frequently metastasize to bone marrow (e.g., small cell lung carcinomas), or ribs with grossly evident or clinically suspected lesions.

1. The rib is described (measurements, color, gross identification as portion of rib) and fixed in formalin. Cartilage may be present at one end if the resection was near the costochondral junction. It is homogeneously pale white, cuts easily with a razor blade, and is not visible on x-ray.
2. If a gross lesion is present that is suspicious for metastatic disease, the specimen is radiographed, serially sectioned, and any soft tissue (i.e., potential tumor) removed prior to decalcification.
3. The remainder of the bone is gently decalcified. Grossly normal bones can be submitted as multiple sections in one cassette. If gross or radiographic lesions are present, submit them in a separate cassette. Do not submit grossly benign cartilage.

Rib squeeze method

The disadvantage of this method is that metastatic tumors and lymphomas may not be easily expressed from the bone marrow due to accompanying marrow fibrosis. However, bone marrow involvement often will have been investigated clinically before surgery is performed, and the finding of malignancy in incidental ribs is very rare.

Table 14-4 Osteosarcoma: Evaluation of treatment response

HISTOLOGIC RESPONSE GRADE

I	No effect identified
IIA	Some necrosis, more than 50% viable tumor remaining
IIB	3% to 50% viable tumor remaining
III	Scattered foci, <3% viable tumor remaining[a]
IV	No viable tumor noted

[a] In some systems, 90% or 95% is used rather than 97%, which is the current standard of the Children's Oncology Group.

The advantage of this method is that it provides better histologic preservation of the bone marrow elements and does not delay the rib in processing. Thus, this is the preferred method with the exceptions noted above.

1. The rib is described as above.
2. The specimen must be fresh and unfixed. Use a bone saw to cut a portion approximately 2 cm in length with marrow present at both ends of the specimen. Use a pliers to squeeze until marrow is expressed from both ends. Collect the marrow in formalin. If very little marrow can be expressed, the bone should be fixed and decalcified as described above. The remainder of the rib is cut longitudinally and examined for gross lesions. Submit any lesions seen. Document in the gross description that the bone was not decalcified.
3. The marrow should be wrapped in paper or placed in a specimen bag and submitted in one cassette.

■ MENISCUS

Menisci are usually removed because of traumatic tears that interfere with articular movement. Occasionally joint mice (loose bodies) may be removed during the same type of procedure. These are fragments of cartilage free in the joint space and often become ossified. The meniscus can also be affected by CPPD, and ochronosis (see "Synovium—Gross differential diagnosis").

Processing the specimen

1. Describe the specimen including size, color (normally white and glistening), texture (smooth, fibrillated), presence of tears.
2. If chalky white deposits are present, a portion of the specimen is processed in absolute ethanol to preserve crystals (see also "Synovium").
3. Submit representative sections in one cassette.

■ SYNOVIUM

Synovium may be biopsied for diagnostic purposes (e.g., inflammatory arthritis) or removed for the treatment of disease (e.g., pigmented villonodular synovitis—giant cell tumor, diffuse type or dialysis-related amyloidosis).

Processing the specimen

1. Record the aggregate dimensions, size range, and approximate number of fragments.

Describe the color and consistency of the synovium:

- Normal: white/tan, delicate, villous.
- Hemochromatosis: brown/green.
- β_2-microglobulin amyloidosis: tan/yellow, firm, and homogeneous.
- Giant cell tumor, diffuse type (pigmented villonodular synovitis or PVNS): red/brown and shaggy (delicate villi with small nodules may be appreciated if the tissue is floated in saline). Necrotic foci may appear yellow due to the presence of histiocytes.
- Gout or chondrocalcinosis: chalky white crystalline material.

If infection is suspected and fresh tissue is received, confirm that cultures have been taken. If not, send sterile tissue to microbiology.

2. Submit up to two cassettes and order one level (H&E). Order special studies as indicated below for specific cases. If the specimen is a small biopsy, submit all the tissue and order three levels.

Special studies

Crystal disease

Chalky white deposits may be present in synovium. Representative sections must be fixed in absolute alcohol. See "Total joint arthroplasty—Special studies."

Amyloidosis

All tissue can be fixed in formalin. Amyloid can be diagnosed using a Congo red stain and polarized light. Immunohistochemistry can be used to identify the type of amyloid present. Dialysis-related amyloidosis of joints is due to β_2-microglobulin.

Infection

Fresh sterile tissue may be sent for culture.

Gross differential diagnosis

Normal synovium. Normal synovium is glistening white with delicate villous projections.

Gout or CPPD. Chalky white or crystalline deposits are present and must be fixed in absolute alcohol. See "Total joint arthroplasty—Special studies" for information on how to process.

Giant cell tumor, diffuse type (pigmented villonodular synovitis, PVNS). The synovium is a rusty red color due to extensive hemosiderin deposition. Coarse villi with occasional attached nodules are present. These areas become more apparent when floated in saline and can be photographed well in this manner. There may be an abundance of tissue with areas of fibrosis.

Detritic synovitis. Changes occurring around an artificial joint can appear very similar to PVNS (see "Revision total joint arthroplasty").

Dialysis-related amyloidosis. There are characteristic yellow/tan plaques that may be superficial, run along tendons, or form large homogeneous nodules.

Synovial chondromatosis. Multiple small nodules of cartilage are present within the synovial tissue. The cartilage may need to be decalcified.

Hemochromatosis. The synovium can become hyperplastic and brown in color due to dense hemosiderin deposition. The appearance can mimic PVNS, but nodules are not present. The cartilage takes on a characteristic greenish-black appearance.

Microscopic sections

Synovium
Up to two cassettes. If the biopsy is small (only enough tissue for one cassette), order three levels.

Sample dictation

Received fresh, labeled with the patient's name, unit number, and "synovium right knee" are multiple fragments of reddish brown soft tissue measuring in aggregate $5 \times 4 \times 1$ cm. Delicate villous projections and small nodules are present.

Cassettes #1 and 2: mult frags, RSS.

■ CARPAL TUNNEL RELEASE (TENOSYNOVIUM)

Most patients present with idiopathic carpal tunnel syndrome and only a small fraction of these patients will show evidence of amyloid on microscopic examination. However, in renal dialysis patients carpal tunnel syndrome is very common and β_2-microglobulin amyloidosis is often present.

These specimens consist of synovium and soft tissue from around the tendons and nerves of the carpal tunnel that are removed during a carpal tunnel release procedure. The specimens may be processed in the same manner as synovium but are examined with one level.

■ INTERVERTEBRAL DISC MATERIAL

Specimens derived from operations on herniated discs consist of small fragments of bone, nucleus pulposus, annulus fibrosus, and ligamentum flavum. These specimens are rarely of diagnostic importance. The specimen is fixed and decalcified, and one representative section is submitted.

Special cases

Metastatic disease. Any soft tissue is dissected away and submitted without decalcification. If the primary site is unknown, and there is sufficient tissue, then consideration should be given to special studies (frozen tissue, EM).

Infection. Any soft tissue is dissected away and submitted without decalcification. If there is sufficient tissue, consideration should be given to sending tissue for cultures. Special stains may be helpful. Aspergillus can invade cartilage without causing an inflammatory response and may not be detectable without fungal stains.

The value of examining "routine" disc specimens has been questioned.[6,7] In the study of Grzybicki et al,[7] if cases with significant clinical histories were excluded (i.e., any indication for surgery other than a benign noninfectious indication for laminectomy), only 3 of 1071 (0.3%) specimens yielded a clinically significant unsuspected diagnosis. All three cases were epidural abscesses that were also diagnosed clinically in the perioperative period. Of 38 cases with a significant clinical history, 21 (55%) resulted in a clinically significant pathologic diagnosis. Thus, if an adequate clinical history is provided, it may not be necessary to examine all such specimens histologically. See Chapter 21 for a discussion of this issue.

REFERENCES

1. Campbell ML, Gregory AM, Mauerhan DR. Collection of surgical specimens in total joint arthroplasty. Is routine pathology cost effective? J Arthroplasty 12:60, 1997.
2. DiCarlo ER, Bullough PG, Steiner G, Bansal M, Kambolis C. Pathological examination of the femoral head (FH). Mod Pathol 7:6A (Abstract 16), 1994.
3. Fechner RE, Mills SE. AFIP Atlas of Tumor Pathology, Tumors of the Bones and Joints, 3rd series, fascicle 8. Washington, D.C., Armed Forces Institute of Pathology, 1993.
4. Weatherby RP, Unni KK. Practical aspects of handling orthopedic specimens in the surgical pathology laboratory. Path Annu 17, part 2:1-31, 1982.
5. Patterson K. The pathologic handling of skeletal tumors. Am J Clin Pathol 109 (Suppl 1):S53-S66, 1998.
6. Daftari TK, Levine J, Fischgrund JS, Herkowitz HN. Is pathology examination of disc specimens necessary after routine anterior cervical discectomy and fusion? Spine 21:2156, 1996.
7. Grzybicki DM, Callaghan EJ, Raab SS. Cost-benefit value of microscopic examination of intervertebral discs. J Neurosurg 89:378-381, 1998.

Breast

15

Carcinomas are the only common clinically significant lesion of the breast, and most surgical procedures are performed to investigate the possibility of carcinoma or to treat a known carcinoma. Breast biopsies are common surgical specimens for the evaluation of palpable masses, mammographic lesions, nipple discharge, or, rarely, inflammatory lesions. Reexcisions for malignant disease may include portions of the breast (lumpectomies and quadrantectomies) or the entire breast. Less commonly, breasts are removed for prophylactic (simple mastectomy) or cosmetic/functional reasons (reduction mammoplasty or gynecomastia).

Relevant clinical history (in addition to age and gender)

See Table 15-1.

Table 15-1 Relevant clinical history (in addition to age and gender)	
HISTORY RELEVANT TO ALL SPECIMENS	HISTORY RELEVANT TO BREAST BIOPSIES
Organ/tissue resected or biopsied	Type of lesion biopsied (e.g., palpable mass, mammographic lesion (density, calcifications, or architectural distortion), or nipple discharge). If the lesion is mammographic, a specimen radiograph with interpretation may be required in order to fully evaluate the specimen
Purpose of the procedure	
Gross appearance of the organ/tissue/lesion sampled	
Any unusual features of the clinical presentation	
Any unusual features of the gross appearance	Current pregnancy or lactation
Prior surgery/biopsies—results	Drug use that could change the appearance of the breast (e.g., oral contraceptives or other hormonal therapy)
Prior malignancy	
Prior treatment (radiation therapy, chemotherapy, drug use that can change the histologic appearance of tissues)	Prior personal or family history of breast carcinoma
Compromised immune system	Collagen vascular disease

■ LARGE CORE NEEDLE BIOPSIES

Large core needle biopsies may be performed for palpable masses (Tru-Cut) without radiologic guidance, under ultrasound guidance to sample masses, or mammographically directed ("stereotactic") for either calcifications or mammographic densities.

Specimen processing

1. Describe the number of cores, color, and size.
2. All tissue cores are aligned in parallel on a flat surface and wrapped in paper. A sponge can be used in the cassette to hold the biopsies flat. Order three levels.

Special studies

Calcifications

If malignancy is present in a breast biopsy for radiologic suspicious calcifications, the carcinoma will either be at the site of the calcifications or within 1 cm in more than 95% of cases. Therefore, it is important for the pathologist to be sure that this area has been examined histologically.

The radiologist documents calcifications in the cores by specimen radiography. If the radiologist submits the cores wrapped in lens paper in a cassette, the likelihood of the calcifications being lost during processing is minimized. Different cassettes may be used for different lesions or cores with or without calcifications. Commercial multicompartment containers are also available.

It may also be useful to have the histology laboratory make shallower initial levels of cores containing calcifications to ensure that all tissue present is adequately sampled.

- **Calcium phosphate crystals** are purple in color and do not polarize. They are commonly seen in association with cysts, sclerosing adenosis, and in hyalinized fibroadenomas, as well as in DCIS and invasive carcinomas.
- **Calcium oxalate crystals** are rhomboidal refractile pale yellow or clear crystals, usually found in apocrine cysts and easily seen under polarized light. They are sometimes seen in stroma adjacent to cysts, with or without a giant cell reaction. When the crystals are numerous in large cysts, they are referred to as "milk of calcium" by radiologists as they line the bottom of cysts in a teacup shape in the medial-lateral-oblique view and change in spatial orientation (flatten) in the cranial-caudal view. Calcium oxalate crystals have not been associated with carcinomas.

If calcifications are not found corresponding to mammographic calcifications after histologic examination, deeper sections are obtained of the blocks with radiologic calcifications. In some cases it may be useful to radiograph the paraffin blocks to localize the calcifications. It can be helpful to radiograph the blocks flat and on edge to determine the depth of the calcifications in the block for the histotechnologist.

Radiographic "calcifications" can rarely be due to surgical debris (at an old biopsy site) that may not be evident histologically. Evidence of an old biopsy site should be present.

Calcifications can also dissolve if left in formalin for over 24 hours.[1] Small biopsies should be processed expeditiously or stored in alcohol if processing will be delayed.

Hormone receptors and HER2/neu

Hormone receptor and HER2/neu status can be determined on carcinomas by immunohistochemistry.

HER2/neu score. The scoring system shown in Table 15-2 is used for evaluating HecepTest®.[2] Many studies of immunoreactivity of breast cancers for HER2/neu have used this system, and use of the same system facilitates comparison of results to other studies. However, it has not been shown to be the optimal system for predicting prognosis or response to trastuzumab (Herceptin).

Only membrane immunoreactivity is scored. Marked cytoplasmic immunoreactivity may make interpretation difficult. FISH studies may be preferred for such cases.

Overall, 20% to 30% of newly diagnosed cases of breast carcinoma show overexpression of HER2/neu.

There is amplification of the HER2/neu gene has been amplified in more than 90% of carcinomas with protein overexpression. In 3% to 5% of cases, protein overexpression can occur due to other mechanisms. In less than 5% of cases, there may be gene amplification without protein overexpression. In general, there is a 20% to 40% response to Herceptin alone in patients with cancers showing gene amplification by FISH, and less than 5% of patients

Table 15-2 HER-2/neu score used to evaluate HecepTest®

SCORE	CRITERIA	PERCENTAGE OF CASES	PERCENTAGE OF CASES THAT SHOW AMPLIFICATION BY FISH
0 (Negative)	No immunoreactivity or immuno-reactivity in <10% of tumor cells	~60%	0 to 3%
1+ (Negative)	Faint weak immunoreactivity in >10% of tumor cells but only a portion of the membrane is positive	~10%	0 to 7%
2+ (Weak positive)	Weak to moderate complete membrane immunoreactivity in >10% of tumor cells	~5–10%	25–35%
3+ (Positive)	Moderate to strong complete immuno-reactivity in >10% of tumor cells	~15–20%	75–90%

respond if their carcinomas do not show amplification. Therefore, FISH studies may be helpful for cases with 2+ positivity or cases that are difficult to interpret (e.g., those with variable positivity or cytoplasmic positivity).

Well and moderately differentiated lobular carcinomas are rarely positive (<5%). However, in some cases there may be edge enhancement of individual tumor cells that may be difficult to interpret. FISH studies may be helpful.

In rare cases, DCIS overexpresses HER2/neu but the accompanying invasive carcinoma does not. This is a source of potential false positive results for IHC or FISH.

Estrogen and progesterone receptor evaluation. Hormone receptors are routinely determined on invasive breast carcinomas and DCIS. ER and PR are weak prognostic markers and are more useful to predict the likelihood of response to hormonal therapies.

Many different methods are currently used to report the results of IHC studies for ER and PR. One method that has been used in multiple studies is the H-score or Allred score method (Table 15-3). Patients with carcinomas with a total score of 3 (<1% of cells with intermediate intensity or 1% to 10% of cells with weak intensity) or above showed improved disease-free survival when treated with endocrine therapy.[3] Patients with carcinomas with a total score of 2 (<1% weakly positive cells) had survival similar to patients with ER-negative carcinomas (total score of 0).

Approximately 80% of DCIS cases are positive for ER using the same method of scoring. Women with ER-positive DCIS were shown to experience fewer local recurrences, contralateral recurrences, and distant recurrences when treated with tamoxifen.[4] Women with ER-negative DCIS did not benefit from tamoxifen.

After optimization of IHC with newer antigen retrieval methods, more than 95% of carcinomas will have scores of 0, 7, or 8.[5] Many laboratories report results as positive or negative. The value of further subdividing positive cases by percent positive cells, H-score, or image analysis for either prognosis or to predict response to tamoxifen has not been demonstrated. Intensity of immunoreactivity is difficult to evaluate as most cases show strong reactivity with optimal assay methods and most carcinomas show considerable variability in intensity.

A possible method for reporting results is shown in Table 15-4. The same system can be used for reporting progesterone receptor results. The use of both ER and PR may be helpful for determining the likelihood of response to tamoxifen, as has been shown with data using the biochemical assay (Table 15-5). Presumably, the presence of the ER-regulated gene product PR is more predictive of an intact ER regulatory pathway.

Table 15-3 H-Score (Allred score)

PROPORTION SCORE (PS)	PERCENTAGE POSITIVE CELLS
0	0
1	<1%
2	1–10%
3	10–33%
4	33–66%
5	>66%

INTENSITY SCORE (IS)	INTENSITY OF POSITIVITY
0	None
1	Weak
2	Intermediate
3	Strong

The PS and IS are added together for a total score

TOTAL SCORE (TS) PS + IS	INTERPRETATION
0, 2	Negative
3, 4, 5, 6, 7, 8	Positive

Table 15-4 Reporting results of ER and PR evaluation

RESULT	PERCENTAGE OF POSITIVE CELLS	PERCENTAGE OF CASES	COMMENTS
Positive	>10% of cells	70–80%	This group corresponds to PS scores of 3 and above. The majority of these carcinomas will have scores of 7 or 8
Borderline or low positive	>0 to 10%	<5–10%	The clinical significance of this group is unclear. This group may be interpreted as "negative" or "positive" by some laboratories depending on the cut-off point chosen. This group could include cases with H-scores of 2, 3, 4, or 5
Negative	0	20–30%	This group corresponds to a TS score of 0

Table 15-5

STATUS OF CARCINOMA	PERCENTAGE OF CARCINOMAS	PERCENTAGE OF PATIENTS RESPONDING TO TAMOXIFEN
ER+ PR+	63%	75–80%
ER+ PR–	15%	25–30%
ER– PR+	5%	40–45%
ER– PR–	17%	<10%

False negative results and, to a lesser extent, false positive results, are potential problems. False negative results may be due to:

- Low sensitivity of the assay
- Errors in performing the assay
- Delayed fixation of tissue
- Over- or underfixation of tissue
- Overheating of tissue (e.g., with cautery during surgery)
- Decalcification of tissue.

Most cases of false negativity can be detected, as the normal breast tissue will also be negative. In such cases, the assay should be repeated on the same block, a different block from the same case, or on another specimen from the patient, if available. If the normal tissue remains negative, the possibility of loss of antigenicity can be mentioned.

False positive results may be due to:

- Entrapped normal ducts or lobules misinterpreted as carcinoma—this can be a difficult issue for DCIS as some ducts or lobules may be only partially involved by DCIS
- Control placed on same slide misinterpreted as the carcinoma
- Sclerosing adenosis (or other benign lesion) misinterpreted as invasive carcinoma
- Cytoplasmic positivity misinterpreted as nuclear positivity.

■ INCISIONAL BIOPSIES

Incisional biopsies are unusual specimens that are almost always performed to evaluate unresectable invasive carcinomas. Often the purpose of the biopsy is to confirm the clinical diagnosis and to ascertain hormone receptor and HER2/neu status.

The specimen usually consists of a single small fragment, or multiple small fragments, of tissue. The entire specimen is submitted. The tissue need not be inked if clearly labeled as an incisional biopsy.

■ EXCISIONAL BIOPSIES

Excisional biopsies are defined as procedures intended for the primary evaluation of a breast lesion with complete removal of the lesion. If there has been a prior diagnosis of malignancy (e.g., by core biopsy), the intent of the procedure is to obtain wide margins. The processing of an excisional biopsy varies depending on the type of lesion resected.

All biopsies must be inked in order to evaluate margins. Fragmented biopsies are inked because the lesion may be located in only one of the fragments.

Orientation.

Some surgeons attempt to minimize cosmetic deformity by only resecting specific positive margins if malignancy is found. In such cases, it is necessary to identify each of six possible margins (superior, inferior, medial, lateral, anterior, posterior) and to evaluate them separately. This can be accomplished if the surgeon provides at least two orienting sutures perpendicular to each other (e.g., "superior" and "lateral"). Orientation can be maintained by taking and labeling sections in relation to the sutures, or by inking each margin with a different color.

The posterior margin always corresponds to the deep margin closest to the chest wall. The superficial (skin) margin is usually anterior but can correspond to any of the other margins depending on the location of the biopsy within the breast.

Excisional biopsies for palpable masses

A primary biopsy without wire localization (see "Excisional biopsies for mammographic lesions with wire localization," below) or a history of nipple discharge (see "Duct dissections/Nipple biopsies," page 266) is usually performed to excise a palpable mass. Invasive carcinoma will be found in approximately 20% of specimens (average size 2 cm), DCIS alone in less than 5%, and fibroadenomas in about 20%. The remainder of the specimens will have a wide variety of benign lesions or other (very rare) malignant lesions.

Specimen processing

1. Record total dimensions and note any orienting sutures. It is helpful to designate the orientation of the dimensions (i.e., distance from medial to lateral, anterior to posterior, and inferior to superior).

   Ink all fragments. Blot the surface dry and change gloves if necessary to avoid introducing ink into the interior of the specimen.

   Unoriented specimens can be inked entirely in black. Oriented specimens may be inked using colored inks to identify specific margins. If there is any ambiguity about specimen orientation (e.g., a suture has fallen off), contact the surgeon before proceeding.

   Serially section the specimen. Do not cut off any orienting sutures. If a suture is inadvertently severed, mark the area by clipping with a cassette.

2. Describe lesions including size (accurate to nearest mm for staging), consistency (rubbery and bulging, soft, firm, hard), growth pattern (well-circumscribed, stellate, invasive, poorly circumscribed), necrosis, and distance from margins. If there are multiple lesions, describe their relationship to each other.

   Sample all gross lesions. For lesions suspicious for malignancy, four to five cassettes of the lesion are adequate. For fibroadenomas, or other grossly benign lesions, one section per 1 cm (two per cassette) of greatest dimension is adequate. If there are multiple lesions, submit a section of tissue in between the two lesions.

   If a gross lesion is not evident, make sure the biopsy was performed for a palpable mass. Most masses palpable to the surgeon will be grossly evident to the pathologist. Occasionally, surgeons biopsy vaguely denser areas of breast tissue without a discrete mass. In such cases, submit at least 10 cassettes, selecting out the most fibrous areas and avoiding pure adipose tissue. If carcinoma in situ or atypical hyperplasia is found in this tissue, then the entire specimen is submitted for histologic examination.[6]

   Never take tissue for special studies or research unless a definitive diagnosis of invasive carcinoma has been established.

3. Submit perpendicular sections of the closest approach of suspicious lesions to all margins of oriented specimens. Up to 12 cassettes (corresponding to two sections from each of the six margins) may be submitted if malignancy is known or highly suspected. Often margins are included in the same cassette with a section of the lesion.

4. If there is additional fibrous parenchyma not included in the cassettes with the lesion or margin, submit at least one cassette. If skin is present, submit one section.

   Most specimens can be submitted in 10 cassettes or less. If the entire specimen is not submitted, the gross description should include a statement estimating the percentage of the lesion and total specimen submitted for histologic examination.

Special studies

Estrogen and progesterone receptors

These studies are performed on formalin-fixed tissues of all invasive breast carcinomas and DCIS and recurrences of invasive carcinoma (see Tables 15-3 to 15-5). The information is used for prognosis as well as for therapeutic decision making.

Hormone receptor antigenicity can be diminished or eliminated by some fixatives (e.g., Bouin's fixative), over- or underfixation in formalin, and decalcification. Thus, these should be avoided if hormone receptors may need to be determined. Delayed fixation or heat (e.g., from surgical cautery) can also result in degradation of receptor proteins.

HER2/neu (c-erb B2)

Overexpression can be determined either by IHC or by FISH on formalin-fixed tissue as more than 95% of tumors with protein overexpression also have gene amplification (see Table 15–2, page 241 "HER2/neu" and Table 7–33.

Flow cytometric analysis

Flow cytometry may be used to determine DNA content and S phase fraction (SPF). Abnormal DNA content and high SPF are poor prognostic factors. These studies are best performed on fresh tissue, but can also be performed on formalin-fixed tissue. See "Analytical cytology," page 166, for more information.

Tissue for research

Tissue can only be removed for research if a diagnosis of invasive carcinoma has been firmly established. In all other cases, all breast tissue may need to be examined microscopically to exclude carcinoma or invasion in cases of DCIS.

Gross differential diagnosis (Fig. 15-1)

Invasive carcinoma usually appears as a very hard white mass with irregular or stellate borders. The consistency when cut through is gritty (like a water chestnut). Pale yellow streaks in the tumor are usually due to elastosis in the desmoplastic response and not necrosis. Some invasive tumors are well circumscribed (e.g., medullary or mucinous carcinomas) and may be firm or soft. Occasionally they are mistaken for fibroadenomas. However, these tumors do not bulge or have clefts, and they may have areas of necrosis. Mucinous carcinoma may have a gelatinous appearance.

Less commonly, lobular carcinomas, as well as some ductal carcinomas, may have a diffusely infiltrating pattern and may be subtle (consisting of diffusely firm white tissue) or occult on gross examination. The size of such tumors can only be estimated using both gross and microscopic appearances.

Inflammatory carcinoma is a diagnosis based on both clinical and pathologic features. The patient presents with diffuse erythema and edema involving the breast and skin. The carcinoma often has a diffusely invasive pattern with little or no desmoplasia and most women do not have a palpable mass. The skin changes correlate with tumor in dermal lymphatics—true inflammation is not present. The erythema and edema are not apparent in the excised breast. Mastectomy is often performed only after the patient has responded to chemotherapy.

Metastatic carcinoma to a lymph node with an occult primary is a rare presentation for breast cancer. A breast mass cannot be found by palpation, mammography, or ultrasonography. Occasionally, breast MRI will identify the primary. A gross lesion is usually not identifiable in the mastectomy if all radiologic studies are negative. Occasionally, evidence of carcinoma (e.g., LVI) will be found by sampling grossly normal tissues. However, the prognosis for the woman is governed by the number of involved lymph nodes and is not altered whether or not a primary is identified.

Ductal carcinoma in situ (DCIS) is most often occult on gross examination due to the lack of a surrounding desmoplastic response. The one exception is comedocarcinoma, which may incite desmoplasia and can have pinpoint areas of necrosis which are extruded when the tissue is gently squeezed. The grossly involved area is often firm but not hard and is not well

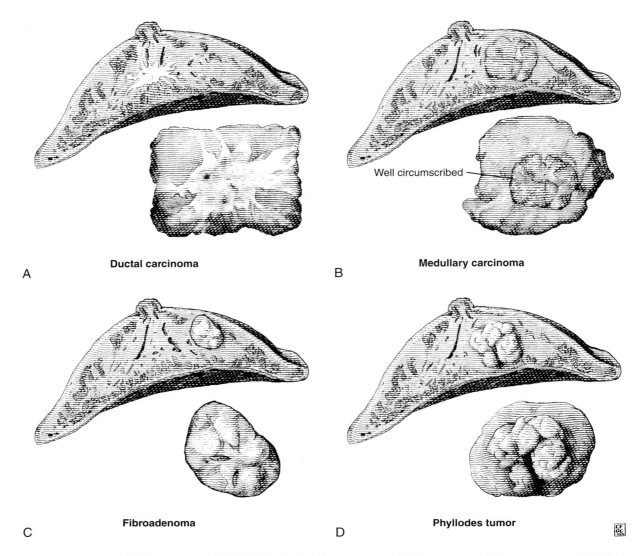

A   **Ductal carcinoma**

B   Well circumscribed ———   **Medullary carcinoma**

C   **Fibroadenoma**

D   **Phyllodes tumor**

Figure 15-1 Gross anatomy of breast lesions.

delimited. Encysted papillary carcinoma in situ may appear as a well-circumscribed mass with a fine papillary surface.

Paget's disease of the nipple is a result of DCIS spreading from a ductal system into the skin of the breast. The normal squamous barrier is disrupted and extracellular fluid can seep onto the surface, resulting in a scale crust. This crust is removed when the skin is cleaned prior to surgery, and the involved nipple usually has a normal gross appearance in the specimen.

Fibroadenomas (FAs) are the most common benign mass-forming lesions of the breast and usually occur in women younger than 40 years of age. The characteristic appearance is of an ovoid or smoothly lobulated mass with a rubbery firm consistency. Clefts are often grossly apparent due to stromal overgrowth surrounded by epithelial lining cells. FAs are firmer than the surrounding tissue and appear to stand up from it and bulge outward. FAs may infarct during pregnancy and appear poorly circumscribed with areas of necrosis and hemorrhage. Numerous other benign lesions have a grossly similar appearance (e.g., hamartomas, adenosis lesions, sclerosing lobular hyperplasia, pseudoangiomatous stromal hyperplasia, fibrous tumors). Well-circumscribed carcinomas should be suspected in women older than 50 years of age and when the lesion is not typical for FA.

Phyllodes tumors may grossly resemble FAs. Phyllodes tumors are usually larger, may have areas of necrosis and hemorrhage, and may be less well circumscribed due to invasion into the surrounding stroma. Most large biphasic stromal lesions (either FAs or phyllodes tumors) will have "leaf-like" protuberances due to areas of stromal overgrowth. Phyllodes tumors are rare and usually present at an older age than FAs.

Fibrocystic changes can occasionally form palpable masses. A single unilocular cyst is generally aspirated and not excised. However, recurrent cysts or cysts that fail to disappear after aspiration (e.g., due to debris within the cyst) may be excised. Tissue may be diffusely firm due to small cysts and fibrosis caused by chronic inflammation. A discrete mass is usually not present.

Complex sclerosing lesions (radial scars) consist of a central hyalinized nidus with radiating arms consisting of epithelial hyperplasia. These lesions are rarely palpable. However, they may present as spiculated mammographic densities closely mimicking invasive carcinomas. The center of the lesion is usually small in relation to the arms, as opposed to invasive carcinomas that have a more solid center. Grossly, they may look stellate but are often soft except for the small firm nidus. Frozen sections should be avoided as the center of the lesion is easily mistaken for an invasive carcinoma and examination of the intact lesion is helpful for diagnosis.

Microscopic sections

Mass
Four to five cassettes of possible carcinomas or 1 section per cm for other grossly identifiable masses. In the absence of a discrete mass, at least 10 cassettes of fibrous tissue are submitted.

Margins
Up to 12 perpendicular sections representing each of the six margins for oriented specimen suspicious for carcinomas (2 cassettes per margin).

Normal tissue
At least one cassette of representative fibrous tissue if not present in the slides above.

Sample dictation

Received fresh, labeled with the patient's name and unit number and "left breast mass," is a 6 (medial to lateral) × 4 (inferior to superior) × 3 (anterior to posterior) cm breast biopsy with two sutures—the long designated "lateral" and the short designated "superior." There is a 2.3 × 2.0 × 1.5 cm very hard white stellate mass that is grossly within 0.1 cm of the medial resection margin. The mass is 1 cm from the superior margin, 1.5 cm from the inferior margin, 4 cm from the lateral margin, 1.5 cm from the posterior margin, and 0.8 cm from the anterior margin. The remainder of the breast tissue consists of grossly unremarkable adipose tissue. The entire tumor and 80% of the entire specimen are submitted for histologic examination. The specimen is inked for the evaluation of margins: posterior = black; anterior = blue; superior = red; inferior = green; lateral = yellow; medial = orange. Sections of margins are submitted for microscopic examination.

Cassettes #1 and 2: Tumor and medial margin, 2 frags, ESS.
Cassettes #3 and 4: Tumor and anterior margin, 4 frags, ESS.
Cassettes #5 and 6: Remainder of tumor, 2 frags, ESS.
Cassettes #7 and 8: Superior margin, 2 frags, RSS.
Cassettes #9 and 10: Inferior margin, 2 frags, RSS.
Cassettes #10 and 11: Lateral margin, 2 frags, RSS.
Cassettes #12 and 13: Posterior margin, 2 frags, RSS.

Pathologic prognostic/diagnostic features sign-out checklist for tumors

See checklist after "Mastectomies," below.

Excisional biopsies for mammographic lesions with wire localization

Mammographic (nonpalpable) lesions are biopsied by placing a wire in the breast at the site of the mammographic abnormality. After excision, the biopsy is sent to mammography for a specimen radiograph and a radiologist confirms the presence of the lesion. The pathologist should receive a copy of the specimen radiograph as well as the interpretation by the radiologist. It is helpful to have the radiologist circle lesions (e.g., faint calcifications) that are not readily apparent.

Biopsies performed for mammographic densities will reveal invasive carcinomas in 20% to 30% of cases (average size 1 cm), DCIS alone in less than 5%, and fibroadenomas in 20% to 30%. The types of mass-forming lesions are similar to those forming palpable masses but are smaller in size.

Biopsies performed for mammographic calcifications without a mass will reveal invasive carcinomas in less than 10% of cases (average size less than 1 cm), DCIS alone in 20% to 30%, and fibroadenomas in 5% to 10%.

Biopsies for architectural distortion are less common and may either correspond to irregular involution, DCIS, or diffusely invasive carcinomas such as invasive lobular carcinoma.

Wide excisions after a core needle diagnosis of malignancy are processed similarly to diagnostic excisional biopsies as the lesion is still within the specimen and is marked with a wire. More extensive sampling (usually submission of the entire specimen) is indicated if a diagnosis of DCIS or ADH has already been established. Important prognostic factors for DCIS are the size of the lesion and distance from the margins (preferably at least 1 cm). In order to optimally evaluate these features, it is usually preferable to submit the entire specimen in consecutive order with oriented margins. If this would require more than 20 blocks, it may be appropriate to examine initial sections before submitting additional tissue.

Specimen processing for mammographic densities

These specimens usually contain the same types of lesions present in biopsies for palpable masses with the exception that the lesions are smaller. They may be processed in a similar fashion if the lesion is grossly evident. Lesions that cannot be identified grossly will require radiologic guidance.

1. Examine the specimen radiograph and the radiologist's report and determine what type of mammographic lesion is present (irregular, well-circumscribed, ill-defined) and its location within the specimen using the shape of the specimen and the wire as guides. Larger masses can often be palpated.

   The specimen can be inked one color if not oriented or multiple colors if oriented.

   The specimen can be bisected along the plane of the wire. In the majority of cases, a gross lesion can be identified corresponding to the radiologic density and the specimen can be processed as for palpable masses.

   In rare cases, if no gross lesion can be identified, it is important to identify the tissue in the area of the radiologic density. It is usually difficult or impossible to find a subtle mass lesion by radiography once the specimen has been sliced. If a gross lesion cannot be identified, all fibrous tissue is processed.

   Never take tissue for special studies or research unless a definitive diagnosis of invasive carcinoma has been established.

2. If the specimen is oriented, oriented margins should be submitted if the lesion is suspicious for malignancy. Up to two cassettes per margin (12 total) may be submitted.

3. If the entire specimen is not submitted, the gross description should include a statement estimating the percentage of the specimen submitted.

Microscopic sections

Mass
Four to five cassettes of possible carcinomas or 1 section per cm for other grossly evident masses. In the absence of an identified mass, all fibrous breast tissue is submitted.

Margins
Up to 12 perpendicular sections representing each of the six margins for oriented specimens suspicious for carcinoma or known to have carcinoma.

Normal tissue
At least one cassette of representative fibrous tissue if not present in the slides above.

Specimen processing for mammographic calcifications or prior needle diagnoses of DCIS or ADH

This type of specimen has the highest probability of revealing DCIS (20% to 30%). Carcinomas are almost always at or very near the area of the calcifications.[7] The lesions are usually not grossly evident and the specimen will consist of benign-appearing breast tissue.

1. Examine the specimen radiograph and the radiologist's report and determine the location of the calcifications or clip within the specimen. Calcifications most likely to be associated with DCIS are small, numerous, clustered, and may be linear or branching. If a core needle biopsy has been performed and has removed most of the calcifications, the radiologist will have placed a small titanium clip at the biopsy site. Large ("popcorn") calcifications are not normally biopsied, but may be present incidental to another mammographic lesion.

    Specimens may be received on radiographic grids, which help to identify the site of radiologic lesions.

    The specimen can be inked one color if not oriented or multiple colors if oriented.

    The specimen may be bisected along the plane of the wire. In the majority of cases, no gross lesion will be present. If a gross lesion is present correlating with the radiologic calcifications (e.g., a small hyalinized fibroadenoma with calcifications, a biopsy site, gel beads corresponding to a core site), the specimen may be processed as for palpable masses. If there is no gross lesion, but the site of the calcifications is identified, the specimen can be processed the same way.

    If there is no gross lesion, and the site of the calcifications cannot be identified (e.g., because the wire had fallen out of the specimen), then the sliced tissue should be re-radiographed. Small specimens (e.g., submitted in <10 cassettes) may be submitted in entirety without additional radiography.

    - **Low suspicion lesion.** The tissue containing the calcifications is completely submitted along with adjacent tissue on either side. The remaining slices may be placed in designated cassettes to maintain orientation, but need not be submitted if the tissue appears grossly benign. The location of this tissue can be marked on the sliced specimen radiograph. If the blocks of the mammographic calcifications reveal atypical hyperplasia or DCIS, all additional fibrous tissue should be examined microscopically.
    - **High suspicion lesion or prior diagnosis of DCIS or ADH by core needle biopsy.** Completely submit all the tissue containing the mammographic calcifications, all fibrous tissue, and at least two representative sections of each margin. If the sections are submitted in order (e.g., from medial to lateral), the size of the area of DCIS can be estimated.

        Never take tissue for special studies or research unless a firm diagnosis of invasive carcinoma has been established.

2. If the entire specimen is not submitted, the gross description should include a statement estimating the percentage of the specimen submitted.

Microscopic sections

Calcifications
All tissue containing the radiologic calcifications and adjacent tissue. Indicate which blocks contain tissue with calcifications. If DCIS or ADH has been diagnosed previously, submit all fibrous tissue, if feasible (e.g., ≤20 cassettes).

Margins
At least 12 cassettes of two perpendicular sections from each of the six margins for oriented specimens with known or suspected carcinoma.

Sample dictation

Received, labeled with the patient's name and unit number and "right breast," is a 5 (medial to lateral) × 3 (inferior to superior) × 2 (anterior to posterior) cm breast biopsy with a localization wire in place and a short suture marking the superior margin and a long suture marking the lateral margin. An accompanying specimen radiograph demonstrates a tight cluster of calcifications and the localization wire. The specimen is inked for the evaluation of margins: posterior = black; anterior = blue; superior = red; inferior = green; lateral = yellow; medial = orange. The tissue consists of dense fibrous parenchyma with multiple small blue dome cysts and a gross lesion at the site of the radiologic calcifications is not seen. The specimen is re-radiographed and the area of calcifications identified. This area is 0.2 cm from the superior margin, 2 cm from the inferior margin, 1 cm from the posterior margin, 0.5 cm from the anterior margin, 3 cm from the medial margin, and 2 cm from the lateral margin. Two sections of each margin are submitted for microscopic examination. The margins consist of unremarkable adipose tissue. 50% of the specimen is submitted including all fibrous tissue. The location of the tissue blocks is recorded on a specimen diagram.

Cassettes #1 and 2: Mammographic microcalcifications with superior margin, 2 frags, ESS.
Cassettes #3 and 4: Closest lateral margin, 1 frag, RSS.
Cassettes #5 and 6: Closest medial margin, 1 frag, RSS.
Cassettes #7 and 8: Closest anterior margin, 1 frag, RSS.
Cassettes #9 and 10: Closest inferior margin, 1 frag, RSS.
Cassettes #11 and 12: Closest posterior margin, 1 frag, RSS.
Cassettes #13–15: Remaining fibrous tissue, 5 frags, ESS.

Pathologic prognostic/diagnostic features sign-out checklist for tumors

See checklist after "Mastectomies," below.

■ REEXCISIONS

Breast reexcision is a general term for a larger excision of an excisional biopsy site when malignancy has been found. Lumpectomies (used loosely because usually a "lump" is no longer present) and quadrantectomies (used to refer to a larger resection of an entire breast quadrant) are examples of this type of specimen. Reexcisions often have a small ellipse of skin (containing the original biopsy scar) that may be oriented with sutures of different lengths. The nipple will not be present. A biopsy cavity must be identified. Separate axillary dissections or sentinel node biopsies are usually performed if invasive carcinoma was diagnosed.

If no gross lesions were found, the entire specimen would need to be submitted to reliably detect every case of residual carcinoma of possible clinical significance. In the study of Abraham et al,[8] submitting one block per cm of maximal tissue dimension detected 88% of lesions of major clinical significance and 81% of lesions with any clinical significance and resulted in a 52% reduction in the number of blocks examined. Submitting two blocks per centimeter resulted in the detection of 97% of lesions of major clinical significance and 95% of lesions with any clinical significance and resulted in a 17% reduction in the number of tissue blocks.

The amount of tissue appropriate to sample will also vary according to the prior diagnosis. Almost all women with a history of invasive carcinoma will receive radiation to the breast, and the purpose of the margin evaluation is to exclude relatively large areas of residual DCIS. Thus, such reexcisions may not need to be sampled in entirety.

Although many women with DCIS alone will also receive radiation to the breast, there may be a subgroup of women with widely clear margins that do not require radiation. Therefore, thorough margin evaluation of the reexcision specimen in these patients is more important for guiding patient management. Even a small amount of DCIS at or near the margin would be treated with either additional surgery or radiation. In addition, if an area of invasion were found in the reexcision, this would change the patient's prognosis and likely her treatment.

1. Record the total dimensions, size and color of skin ellipse, size and condition (well-healed, recent) of scar.

   Ink the entire specimen except for the skin. Different colors of ink can be used if this will help in identifying margins.

   Serially section the specimen without cutting through the skin or any sutures. Carefully palpate the specimen, locating the biopsy cavity and any other lesions.

   Describe the size of the indurated area around the cavity, the diameter and contents of the cavity, thickness (range) of cavity wall, size of any areas suspicious for residual tumor. Describe the nearest approach of the biopsy cavity and firm surrounding areas to the margins. Large specimens should be fixed overnight in formalin with gauze between the sections.

2. Submit up to four sections of the biopsy cavity, selecting areas that are most suspicious for tumor and that are close to margins.

   More extensive sampling of suspicious areas around the biopsy site and in the remaining breast is indicated for patients in whom only DCIS has been diagnosed. Invasive carcinoma may be difficult to detect due to the fibrosis of the prior biopsy cavity.

3. Sample all margins, giving orientation if provided. Twelve cassettes (corresponding to two sections of each of the six margins) are usually adequate unless there are multiple suspicious areas. Cases of DCIS alone should be sampled more thoroughly or completely submitted if possible.

4. Sample the skin to evaluate possible dermal lymphatic involvement or direct skin invasion.

5. If the entire specimen is not submitted, give an estimate of the amount of tissue submitted for histologic examination.

6. If an axillary tail is submitted, see "Axillary dissections," below, for instructions on processing.

Occasionally, wire localization is performed in addition to a reexcision to remove a mammographic lesion close to a prior biopsy site. These specimens are processed as wire localization biopsies (see above).

Special studies

Special studies are usually not indicated because the primary tumor has been removed. If gross tumor is present, it is prudent to determine whether studies have been performed on a prior specimen and consider determining hormone receptor status and HER2/neu on fixed tissue.

Microscopic sections

Biopsy cavity
At least four cassettes including any areas suspicious for residual carcinoma.

Margins
At least 12 cassettes corresponding to two sections of six margins (if no skin is present) or five margins (if skin is present). Take additional sections for women with only DCIS. Submit entire specimen or all fibrous tissue if feasible in these cases.

Skin
One cassette.

Sample dictation

The specimen is received fresh in two parts, labeled with the patient's name and unit number.

The first part, labeled "#1, right lumpectomy," consists of a 10 (medial to lateral) × 9 (inferior to superior) × 7 (anterior to posterior) cm reexcision specimen with a 4 × 1 cm white skin ellipse containing a 3.5 cm well-healed surgical scar and two orienting sutures designated "medial" and "superior." The specimen is inked for the evaluation of margins: posterior = black; anterior = blue; superior = red; inferior = green; lateral = yellow; medial = orange. Two cm deep to the skin there is a 3 × 3 × 2 cm biopsy cavity filled with blood clot and surrounded by dense white tissue (approximately 1 cm in greatest thickness) and areas of fat necrosis. No areas grossly suspicious for invasive carcinoma are seen. The biopsy cavity is 0.5 cm from the deep margin, which is the closest margin. The remaining margins are at least two cm from the cavity and are taken as perpendicular sections for microscopic examination. The remainder of the specimen consists of yellow/white adipose tissue. Approximately 70% of the specimen is submitted for histologic examination.

Cassettes #1–4: Biopsy cavity, 4 frags, RSS.
Cassettes #5 and 6: Biopsy cavity and deep margin, 2 frags, RSS.
Cassettes #7 and 8: Inferior margin, 2 frags, RSS.
Cassettes #9 and 10: Medial margin, 2 frags, RSS.
Cassettes #11 and 12: Superior margin, 2 frags, RSS.
Cassettes #13 and 14: Lateral margin, 2 frags, RSS.
Cassette #15: Skin, 3 frags, RSS.
Cassette #16: Representative fibrous tissue away from the biopsy cavity, 2 frags, RSS.

The second part, labeled "#2, axillary nodes," consists of a 6 × 5 × 3 cm fragment of adipose tissue containing 12 possible lymph nodes. The largest lymph node measures 1.2 cm in size and is firm tan/white with irregular borders.

Cassette #13: Largest lymph node, 3 frags, ESS.
Cassette #14: Three lymph nodes, 3 frags, ESS.
Cassettes #15–18: Two lymph nodes per cassette, uninked or inked, 8 frags, ESS.
Cassette #19: Possible small lymph nodes, 5 frags, ESS.

■ SHAVE MARGINS

To provide better cosmetic results, surgeons may selectively remove tissue from a portion of the breast if only some margins were positive on the original excision. These specimens are usually flattened pieces of tissue with one side marked with a suture as the new margin. The new margin should be inked in black and the old margin in blue. Sections are taken perpendicular to the new margin. At least one section per 1 cm of length should be submitted. Additional sampling is indicated for women with DCIS alone (preferably the entire specimen unless it is quite large).

■ MASTECTOMIES FOR MALIGNANCY

There are several types of mastectomy:

- Subcutaneous (without skin, only performed in males for gynecomastia)
- Simple (without an axillary dissection)—a sentinel node biopsy may be performed
- Modified radical (a simple mastectomy with an axillary dissection; Fig. 15-2)
- Skin sparing (removes only the nipple and a rim of surrounding skin along with the breast tissue)
- Radical (includes pectoralis muscles)—performed only in exceptional cases with chest wall invasion
- Prophylactic (a simple mastectomy in a woman at high risk for carcinoma).

Most women can be treated by breast conservation. Women going to mastectomy are more likely to have the following:

- Multiple cancers that cannot be resected in a single excision. If the cancers were diagnosed by core needle biopsy, radiologic examination of the specimen may be necessary to find the involved areas.
- Locally advanced cancers, often with chest wall or skin invasion. Some of these women will have received preoperative therapy.
- Inflammatory cancer—most of these women will have received preoperative therapy.
- Metastatic carcinoma to a lymph node with an occult primary.

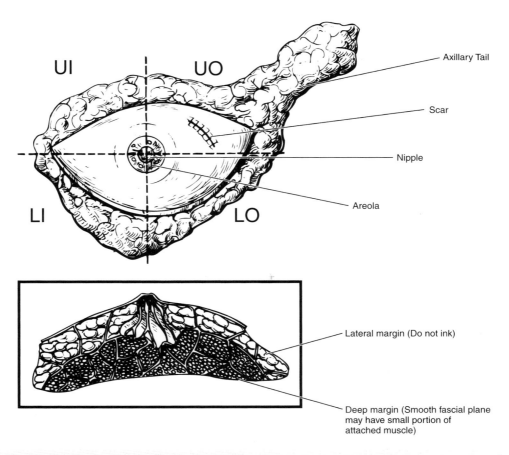

Figure 15-2 Modified radical mastectomy (left side).

- Recurrent cancer in patients previously treated with radiation.
- Women at high risk for additional carcinomas (e.g., due to *BRCA1* or *BRCA2* mutations).

Thus, these tend to be complicated specimens. Unless a good history is provided ("Breast cancer" does *not* constitute a good history), it may be helpful prior to gross examination of the specimen to contact the clinician or review the medical record to determine the number and type of lesions present, as well as any preoperative therapy.

Additional important information can be derived from mastectomies after excision of an invasive carcinoma (e.g., increase in tumor size, deep margin involvement, lymphatic invasion, skeletal muscle invasion, skin invasion) or DCIS (e.g., unsuspected areas of invasion). Mastectomy specimens require meticulous gross examination as only a small proportion of the specimen is examined microscopically. In one study, 83% of major diagnostic discrepancies in breast specimens resulted from inadequate sampling of tissue from mastectomies.[9]

Difficult cases

Mastectomies after core needle biopsy are often problematic as it may be difficult to find the site of the original lesion because the biopsy site may not be visible. If the biopsy was performed for a palpable mass or a mammographic density, most lesions can be found by careful gross examination. If the biopsy was performed for calcifications, it is helpful to radiograph the specimen prior to sectioning to locate the area of calcifications and any clips placed by the radiologist. Additional radiographs after sectioning of the specimen may be helpful to guide selection of tissue.

Mastectomies after chemotherapy can be problematic as the area of the prior carcinoma may be difficult to detect. The extent of residual carcinoma (viable or nonviable) is an important prognostic factor and must be documented. Women with a complete response (no residual carcinoma) have a better prognosis than women with a partial or no response.

If the carcinoma was originally palpable, the surgeon can indicate the site with a suture or a description. If there were mammographic findings associated with the carcinoma (e.g., calcifications or a clip placed prior to treatment), the specimen can be radiographed. Calcifications generally do not disappear with therapy. Once the site of the prior carcinoma is identified, it is helpful to take a series of consecutive sections: for example, one tissue section per cm from medial to lateral in the area of a previously palpable 5 cm carcinoma.

Processing the specimen

1. Describe:

   Weight. Entire specimen.

   Dimensions. Total size of breast, size of axillary dissection.

   Skin ellipse. Size, color, presence of skin retraction, presence of ulceration over tumors, skin lesions. Occasionally there will be red oval-shaped marks that are often associated with detachment of the overlying epidermis at the edges of the skin ellipse. These are clamp marks made during the procedure and need not be sampled.

   Nipple. Size of nipple (i.e., the area where the ducts emerge, not the pigmented areola), retraction, inversion, irregular or crusted surface (may indicate Paget's disease of the nipple).

   Scar. Size and condition (well-healed, recent, sutured) of surgical incision or scar, location (quadrant—most commonly upper outer) of incision and distance from nipple. Scars are most easily found when the specimen is fresh. Semicircular scars around the areola may be difficult to see. Scars can be distinguished from marks on the skin by making an incision and looking for the area of underlying dermal fibrosis. A scar may be absent if the mastectomy was performed for prophylactic reasons, if the original diagnosis was made with a needle biopsy, or if a "skin sparing" mastectomy is performed. If a scar or a biopsy cavity cannot be found and the reason for the mastectomy is unclear, the surgeon should be called.

Deep margin. Usually consists of a smooth fascial plane overlying the pectoralis muscle. Areas of irregularity or attached portions of skeletal muscle are documented (size and location).

If the prior procedure was a core needle biopsy for a nonpalpable lesion, it may be useful to radiograph the intact specimen.

2. Ink the deep fascial margin black but not the lateral soft tissue margins. The adipose tissue not at the deep margin abuts subcutaneous tissue in the patient. Although breast ducts can sometimes be present in subcutaneous tissue, this tissue is not generally considered to be a true margin and a positive margin in this area is of unknown clinical significance. If this tissue is inked, it should be in a different color than the deep fascial margin and reported separately.

3. Separate the axillary tail and fix in a separate container. If removing the tail will make the specimen difficult to orient, cut a notch in the skin at the site of the tail. See the section on "Axillary dissections," below, for processing.

     Lymph nodes *must* be searched for even in specimens designated "simple mastectomies." Often one or two low lymph nodes (but occasionally many more than this) are included and are often the most important tissue to examine.

4. Serially section the specimen at approximately 0.5 cm intervals but do not cut through the skin. Carefully palpate all sections and locate the biopsy cavity and any other suspicious lesions. This must be done in the fresh state because formalin hardens tissues, and small lesions may be missed.

     Describe size, location (quadrant), and distance from the deep margin and skin of any lesions including the biopsy cavity. If tumor is present, also describe color, borders (infiltrating, well-circumscribed, ill-defined), consistency (firm, hard), relationship, if any, to biopsy cavity and nipple, and distance from skin, deep margin, and other margins (e.g., lateral) if involved.

     The deep margin is always taken as a perpendicular margin because this is a true tissue plane and even a thin rim of tissue (e.g., less than 0.1 cm) would be considered a negative margin. Any skeletal muscle present is sampled to look for muscle invasion.

     If multiple lesions are present, describe their relationship to each other and submit a cassette of tissue in-between the lesions.

     The remainder of the non-lesional breast tissue is described (e.g., predominantly fatty, firm, white, cysts—size, gross calcifications, etc.).

     If a grossly inapparent radiographic lesion is present (e.g., calcifications), it is usually useful to radiograph the sliced specimen to ensure that the lesion is sampled.

5. Fix the specimen overnight in a large container filled with formalin. Gauze is used to separate the sections and placed underneath the specimen.

6. The following day, tissue blocks are taken from the mastectomy at the sites noted (see below).

     Nipple. In the usual nipple examination, one perpendicular section is taken. This type of section will only examine one to four of the main nipple ducts. If there is a reason to examine the nipple more thoroughly (e.g., the nipple is grossly abnormal or there is a clinical history of Paget's disease), additional sections may be taken (Fig. 15-3). The nipple is amputated in a plane parallel to the skin surface. A second, deeper, section is taken in the same plane. This section will demonstrate all the major ducts as they approach the nipple. The more superficial section is serially sectioned perpendicular to the skin surface and all these slices are submitted. These sections will demonstrate most of the nipple ducts as they empty onto the skin surface.

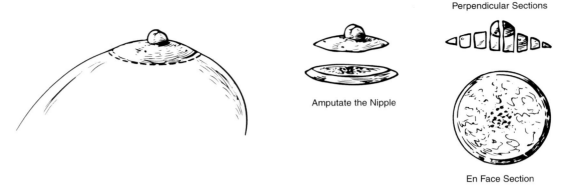

Perpendicular Sections

Amputate the Nipple

En Face Section

Figure 15-3 Nipple sectioning diagrams.

Sample dictation

Received fresh, labeled with the patient's name and unit number and "MRM—left," is an 850-g left modified radical mastectomy specimen (15 × 10 × 5.5 cm) with a white/tan skin ellipse (14 × 7 cm) and an attached axillary tail (7 × 6 × 3 cm). There is a 3.4 cm well-healed surgical scar in the upper outer quadrant, 2 cm from the unremarkable 0.5 cm nipple. One cm deep to this scar is a firm white area (4.5 × 4.0 × 2.0 cm) containing a recent biopsy cavity (3.0 cm in diameter) filled with organizing red/tan clot, 1.5 cm from the deep margin which is a smooth fascial plane without skeletal muscle present. The wall of the cavity is firm and white to yellow, ranging from 0.5 to 1 cm in thickness, without gross tumor present. The remainder of the breast parenchyma is predominantly white and firm with small cysts measuring up to 0.3 cm in greatest dimension. There are 15 tan lymph nodes in the axillary tail, the largest measuring 0.8 cm in greatest dimension. Lymph nodes placed in the same cassette are differentially inked.

Cassettes #1–4: Biopsy cavity, 4 frags, RSS.
Cassette #5: Deep margin of biopsy cavity, perpendicular section, 1 frag, RSS.
Cassette #6: Skin with scar, 2 frags, RSS.
Cassette #7: Upper outer quadrant, 1 frag, RSS.
Cassette #8: Upper inner quadrant, 1 frag, RSS.
Cassette #9: Lower outer quadrant, 1 frag, RSS.
Cassette #10: Lower inner quadrant, 1 frag, RSS.
Cassette #11: Nipple, 1 frag, RSS.
Cassettes #12–16: Lymph nodes, 3 per cassette, 15 frags, ESS.

Microscopic sections

Biopsy cavity
At least four sections. More sampling is indicated in cases of DCIS alone (to look for foci of invasion), fewer in cases of known large invasive carcinomas.

Invasive carcinomas
Residual tumor may be present if the prior procedure was an incisional biopsy or a core needle biopsy. Four to five cassettes of tumor, including the relationship to skin and deep margin, should be submitted.

Radiologic lesions
Mastectomies may be performed after a prior diagnosis of DCIS or invasive carcinoma by core needle biopsy. The calcifications, density, and/or clip should be located by radiographing the specimen if not grossly evident. The entire area of involved tissue is submitted.

Skin

One section of biopsy scar. Additional sections should be submitted of skin lesions, carcinoma involving skin, or if there was a clinical history of inflammatory carcinoma (i.e., carcinoma involving dermal lymphatics).

Deep margin

One section if grossly not involved. Take at the biopsy cavity and near any other gross lesions. Always take as a perpendicular margin. Do not routinely sample other deep margins (e.g., from quadrants) unless grossly abnormal. Skeletal muscle at the deep margin is sampled using perpendicular sections.

Other margins

One perpendicular section may be taken if the biopsy site or a gross lesion is very close to a non-deep (subcutaneous tissue) margin. The clinical significance of such margin involvement is unknown and such sections must be clearly distinguished from the deep margin.

Nipple

One section. Two sections (perpendicular and deep en face) if gross lesions are present or if there is a clinical history of Paget's disease.

Representative

One section from each quadrant (upper outer, upper inner, lower quadrants outer, lower inner). These sections should be away from any other lesions sampled (e.g., the biopsy cavity). If they are not, this is noted in the gross description. They are taken of fibrous breast parenchyma (not adipose tissue).

Lymph nodes

Each thinly sliced (0.2 to 0.3 cm) and entirely submitted. More than one lymph node can be placed in one cassette if selectively inked in different colors.

■ AXILLARY DISSECTIONS

Axillary dissections are performed for the staging of women with invasive carcinoma. The number of lymph nodes with metastases is the most important prognostic factor for women with breast carcinoma. Treatment protocols may require a minimum number of examined lymph nodes for entry (typically 6 or 10) to avoid enrolling women misclassified because of inadequate sampling.

See Chapter 27, page 521 for instructions on processing. All lymph nodes are thinly sliced and are completely submitted. The number of lymph nodes with metastases is important for prognosis and for treatment protocols. In order to count the nodes, a single node should be placed in each cassette, or multiple lymph nodes may be placed in the same cassette if differentially inked to avoid confusing fragments of the same lymph node with separate nodes.

Record the total number of lymph nodes, the size of the largest lymph node, and the presence of any lymph nodes with areas suspicious for metastatic tumor (firm white lymph nodes or those with irregular borders). If there is extensive extranodal extension with matting of lymph nodes, estimate the probable total number of lymph nodes involved.

Most axillary dissections should yield between 10 and 20 lymph nodes. If fewer than 10 nodes are found grossly, reexamine the specimen and submit any areas that may represent lymph nodes. Nodes largely replaced by fat may be difficult to recognize but will have a firm rim of tissue around the fatty center. If the specimen was not fixed in Bouin's, post fixation can help to identify nodes. Finally, the entire axillary tail may not have been identified on a mastectomy specimen and additional nodes in the lateral portion of the specimen should be sought.

If the mastectomy was performed for a diagnosis of extensive DCIS, some surgeons perform a low axillary lymph node dissection. There may be fewer nodes in such specimens.

Although simple mastectomies do not specifically remove axillary nodes, a few low nodes are sometimes removed. Nodes should always be searched for in lateral tissue and their presence or absence documented.

If a portion of pectoralis minor muscle is attached, the level of the nodes can be determined. Level I nodes are inferior, level II posterior, and level III superior (these latter nodes are often not resected because of the greater morbidity involved). The nodes are submitted in cassettes designated as to the levels and labeled this way in the final report.

Sentinel node biopsy is a common procedure for breast carcinoma staging. See Chapter 27, "Sentinel lymph nodes," for instructions on processing.

Pathologic prognostic/diagnostic features sign-out checklist for breast tumors

Specimen type*
Needle core biopsy (ultrasound-guided—masses, stereotactic—calcifications, density, architectural distortion, or for palpable mass), incisional biopsy, excisional biopsy for palpable mass, excisional biopsy for mammographic lesion (calcifications, density, architectural distortion), nipple duct excision, reexcision, simple mastectomy, skin-sparing mastectomy, modified radical mastectomy.

Lymph node sampling*
No lymph node sampling, sentinel lymph node(s) only, sentinel node with axillary dissection, axillary dissection.

Specimen size*
The greatest dimension of the specimen should be provided, if the procedure is less than a mastectomy. The size in three dimensions may also be given.

Laterality*
Right, left breast, unspecified.

Tumor site*
Upper outer, lower outer, upper inner, lower inner, central, not specified.

Size*
Invasive: Greatest dimension to nearest 1 mm based on gross and microscopic findings. Description as "small" or "microscopic" is inadequate for staging (see below). If an exact size cannot be given (e.g., due to fragmentation) an estimate or minimal size is clinically useful. Do not include adjacent areas of DCIS in the overall size.
DCIS: Greatest dimension encompassing all foci if on one slide or number of slides if present in multiple slides. If the biopsy has been submitted as sequential sections the total area involved can be estimated.
LCIS need not be quantified.

Histologic type*
Invasive carcinoma: ductal (no special type), lobular, mucinous, tubular, medullary, other rare types.
Ductal carcinoma in situ, lobular carcinoma in situ.
In situ carcinoma with microinvasion (foci of invasive carcinoma measuring less than 0.1 cm in size).

Single versus multiple Invasive carcinomas
If multiple carcinomas are present, describe each separately and give size for each.
The aggregate size of grossly evident invasive carcinomas correlates better with the risk of lymph node metastases than the size of the largest carcinoma.[10] However, sizes should not be added together for T classification. The presence of multiple invasive carcinomas is denoted by "m" or the number of foci of invasion in parentheses.

Extensive intraductal component (EIC)

A carcinoma is EIC positive if DCIS is prominent within the main tumor mass and is present outside the mass or the tumor is primarily intraductal with only focal invasion.

EIC-positive carcinomas are more likely to have residual carcinoma in the breast if margins are positive or close when compared to EIC-negative carcinomas.

Histologic grade*

A specific grading system is not mandated, but the system used should be specified.

Invasive: May be graded using the Nottingham Histologic Score (the Elston–Ellis modification of the Scarff–Bloom–Richardson grading system, Table 15-7). CAP recommends reporting all three components, if the Nottingham Histologic Score is used.

Grade all histologic subtypes of carcinoma. Necrosis is a poor prognostic indicator if extensive (≥1 HPF).

DCIS: Nuclear grade (low, intermediate, high), presence or absence of necrosis. Necrotic areas should contain ghost cells and karyorrhectic debris to distinguish necrosis from secretory material.

Extent of invasion*

Confined to breast parenchyma, extension to chest wall (not including pectoralis muscle), edema (including peau d'orange) or ulceration of the skin of the breast or satellite skin nodules confined to the same breast.

Regional lymph nodes*

Number of nodes examined (intramammary nodes are included), number with metastases (tumor nodules in axillary fat without an identifiable lymph node can be counted as positive nodes).

Method of examining lymph nodes (H&E levels, IHC, RT-PCR).

Size of largest metastasis.

Extranodal invasion.

If sentinel nodes are received, the method of examination should be stated (e.g., number of levels examined, immunohistochemical studies). Metastases found only by immunohistochemistry (i.e., cells are inapparent on H&E sections) should be specified.

Distant metastasis*

Absent, present (specify site if known).

Margins*

The method of evaluating and reporting margins has not been standardized. If shave margins (parallel to the margin) are taken, this must be specified. Perpendicular margins are recommended.

Invasive carcinoma: Positive margins (= ink on tumor), give distance to closest margin.

Describe extent of margin involvement (e.g., unifocal, multifocal, extensive, or give number of slides with margin involvement). Give orientation of positive margins if the specimen was oriented.

DCIS: A positive margin is ink on tumor. Give the closest approach of DCIS to each margin if oriented. Quantify the amount of DCIS at or near margins (e.g., unifocal, multifocal, extensive, or give number of slides with margin involvement).

LCIS: Margins are not given (recognized to be multifocal and bilateral).

Venous/lymphatic (large/small vessel) invasion (lymphovascular invasion = LVI)

Absent, present. Use criteria of Rosen (Box 15-1).

Dermal lymphovascular invasion is usually present in carcinomas presenting clinically as inflammatory carcinoma.

CAP recommends that LVI be reported, but it is not mandated.

Perineural invasion

Present or absent. This feature is of uncertain prognostic significance and is optional to report.

Microcalcifications

It is important to correlate with carcinomas if the biopsy contained radiographically suspicious calcifications.

Present in DCIS, present in invasive carcinoma, present in nonneoplastic tissue, present in both tumor and nonneoplastic tissue

Biopsy cavity

Absent, present. This is important to document in specimens with a prior needle core biopsy or excision.

Relationship to any residual tumor.

Special studies

Hormone receptors: Determined on all carcinomas.

HER2/neu: Often determined on all invasive carcinomas.

Flow cytometry: Requested by some oncologists.

Prior treatment

If the patient has received preoperative therapy, the status of the residual carcinoma is a prognostic factor.

Complete response: No tumor identified. However, make sure the prior tumor site has been identified and changes consistent with treated tumor are present (stromal fibrosis, chronic inflammation, often residual DCIS and/or calcifications).

Partial response: Often not grossly identifiable or only a vague firmer area. Microscopically, the tumor consists of small islands of viable-appearing tumor cells within a larger area of fibrosis.

No or minimal response: Grossly evident tumor with little or no evidence of treatment effect.

It is also helpful to describe the number of lymph nodes with metastases as well as the number of lymph nodes with areas consistent with treated tumor (e.g., areas of fibrosis or necrosis).

Nonlesional breast tissue

Relevant findings such as ADH, ALH, benign calcifications, radiation changes, etc.

This list incorporates recommendations from the Association of Directors of Anatomic and Surgical Pathology (www.panix.com/~adasp/) and CAP (www.cap.org). The asterisked elements are considered to be scientifically validated or regularly used data elements that must be present in reports of cancer-directed surgical excisions from ACS CoC-approved cancer programs. The details of reporting these elements may differ among institutions.

■ PROPHYLACTIC MASTECTOMIES

Prophylactic mastectomies are simple mastectomies performed on women without a diagnosis of breast cancer. Unilateral procedures may be performed on women with contralateral carcinoma. Bilateral procedures may be performed on women at high risk for developing invasive carcinoma due to either a diagnosis of LCIS or an inherited susceptibility to breast cancer (*BRCA1* or *BRCA2* carriers). Occult carcinomas were found in 15% of prophylactic mastectomies from women with a family history of breast carcinoma and contralateral carcinoma.[17]

If there is a known palpable or radiographic abnormality, the examination should be directed towards finding and examining this area.

In the absence of a known abnormality, the breast is thinly sectioned and examined in the fresh state. All areas grossly suspicious for in situ or invasive carcinoma should be submitted. In the absence of grossly suspicious areas, one to two blocks of tissue per quadrant and one section of the nipple may be submitted for microscopic examination. Lymph nodes should not be present but should be searched for and submitted if present.

Table 15-6 AJCC (6th edition) classification of breast carcinomas

Tumor	TX	Primary tumor cannot be assessed
	T0	No evidence of primary tumor
	Tis	Carcinoma in situ: Intraductal carcinoma, lobular carcinoma in situ, or Paget's disease of the nipple without an invasive carcinoma
	T1	Tumor 2 cm or less in greatest dimension
	T1mic	Microinvasion 0.1 cm or less in greatest dimension
	T1a	>0.1 cm but ≤0.5 cm
	T1b	>0.5 cm to ≤1 cm
	T1c	>1 cm to ≤2 cm
	T2	>2 cm to ≤5 cm
	T3	>5 cm
	T4	Tumor of any size with direct extension to (a) chest wall or (b) skin, only as described below
	T4a	Invasion of ribs, intercostal muscles, or serratus anterior muscle. Invasion of the pectoral muscle is not included
	T4b	Edema (including peau d'orange) or ulceration of the skin of the breast or satellite skin nodules confined to the same breast
	T4c	Both T4a and T4b
	T4d	Inflammatory carcinoma. This is a clinical diagnosis and usually is correlated with dermal lymphatic invasion. However, the pathologic finding of dermal lymphatic invasion in the absence of the clinical appearance of inflammatory carcinoma is insufficient for this classification

Note: The pathologic tumor size includes only the invasive component. The largest focus of invasion or microinvasion is used for classification. Do not add the sizes of separate foci. If multiple macroscopic foci of invasion are present this should be noted. If macroscopic tumor is present at the margin, the tumor is classified as TX as the actual tumor size may be larger than evident in the specimen.
The best size is based on gross, microscopic, and imaging findings.
Bilateral synchronous carcinomas should each be given a separate stage.

Regional lymph nodes (including intramammary nodes)	pNX	Regional lymph nodes cannot be assessed
	pN0	No regional lymph node metastasis. Metastases <0.02 cm in size (approximately 20 cells end to end) are classified as N0 and can be further described as follows: pN0(i+) isolated tumor cells detected by H&E or IHC pN0 (mol+) tumor cells detected by RT-PCR
	pN1	Metastasis in 1 to 3 axillary lymph nodes, and/or internal mammary nodes with microscopic disease detected by sentinel lymph node dissection but not clinically apparent
	pN1mi	>0.02 cm but not more than 0.2 cm
	pN1a	Metastasis to one to three axillary lymph nodes, at least one >0.2 cm
	pN1b	Metastasis in internal mammary nodes. Nodes with microscopic disease detected by sentinel lymph node dissection but not clinically apparent
	pN1c	Metastasis in 1 to 3 axillary lymph nodes and metastasis in internal mammary nodes. Nodes with microscopic disease detected by sentinel lymph node dissection but not clinically apparent. If there are more than 3 positive axillary nodes, the internal mammary nodes are classified as pN3b to reflect increased tumor burden
	pN2	Metastasis to 4 to 9 axillary lymph nodes or in clinically apparent internal mammary lymph nodes in the absence of axillary lymph node metastasis
	pN2a	Metastasis to 4 to 9 axillary lymph nodes (at least one >0.2 cm)
	pN2b	Metastasis in clinically apparent internal mammary nodes in the absence of axillary lymph node metastasis
	pN3	Metastasis in 10 or more axillary lymph nodes, or in infraclavicular nodes, or in clinically apparent ipsilateral internal mammary nodes in the presence of one or more positive axillary nodes, or in more than 3 axillary nodes with clinically negative microscopic metastasis in internal mammary nodes, or in ipsilateral supraclavicular nodes
	pN3a	Metastasis in 10 or more axillary nodes or metastasis to the infraclavicular nodes

Table 15-6 AJCC (6th edition) classification of breast carcinomas—*cont'd*

	pN3b	Metastasis in clinically apparent ipsilateral internal mammary nodes in the presence of one or more positive axillary nodes, or in more than 3 axillary nodes and in internal mammary nodes with microscopic disease detected by sentinel lymph node dissection but not clinically apparent
	pN3c	Metastasis in ipsilateral supraclavicular lymph nodes

Sentinel nodes can be indicated by adding (sn) to the classification.

Clinically apparent is defined as metastases detected by imaging studies (excluding lymphoscintigraphy) or by clinical examination.

Foci of cancer in fat adjacent to the breast without histologic evidence of residual lymph node tissue are classified as regional lymph node metastasis.

The axillary node staging is simplified to the following in the absence of information about other nodal groups based on H&E examination:

	pN0	No tumor cells >0.02 cm in size
	pN1mi	Micrometastasis >0.02 cm to 0.2 cm
	pN1a	Metastasis to 1 to 3 axillary nodes, at least one >0.2 cm
	pN2a	Metastasis to 4 to 9 axillary nodes, at least one >0.2 cm
	pN3a	Metastasis to 10 or more axillary nodes, at least one >0.2 cm
Distant metastasis	MX	Distant metastasis cannot be assessed
	M0	No distant metastasis
	M1	Distant metastasis including contralateral internal mammary nodes or cervical lymph node(s)

Table 15-7 Nottingham combined histologic grade (the Elston–Ellis modification of the Scarff–Bloom–Richardson grading system) for invasive breast carcinomas

FEATURE	SCORE
Tubule formation	
Majority of tumor (>75%)	1
Moderate degree (10–75%)	2
Little or none (<10%)	3
Clear lumina must be present to be scored	
Nuclear pleomorphism	
Small, regular uniform cells	
Size of normal cells, uniform chromatin	1
Moderate increase in size and variability	2
Open, vesicular nuclei with visible nucleoli	3
Marked variation, especially large and bizarre nuclei	
Vesicular with prominent, often multiple nucleoli	

Mitotic counts with a 40× objective

Field diameter 0.44 (area 0.152 mm^2)	*Field diameter 0.59 (area 0.24 mm^2)*	
0–5 mitoses per 10 HPF	<10 mitoses per 10 HPF	1
6–10 mitoses per 10 HPF	10–20 mitoses per 10 HPF	2
>10 mitoses per 10 HPF	>20 mitoses per 10 HPF	3

Assess mitotic counts at the periphery of the tumor, in the most mitotically active area. Only clearly identifiable mitotic figures are counted—do not include hyperchromatic, karyorrhectic, or apoptotic nuclei. Count at least 10 fields. The number of mitoses per 10 HPFs is used to determine the score. The size of a 40 field varies widely with microscope type and with modifications (e.g., multiheaded microscopes and built-in polarizers). The size of the field should be measured with a stage micrometer and the mitotic counts adjusted. See Chapter 9 for information on measuring field sizes.

Overall tumor grade		
3–5 points	Grade I	Well-differentiated
6–7 points	Grade II	Moderately differentiated
8–9 points	Grade III	Poorly differentiated

Note: All tumors should be graded regardless of histologic type. Overall, approximately 20% of cancers should be grade I, 40% grade II, and 40% grade III. All tubular carcinomas are well differentiated and all medullary carcinomas are poorly differentiated. Other histologic types vary in grade.
See also references 12 and 13.

Table 15-8 Nuclear grade of ductal carcinoma in situ[14]

FEATURE	LOW GRADE	INTERMEDIATE GRADE	HIGH GRADE
Pleomorphism	Monomorphic	Intermediate	Marked
Size	1.5 to 2 times larger than RBC or size of normal duct epithelial cell nucleus	Intermediate	>2.5 RBC or size of normal duct epithelial cell nucleus
Chromatin	Diffuse, finely dispersed	Intermediate	Vesicular with irregular chromatin
Nucleoli	Only occasional	Intermediate	Prominent, often multiple
Mitoses	Only occasional	Intermediate	May be frequent
Oriented	Polarized towards luminal spaces	Intermediate	Usually not oriented

Table 15-9 Fibroadenoma and grading of phyllodes tumors[a]

FEATURE	FIBROADENOMA	LOW GRADE ("BENIGN")	INTERMEDIATE GRADE ("BORDERLINE")	HIGH GRADE ("MALIGNANT")
Stromal cellularity	Paucicellular to mild	Mildly to moderately cellular	Moderate to markedly cellular	Usually highly cellular
Nuclear pleomorphism	Minimal	Minimal to mild	More evident	May be marked
Mitotic rate[b]	Usually absent or very rare	Usually present but infrequent (e.g., 0–1/10 HPF)	Slightly increased (e.g., 2–5/10 HPF)	Frequently have a high mitotic rate (e.g., >5/10 HPF)
Stromal overgrowth (absence of epithelium in cellular areas)	Absent (but may be hyalinized with atrophic or absent epithelium)	Absent or focal	Often present	Often marked (may be difficult to distinguish from a sarcoma)
Borders	Circumscribed (fibroadenomatoid changes may be ill defined)	Usually circumscribed and pushing	Usually has some invasion into stroma	Usually has marked invasion into stroma
Heterologous elements	May have benign lipomatous and osseous metaplasia	May have benign lipomatous and osseous metaplasia	May have benign lipomatous and osseous metaplasia	May have malignant stromal components (e.g., rhabdomyosarcoma, liposarcoma, angiosarcoma)

[a] There is no generally accepted grading system for phyllodes tumors. The WHO system uses a three-category system (benign, borderline, and malignant) based on the features in the table.[15]
Due to the fact that rare "benign" phyllodes tumors have been reported to have metastasized and resulted in the death of patients and because the majority of "malignant" or high-grade lesions are cured by local therapy, diagnostic terms implying clinical behavior should be used with caution.[16] Some pathologists prefer to separate phyllodes into three grades (low, intermediate, and high).
[b] In published series, mitotic rates have not been standardized for the size of the microscopic field.

Box 15-1   Rosen criteria for lymphovascular invasion (LVI)[11]

1. Lymphatic invasion must be diagnosed outside the border of the invasive carcinoma. The most common area to find LVI is within 0.1 cm of the edge of the carcinoma.
2. The tumor emboli usually do not conform exactly to the contours of the space in which they are found. In contrast, invasive carcinoma with retraction artifact mimicking LVI will have exactly the same shape.
3. Endothelial cell nuclei should be seen in the cells lining the space.
4. Lymphatics are often found adjacent to blood vessels and often partially encircle a blood vessel.

LVI may be seen in stroma between uninvolved lobules and can sometimes be mistaken for DCIS. Immunohistochemical studies for vascular antigens have not been found to be superior to the histologic evaluation of LVI.

■ REDUCTION MAMMOPLASTY

Reduction mammoplasties are almost always bilateral and consist of fragments of breast tissue with attached skin. The nipples are not present. The procedure is considered therapeutic if the specimen weighs over 300 g (e.g., to relieve back pain) but cosmetic if the specimen weighs less than this. The weight is important to document, as some insurance policies will not pay for cosmetic surgery.

Incidental carcinomas are found rarely (approximately 2 to 4 per 1000 cases). The two sides must be clearly labeled and designated tissue submitted separately from each side. If the side is not specified, the woman may require bilateral mastectomies if an incidental carcinoma is found.

A unilateral reduction mammoplasty is occasionally performed to obtain a balanced cosmetic result in a woman who has had surgery for carcinoma on the contralateral side. Additional sections should be taken from such specimens because of the increased risk of carcinoma in these patients. Approximately one third of these patients will have a contralateral carcinoma (in most cases DCIS or LCIS).

1. Weigh the specimen. Measure the entire specimen in aggregate. Record the total number of fragments, number of fragments with skin, skin color, and range of greatest dimension of fragments.
2. Section and palpate each fragment for lesions.
3. Submit two sections per side including breast parenchyma and skin. Any suspicious areas are sampled.

Additional sections are submitted if the patient has risk factors for breast carcinoma (e.g., a previous history of breast cancer or a strong family history). Be suspicious if one side is markedly different in size than the other or if only one side is submitted. This may indicate that a prior surgical procedure for cancer has been performed.

Sample dictation

The specimen is received fresh in two parts, each labeled with the patient's name and unit number. The first part, labeled "Left breast," is a 350-g specimen consisting of five fragments of breast parenchyma with three of the fragments containing white/tan skin (in aggregate 25 × 10 × 10 cm; skin measuring up to 4 cm in size). A nipple is not present. The breast parenchyma consists of approximately 60% dense white tissue and the remainder yellow/white unremarkable adipose tissue. No gross lesions are present.

Cassettes #1 and 2: Breast parenchyma and skin, 4 frags, RSS.

The second part, labeled "Right breast," is a 375-g specimen consisting of six fragments of breast parenchyma with three of the fragments bearing white/tan skin (in aggregate (27 × 11 × 10 cm; skin measuring up to 5 cm in size). A nipple is not present. There is a 2 cm area of small simple cysts measuring up to 0.4 cm in size in the breast tissue. The remainder of the breast tissue consists of approximately 60% dense white tissue and the remainder unremarkable yellow/white adipose tissue.

Cassette #3 and 4: Breast parenchyma including area of cysts and skin, 5 frags, RSS.

■ DUCT DISSECTIONS/NIPPLE BIOPSIES

Duct dissections are usually performed to evaluate nipple discharge without a palpable mass. The most common lesion found is a large duct papilloma, but occasionally papillary or micropapillary DCIS may be found. A duct dissection specimen is usually small, and large ducts may be grossly visible. Ducts look like flaccid white tubes approximately 0.2 to 0.3 cm in diameter. Large papillomas may be evident grossly as lobulated outgrowths from the duct wall. Ink the outer portion of the specimen. If a ductal lesion is evident grossly, submit the ductal margin. Take cross-sections across the duct(s) and submit the entire specimen. Orient all sections if orientation is provided.

A nipple wedge excision (which includes skin) may be performed to treat a recurrent subareolar abscess.[18]

A nipple biopsy may be performed to evaluate possible Paget's disease (see page 87, "Nipple lesions").

Small skin biopsies may be performed to evaluate possible inflammatory breast carcinoma. If carcinoma is not seen and another cause for the clinical appearance is not found (e.g., infection or an inflammatory dermatitis), inflammatory carcinoma cannot be excluded as dermal lymphatic involvement by carcinoma in such cases can be very focal.

■ BREAST IMPLANTS

Explanted permanent implants should be well documented in the surgical pathology report due to the concern over possible long-term complications. The Safe Medical Devices Act (SMDA) went into effect in August of 1993. This act requires that certain medical devices (including breast implants) used after this date must be tracked by the manufacturer as well as by physicians and hospitals. Current information about implants can be found at www.fda.gov/cdrh/breastimplants/.

Implants are of two general types:

Tissue expanders are placed temporarily after a surgical procedure for malignancy. They are removed within days to weeks. These implants are almost always filled with saline and have a textured surface and a large port (a circular metallic disc) for changing the volume. These implants are unlikely to be involved in litigation and do not need to be photographed unless they were removed due to a complication (most likely infection).

Permanent implants are commonly placed for cosmetic reasons, are usually bilateral, and are filled with either silicone or saline. These implants may be removed because of complications (rupture, calcification, capsular contracture, infection), systemic complaints attributed to the implant, or patient concerns over safety. Implants that are removed may be requested for litigation. All such implants should be photographed.

The gross description includes:

Size. Three dimensions.

Shape. Usually ovoid. If permanent folds or creases are present, these are documented in the dictation and photographs taken.

Surface appearance. Smooth or textured, presence or absence of calcifications and/or adherent tissue. A tacky (sticky) surface is usually indicative of silicone bleed through an intact shell. Implants with thicker shells or saline implants will have a dry smooth surface. The shell for both saline and silicone implants is most commonly made of silicone polymers.

Contents. Silicone is more viscous than saline. Saline will freeze if placed in a freezer whereas silicone will not. However, this should not be used to distinguish the two because the shell may be damaged by freezing.

Color of contents. Usually translucent or with a slight yellowish cast. If the contents are opaque, cloudy, or colored (e.g., red or brown) this is an unusual finding that may indicate infection or degradation.

Single or double lumen. Some implants have an inner and an outer chamber. One may be filled with silicone and the other with saline.

Presence of a patch. A Dacron patch was present on some of the earliest implants.

Presence of a fill port. Some saline implants have a large port (if intended for temporary use), others a small port (if intended for permanent use) that can be used to alter the total volume. Silicone implants do not have a port.

Gross evidence of leakage. A leaking saline implant will be completely collapsed and the surface will not be sticky. A leaking silicone implant may be intact or completely ruptured. In the latter case the specimen may consist of thick, viscous, sticky silicone gel with portions of the shell floating within it.

Source of leakage. Tacky surface, pinpoint holes, or gross tears. Give the size of any tears present.

Identifying marks. Most implants were not identified with the manufacturer's name. Some will have a name, number, or design.

Take three pictures (more if necessary) demonstrating identifying marks and gross abnormalities of permanent implants (not tissue expanders).

Soft tissue removed with the implant is carefully examined for gross evidence of foreign material. Essentially all implants release small amounts of silicone (i.e., "gel bleed"), even if leakage is not apparent grossly. Submit one to two cassettes and sample all tissue with grossly different appearances. Tumors may be difficult to detect clinically and radiologically in the presence of implants and must be diligently searched for in these specimens. Silicone granulomas can be very hard, gritty, nodular masses that closely simulate the gross appearance and texture of carcinoma.

Some older implants were covered with a polyurethane shell. This shell is textured and rapidly becomes incorporated into the surrounding fibrous capsule. The capsular material may appear shiny if this material is present.

Sample dictation

The specimen is received fresh, labeled with the patient's name and unit number, in four parts.
The first part, labeled "right implant," consists of an ovoid implant with a smooth dry surface and viscous translucent contents (9 × 9 × 4 cm). No gross ruptures, adherent tissue, or identifying marks are present. Photographs are taken.
The second part, labeled "right capsule," consists of six fragments of tan/white fibrous tissue measuring in aggregate 7 × 5 × 4 cm. Most of the fragments have a smooth surface and an opposite surface which is irregular and is comprised of yellow/tan soft tissue. The fibrous areas measure up to 0.8 cm in thickness.

Cassettes #1 and 2: four frags, RSS.

The third part, labeled "left implant, ruptured," consists of three portions of synthetic translucent material measuring 9 × 9 × 0.3 cm, 9 × 7 × 0.3 cm, and 3 × 2 × 2 cm grossly consistent with the outer shell of a breast implant. No identifying marks are present. Associated with these fragments is viscous tacky translucent material measuring approximately 9 × 9 × 4 cm. Photographs are taken.

The fourth part, labeled "left capsule," consists of approximately 15 fragments of tan/white soft tissue (in aggregate 6 × 5 × 5 cm). Two of the fragments have poorly circumscribed areas that are tan/gray, gritty in consistency, and measure 0.8 cm in greatest dimension. Some of the remainder of the fragments have a smooth surface and are grossly consistent with portions of the capsule.

Cassettes #3 and 4: gritty areas, four frags, ESS.
Cassettes #5 and 6: areas of capsule, RSS.

■ GYNECOMASTIA

The specimens are usually unilateral subcutaneous (without skin present) mastectomies. The specimen is weighed and measured. Serially section the specimen and carefully palpate for gross lesions. Two sections are submitted unless gross lesions are present. If a mastectomy is performed in a male for breast carcinoma, it is processed as for a mastectomy in a female (see previous section).

REFERENCES

1. Moritz JD, Luftner-Nagel S, Westerhof JP, Oestmann J-W, Grabbe E. Microcalcifications in breast core biopsy specimens: disappearance at radiography after storage in formaldehyde. Radiology 200:361-363, 1996.
2. www.dakocytomation.us/index/support_infocenter
3. Harvey JM, Clark GM, Osborne CK, Allred DC. Estrogen receptor status by immunohistochemistry is superior to the ligand-bound assay for predicting response to adjuvant endocrine therapy in breast cancer. J Clin Oncol 17:1474-1481, 1999.
4. Fisher B, Dignam J, Wolmark N, et al. Tamoxifen in treatment of intraductal breast cancer: National Surgical Adjuvant Breast and Bowel Project B-24 randomised controlled trial. Lancet 353:199-2000, 1999.
5. Botero M, Jacobs T, Connolly J, Schnitt S. Mod Pathol 15:29A, Abstract 109, 2002.
6. Schnitt SJ, Wang HH. Histologic sampling of grossly benign breast biopsies. How much is enough? Am J Surg Pathol 13:505-512, 1989.
7. Owings DV, Hann L, Schnitt SJ. How thoroughly should needle localization breast biopsies be sampled for microscopic examination: A prospective mammographic/pathologic correlative study. Am J Surg Pathol 14:578-583, 1990.
8. Abraham SC, Fox K, Fraker D, Solin L, Reynolds C. Sampling of grossly benign breast reexcisions. A multidisciplinary approach to assessing adequacy. Am J Surg Pathol 23:316-322, 1999.
9. Wiley EL, Keh P. Diagnostic discrepancies in breast specimens subjected to gross reexamination. Am J Surg Pathol 23:876-879, 1999.
10. Andea AA, Bouwman D, Wallis T, Visscher DW. Correlation of tumor volume and surface area with lymph node status in patients with multifocal/multicentric breast carcinoma. Cancer 100:20-27, 2004.
11. Rosen PP. Tumor emboli in intramammary lymphatics in breast carcinoma: Pathologic criteria for diagnosis and clinical significance. Pathol Annu 18(pt 2):215-232, 1983.
12. Elston E, Ellis IO. Pathological prognostic factors in breast cancer. Histopathology 19:403, 1991.
13. Elston E, Ellis IO. The Breast, Vol. 13, NY, Churchill Livingstone 1998, p 365.
14. Consensus conference on the classification of ductal carcinoma in situ, the Consensus Conference Committee. Cancer 80:1798-1802, 1997.
15. The World Health Organization. Tumours of the Breast and Female Genital Organs. WHO, Geneva, 2003.
16. Reinfuss M, Mitus J, Duda K, Stelmach A, Rys J, Smolak K. The treatment and prognosis of patients with phyllodes tumor of the breast. An analysis of 170 cases. Cancer 77:910-916, 1996.
17. Khurana KK, Loosmann A, Numann PJ, Khan SA. Prophylactic mastectomy. Pathologic findings in high-risk patients. Arch Pathol Lab Med 124:378-381, 2000.
18. Mequid MM, Oler A, Numann PJ. Subareolar breast abscess: the penultimate stage of the mammary duct-associated inflammatory disease sequence. In: Bland KI, Copeland EM III (eds): The Breast, Comprehensive Management of Benign and Malignant Diseases, 2nd edn. Saunders, Philadelphia, 1998, Chapter 6, p. 109.

Cardiovascular specimens

16

Information gained from the gross examination of some cardiac tissues (e.g., valves and hearts) is often of considerable diagnostic importance; gross findings are often more critical than microscopic features to render a specific etiologic diagnosis. For more information, see Schoen[1] and Silver et al.[2]

■ ENDOMYOCARDIAL BIOPSIES

Right, or occasionally left, heart biopsies taken by catheter are most often performed to evaluate graft status in cardiac transplant patients and less commonly to evaluate cardiomyopathies. Rarely, an endomyocardial biopsy is performed to diagnose an intracavitary or myocardial tumor.

Processing the specimen

1. Describe the specimen, including the number of fragments (carefully check the lid and sides of the container), size, and color (myocardium is tan, scar is white, clot is red to brown).

   Four tissue samples, each consisting of at least 50% myocardium, are required for adequate assessment.

2. Wrap in lens paper and submit in one cassette.

   Transplant recipients. Order three H&E sections and one unstained section. Tissue is saved for special studies (e.g., EM) only by request.

   All others. Order three H&E, one Masson's trichrome, and two unstained sections (to be available for iron or amyloid stains if needed). A piece of tissue may be submitted for EM if received in glutaraldehyde (Karnovsky fixative). A good sampling consists of four fragments for light microscopy, one fragment for EM, and an additional fragment for freezing if a metabolic disease is suspected. When evaluation for Adriamycin toxicity is the major consideration, all tissue is submitted to the EM laboratory for embedding in plastic.

Special studies

Anthracycline (Adriamycin) cardiotoxicity

Semithin (plastic) sections prepared prior to electron microscopy are necessary for the evaluation of myocyte vacuolization and myofibrillar lysis.

Amyloidosis

The diagnosis can be made on formalin-fixed tissues with Congo red or sulfated Alcian blue (SAB) stain. Sulfated Alcian blue may be preferred, as polarization is not necessary to visualize the green-staining amyloid. EM is usually unnecessary but can also confirm the presence of amyloid. Immunohistochemistry on fixed tissue can be used to subtype the amyloid (e.g., light chains in cases secondary to multiple myeloma).

Hemochromatosis and hemosiderosis

Iron deposition can be diagnosed using iron stains on fixed tissue.

Metabolic disease

Frozen tissue may be useful for the evaluation of cases of metabolic disease.

Mitochondrial myopathies

EM is necessary for evaluation.

Pathologic features sign-out checklist for endomyocardial biopsies: Non-transplant

Site
Right or left ventricle.

Adequacy
Should have at least 4 fragments of evaluable myocardium.

Myocyte hypertrophy
Present or absent, mild, moderate, or severe.

Interstitial and/or perivascular fibrosis
Present or absent, mild, moderate, or severe.

Subendocardial myocyte vacuolization
Present or absent, focal or diffuse (suggestive of chronic ischemia).

Replacement fibrosis
Present or absent (consistent with healed ischemic injury).

Myocardial infarction
Present or absent, acute or organizing.

Scattered necrotic myocytes and inflammation
Present or absent (consistent with catecholamine effect).

Endocardial thickening
Present or absent, focal or diffuse.

Active myocarditis
Present or absent, focal lymphocytic, diffuse lymphocytic, toxoplasma, CMV, granulomatous.

Mesothelial cells
Present or absent, indicates cardiac perforation.

Other
Amyloid, iron deposition, arrhythmogenic right ventricular dysplasia, carcinoid plaque, anthracycline cardiotoxicity.
Old biopsy site, contraction bands, thrombus.

Pathologic features sign-out checklist for endomyocardial biopsies: Transplant

Site
Right ventricle or left ventricle.

Adequacy
At least 4 fragments of evaluable myocardium should be present.

Time since transplantation
Interval since operation.

Rejection
Give ISHLT grade (Table 16-1).

Coagulation necrosis
Present or absent, focal, multifocal, confluent.

Healing ischemic injury
Present or absent, focal, multifocal, confluent.

Subendocardial myocyte vacuolization
Present or absent, mild, moderate, or severe (suggestive of chronic ischemia).

Endocardial infiltrate
Quilty A or Quilty B.

Mesothelial cells
Present or absent, indicates cardiac perforation.

Other
Old biopsy site, fat necrosis, foreign body giant cell reaction, dystrophic calcification.

Sample sign-out: Right ventricular endomyocardial biopsy

Six months S/P cardiac transplantation.
No evidence of rejection; ISHLT grade 0.
Old biopsy site.
Four fragments of diagnostic myocardium.

Sample sign-out: Right ventricular endomyocardial biopsy

Four weeks S/P cardiac transplantation.
Multifocal interstitial infiltrate with associated myocyte damage (ISHLT grade 3A).
Focal healing ischemic injury.
Four fragments of diagnostic myocardium.
One fragment of blood clot.

Sample sign-out: Right ventricular endomyocardial biopsy

Clinical: Idiopathic dilated cardiomyopathy.
Diffuse moderate and focally bizarre hypertrophy.
Cellular degenerative changes, including moderate lipofuscin deposition.
Mild interstitial and endocardial fibrosis; focal replacement fibrosis.
Diffuse subendocardial myocyte vacuolization.
No evidence of amyloid or iron (Congo red and iron stains examined).
No evidence of active myocarditis or acute or recent myocardial infarction.
Four fragments of diagnostic myocardium.

Note: These findings are entirely nonspecific and could result from right-sided changes secondary to left-sided heart disease of numerous etiologies (e.g., ischemic heart disease, valvular heart disease), a global cardiac process such as idiopathic dilated cardiomyopathy, or right-sided changes secondary to primary pulmonary disease.

Table 16-1 International Society for Heart and Lung Transplantation (ISHLT) grading of cardiac rejection[3]

LEVEL	DIAGNOSIS
0	No rejection
IA	Focal (perivascular or interstitial) infiltrate without myocyte damage
IB	Diffuse but sparse infiltrate without myocyte damage
2	One focus only with aggressive infiltrate and/or focal myocyte damage
3A	Multifocal aggressive infiltrates and/or myocyte damage
3B	Diffuse inflammatory process with myocyte damage
4	Diffuse aggressive polymorphous infiltrate ± edema, ± hemorrhage, ± vasculitis

"Resolving" rejection is denoted by a lesser grade.
"Resolved" rejection is denoted by grade 0.

■ CARDIAC VALVES

Critical information about removed valves is obtained from the gross examination and dissection of the specimens. Although all specimens (excluding mechanical valves) are sectioned, histologic study is particularly valuable to address specific questions such as endocarditis. All prosthetic valves, intact native valves, and any unusual lesions (vegetations, endocardial fibroelastomas) should be photographed, as close up as possible. Both acute and underlying chronic lesions should be documented.[4]

Native mitral and aortic valves

Native aortic valves are generally replaced because of calcific degeneration (valves with either two or three cusps). Mitral valves are replaced because of rheumatic valve disease or because the valve is myxomatous. In most cases, the most important diagnostic information is derived from the gross examination of the specimen (Figs 16-1, 16-2, 16-3, Tables 16-2, 16-3).

Specimen examination, dictation, and processing

1. Examine the specimen grossly and determine the type of valve (aortic or mitral).

   Leaflets or cusps. Assess the number of recognizable leaflets (atrioventricular valves) or cusps (semilunar valves), size, consistency (thickened, fibrotic, calcified, thinned, redundant [ballooned], perforated), and additional fragments. If an abnormality is present, describe the distribution (focal or diffuse), surface (atrial or ventricular or both), and location (free edge or base).

   Commissures. Describe their relationship to each other (completely fused, partially fused).

   Chordae tendineae (tendinous cords). Determine their length (shortened, elongated) and status (intact, thickened, ruptured, fused). Mitral valves have cords; aortic valves do not.

   Papillary muscles. Record dimensions and abnormalities (hypertrophied, elongated, scarred).

   Vegetations. Assess color, size, location, consistency (firm or friable), and destruction of underlying tissue.

   Endocarditis is a life-threatening disease, and any indication that acute endocarditis is present should immediately be brought to the attention of the clinician. Order Gram stain and MSS if a diagnosis of endocarditis seems possible, either from clinical information or after gross or histologic examination.

2. Submit one cassette with representative sections taken from the free edge to the anulus. It may be necessary to decalcify some specimens.

Gross differential diagnosis (Fig. 16-1)

Degenerative calcific aortic valve stenosis. Calcific deposits are present within the cusps, primarily at the base. The free cuspal edges are usually not involved. The cusps may be heavily fibrosed and thickened but are not fused. Congenital bicuspid valves are predisposed to degenerative calcification. Usually one of the cusps is larger with a midline raphe resulting from the incomplete separation of two cusps. Less frequently the cusps may be of equal size. The raphe is often the site of extensive calcification.

Mitral annular calcification. Calcifications occur in the annulus of the mitral valve. The chordae are uninvolved.

Myxomatous degeneration of the mitral valve. The leaflet is enlarged and redundant. The cords may be elongated and thinned and sometimes rupture.

Aortic postinflammatory scarring (rheumatic type). The cusps are fused. There is diffuse thickening, and calcification is rather evenly distributed and includes the free cuspal edges. The mitral valve is virtually always involved as well.

Mitral postinflammatory scarring (rheumatic type). The leaflets are thickened and there is commissural fusion and shortening. The cords are thickened and fused. Calcification is often present.

Endocarditis. Large friable vegetations are found on the valves in acute bacterial endocarditis and may be single or multiple. They may extend onto the chordae. There is often perforation or erosion of the underlying valve. The vegetations of nonbacterial thrombotic endocarditis (NBTE) are small and bland and are attached at the line of closure. Systemic lupus may be associated with small bland vegetations that may be located on both surfaces of the valve or on the cords (Libman–Sacks endocarditis).

Sample dictation for calcific degeneration of the aortic valve

The specimen, received fresh, labeled with the patient's name, unit number, and "aortic valve" consists of three semilunar valve cusps, measuring 2.5, 2.6, and 2.3 cm along the free edges and 1.0 cm from free edge to base. The outflow surfaces of all three cusps contain numerous irregular yellow/tan calcific deposits up to 1.0 cm. There is no evidence of commissural fusion. No vegetations are present. The specimen is fixed and decalcified prior to processing.

Cassette #1: Aortic valve cusp, 3 frags, RSS.

Sample dictation for myxomatous degeneration of the mitral valve (posterior leaflet)

The specimen, received fresh, labeled with the patient's name, unit number, and "mitral valve leaflet," consists of an atrioventricular valve leaflet measuring 4.0 cm along the free edge and 1.4 cm from free edge to base. There is diffuse myxomatous thickening of the leaflet, which appears billowing and redundant. The chordae are thin and elongated and there is rupture of one chorda.

Cassette #1: Mitral valve leaflet, 3 frags, RSS.

Sample dictation for rheumatic mitral valve (anterior leaflet)

The specimen, received fresh, labeled with the patient's name, unit number, and "mitral valve leaflet," consists of an atrioventricular valve leaflet measuring 3.5 cm along the free edge and 1.5 cm from free edge to base. The leaflet is diffusely thickened to 0.4 cm and fibrotic. The surface of the leaflet is white/tan and smooth without vegetations or perforations. Focal calcific deposits are located toward the annulus. The attached chordae are thickened, measuring up to 1.8 cm in length and 0.2 cm in thickness, and are focally fused.

Cassette #1: Mitral valve leaflet, 3 frags, RSS.

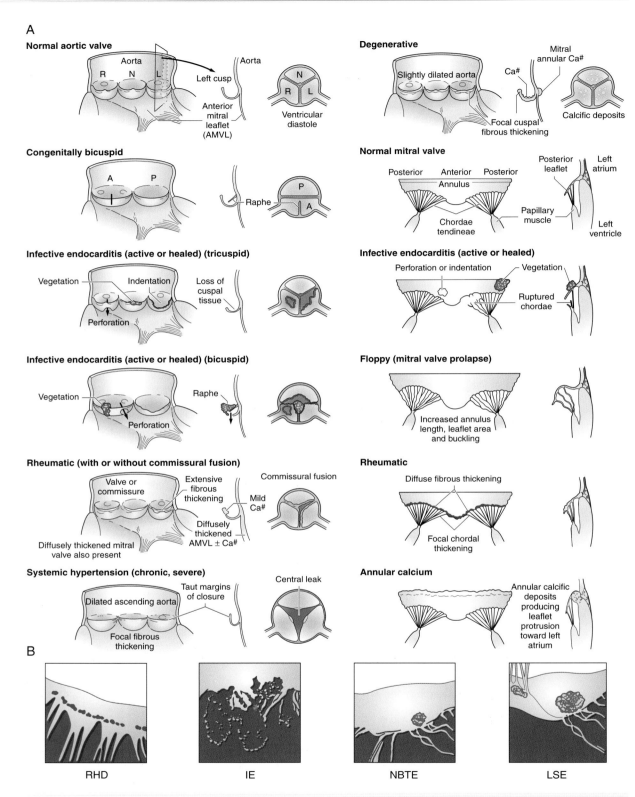

Figure 16-1 A, B Evaluation of operatively excised cardiac valves: etiologic determination of valvular heart disease. RHD, rheumatic heart disease; IE, infective endocarditis; NBTE, nonbacterial thrombotic endocarditis; LSE, Libman–Sacks endocarditis. (**A,** Modified from Waller BF et al. Cardiol Clin 2:687, 1984; **B,** modified from Schoen FJ. The heart. In Cotran RS, Kumar V, Robbins SL (eds): Robbins Pathologic Basis of Disease, 5th edn. Philadelphia, W.B. Saunders, 1994, p. 554.)

Pathologic features sign-out checklist for native valves

Type of valve
Aortic, congenital bicuspid aortic valve, mitral, tricuspid.

Disease process
Calcific degeneration; myxomatous degeneration; postinflammatory scarring, rheumatic type; endocarditis.

Papillary muscle
Infarcted or scarred.

Vegetations
Present or absent, type.

Sample sign-outs

Aortic valve

Calcific degeneration of bicuspid aortic valve.

Aortic valve

ENDOCARDITIS, ACTIVE, ON BICUSPID AORTIC VALVE.
Valve with extensive necrosis, acute inflammation, and neovascularization.
Gram-positive cocci identified.
Congenital bicuspid aortic valve. (Fig. 16-2)

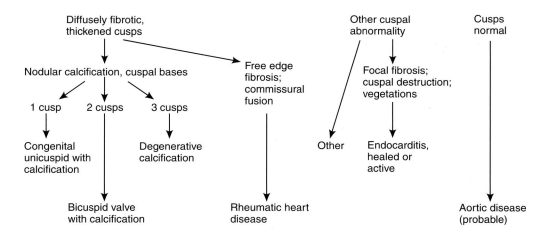

Figure 16-2 Overview of major diagnostic considerations in aortic valve disease. (From Schoen FJ. Evaluation of surgically removed natural and prosthetic heart valves. In Virmani R, Fenoglio JJ (eds): Cardiovascular Pathology. Philadelphia, W.B. Saunders, 1991, p. 404).

Table 16-2 Etiologic assessment of valvular heart disease[4]

	SENILE DEGENERATION	MYXOMATOUS DEGENERATION	RHEUMATIC	INFECTIVE	SECONDARY
Gross features					
Leaflet/cuspal thickening	0	0/+	+	0	0
Calcification	+	0	0/+	0	0
Commissural/chordal fusion	0	0	+	0	0
Leaflet/cuspal redundancy	0	+	0	0	0
Leaflet/cuspal defects	0	0	0	+	0
Chordal rupture	0	0/+	0	0	0
Histologic features		*			
Preservation of layered architecture	+	+	0	0/+	+
GAG accumulation in spongiosa	0	+	0	0	0/+
Thinned fibrosa	0	+	0	0	0
Neovascularization	0	0	0/+	0/+	0
Superficial fibrosis only	0/+	0/+	0	0/+	0/+

Table 16-3 Gross morphologic assessment of abnormal cardiac valvular function[4]

PATHOLOGIC FEATURE	STENOTIC VALVE	PURELY REGURGITANT VALVE
For all valves		
Valve weight	Increased	Normal or slightly increased or decreased
Fibrous thickening	Diffuse	Diffuse, focal, or none
Calcific deposits	Heavy	Minimal (if any)
Tissue loss (perforation, indentation)	None	May be present
Vegetations	Minimal	May be present
Commissural fusion	May be present	Minimal (if any)
Annular circumference	Normal	Normal or increased
For aortic valves		
Number of cusps	1, 2, or 3	2 or 3
For mitral (or tricuspid) valves		
Abnormal papillary muscles	No	May be present
Chordae tendineae fusion	Usually present	Absent
Elongation	Absent	May be present
Shortening	Usually present	May be present
Rupture	Absent	May be present

Mitral valve

Diffuse leaflet thickening, commissural fusion, and chordae fibrosis; transmural fibrosis and neovascularization, consistent with postinflammatory scarring, rheumatic type. (Fig. 16-3)

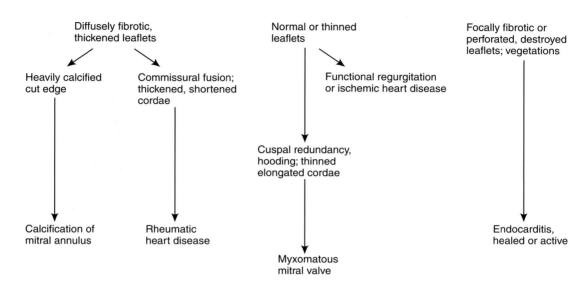

MITRAL VALVE DISEASE

Figure 16-3 Overview of major diagnostic considerations in mitral valve disease. (From Schoen FJ. Evaluation of surgically removed natural and prosthetic heart valves. In Virmani R, Fenoglio JJ (eds): Cardiovascular Pathology. Philadelphia, W.B. Saunders, 1991, p. 404).

Prosthetic valves

The gross examination of the valve can identify the type of valve and any defects present (Figs 16-4, 16-5, 16-6, 16-7, Table 16-4). For good references on the examination of valves, see references 5 and 6.

Processing the specimen

1. Identify the type of prosthesis using Figures 16-4 to 16-7. Measure the external diameter of the outside sewing ring. The type of valve is included in the diagnosis. Commonly used valves are either Hancock or Carpentier–Edwards porcine bioprostheses, St. Jude bileaflet (all carbon), or Björk–Shiley tilting disk (carbon disk with a metal frame) valves.
2. Describe any tissue overgrowth of the sewing ring.
3. For mechanical valves, also describe any asymmetry, notches, or cracks of any of the components. Describe any impairment in motion of the components.
4. For tissue valves, describe any tears or perforations of the cusps and/or any impairment of cusp motion.
5. Describe any tissue overgrowth, vegetations including color, site (surface of valve, sewing ring), size, consistency (firm or friable), and destruction to underlying material.
6. Describe any calcific deposits and their location. Calcification will be graded on a scale from 0 to 4 using the specimen radiograph.
7. Photograph all valves. Radiograph all tissue valves. Mechanical valves do not require radiographs. The developed radiograph is kept with the slides for sign-out.
8. Submit a portion of bioprosthetic valve cusps for histologic examination. Submit tissue on the sewing ring adjacent to all valve prostheses. In cases of suspected endocarditis, Gram and fungal (methenamine silver) stains are ordered in advance.

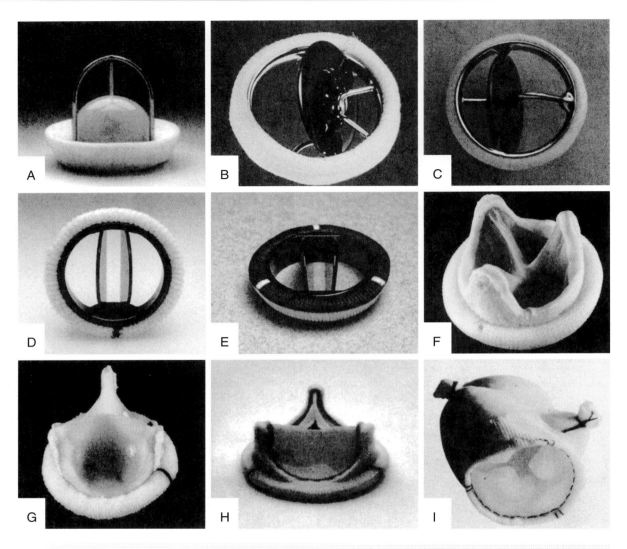

Figure 16-4 Representative prosthetic heart valves: **A,** Starr–Edwards caged ball valve; **B,** Björk–Shiley tilting disk valve; **C,** Medtronic-Hall tilting disk valve; **D,** St. Jude Medical tilting disk valve; **E,** CarboMedics (CPHV) bileaflet tilting disk valve; **F,** Hancock porcine aortic valve bioprosthesis; **G,** Ionescu–Shiley bovine pericardial bioprosthesis; **H,** Carpentier–Edwards bovine pericardial bioprosthesis; **I,** Medtronic Freestyle stentless porcine aortic valve bioprosthesis.

Sample dictation for mechanical valves

The specimen received fresh, labeled with the patient's name, unit number, and "aortic valve," consists of a St. Jude bileaflet tilting-disk prosthesis with an external sewing ring diameter of 21 mm. The prosthesis is intact. There is focal tissue overgrowth of the sewing ring. The leaflets move freely and open and close completely. No thrombi or vegetations are present. Also present in the same container are multiple detached fragments of tan soft tissue measuring in aggregate 3.0 × 2.5 cm. The specimen is photographed.

Cassette #1: Tissue from sewing ring and detached tissue fragments, mult frags, ESS.

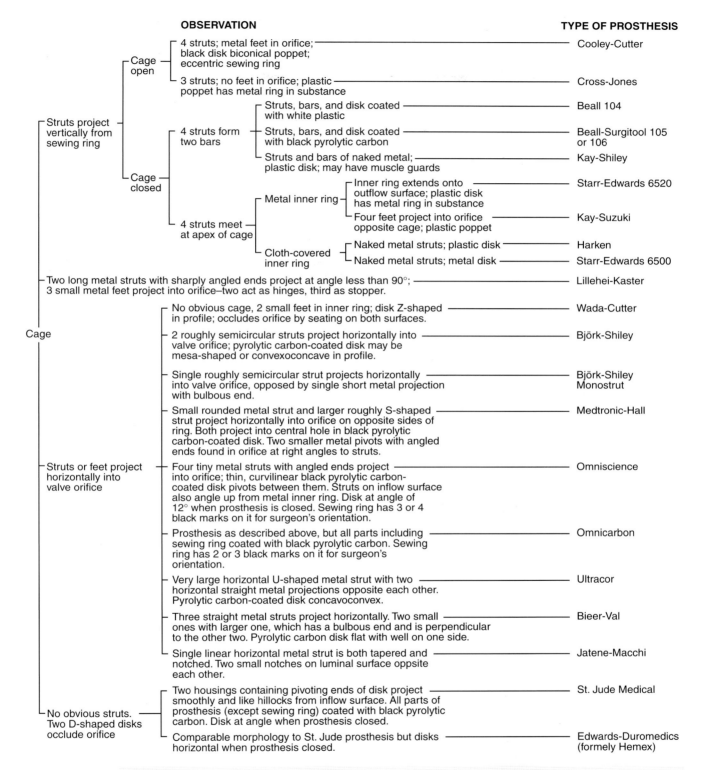

OBSERVATION   **TYPE OF PROSESIS**

Cage

Struts project vertically from sewing ring

Cage open
- 4 struts; metal feet in orifice; black disk biconical poppet; eccentric sewing ring —— Cooley-Cutter
- 3 struts; no feet in orifice; plastic poppet has metal ring in substance —— Cross-Jones

Cage closed

4 struts form two bars
- Struts, bars, and disk coated with white plastic —— Beall 104
- Struts, bars, and disk coated with black pyrolytic carbon —— Beall-Surgitool 105 or 106
- Struts and bars of naked metal; plastic disk; may have muscle guards —— Kay-Shiley

4 struts meet at apex of cage

Metal inner ring
- Inner ring extends onto outflow surface; plastic disk has metal ring in substance —— Starr-Edwards 6520
- Four feet project into orifice opposite cage; plastic poppet —— Kay-Suzuki

Cloth-covered inner ring
- Naked metal struts; plastic disk —— Harken
- Naked metal struts; metal disk —— Starr-Edwards 6500

Two long metal struts with sharply angled ends project at angle less than 90°; 3 small metal feet project into orifice–two act as hinges, third as stopper. —— Lillehei-Kaster

Struts or feet project horizontally into valve orifice
- No obvious cage, 2 small feet in inner ring; disk Z-shaped in profile; occludes orifice by seating on both surfaces. —— Wada-Cutter
- 2 roughly semicircular struts project horizontally into valve orifice; pyrolytic carbon-coated disk may be mesa-shaped or convexoconcave in profile. —— Björk-Shiley
- Single roughly semicircular strut projects horizontally into valve orifice, opposed by single short metal projection with bulbous end. —— Björk-Shiley Monostrut
- Small rounded metal strut and larger roughly S-shaped strut project horizontally into orifice on opposite sides of ring. Both project into central hole in black pyrolytic carbon-coated disk. Two smaller metal pivots with angled ends found in orifice at right angles to struts. —— Medtronic-Hall
- Four tiny metal struts with angled ends project into orifice; thin, curvilinear black pyrolytic carbon-coated disk pivots between them. Struts on inflow surface also angle up from metal inner ring. Disk at angle of 12° when prosthesis is closed. Sewing ring has 3 or 4 black marks on it for surgeon's orientation. —— Omniscience
- Prosthesis as described above, but all parts including sewing ring coated with black pyrolytic carbon. Sewing ring has 2 or 3 black marks on it for surgeon's orientation. —— Omnicarbon
- Very large horizontal U-shaped metal strut with two horizontal straight metal projections opposite each other. Pyrolytic carbon-coated disk concavoconvex. —— Ultracor
- Three straight metal struts project horizontally. Two small ones with larger one, which has a bulbous end and is perpendicular to the other two. Pyrolytic carbon disk flat with well on one side. —— Bieer-Val
- Single linear horizontal metal strut is both tapered and notched. Two small notches on luminal surface oppsite each other. —— Jatene-Macchi

No obvious struts. Two D-shaped disks occlude orifice
- Two housings containing pivoting ends of disk project smoothly and like hillocks from inflow surface. All parts of prosthesis (except sewing ring) coated with black pyrolytic carbon. Disk at angle when prosthesis closed. —— St. Jude Medical
- Comparable morphology to St. Jude prosthesis but disks horizontal when prosthesis closed. —— Edwards-Duromedics (formely Hemex)

Figure 16-5 Key for identifying caged-disk and tilting prostheses. (Modified from Silver MD, Wilson JG. Pathology of cardiovascular prostheses including coronary artery bypass and other vascular grafts. In Silver MD, ed: Cardiovascular Pathology. New York, Churchill Livingstone, 1991.)

CAGED-BALL PROSTHESIS

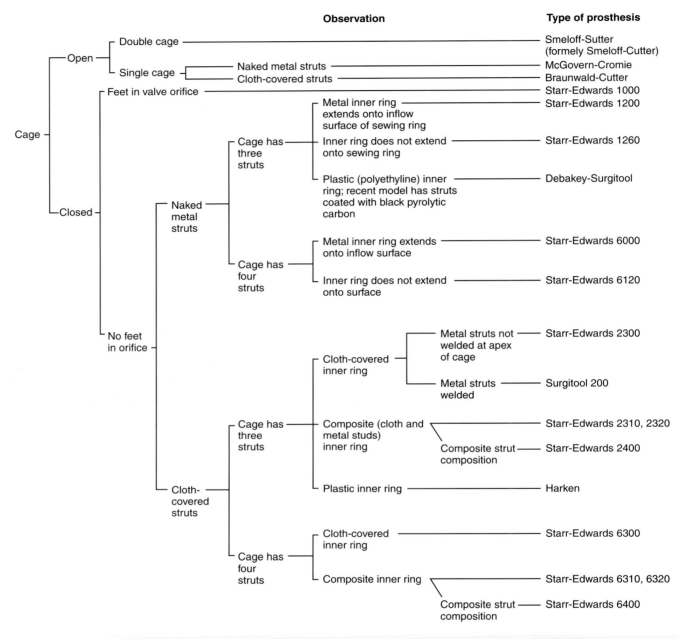

Figure 16-6 Key for identifying caged-ball prostheses. (Modified from Silver MD, Wilson JG. Pathology of cardiovascular prostheses including coronary artery bypass and other vascular grafts. In Silver MD, ed: Cardiovascular Pathology. New York, Churchill Livingstone, 1991.)

BIOPROSTHESES

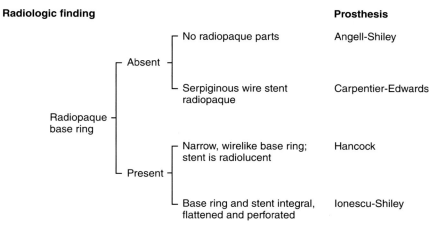

Figure 16-7 Key for identifying bioprostheses. (Modified from Silver MD, Wilson JG. Pathology of cardiovascular prostheses including coronary artery bypass and other vascular grafts. In Silver MD, ed: Cardiovascular Pathology. New York, Churchill Livingstone, 1991.)

Sample dictation for bioprosthetic valves

The specimen received fresh, labeled with the patient's name, unit number, and "mitral valve," consists of a bioprosthetic valve with an external sewing ring diameter of 31 mm. The valve cusps are moderately stiffened and there is focal commissural calcification. One of the cusps contains a single 0.4 cm linear tear near the commissure involving the cuspal free edge. The remaining cusps are intact. No thrombi or vegetations are present. Also present in the same container are six detached irregular fragments of tan–yellow soft tissue, measuring in aggregate 2.0 × 1.5 cm. The specimen is photographed and radiographed.

Cassette #1: Valve cusp and detached fragments, mult frags, RSS.

Pathologic features sign-out checklist for prosthetic valves

Site
Aortic or mitral.

Type of valve
Use Figures 16-4 to 16-7 to identify the type of valve.

Calcifications
Grade 1+ to 4+ using specimen radiograph.

Cuspal tears
Present or absent, size.

Mechanical degeneration
Type, location.

Tissue degeneration
Present or absent.

Tissue overgrowth
Focal or extensive.

Overhanging suture
Present or absent.

Endocarditis
Present or absent.

Vegetations
Present or absent.

Cuspal perforation
Present or absent.

Sample sign-out: Bioprosthetic mitral valve

Hancock porcine mitral valve bioprosthesis.
Calcification (2+/4+ by radiograph).
Cuspal tear near commissure, 4 mm long, involving cuspal free edge.
Microscopic severe degeneration and mineralization.
There is no evidence of endocarditis.

■ HEART TRANSPLANTS

Patients receiving heart transplants usually are in end-stage cardiac failure due to ischemic heart disease or idiopathic cardiomyopathy. The specimen usually consists of both ventricles and atria amputated above the ventricles. Occasionally small portions of the donor heart (e.g., auricular appendages) will also be received.

Processing the specimen

1. Weigh the specimen. Normal weights for the entire heart are 270 to 360 g for males and 250 to 280 g for females.
2. Describe the epicardial surface, including pericardial fat (abundant or scant), petechiae, and adhesions.
3. In general, hearts are cut after fixation in a manner dictated by the pathology to be demonstrated (Fig. 16-8).

Table 16-4 Pathologic analysis of bioprosthetic valves

GROSS EXAMINATION	HISTOLOGY	RADIOGRAPHY
Thrombi	Vegetations and organisms	Valve type identification
Vegetations	Thrombi	Calcification
Paravalvular leak	Host cell interactions	Degree
Tissue overgrowth	Endothelialization	Localization
Cuspal stiffness	Pannus overgrowth	Ring or stent fracture
Cuspal hematomas	Degeneration	
Calcification	Calcification	
Cuspal fenestrations and tears	Degree	
Cuspal abrasions	Morphology	
Cuspal stretching	Location	
Strut relationships		
Extrinsic interference or damage		
Tissue separation from strut		

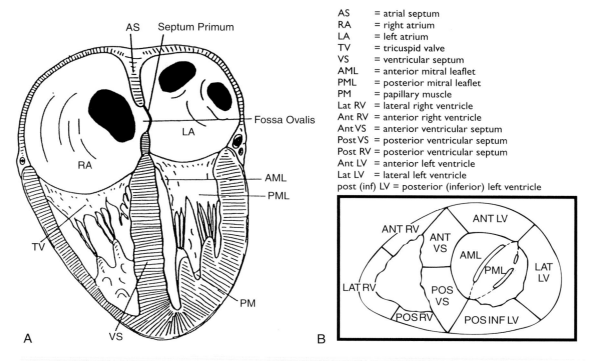

AS = atrial septum
RA = right atrium
LA = left atrium
TV = tricuspid valve
VS = ventricular septum
AML = anterior mitral leaflet
PML = posterior mitral leaflet
PM = papillary muscle
Lat RV = lateral right ventricle
Ant RV = anterior right ventricle
Ant VS = anterior ventricular septum
Post VS = posterior ventricular septum
Post RV = posterior ventricular septum
Ant LV = anterior left ventricle
Lat LV = lateral left ventricle
post (inf) LV = posterior (inferior) left ventricle

Figure 16-8 Cardiac anatomy: **A,** longitudinal cut; **B,** transverse cut. (**A,** From Virmani R, Ursell PC, Fenoglio JJ. Examination of the heart. In Virmani R, Atkinson JB, Fenoglio JJ (eds): Cardiovascular Pathology. Philadelphia, W.B. Saunders, 1991, p. 9.)

Hearts with dilated cardiomyopathy are cut longitudinally from apex to base, bivalving both ventricles and bisecting tricuspid and mitral valves ("apical 4-chamber" cut).

Hearts with ischemic heart disease are cut similarly or, more often, transversely at approximately 1- to 2-cm intervals beginning at the apex to the level of the mitral valve ("serially sectioned"). The base of the heart may be cut longitudinally or opened according to the lines of flow.

4. Describe each ventricle separately, including hypertrophy or dilatation, fibrosis (endocardial, epicardial, transmural, location and degree), infarcts (old or recent, size, location, transmural or subendocardial), trabeculation, papillary muscles (hypertrophied, thinned, scarred, infarcted), and presence of mural thrombus. Measure the wall thickness of both ventricles. The normal thickness of the left ventricle is 0.9 to 1.5 cm and that of the right ventricle 0.25 to 0.3 cm. Figure 16-8 may facilitate documentation of findings.

5. Describe the atria if there are any endocardial lesions.

6. Describe any valve lesions as in "Cardiac valves" (native or prosthetic).

7. Atherosclerotic coronary arteries are dissected from the heart, fixed and decalcified, and sectioned transversely at 3- to 5-mm intervals. Soft, unobstructed coronary arteries may be carefully cut in transverse sections on the fixed heart at 3-mm intervals. Describe the arteries including dominance (right or left), percentage of luminal compromise, location, recent thrombi or plaque hemorrhage, and the locations of these lesions.

8. Describe any bypass grafts including type (saphenous vein, left internal mammary), location of graft to native vessel, and patency. Remove the junction of the graft and native vessel as a block of tissue from the epicardial surface. Serially section perpendicular to the vessels to look for luminal obstructions.

9. Submit sections according to "Microscopic sections".

Microscopic sections

Left ventricular free wall
Two sections (apex and base) in one cassette. Order a Masson's trichrome on a representative section of myocardium.

Right ventricular free wall
Two sections (apex and base) in one cassette.

Septum
Two sections (apex and base) in one cassette.

Native coronary arteries
Up to four cassettes if abnormalities are present in the left main (LMA), left anterior descending (LAD), left circumflex (LCX), and right coronary artery (RCA) including areas of obstruction.

Bypass grafts
One cassette of each graft.

Other lesions
Representative sections.

Gross differential diagnosis

Ischemic heart disease. By the time a patient comes to cardiac transplantation, extensive damage is usually present. There may be fibrous scars and pericardial adhesions due to previous healed infarcts. Aneurysms may be present. The vessels usually demonstrate extensive atherosclerosis, and bypass grafts are often present.

Idiopathic dilated cardiomyopathy. The heart is usually enlarged (two to three times the normal weight) and all four chambers are enlarged. The ventricular wall thickness can be thin, thick, or normal, depending on the balance of hypertrophy and dilatation. There may be small patchy subendocardial fibrous scars in the left ventricle. Endocardial plaques may be present. Mural thrombi are commonly found near the apex of the ventricles. The valves and coronary arteries are generally normal.

Sample dictation for idiopathic dilated cardiomyopathy

The specimen, received fresh, labeled with the patient's name and unit number, consists of a heart weighing 650 g. The atria have been severed approximately 3 cm above the ventricles. The epicardial surface is smooth and glistening without adhesions. The major epicardial coronary arteries arise in their usual configuration in a right dominant system and show no gross atherosclerosis. Sectioning the heart longitudinally reveals severe biventricular dilatation and hypertrophy. There is patchy fibrous thickening of the endocardium. No mural thrombi are present. The valves are grossly of normal configuration. The left ventricular myocardium is 1.3 cm in thickness; the right ventricular myocardium is 0.3 cm in thickness. There is no evidence of myocardial discoloration or necrosis.

Cassette #1: Left ventricle, base and apex, 2 frags, 1 cass.
Cassette #2: Interventricular septum, base and apex, 2 frags, RSS.
Cassette #3: Right ventricle, base and apex, 2 frags, RSS.

Sample dictation for atherosclerotic coronary artery and ischemic heart disease with bypass grafts

The specimen received fresh, labeled with the patient's name, unit number, and "heart," consists of a heart weighing 485 g. The atria have been severed approximately 3 cm above the ventricles. The epicardial surface contains dense fibrous adhesions, which are most extensive over the base of the heart. Within these adhesions, segments of bypass grafts inserting into the left anterior descending, circumflex, and right coronary arteries are identified. The graft to the left anterior descending artery is totally occluded by thrombus. The graft to the circumflex has a circumferentially thickened wall but remains patent. The graft to the right coronary artery is widely patent. Examination of the native epicardial coronary arteries reveals a right dominant system with severe, diffuse atherosclerosis. The left main coronary artery is approximately 50% occluded by atheromatous plaque. The left anterior descending coronary artery is 100% occluded by atheromatous plaque. The left circumflex and right coronary arteries are each approximately 70% occluded by atheromatous plaque. There are no acute plaque changes. Sectioning the heart transversely reveals biventricular dilatation with aneurysmal dilatation to 4 cm of the anterior left ventricle at the apex. The anterior left ventricular myocardium is replaced by dense white transmural fibrous scarring and measures 0.3 cm in thickness. The lateral, posterior, and septal walls contain focal areas of fibrous scarring up to 1 cm. The endocardium of the anterior wall is thickened, measuring 0.2 cm. No mural thrombus is present. The right ventricular myocardium measures 0.3 cm and shows no evidence of scarring or necrosis. The valves are grossly of normal configuration. The coronary arteries are removed from the specimen and decalcified prior to processing.

Cassette #1: Left ventricle anterior, 1 frag, RSS.
Cassette #2: Left ventricle lateral, 1 frag, RSS.
Cassette #3: Left ventricle posterior, 1 frag, RSS.
Cassette #4: Interventricular septum, 1 frag, RSS.
Cassette #5: Right ventricle, 2 frags, RSS.
Cassette #6: Left main coronary artery, 3 frags, RSS.
Cassette #7: Left anterior descending coronary artery, 3 frags, RSS.
Cassette #8: Left circumflex coronary artery, 3 frags, RSS.
Cassette #9: Right coronary artery, 3 frags, RSS.
Cassette #10: Bypass graft to left anterior descending, 3 frags, RSS.
Cassette #11: Bypass graft to left circumflex, 3 frags, RSS.
Cassette #12: Bypass graft to right coronary artery, 3 frags, RSS.

Pathologic features sign-out checklist for hearts

Size
Weight in grams.

Hypertrophy
Present or absent, degree (mild, moderate, or severe), gross or microscopic.

Dilatation
Present or absent, degree (mild, moderate, or severe).

Asymmetric septal hypertrophy
Present or absent.

Atrial septal defect
Present or absent, size.

Ventricular septal defect
Present or absent, size.

Foramen ovale
Describe if patent.

Previous surgical sites
If present, describe (e.g., stents present).

Myocardial infarcts
Acute, remote, location, size, extent (transmural).

Aneurysm
Location, size.

Mural thrombus
Location, size.

Subendocardial myocyte vacuolization
Focal or diffuse (suggestive of chronic ischemia).

Replacement fibrosis
Focal or diffuse.

Myofiber disarray
Present or absent in septum.

Endocardial fibrosis
Present or absent, degree (focal, multifocal, diffuse).

Endocarditis
Present or absent.

Pericardium
Fibrous or fibrinous pericarditis.

Coronary arteries
Atherosclerosis, location, degree (percent occlusion), thrombosis, acute plaque change.

Bypass grafts
Present or absent, location, intimal hyperplasia (percent luminal narrowing).

Valves
Report as for native or prosthetic valves as appropriate.

Devices
Pacemaker wire, defibrillator patches, ventricular assist device.

Sample sign-out: Heart (510 g)

IDIOPATHIC DILATED CARDIOMYOPATHY
Biventricular hypertrophy and dilatation, moderate.
Microscopic generalized hypertrophy, focally bizarre.
Mild to moderate interstitial and perivascular fibrosis with focal replacement fibrosis.
Multifocal fibrous endocardial thickening.
Coronary arteries with chronic, focal 60% narrowing of mid right coronary artery; otherwise no obstruction greater than 40%.

No evidence of active myocarditis, acute infarction, or primary valvular disease.

Sample sign-out: Heart (450 g)

ATHEROSCLEROTIC CORONARY ARTERY AND ISCHEMIC HEART DISEASE
Large, remote, myocardial infarct involving anterior, anterolateral, and septal myocardium, transmural, with aneurysm (3 × 2 cm).
Small apical mural thrombus, unorganized, bland.
Biventricular hypertrophy and dilatation with microscopic global myocyte hypertrophy in noninfarcted regions. Mild perivascular and interstitial fibrosis.
Severe transmural replacement fibrosis involving infarcted areas.

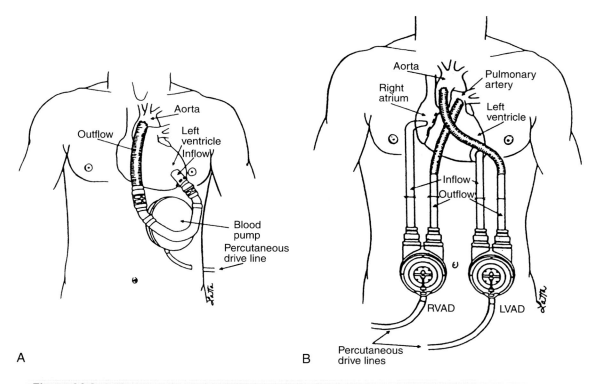

Figure 16-9 A, The HeartMate implantable pneumatic left ventricular assist system. **B,** The Thoratec ventricular assist system in the biventricular support configuration. RVAD, right ventricular assist device; LVAD, left ventricular assist device. (**A, B** From Hunt SA, Frazier OH. Mechanical circulatory support and cardiac transplantation. Circulation 97:2079-2090, 1998.)

Diffuse subendocardial myocyte vacuolization suggestive of severe chronic ischemia.
Coronary artery occlusions:

Left anterior descending coronary, with 95% chronic occlusion.
Right coronary artery with 100% occlusion by chronic atherosclerosis, with acute plaque change and completely occlusive recent coronary thrombosis.
No evidence of myocarditis, primary valvular disease, or acute infarction.
Mitral annuloplasty ring, intact.
Right ventricular transvenous pacemaker wire near apex, well healed.

■ VENTRICULAR ASSIST DEVICES

Ventricular assist devices (VAD; Fig. 16-9) may be used to provide mechanical support as a bridge to transplantation and are sometimes received with an explanted heart. Either the entire device or parts of the device attached to the heart may be received.

VAD can totally replace ventricular function for extended periods and may be inserted into the left ventricle (LVAD), right ventricle (RVAD), or both ventricles (BiVAD). The device is connected from the atrium or ventricle to the pump via the inflow (inflow to the pump) cannula and from the pump to the aorta or pulmonary artery via the outflow (outflow from the pump) cannula. Prosthetic valves are present within the metal connectors of both cannulae.

For additional information, including a more detailed discussion of pathologic analysis and device complications, see references 7 to 9.

■ ATRIAL OR VENTRICULAR MYOCARDIUM

Portions of the heart may be removed during open-heart surgery (e.g., repair of ventricular aneurysms, hypertrophic cardiomyopathy septal resection, or removal of atrial myxomas). An apical core may be removed during insertion of a cardiac assist device. Describe the specimen including size, variations in the thickness of the wall, presence of scarring (transmural or not), necrotic tissue, calcification, or mural thrombus (organized or unorganized), hemorrhage, color and thickness of epicardium, and color and thickness of endocardium.

Two to three sections in one cassette are usually sufficient. For hypertrophic cardiomyopathy, submit two to three cassettes and order Masson's trichrome and H&E stains. For atrial myxomas, submit two to three cassettes.

Sample sign-out: Ventricular aneurysm

Transmural replacement fibrosis, with entrapped residual viable hypertrophied myocytes and subendocardial myocyte vacuolization; focal healing myocyte necrosis, 2 to 3 weeks in duration, with central mummification; complicated by calcification in fibrous tissue; and mural thrombus, bland, organizing, of at least 3 weeks' duration.

■ BLOOD VESSELS

Typical specimens include endarterectomies of the carotid bifurcation, abdominal aortic aneurysm repairs, revision of vascular grafts, and varicose veins. Temporal artery biopsies are performed for the diagnosis of arteritis.

Aorta (with or without dissection)

An aortic dissection results in a medial hematoma that usually has an associated intimal flap entrance site and often has either an intimal reentrant site or an adventitial rupture site. These specimens may be labeled "ascending aortic aneurysm" or "thoracic aortic aneurysm." Specimens taken during aortic aneurysm repair consist of the inner media only or both inner and outer media. Increasingly, fragments of aorta from aortic valve replacements or from bypass cannula sites are also submitted and may be of diagnostic importance.

In cases of dissections, sections are taken from areas of medial separation. Representative sections (three to four in one cassette) are also taken of grossly normal tissue. It is important to characterize the location of any dissection, its age, medial flaps, the presence of prior dissection, and underlying vessel wall pathology as the etiology of the dissection. Request that the histology laboratory carefully orientate the specimens on edge, to ensure that the entire wall thickness may be assessed. Stain one section for elastin in addition to the routine H&E sections. The sign-out diagnosis should include a statement regarding the presence or absence of acute aortitis or other pathologic lesions.

Sample sign-out: Aorta, aortic dissection

Aortic medial tear, adventitial hemorrhage and dissecting hematoma, acute; consistent with aortic dissection.
Focal chronic dissection with intimal hyperplasia.
Severe fragmentation of elastic lamellae and acute accumulation of amorphous extracellular matrix material ("cystic medial degeneration").
No evidence of active aortitis.

Abdominal aortic aneurysm

During the surgical repair the aneurysm is opened, the clot removed, and the graft sewn inside of the aorta. The aorta is then closed around the graft. The specimen usually consists of laminated thrombus, with or without calcified plaque. It is relatively unusual to receive portions of the aortic wall. Portions of the wall can usually be identified because they have more consistency (i.e., they are less "flaky" and friable) than thrombus.

The thrombus is serially sectioned grossly to look for the rare mycotic (infected) aneurysm, or tumor metastasis — this has happened!. Describe the overall dimensions, color, consistency (rubbery), and presence of calcifications. Several representative sections of thrombus in one cassette are adequate. If aortic wall is present, additional sections are submitted.

Atherectomy specimens

Techniques are now available for the removal of atherosclerotic plaque via a catheter; this takes place in the cardiac catheterization laboratory. The most widely used method, rotational atherectomy, uses a catheter with a cylindrical cutting blade at its end; this results in multiple strips of fibrous and calcified plaque that defy orientation as pathologic specimens. These pieces are submitted in their entirety.

Endarterectomy specimens

Endarterectomy specimens consist of the luminal plaque with portions of the intima and media attached. The adventitia is not removed. Often the specimen retains the shape of the bifurcation. Open the specimen longitudinally if it is intact. Describe the shape (" -shaped fragment consistent with carotid bifurcation"), color, size, presence of calcifications, degree of stenosis, and acute plaque change. One section is adequate. Most specimens require decalcification.

Vascular grafts

Grafts are generally removed because of thrombosis, fibrous obstruction, or infection. Cultures may be requested for bacteria (aerobic and anaerobic), fungi, and AFB. Describe the dimensions (length and diameter), integrity (any holes or tears), color (usually white and not discolored), type of graft (e.g., saphenous vein, Gore-Tex, Dacron, see below), and soft tissue present in the lumen.

Gore-Tex (expanded polytetrafluoroethylene) is smooth surfaced and homogeneous, approximately 0.5 mm thick. It does not appear woven or corrugated. In contrast, Dacron polyester is a fabric with a grossly visible weave; it has a rough surface and it is corrugated. Tissue grafts are usually derived from large veins and are easily distinguished from synthetic material.

Any soft tissue is submitted for histologic examination, as infection is frequently occult. The graft is also submitted. Saphenous vein and Gore-Tex grafts cut easily with a scalpel blade and are easily sectioned for slides. Dacron grafts are difficult to section with a scalpel and feel "gritty" to the blade. When Dacron graft material is submitted it is helpful to notify the histology laboratory. A Gram stain is ordered for any graft for which there is a clinical history of infection or a request to rule out infection.

Coronary bypass grafts

Saphenous vein or internal mammary artery grafts may occasionally be removed during a second coronary artery bypass operation. Describe the length, average diameter, presence of atherosclerosis or intimal hyperplasia, acute plaque change, thrombus, and presence and extent of occlusions. One cassette per graft, containing multiple cross-sections of the specimen, is usually sufficient.

Table 16-5 Scoring system for temporal arteritis

SCORE	HISTOLOGIC FEATURES
Positive	Inflammatory infiltrate with giant cells
Probable	Lymphohistiocytic infiltrate involving the arterial wall transmurally or constituting 25% or more of the arterial wall without giant cells, or evidence of healed arteritis (transmural fibrosis)
Healed arteritis	Disruption of the elastica for at least one third of the circumference of the vessel with transmural fibrosis
Negative	No inflammatory infiltrate or giant cells or evidence of healed arteritis

Adapted from reference 10.

Varicose veins

Varicose veins are flaccid veins from the lower extremities. They are often inverted during removal. Describe the length, average diameter, and any unusual features such as obvious thrombus, tortuosity, thickening of the wall, or nodularities. One transverse section is sufficient.

Temporal arteries

Temporal arteries are biopsied (approximately 1 cm) to evaluate patients for temporal, or giant cell, arteritis (Table 16-5). Describe the dimensions (length and diameter), color, and any additional soft tissue. Do not cut the specimen! Orientation is very important for proper evaluation and cannot be accomplished with small cross-sections. Wrap the entire specimen in lens paper. The specimen should be cut into cross-sections by the histotechnologist after processing and just before embedding. Three levels and two elastic stains are ordered.

REFERENCES

1. Schoen FJ. Interventional and Surgical Cardiovascular Pathology: Clinical Correlations and Basic Principles. Philadelphia, W.B. Saunders, 1989.
2. Silver MD, Gotlieb AI, Schoen FJ (eds). Cardiovascular Pathology, 3rd edn. Philadelphia, W.B. Saunders, 2001.
3. Billingham ME, Cary NRB, Hammond ME, et al. A working formulation for the standardization of nomenclature in the diagnosis of heart and lung rejection: Heart rejection study group, The International Society for Heart Transplantation. J Heart Transplant 9:587–593, 1990.
4. Schoen FJ. Surgical pathology of removed natural and prosthetic cardiac valves. Hum Pathol 18:558–567, 1987.
5. Schoen FJ. Approach to the analysis of cardiac valve prostheses as surgical pathology or autopsy specimens. Cardiovasc Pathol 4:241–255, 1995.
6. Schoen FJ. Role of device retrieval and analysis in the evaluation of substitute heart valves. In Witkin KB (ed): Clinical Evaluation of Medical Devices: Principles and Case Studies. Totowa, NJ, Humana, pp 209–231, 1998.
7. Schoen FJ, Anderson JM, Didisheim P, et al. Ventricular assist device (VAD) pathology analysis: Guidelines for clinical studies. J Appl Biomater 1:49–56, 1990.
8. Hunt SA, Frazier OH. Mechanical circulatory support and cardiac transplantation. Circulation 97:2079–2090, 1998.
9. Goldstein DJ, Oz MC, Rose EA. Implantable left ventricular assist devices. N Engl J Med 339:1522–1533, 1998.
10. Robb-Nicholson C, Chang RW, Anderson S, et al. Diagnostic value of the history and examination in giant cell arteritis: A clinical pathological study of 81 temporal artery biopsies. J Rheumatol 15:1793-1796, 1988.

Cytology specimens

17

Cytology specimens may be obtained from fluids (e.g., sputum, pleural fluid, urine, CSF), fine needle aspiration (FNA) of solid masses, smears and scrapes of superficial lesions (e.g., PAP smear), or after surgical excision (e.g., touch preparations). Cytologic specimens have advantages over excisional specimens or large core biopsies:

- There is minimal or no morbidity to the patient.
- There is excellent cytologic preservation (e.g., crush and cautery artifacts are absent).
- Large areas can be sampled.
- Cells and nuclei are intact—this is an advantage for certain studies such as FISH.
- Specimen acquisition, preparation, and examination can be performed in a short period of time.

■ CELL BLOCKS

Cells suspended in fluids may be used to make smears, cytospins, Thin Preps®, or cell blocks. The cell block is the leftover sediment fixed (in formalin or Bouin's), embedded in paraffin, and sectioned like a biopsy. Cell blocks can provide multiple sections of the same group of cells to be used for histochemical stains and/or immunoperoxidase studies.

Processing the specimen

Fluids

1. Record the volume of fluid, color, and the size of any particulate matter in the specimen. Remove any clots, wrap in filter paper, and submit as cell blocks.
2. Centrifuge 80 mL (in two 50 mL tubes) for 20 minutes at maximum speed. If the sediment is scanty, decant the fluid, refill the tubes with more specimen fluid, and recentrifuge.
3. The fluid is decanted, being careful not to lose any of the pellet or particulate matter. Make about four smears on previously labeled glass slides. Use a wooden applicator or spatula to transfer a small portion of the pellet to one end of the slide. Use a second slide to make a smear. Immediately fix in 95% alcohol.
4. The pellet is transferred and wrapped in lens paper. Alternatively, the pellet may be resuspended in a small amount of fluid and poured through a nylon specimen bag. Do this over a clean specimen cup in order to be able to retrieve any spilled fluid.
   Order one H&E stain as well as other special stains as indicated.
5. If the quantity of fluid is small and appears clear or yields essentially no sediment, the specimen may require processing by cytospin or Millipore filtration.

Bronchoalveolar lavage is a method in which small quantities of fluid are introduced into the bronchial tree via a fiberoptic bronchoscope and then aspirated for analysis of cells and secretions from the distal airways. It is a useful method to recover pathogenic organisms (*Pneumocystis*, fungi, bacteria, mycobacteria, and CMV) from immunocompromised patients. These cases are treated as potentially infectious. Masks, gloves, and aprons should be worn.

The specimen should be handled gently to avoid aerosolization of organisms. All instruments and surfaces should be cleaned with bleach.

Fine needle aspirations

The following equipment should be assembled in a kit:

- Blank slides
- Pencil
- Spray fixative
- A 50 mL Falcon tube with normal saline ("normosol" = 0.9% saline); store in a refrigerator when not in use
- Empty container or tube holder
- Slide tray.

After the FNA is performed the specimen is prepared as follows:

1. Take the needle and syringe and express a small drop on each of two slides (using a stylet if the material is stuck in the needle). Stand the needle/syringe in the Falcon tube.
2. Immediately take one slide with material and spread the drop with a blank spreader slide *gently* but quickly.
3. Spray fix these two slides *immediately* or they will air dry within seconds, rendering the nuclear detail less distinct and difficult to interpret.
4. Take the other slide with a drop of material and spread it with yet another blank spreader slide but allow these two to thoroughly air dry. Cytoplasmic and extracellular material are seen well in air dried slides.
5. Rinse the needle/syringe in the Falcon tube, backwashing 2 to 3 times.
   The needle rinsings (in saline) are critical for special studies (e.g., flow cytometry, ThinPreps®, cell blocks).

Lymphoma: The specimen may be sent for flow cytometry.
Infection: If an infectious process is suspected, notify the radiologist, who will usually take a separate aspiration for multiple cultures.
Cell block: The remainder of the specimen can be used to prepare a cell block.
The slides may be stained with Diff-Quik or PAP stains if the adequacy of the specimen is to be assessed or a diagnosis is to be made at the time of the procedure.

■ STORAGE OF CYTOLOGY SPECIMENS

Cytology specimens obtained at night or during the weekend may need to be stored before processing. Most fluids are reasonably preserved for 48 to 72 hours in the refrigerator without fixation, especially pleural fluids. Other fluids (urine, CSF) may deteriorate after 24 hours even if refrigerated. This can be prevented by adding an equal volume of 50% ethanol (final concentration, 25%) to the fluid and refrigerating. Note that the addition of ethanol precludes the preparation of air-dried slides, which are especially useful in the evaluation of lymphoma and leukemia.

Dermatopathology

18

Of all organ systems, the skin has the greatest number of lesions described, perhaps because the skin is subject to a wide variety of environmental exposures and no special procedures are necessary to visualize its surface.

Relevant clinical history (in addition to age and gender)

See Table 18.1.

Table 18-1 Relevant clinical history (in addition to age and gender)	
HISTORY RELEVANT TO ALL SPECIMENS	HISTORY RELEVANT TO DERMATOPATHOLOGY SPECIMENS
Organ/tissue resected or biopsied	Site, duration, and appearance of the lesion (especially for incisional biopsies)
Purpose of the procedure	
Gross appearance of the organ/tissue/lesion sampled	Systemic diseases that affect the skin
Any unusual features of the clinical presentation	Clinical differential diagnosis
Any unusual features of the gross appearance	Family history (see Table 7.36, page 164, "Hereditary tumor syndromes")
Prior surgery/biopsies—results	Previous similar lesions
Prior malignancy	
Prior treatment (radiation therapy, chemotherapy, drug use that can change the histologic appearance of tissues)	
Compromised immune system	

General considerations

The ability to clearly visualize the entire epidermis in a perpendicular section is important for diagnosis and at times for prognosis (e.g., malignant melanoma). Therefore, try to maintain vertical orientation at all times in sections. Any specimen that is labeled "excision," regardless of the type of specimen, must have the margins evaluated by inking and submission of appropriate sections. Diagrams are used for any difficult or complicated specimens.

Never cut through small vesicular lesions in any type of specimen. The overlying tissue layer is important for diagnosis but is fragile and easily detached and lost. Cut the specimen so as to leave the vesicle intact or submit small specimens whole and request that the histotechnologist bisects the specimen after processing.

Special studies

Immunofluorescence, electron microscopy, or frozen tissue

Occasionally, fresh or frozen specimens (usually punch biopsies) are submitted for special studies such as immunofluorescence (e.g., for lupus erythematosus, bullous pemphigoid, or pemphigus), immunophenotyping (e.g., leukemias and lymphomas), or electron microscopy (epidermolysis bullosa, other blistering diseases, some melanomas [e.g. S100-negative tumors], unusual tumors, amyloid). See Chapter 7.

Operating Room consultations with frozen sections

Frozen-section examination may be requested in cases of suspected toxic epidermal necrolysis (TEN) or staphylococcal scalded skin syndrome (SSSS). Skin stripping or a sloughed specimen ("jelly roll") may be submitted for frozen section to determine the level of cleavage and degree of necrosis in the epidermis. Frozen-section examination of skin may also be helpful in the early diagnosis of necrotizing fasciitis. See Chapter 6 for additional information.

■ SKIN PUNCH BIOPSIES

Punch biopsies are performed to completely excise small lesions, sample large lesions, or evaluate an inflammatory process or a systemic disease (e.g., pustular psoriasis). Punch biopsies can be 2, 3, 4, 5, or 8 mm in diameter.

Processing the specimen (Fig. 18-1)

1. Describe the type of specimen ("punch biopsy") including diameter and depth and skin color. Describe any lesions including size, type (macular, papular, vesicular, plaque), borders (well-circumscribed, irregular), color (brown, black, variegated), shape (verrucous, lobulated), and distance from the closest margin.

   Ink all punch biopsies.

2. Punch biopsies 3 mm or smaller are submitted uncut in entirety. These specimens can be bisected by the histology laboratory.

   Punch biopsies larger than 4 mm are bisected or trisected, depending on size. If there is a discrete lesion, cut in a plane to demonstrate the closest margin. If the lesion is very small (i.e., leveling the block might remove the lesional tissue), cut the punch biopsy on either side of the lesion. Do not section through vesicles or blisters; submit whole and request sectioning by the laboratory.

3. Request three levels.

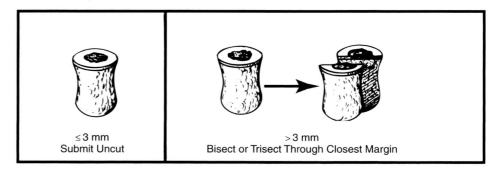

≤ 3 mm
Submit Uncut

> 3 mm
Bisect or Trisect Through Closest Margin

Do Not Bisect Specimens with Vesicles or Blisters
Ink if Labeled "Excision"

Figure 18-1 Punch biopsy of the skin.

Received in formalin, labeled with the patient's name and unit number and "5 mm punch, left leg," is a 5 mm in diameter by 5 mm (depth) punch biopsy with tan/white skin. There is a flat homogeneously brown lesion with slightly irregular margins on the skin surface which approaches to within 1 mm of the nearest margin, but does not grossly involve the margin.

Cassette: bisected, 2 frags, ESS.

■ SKIN SHAVE BIOPSIES

Shave biopsies are usually performed to remove nonmalignant lesions (seborrheic keratoses, actinic keratoses, fibroepithelial polyps, etc.) or for diagnosis of basal cell carcinomas. Shave biopsies of pigmented lesions should be strongly discouraged and interpreted with caution. The diagnosis of melanoma may be difficult in such a specimen due to limited sampling, and the depth of invasion may be impossible to assess. Specimens are inked if designated "excision."

Processing the specimen

1. Describe the specimen type ("shave biopsy"), the dimensions (including depth), and the surface appearance. The specimen is usually oval and relatively flat. The edges may curl due to retraction of the dermis. Specimens greater than 3 to 4 mm in diameter may be bisected or trisected. Try to maintain the vertical orientation in sections by making one or more cuts perpendicular to the surface at 2 to 3 mm intervals.
2. Submit in entirety and order three levels.

■ SKIN CURETTINGS

Skin curettings are usually skin scrapings of seborrheic or actinic keratosis or basal cell carcinoma.

Processing the specimen

1. Describe the specimen including number fragments (or estimate), color, and size in aggregate.
2. Submit entirely using a nylon specimen bag or lens paper to wrap the fragments. Check the sides of the container and lid for small pieces. Orientation is usually not possible. Margins cannot be evaluated due to the specimen fragmentation. Order three levels.

■ SKIN ELLIPSES

Skin ellipses are excisions of malignant tumors (squamous cell carcinoma or basal cell carcinoma), typical or atypical melanocytic nevi (and to rule out melanoma), or large benign lesions (e.g., epithelial inclusion cysts). Occasionally, ellipses are submitted for the evaluation of panniculitis or large vessel vasculitis.

Processing the specimen (Fig. 18-2)

1. Record the dimensions (length, width, and depth) and describe the skin color. Describe any lesions including color, borders, ulceration, shape, and distance from margins. Describe any scars from prior biopsies (length, recent or well-healed).

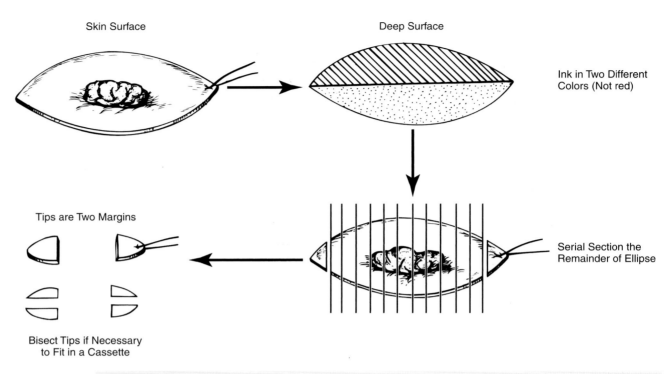

Skin Surface

Deep Surface

Ink in Two Different Colors (Not red)

Tips are Two Margins

Serial Section the Remainder of Ellipse

Bisect Tips if Necessary to Fit in a Cassette

Figure 18-2 Skin ellipses.

2. If an orienting suture is present, use the clinical designation or (lacking this) designate it 12 o'clock. Use two different colors of ink (but not red ink because this color is harder to see histologically) to mark the two longitudinal halves of the specimen and dictate the location of the inks (e.g., "the 12 o'clock margin is inked green and the 6 o'clock margin is inked blue"). Green and blue inks are recommended as these colors are easier for the histotechnologist to see during embedding and sectioning the tissue.

   Serially section the entire specimen along the short axis at 2 to 3 mm intervals.

   Submit the most distal sections ("tips") as two of the margins in two cassettes. If the ellipse is unoriented, only one color of ink can be used and the tip margins can be submitted together in one cassette. The tips should be taken as a thin section of tissue, narrow enough to fit into a cassette without bisecting.

   Submit the remainder of the specimen in one or more cassettes.

   A simple diagram showing orientation and sections is very helpful in interpreting the sections histologically. This is especially true for large or irregularly shaped skin excisions.

   For pigmented lesions, the initial cut is made through the thickest or darkest portion of the lesion (the area most likely to have deep invasion). Describe the gross depth of invasion or involvement of subcutaneous tissues.

3. Very large ellipses (several centimeters) are usually reexcisions. The central scar is serially sectioned and representative sections taken including the deep margin. Representative sections are taken of the 3, 6, 9, and 12 o'clock margins.

Gross differential diagnosis

Seborrheic keratosis. This is a rounded, raised lesion that is sharply demarcated from any surrounding skin and has a "stuck on" appearance. The color is usually dark brown, black, or gray, and the lesion has a dirty appearance due to the presence of horn cysts containing keratinous debris.

Epidermal inclusion cyst. These cysts are often received in multiple fragments. The wall of the cyst is thin (1 to 2 mm) and has a smooth inner lining. The cyst is filled with white or yellow friable, often malodorous, material corresponding to keratinaceous debris. Some cysts are caused by the traumatic or iatrogenic introduction of keratinizing epithelium into deep soft tissues. If located near the nipple, the lesion may be in a lactiferous sinus (squamous metaplasia of lactiferous ducts or recurrent subareolar abscess).

Fibroepithelial polyp (acrochordon). This is a flesh-colored papule often designated a "skin tag" by the clinician.

Basal cell carcinoma. The lesion is a translucent papule or plaque with a yellow or pearly hue. Central ulceration with a rolled border is common in larger lesions. The outer margin tends to be sharply demarcated from the surrounding skin.

Squamous cell carcinoma. This is a raised irregular flesh-colored lesion that is often centrally ulcerated.

Nevus. Nevi are pigmented or flesh-colored flat or raised lesions. Dysplastic nevi have some of the characteristics of melanoma such as an irregular shape and some variation in pigmentation.

Malignant melanoma. The most common appearance of malignant melanoma is as a pigmented lesion with irregular or notched borders. The pigmentation is often variable and may be very dark. Nodules or ulcers within the lesion are usually indicative of invasion.

Microscopic sections

Small ellipses (<2 cm)
The lesion is entirely submitted in the first cassette(s). Order three levels.
Submit tips in one cassette (if unoriented) or in two cassettes (if oriented). Order three levels.

Larger ellipses (>2 cm)
Representative sections of the lesion and margins are submitted. Reexcisions must have the margins carefully evaluated. Order one level.

Sample dictation

Received in formalin, labeled with the patient's name, unit number, and "right shoulder," is a 2.5 × 1 × 0.8 cm (depth) skin ellipse with tan/brown skin and an orienting suture at one tip (designated by the surgeon as 12 o'clock). There is a variegated brown and black lesion (1 × 0.8 cm) with markedly irregular borders with notching located in the center of the ellipse. Within the lesion there is a raised black nodule (0.3 × 0.3 cm) that grossly appears to extend through the epidermis into the dermis and is 0.2 cm from the deep resection margin. The closest margin is the 3 o'clock margin, which is 0.1 cm from the lesion. The 3 o'clock margin is inked black and the 9 o'clock margin is inked blue.

Cassette #1: 12 o'clock margin, 1 frag, ESS.
Cassette #2: 6 o'clock margin, 1 frag, ESS.
Cassette #3: Cross-sections from 3 to 9 o'clock, 4 frags, ESS.

Pathologic prognostic/diagnostic features sign-out checklist for skin carcinomas

Specimen type*
Punch biopsy, shave biopsy, curettings, excisional biopsy (ellipse).

Tumor site*
Specify, if known.

Tumor size*
Greatest dimension (additional dimensions optional).
For staging: ≤2, ≤5, >5 cm.

Tumor features*
Raised, flat, ulcerated, unpigmented, pigmented, necrosis, hemorrhage, indeterminate.

Histologic type*
Squamous cell (subtypes: acantholytic, adenosquamous, basaloid, spindle cell, undifferentiated (lymphoepithelioma, verrucous)), basal cell, adenocarcinomas of sweat and sebaceous glands.

Histologic grade* (Table 18-3)
Well, moderate, poor, or undifferentiated.

Extent of invasion*
Carcinoma in situ, limited to dermis, invasion of subcutis, invasion of deep extradermal structures (cartilage, skeletal muscle, or bone).
Depth of invasion:
≤0.2 cm in thickness
>0.2 cm in thickness but ≤0.6 cm in thickness
>0.6 cm in thickness

Regional lymph nodes*
Metastases absent, present (number involved, number examined).
Optional:
Size of largest metastatic deposit. Extracapsular invasion present or absent.

Distant metastasis*
Absent, present—specify site(s) if known.

Margins*
Radial ("lateral:" or non-deep):
uninvolved (optional: distance from closest margin), involved (specify location if possible). Specify if carcinoma in situ or invasive carcinoma at margin.
Deep:
uninvolved (optional: distance from closest margin), involved (specify location if possible).

Lymphatic (small vessel) invasion
Present or absent.

Venous (large vessel) invasion
Present or absent.

Perineural invasion
Present or absent.

Adjacent epithelium
Dysplasia, grade (mild, moderate, severe/CIS), extent (focal, multifocal, extensive), proximity to invasive carcinoma (adjacent or distant).

This checklist incorporates information from the CAP Cancer Committee protocols for reporting on cancer specimens (see www.cap.org/). The asterisked elements are considered to be scientifically validated or regularly used data elements that must be present in reports of cancer-directed surgical excisions from ACS CoC-approved cancer programs. The details of how the elements are reported may vary among institutions.
AJCC classification is given in Table 18-2.

Table 18-2 AJCC (6th edition) classification: Skin carcinomas[a]

Tumor	TX	Primary tumor cannot be assessed
	T0	No evidence of primary tumor
	Tis	Carcinoma in situ
	T1	Tumor ≤2 cm in greatest dimension
	T1a	Limited to dermis or 0.2 cm or less in thickness
	T1b	Limited to dermis and >0.2 cm in thickness, but ≤0.6 cm in thickness
	T1c	Invading the subcutis and/or >0.6 cm in thickness
	T2	Tumor >2 cm to ≤5 cm in greatest dimension
	T2a	Limited to dermis or ≤0.2 cm in thickness
	T2b	Limited to dermis and > 0.2 cm in thickness, but ≤0.6 cm
	T2c	Invading the subcutis and/or more than 0.6 cm in thickness
	T3	Tumor >5 cm in greatest dimension
	T3a	Limited to dermis or ≤0.2 cm in thickness
	T3b	Limited to dermis and >0.2 cm in thickness, but ≤0.6 cm
	T3c	Invading the subcutis and/or more than 0.6 cm in thickness
	T4	Tumor invades into deep extradermal structures (i.e., cartilage, skeletal muscle, or bone)
	T4a	≤0.6 cm in thickness
	T4b	>0.6 cm in thickness

Note: If there are multiple simultaneous tumors, the tumor with the highest T category will be classified and the number of separate tumors will be indicated in parentheses, e.g., T2 (5).
The "a," "b," and "c" subdivisions are optional but are suggested in the TNM supplement.[1]

Regional lymph nodes	NX	Regional lymph nodes cannot be assessed
	N0	No regional lymph node metastasis
	N1	Regional lymph node metastasis
Distant metastasis	MX	Distant metastasis cannot be assessed
	M0	No distant metastasis
	M1	Distant metastasis

[a] Used for squamous cell and basal cell carcinomas of the skin and adenocarcinomas developing from sweat or sebaceous glands. This classification is not used for carcinomas of the vulva, eyelid, or penis.

Table 18-3 Histologic grade (squamous cell carcinoma and adnexal carcinoma)

Grade 1	Well differentiated
Grade 2	Moderately differentiated
Grade 3	Poorly differentiated
Grade 4	Undifferentiated

Pathologic prognostic/diagnostic features sign-out checklist for melanoma of the skin

Specimen type*
Punch biopsy, shave biopsy, excisional biopsy, reexcision, lymphadenectomy (sentinel or regional nodes).

Macroscopic tumor*
Absent, present.

Tumor site*
Specify (if known).

Lesion size*
Greatest dimension (optional: additional dimensions).

Satellite nodules*
Absent, present (specify).
Distance from primary tumor

Pigmentation
Absent, present, diffuse, present, patchy/focal, indeterminate.

Histologic type*
Lentigo maligna, superficial spreading, nodular, acral lentiginous, desmoplastic, other.

Ulceration*
Absent, present.
Post-traumatic ulceration (e.g., due to prior surgery) should be distinguished from ulceration due to invasion by tumor when possible. The width of the ulcerated area should be reported.

Depth and extent of invasion*
Specify in millimeters.
Prognosis is primarily related to the depth of invasion measured vertically in mm from the granular cell layer of the epidermis (or the base of the ulcer, if ulcerated) to the deepest point of tumor penetration, excluding tumor surrounding skin appendages (Breslow depth of invasion, Box 18-1).[2] If satellite lesions are used in this measurement, this should be recorded. An ocular micrometer should be used for measurements. The depth of invasion may also be given relative to anatomical landmarks (Clark's level, Box 18-2).

Regional lymph nodes*
Number and percentage of nodes involved, size of the largest metastatic deposit, extracapsular invasion. Sentinel nodes may be examined by multiple H&E levels and immunoperoxidase studies; a standard protocol for all institutions has not been established. Typically, three H&E levels and one to three immunohistochemical studies on intervening levels are examined. S100 is sensitive but other markers are more specific (Table 18-4). The significance of small metastases <0.2 cm in size is unknown, but is currently being investigated.

Distant metastasis*
Absent, present (skin, subcutaneous tissue, distant lymph nodes, lung, other visceral sites, or associated with elevated serum lactate dehydrogenase).

Margins*
Lateral and deep:
Involved or free, positive = ink on tumor. The distance to the closest margins should be given. Specify if melanoma in situ or invasive melanoma.

Venous (large vessel) invasion
Absent, present.

Perineural invasion
Absent, present.

Tumor infiltrating lymphocytes (TILs)
Absent, non-brisk, brisk.
TILs absent: no lymphocytes present, or present but do not infiltrate tumor.
TILs non-brisk: lymphocytes infiltrate melanoma only focally or not along the entire base of the vertical growth phase.
TILs brisk: lymphocytes diffusely infiltrate the entire invasive component of the melanoma or the entire base of the vertical growth phase.

Tumor regression
Absent, present involving <75%, present involving 75% or more of lesion.

Partial or complete obliteration of melanoma by host response (fibrosis, lymphocytes, and macrophages).

Mitotic index

<1 mitotic figure per mm^2

$\geq$1 mitotic figure per mm^2

The size of a microscopic field depends on the microscope (see Chapter 9, "Measuring with the microscope").

Assessed in the vertical growth phase (not the intraepidermal component).

Radial growth phase

Present or absent, type (lentigo maligna, acral lentiginous, superficial spreading).

The tumor is generally of uniform cytologic appearance and is wider than it is deep.

Vertical growth phase

Present or absent, type (epithelioid, spindle, or mixed)

Expansile nests of tumor cells are present in the papillary and/or reticular dermis.

Precursor nevus

Present or absent.

This list incorporates recommendations from the ADASP (see www.panix.com/~adasp/) and information from the CAP Cancer Committee protocols for reporting on cancer specimens. The asterisked elements are considered to be scientifically validated or regularly used data elements that must be present in reports of cancer-directed excisional specimens from ACS CoC-approved cancer programs. The details of reporting the elements may vary among institutions.

AJCC classification is given in Table 18-5.

Box 18-1 Breslow depth of invasion[2]

Measurements should be performed with an ocular reticule.

Nonulcerated lesions: Measure from the top of the granular layer to the deepest point of invasion.

Ulcerated lesions: Measure from the ulcer base overlying the deepest point of invasion.

Difficult cases:

- Melanocytes in junctional nests (i.e., not invasive into stroma) are not included in the measurement. This includes junctional involvement of skin appendages.
- Microscopic satellite lesions in reticular dermis are sometimes used in measurements. It is usually preferable to measure a contiguous area of invasion from the surface. If satellite lesions are used, this can be described in the report.
- If there is marked epidermal hyperplasia (resulting in a thickened granular layer), then the measurement may overestimate the thickness of the melanoma. This situation can be described in the report.
- Lesions with tangential sectioning or curetted lesions cannot have the depth measured accurately.

Box 18-2 Clark's level[3]

Level I: melanoma confined to the epidermis and epidermal appendages

Level II: extension into the papillary dermis by single cells with, at most, only a few cells extending to the interface between the papillary and reticular dermis

Level III: extension of tumor cells throughout the papillary dermis, filling it and impinging upon the reticular dermis but not invading it

Level IV: invasion of the reticular dermis

Level V: invasion of the subcutaneous fat

Table 18-4 Immunohistochemical melanoma markers

TYPE OF CELL	S100	HMB-45	MART-1
Metastatic melanoma	POS	High[a]	High[a]
Nevus cells	POS	neg/weak	POS
Dendritic cells	POS	neg	neg
Nerves, ganglion cells	POS	neg	neg

[a] Approximately 20% of metastatic melanomas are negative for HMB-45 and MART-1.

■ LARGE SKIN EXCISIONS

Large resections are usually carried out after the lesion has been biopsied and a diagnosis made.

Processing the specimen

1. Record the dimensions (length, width, depth), skin color, lesions, scars (presence of a prior biopsy scar), and deep margin (soft tissue, fascia, muscle). Describe the closest approach of the lesion to a margin.

2. Ink all margins, excluding skin surfaces. All sections taken must be thin to allow for adequate fixation of the fatty subcutaneous tissue.

3. There is usually an orienting suture with a designated "o'clock." If there are no orienting sutures, try to pick an identifiable area to designate 12 o'clock. Document in the gross description that the specimen is unoriented and the o'clock designations are arbitrarily assigned. Take four perpendicular sections of the margin at 12 o'clock, 3 o'clock, 6 o'clock, and 9 o'clock but including the closest approach of tumor to the margin(s). This is adequate unless the lesion is grossly at or near the margin. More sections are taken in these areas.

   Even the smallest ellipses must be cross-sectioned perpendicular to the scar (i.e., do not bisect longitudinally) in order to evaluate the closest (lateral) margins.

4. Block out the lesion or the biopsy scar and submit the entire lesion or biopsy site. If these sections do not include the deep margin, separate sections of the deep margin should be submitted.

5. Carefully section through soft tissue looking for lymph nodes. Submit all lymph nodes found.

Table 18-5 AJCC (6th edition) classification: Melanomas[a]

Tumor	pTX		Primary tumor cannot be assessed
	pT0		No evidence of primary tumor
	pTis		Melanoma in situ
	pT1		≤0.1 cm in thickness with or without ulceration
		pT1a	≤1 mm in thickness and level II or III, without ulceration
		pT1b	≤1 mm in thickness and level IV or V with ulceration
	pT2		1.01 to 2 mm in thickness with or without ulceration
		pT2a	1.01 to 2 mm in thickness without ulceration
		pT2b	1.01 to 2 mm in thickness with ulceration
	pT3		2.01 to 4 mm in thickness with or without ulceration
		pT3a	2.01 to 4 mm in thickness without ulceration
		pT3b	2.01 to 4 mm in thickness with ulceration
	pT4		>4 mm in thickness with or without ulceration
		pT4a	>4 mm in thickness without ulceration
		pT4b	>4 mm in thickness with ulceration
	Ulceration: The absence of an intact epidermis overlying the primary melanoma		
Regional lymph nodes (for definitions, see Box 18-3)	NX		Regional lymph nodes cannot be assessed
	N0		No regional lymph node metastasis
	N1		Metastasis in one lymph node
		N1a	Clinically occult (microscopic) metastasis
		N1b	Clinically apparent (macroscopic) metastasis
	N2		Metastasis in two to three regional nodes or intralymphatic regional metastasis without nodal metastases
		N2a	Clinically occult (microscopic) metastasis
		N2b	Clinically apparent (macroscopic) metastasis
		N2c	Satellite or in-transit metastasis without nodal metastasis
	N3		Metastasis in four or more regional nodes, or matted metastatic nodes, or in-transit metastasis with metastasis in regional nodes
Distant metastasis	MX		Distant metastasis cannot be assessed
	M0		No distant metastasis
	M1		Distant metastasis
		M1a	Distant metastasis in skin, subcutaneous tissue, or lymph node(s) beyond the regional lymph nodes
		M1b	Metastasis to lung
		M1c	Metastasis to all other visceral sites or distant metastasis at any site associated with an elevated serum lactate dehydrogenase (LDH)

[a] This classification is not used for melanomas of sites other than skin (e.g., ocular, mucosal, urethral).

Box 18-3 Definitions

Satellite metastasis: Intralymphatic metastases occurring within 2 cm of the primary melanoma.

In-transit metastasis: Intralymphatic metastases occurring more than 2 cm from the primary melanoma but before the first echelon of regional lymph nodes.

Regional nodal metastases: One nodal basin or two contiguous nodal basins (e.g., femoral/iliac, axillary/supraclavicular, cervical/supraclavicular, axillary/femoral, or bilateral axillary or femoral metastases).

Microscopic metastasis: Metastasis in a node not detected by clinical or radiologic examination.

6. Draw a diagram of the specimen that includes the location of all sections taken and a key to the corresponding cassettes in which they are submitted. This is particularly important for irregularly shaped specimens.

■ LIP EXCISIONS

Squamous cell carcinoma is the most common neoplasm of the lip. The specimens are more complicated because there is often both a mucosal and skin surface (Fig. 18-3). There are three margins: both lateral margins (or a lateral and a medial margin) and a deep margin.

Processing the specimen

1. Describe the specimen including overall dimensions and dimensions of mucosal and skin surfaces.
2. Describe any lesions including size, color, quality (exophytic, verrucous, polypoid, ulcerated), and location (with respect to skin, mucosa, and vermilion border, and distance from margins).
3. Ink the lateral, medial, and deep surgical margins.
4. Serially section the specimen. Note the depth of invasion of the tumor. Submit sections demonstrating the tumor and its deepest extent, relationship to skin and mucosa, and relationship to all margins.
5. Draw a diagram showing the location of the lesion and provide a key to the location of tissue sections and the corresponding cassettes.

■ FORESKIN

The foreskins of newborn infants are not submitted for histologic examination unless there are gross abnormalities. Circumcisions of older males are performed in two age groups: young adults (18 to 25 years old) and men older than 50. In the younger age group, the procedure is performed for phimosis, usually due to a subtle anatomic defect (e.g., minimal hypospadias), and the only histologic finding is slight nonspecific chronic balanitis. In the older age group, a

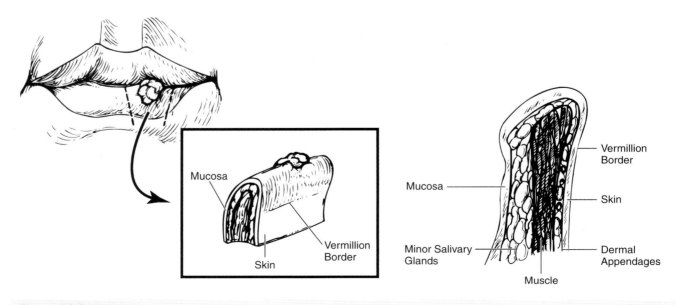

Figure 18-3 Lip resection.

specific inflammatory or neoplastic lesion is usually found. Common lesions of the foreskin are condylomata, balanitis xerotica obliterans (lichen sclerosus), balanitis circumscripta plasmacellularis (Zoon's balanitis), squamous cell carcinoma in situ, and invasive squamous cell carcinomas. If no lesion is detected on the initial sections, and the clinical history is not provided, call the clinician to find out the reason for the circumcision.

Processing the specimen

1. Measure length, width, and thickness. The specimen usually consists of a rectangle of tissue including skin and mucosa on the surface with underlying loose areolar tissue. It is usually not possible to orient the specimen as to proximal and distal margins.
2. Examine the surface carefully for any epidermal lesions. If any are present, describe size, appearance (verrucous, papillary, ulcerated), depth of invasion, and distance from the nearest cut edge. Ink margins if a focal lesion is present.
   Describe the uninvolved skin including color and texture (rugose, atrophic, thickened).
3. The specimen is sectioned longitudinally including both skin and mucosa. One cassette with representative sections is adequate if there are no gross lesions and the foreskin is removed in the clinical context of phimosis. Additional cassettes are submitted to document all lesions and adjacent margins.

■ FINGERNAILS AND TOENAILS

Clippings

Toenail clippings may be sent for the evaluation of fungal infection. Inform the histology laboratory that the specimen consists of a nail as these specimens are usually very difficult to section and may require special techniques for softening.[4,5] Order a PAS stain (for fungi).

Nail bed biopsies are usually submitted for the evaluation of pigmented lesions. Do not order a PAS stain on these specimens (see below).

Tumor

Subungual melanomas occur in all ethnic groups but are proportionately more common in persons of color. These lesions may present as linear pigmented streaks of the nail if the melanoma cells involve the nail matrix. Specimens consisting of only the nail (and not the matrix) will not be diagnostic because melanocytes are not present. The appropriate specimen is a punch biopsy of the nail matrix. If a nail with a pigmented area is received, it is submitted for microscopic examination for evaluation of an atypical melanocytic lesion or melanoma.

REFERENCES

1. Wittekind C, et al, eds. TNM Supplement. A Commentary on Uniform Use, 2nd edn. New York, Wiley-Liss, 2001.
2. Breslow A. Thickness, cross-sectional areas, and depth of invasion in the prognosis of cutaneous melanoma. Ann Surg 172:902-908, 1970.
3. Clark WH Jr, From L, Bernardino EH, et al. Histogenesis and biologic behavior of primary human malignant melanoma of the skin. Cancer Res 29:705-727, 1969.
4. Shapiro L. Softening hard keratin in specimens for microscopic sections. Am J Clin Pathol 54:773-774, 1970.
5. Lewin K, DeWit SA, Lawson R. Softening techniques for nail biopsies. Arch Dermatol 107:223-224, 1973.

Gastrointestinal specimens (including hepatobiliary and pancreatic specimens)

19

Specimens from the gastrointestinal tract are common. Endoscopic biopsies are often performed to evaluate patients with symptoms (bleeding, diarrhea, malabsorption) and to look for pathogens, as well as to evaluate mass lesions (polyps and tumors). Resections are commonly performed for tumors but are also performed for inflammatory bowel disease, diverticulosis, and ischemic bowel.

■ ESOPHAGUS

Relevant clinical history (in addition to age and gender)

See Table 19.1.

Table 19-1 Relevant clinical history (in addition to age and gender)	
HISTORY RELEVANT TO ALL SPECIMENS	HISTORY RELEVANT TO ESOPHAGEAL SPECIMENS
Organ/tissue resected or biopsied	Gross appearance of lesions (e.g., raised masses, ulcers, strictures)
Purpose of the procedure	
Gross appearance of the organ/tissue/lesion sampled	Location of biopsies in the esophagus
Any unusual features of the clinical presentation	→ for example, a history of reflux or lye ingestion
Any unusual features of the gross appearance	
Prior surgery/biopsies—results	→ for example, a history of Barrett's esophagus
Prior malignancy	
Prior treatment (radiation therapy, chemotherapy, drug use that can change the histologic appearance of tissues)	
Compromised immune system	→ for example thrush, HIV, bone marrow transplant

Biopsies

Biopsies are commonly performed for the evaluation of heartburn (e.g., due to reflux or ulcers in immunocompromised patients), for the evaluation of dysphagia (usually secondary to strictures or tumors), or in the surveillance for dysplasia in patients known to have Barrett's esophagus. These biopsies are submitted as described in Chapter 13.

Esophagectomies

The esophagus is usually removed with the proximal stomach for severe dysplasia or for adenocarcinoma arising in a background of Barrett's esophagus. Patients with squamous cell carcinomas are often treated with chemotherapy and radiation therapy prior to resection.

Processing the specimen

1. Stapled margins are removed by cutting away the staple line (as close as possible to the staples) with a pair of scissors. Locate the lesion by gently palpating the gastroesophageal (GE) junction with one finger in the lumen. Open the specimen longitudinally. Avoid cutting across any palpable lesions.

2. Record the length, circumference, and wall thickness of the esophagus and of the stomach. Record the size of any lesions and the distance to distal and proximal margins.

3. Ink the proximal and distal margins and the deep margin underneath the tumor. Pin out on a board. If the tumor is large, make one to three longitudinal cuts into the tumor to aid in fixation. The specimen is fixed in formalin overnight.

   Describe the lesion and/or area of ulceration (if no gross tumor is present after preoperative therapy) including size, color, tumor configuration (exophytic or polypoid, ulcerated, or infiltrative), depth of invasion, location (including relationship to squamocolumnar junction), percentage of circumference involved, luminal diameter at the site of the tumor, and proximal dilatation.

   The distance from the margins (distal, proximal, and deep) should be measured as soon as possible on the fresh specimen as considerable retraction occurs after excision.

   The squamocolumnar junction (Z line) is the intersection of glandular and squamous mucosa. The GE junction is defined as the junction of the tubular esophagus and the sack-shaped stomach, irrespective of the type of mucosa present. In normal individuals, this point usually corresponds to the proximal extent of the gastric folds. Proximal displacement of the Z line above the GE junction is indicative of columnar-line (Barrett's) esophagus.

4. Describe uninvolved mucosa.
   - Normal esophagus (squamous): glistening smooth white mucosa.
   - Normal stomach (glandular): velvety pink/red mucosa with rugal folds.
   - Barrett's mucosa (glandular): pale pink, finely granular, and may be patchy.

5. The adventitial soft tissue away from the tumor can be stripped and placed in Bouin's to aid in identifying lymph nodes. Nodes are virtually always present and may be located very close to the esophagus or stomach. Even small areas of attached adipose tissue need to be searched for lymph nodes.

6. Submit sections after fixing the specimen overnight. Section through the fat and submit all lymph nodes.

Gross differential diagnosis (Fig. 19-1)

Adenocarcinomas of the esophagus are usually present at or just above the GE junction and have a gross appearance similar to colonic adenocarcinomas. The main tumor is often tan/pink, polypoid, and may have an ulcerated center. These tumors often tunnel underneath the proximal noninvolved squamous mucosa and may be present at the proximal or distal margins in the submucosa. This is of great importance when evaluating margins intraoperatively. A section that includes the full thickness of the esophageal or gastric wall should be taken.

Occasionally gastric tumors arising in the proximal stomach may be removed using a similar procedure. Note the location of the center of the tumor in relation to the GE junction to help discriminate between esophageal and gastric origin.

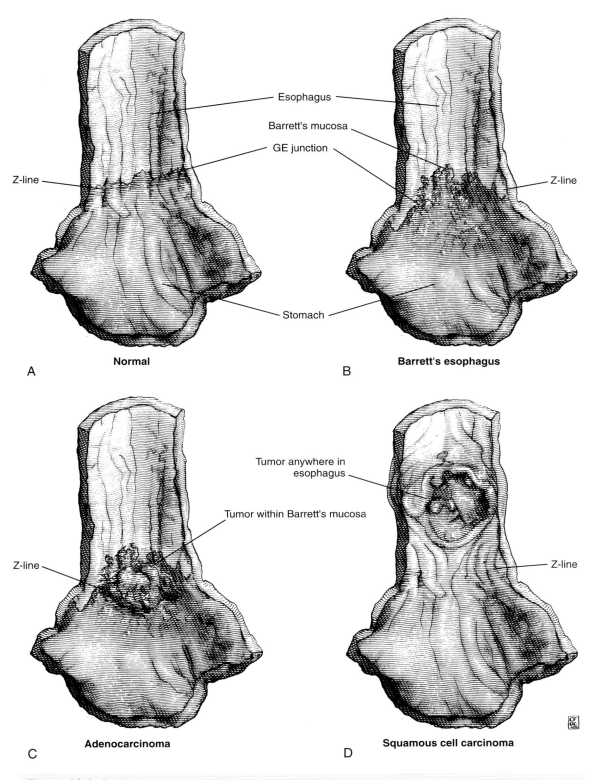

Figure 19-1 Esophagectomy specimens.

Barrett's mucosa is pale pink, finely granular, and may be patchy. It is distinct from the normal esophageal squamous mucosa, which is white, smooth and glistening. Barrett's mucosa is found extending proximally from the GE junction. It is often seen in association with esophageal adenocarcinomas, although the tumor may have obliterated the precursor lesion.

Squamous cell carcinomas can occur at any level of the esophagus. These tumors may be exophytic (intraluminal), ulcerating, or present as a diffuse thickening with narrowing of the lumen. In most cases, preoperative radiation therapy will have been given. The residual tumor may be difficult to appreciate grossly and may consist of areas of shallow ulceration or irregular/granular appearing squamous mucosa. Intraoperatively the margins should be evaluated for carcinoma in situ in the squamous mucosa.

Tumors after treatment. The main tumor mass may be absent, and only a shallow ulceration present at its former site. Post-radiation changes, including fibrosis and esophageal mucosal erosions, may be present.

Leiomyomas of the esophagus almost always arise from the muscularis propria and only rarely from the muscularis mucosae. The tumors are well circumscribed, pink to white, and have a whorled appearance, similar to uterine leiomyomas. Most are present within the wall, but some may project into the lumen as a polypoid mass.

Microscopic sections

Tumor
Four or fewer sections including maximal depth of invasion, relationship to esophagus and stomach. Longitudinal sections are usually best.

If no gross tumor is present, block out the ulcerated/fibrosed area and submit four sections.

Margins
Up to three sections of proximal, distal, and deep margins. The deep margin can usually also be one of the tumor blocks. Use en face (not perpendicular) sections of the proximal margins unless tumor and margin can be included in multiple perpendicular sections.

Esophagus and stomach
Document normal esophageal and gastric mucosa if not included in margins.

Other lesions
Submit sections of all other gross lesions including a representative area of Barrett's mucosa.

Lymph nodes
Submit all lymph nodes found (see Chapter 27).

Sample dictation

Received fresh, labeled with the patient's name and unit number and "esophagus," is an esophagectomy and partial gastrectomy specimen consisting of esophagus (15 cm in length × 4 cm in circumference) and stomach (5 cm in length × 12 cm in circumference). There is a 3.5 × 3 cm tan/pink firm centrally ulcerated tumor mass arising just proximal to, and partially involving, the gastroesophageal junction. The tumor invades into and focally through the muscularis propria into adjacent soft tissue. Tumor is present 0.1 cm from the deep margin, which is inked. The tumor is 12 cm from the proximal margin and 5 cm from the distal margin. The esophageal mucosa adjacent to the tumor is tan/pink and finely granular and extends to within 5 cm of the proximal resection margin. The remainder of the mucosal surfaces is unremarkable. Five lymph nodes are found in the surrounding soft tissue, the largest measuring 1 cm in greatest dimension. This node is very firm and white. The specimen is photographed.

Cassettes #1 and 2: Tumor and deepest extent of invasion and deep margin, 2 frags, ESS.
Cassette #3: Tumor and adjacent esophageal mucosa, 1 frag, RSS.
Cassette #4: Tumor and adjacent gastric mucosa, 1 frag, RSS.

Cassette #5: Proximal margin, en face, 1 frag, RSS.
Cassette #6: Distal margin, en face, 1 frag, RSS.
Cassette #7: Abnormal esophageal mucosa, 1 frag, RSS.
Cassette #8: Largest lymph node, 3 frags, ESS.
Cassette #9: Four lymph nodes, 4 frags, ESS.

Pathologic prognostic/diagnostic features sign-out checklist for esophageal carcinomas

Specimen type*
Esophagectomy, esophagogastrectomy, other.

Tumor site*
Center of tumor and extent of tumor:
GE junction, stomach, location in esophagus (distance from GE junction; upper, middle, lower third).
Subsite:
Circumferential, anterior, posterior, right lateral, left lateral, across GE junction (measure proportion of tumor in esophagus and stomach).
If more than 50% of the carcinoma is in the esophagus, it is classified as esophageal. If more than 50% of the carcinoma involves the stomach, it is classified as gastric. Carcinomas that equally span the GE junction, or are centered at the GE junction, are designated as follows depending on the histologic type:

- Esophageal: squamous, small cell, and undifferentiated carcinomas
- Gastric: adenocarcinomas and signet-ring cell carcinomas.

Tumor size*
Greatest dimension.

Histologic type*
Adenocarcinoma (including mucinous (> 50% mucinous), signet ring cell (> 50% signet ring cells) types), squamous cell carcinoma (including verrucous, spindle cell, and basaloid types), adeno-squamous carcinoma, small cell carcinoma, undifferentiated carcinoma, other rare types. The WHO classification is recommended.

Histologic grade*
Well, moderately, poorly differentiated, or undifferentiated (Boxes 19-1, 19-2)

Configuration
Exophytic, ulcerating (endophytic), diffusely infiltrative.

Extent of invasion*
In situ, invasion into lamina propria (T1a), invasion into submucosa (T1b), invasion into muscularis propria (T2a), invasion into subserosa (T2b), invasion into adventitia (T3), invasion into adjacent structures (T4).

Regional lymph nodes*
The total number and location of nodes examined should be specified, when possible.
The nodes around the stomach and esophagus are considered regional nodes.
Mediastinal nodes are regional nodes for the intrathoracic esophagus.
Cervical and supraclavicular nodes are regional nodes for the cervical esophagus.
Number of positive lymph nodes.
Presence or absence of extranodal invasion.

Distant metastasis*
Presence or absence of distant metastasis.

Margins*
Proximal, distal, and radial or adventitial (soft tissue at deepest extent of tumor), involved or not involved, distance from closest margin, involvement (in cm), type of mucosa at margin. Margins are also evaluated for the presence of dysplasia and/or Barrett's mucosa.

Box 19-1 Grading system for esophageal adenocarcinomas

Grade X	Grade cannot be assessed
Grade 1	Well differentiated (>95% gland forming, includes tubular)
Grade 2	Moderately differentiated (50–95% of tumor composed of glands)
Grade 3	Poorly differentiated (5–49% of tumor composed of glands, includes signet ring cell carcinomas)
Grade 4	Undifferentiated (<5% of tumor composed of glands) (cannot be categorized as squamous cell carcinoma or adenocarcinoma) (includes small cell carcinoma)

The tumor is given the grade of the least differentiated part.
Mucoepidermoid carcinomas and adenoid cystic carcinomas are not usually graded.
See also reference 1.

Box 19-2 Grading system for esophageal squamous cell carcinomas

Grade X	Grade cannot be assessed
Grade 1	Well differentiated
Grade 2	Moderately differentiated
Grade 3	Poorly differentiated
Grade 4	Undifferentiated (cannot be categorized as squamous cell carcinoma or adenocarcinoma)

The tumor is given the grade of the least differentiated part.

Lymphatic (small vessel) invasion (L)
Present or absent.

Venous (large vessel) invasion (V)
Present or absent.

Perineural invasion
Present or absent.

Nonlesional mucosa
Barrett's mucosa (intestinal metaplasia, dysplasia), esophagitis (type), gastritis (type), H. pylori, ulceration, granulomas

Response to therapy
Residual tumor present or absent (none (R0), microscopic (R1), macroscopic (R2), viability

Post-treatment changes
Location and extent of residual tumor.
Note location of acellular mucin pools in wall and at margins.
Note post-treatment inflammatory changes: esophagitis with or without ulceration, epithelial or stromal atypia, obliterative vasculopathy.

This checklist incorporates information from the ADASP (see www.panix.com/~adasp) and the CAP Cancer Committee protocols for reporting on cancer specimens (see www.cap.org/). The asterisked elements are considered to be scientifically validated or regularly used data elements that must be present in reports of cancer-directed surgical resection specimens from ACS CoC-approved cancer programs. The specific details of reporting the elements may vary among institutions.

Table 19-2 AJCC (6th edition) classification of esophageal carcinomas

Tumor	TX	Primary tumor cannot be assessed
	T0	No evidence of primary tumor
	Tis	Carcinoma in situ (including high-grade dysplasia)
	T1	Tumor invades lamina propria or submucosa
	T1a[a]	Tumor invades lamina propria
	T1b[a]	Tumor invades submucosa
	T2	Tumor invades muscularis propria
	T3	Tumor invades adventitia
	T4	Tumor invades adjacent structures
Regional lymph nodes	NX	Regional lymph nodes cannot be assessed
	N0	No regional lymph node metastasis
	N1	Regional lymph node metastasis
	N1a[a]	1 to 3 nodes involved
	N1b[a]	4 to 7 nodes involved
	N1c[a]	>7 nodes involved
Distant metastasis	MX	Distant metastasis cannot be assessed
	M0	No distant metastasis
	M1	Distant metastasis

Tumors of the lower thoracic esophagus (distal approximately 8 cm including the esophagogastric junction)

	M1a	Metastasis in celiac lymph nodes
	M1b	Other distant metastasis

Tumors of the midthoracic esophagus

	M1a	Not applicable
	M1b	Non-regional lymph nodes and/or other distant metastasis

Tumors of the upper thoracic esophagus

	M1a	Metastasis in cervical nodes
	M1b	Other distant metastasis

[a] These categories are not yet part of the AJCC staging system but differ in the incidence of lymph node metastasis (T categories) and 5-year survival rates (T and N categories).
Note: Clinical information may be necessary to distinguish midthoracic from upper thoracic esophageal carcinomas.

◼ STOMACH

The stomach is commonly affected by inflammatory processes (i.e., gastritis) as well as primary malignant tumors.

Relevant clinical history

See Table 19-3.

Biopsy

Biopsies can be processed as described in Chapter 13. Special stains (e.g., Alcian yellow, Diff-Quik, Giemsa, or Steiner) may be used to evaluate the biopsy for *Helicobacter pylori*.

If lymphoma is suspected, an unfixed biopsy specimen may be submitted. This tissue may be frozen for use for hematopathology markers.

Gastrectomy

Stomachs are resected for primary tumors (carcinoma or lymphoma, rarely partial resections for a gastrointestinal stromal tumor), less commonly for benign ulcers, and as part of larger resections (esophagogastrectomies or Whipple procedures).

Gastrectomies may be total but usually are partial. Look carefully at the margins to determine whether duodenal or esophageal mucosa is present.

Table 19-3 Relevant clinical history (in addition to age and gender)

HISTORY RELEVANT TO ALL SPECIMENS	HISTORY RELEVANT TO STOMACH SPECIMENS
Organ/tissue resected or biopsied	Gastritis (Helicobacter pylori or atrophic gastritis)
Purpose of the procedure	
Gross appearance of the organ/tissue/lesion sampled	
Any unusual features of the clinical presentation	
Any unusual features of the gross appearance	
Prior surgery/biopsies—results	→ Gastric surgery (e.g., Billroth)
Prior malignancy	→ History of gastric dysplasia, location of biopsy
Prior treatment (radiation therapy, chemotherapy, drug use that can change the histologic appearance of tissues)	
Immunocompromise	

Processing the specimen

1. Examine the outer surface of the specimen for evidence of tumor invasion through the wall and describe the serosa (color, glistening, dull, indurated, retracted, nodules). Carefully ink the proximal and distal resection margins without getting ink on the mucosa. Once the specimen is opened, the mucosal edges tend to curl under, and it is sometimes difficult to identify the resection margins. The ink can help with this identification.

2. Very gently palpate the mucosa and wall to locate the lesion. The mucosa is very delicate and should be touched as little as possible. Open the stomach along the greater curvature, unless a lesion is present at that site. Record the length of the greater curvature, lesser curvature, proximal resection margin (circumference—look for esophageal mucosa), distal resection margin (circumference—look for duodenal mucosa), and the thickness of the wall. Cassettes can be clipped to the edges of the margins to help to identify them after the stomach is opened.

3. Identify mucosal lesions and describe:
    *   Size (including depth of invasion). Ink the deep margin of any lesions and make several cuts to evaluate the depth of penetration into the wall.
    *   Color.
    *   Shape (ulcerating, polypoid, diffuse, exophytic).
    *   Consistency (hard, firm, soft).
    *   Margins of ulcers (irregular, rolled, puckered).
    *   Location (cardia, fundus, antrum, greater or lesser curvature, anterior or posterior wall).
    *   Perforation of wall.
    *   Relationship to resection margins. The distance to margins should be measured on the fresh specimen as soon as possible after resection, as considerable contraction of the specimen can occur.
    *   Relationship to the visceral peritoneum. Tumor penetration of the visceral peritoneum (grossly corresponding to tumor present at the surface of the perigastric adipose tissue)

is classified as T3, whereas tumor that invades into perigastric soft tissue (e.g., greater omentum) but not through visceral peritoneum is classified as T2.

If the nature of the lesion (i.e., carcinoma vs lymphoma) has not been established (e.g., by previous biopsy) and is not evident from the gross examination, a frozen section or cytologic preparation (e.g., a touch preparation) may be useful to aid in apportioning tissue (e.g., saving tissue for hematologic studies if lymphoma is suspected).

Describe the uninvolved mucosa including color, texture (glistening, hemorrhagic, granular, flattened, fibrotic, constricted), and the preservation of rugal folds.

4. Remove the adventitial soft tissue except at the deep margin of lesions and place in Bouin's fixative, if desired, to better visualize lymph nodes.

5. Pin out the stomach and fix overnight in formalin. The following day, submit microscopic sections of stomach and lesions. Section through soft tissue and submit all lymph nodes. Describe, including size of largest node, evidence of metastasis (white, hard).

Gross differential diagnosis (Fig. 19-2)

Benign ulcers tend to be sharply delineated with converging mucosal folds. The edges are usually flat or only slightly heaped up. Approximately 10% of ulcers thought to be clinically benign are shown to be malignant after pathologic examination. Malignancy is more common in ulcers over 2 cm in size.

Gastric carcinomas of intestinal type are similar in appearance to colonic adenocarcinomas and usually arise in the antrum. The edges are usually heaped up and serpiginous with a central ulcer bed. Polypoid and villous architecture may be present. Nodularity around the edge of an ulcer or an exophytic component is more common in carcinomas. However, some tumors may be ulcerating and lack a heaped up border. Radial mucosal folds are usually absent. Intestinal type carcinomas are associated with chronic atrophic gastritis that causes marked thinning and flattening of the surrounding mucosa. This type of carcinoma is more common in males than females.

Diffuse type (signet ring cell carcinomas) are usually located in the prepyloric region or body of the stomach and can have minimal or absent superficial mucosal involvement. The only sign of an early lesion may be subtle mucosal effacement or erosion, which may be better appreciated in a fixed, pinned-out specimen. In advanced lesions the wall of the stomach is markedly thickened due to the infiltrative nature of the malignant cells (linitis plastica) but the muscularis propria can still be identified and appears thickened and hypertrophic. It may be difficult to determine the extent of the tumor grossly. There is a similar incidence in males and females.

Lymphomas can have a gross appearance very similar to signet ring cell carcinomas with little or no mucosal involvement (i.e., ulceration). Although they also commonly present in the distal stomach, they rarely involve the pyloric region. The gross appearance may resemble hypertrophied mucosal folds or may appear to be a large mass, sometimes with perforation. The wall may appear diffusely thickened (linitis plastica).

Microscopic sections

Lesion
Four or fewer sections including deepest penetration of wall and radial sections of ulcers.

Margins
Representative proximal margin, distal margin, and deep margin (three sections). If esophagus is included, take an en face (not transverse) section of that margin. Take stomach margin en face if the tumor is far from this margin. Take sections perpendicular to the margin (and through the tumor if possible) if the tumor is close to the margin.

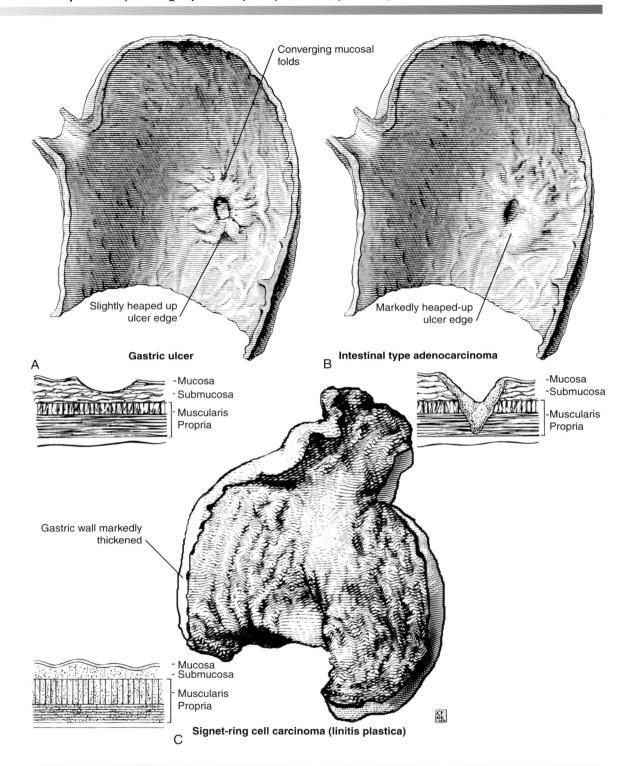

Converging mucosal folds

Slightly heaped up ulcer edge

Gastric ulcer

A

- Mucosa
- Submucosa
- Muscularis Propria

Markedly heaped-up ulcer edge

Intestinal type adenocarcinoma

B

- Mucosa
- Submucosa
- Muscularis Propria

Gastric wall markedly thickened

- Mucosa
- Submucosa
- Muscularis Propria

Signet-ring cell carcinoma (linitis plastica)

C

Figure 19-2 Gross appearances of stomach lesions.

Stomach
Representative sections of cardia, fundus, and antrum if not included in other sections.

Lymph nodes
Submit all lymph nodes.

Sample gross description

Received fresh, labeled with the patient's name and unit number and "stomach," is a 20 (greater curvature) × 15 (lesser curvature) × 15 (circumference of proximal margin) × 5 cm (circumference of distal margin) total gastrectomy specimen with attached portion of duodenum (1.5 cm in length × 5 cm in circumference). The maximal wall thickness is 1.2 cm. There is a 3 × 2.5 cm firm tan/pink polypoid tumor with central ulceration located on the lesser curvature, which is 5 cm from the proximal margin and 7 cm from the distal margin. The tumor grossly invades through the muscularis propria into perigastric soft tissue, but is 0.2 cm from the deep (serosal) inked margin. The remainder of the mucosal surface is unremarkable. The gastric wall is not thickened away from the tumor (average thickness 0.5 cm). There is a small amount of attached adipose tissue (approximately 10 × 1 × 1 cm). A single hard white lymph node measuring 1 cm in greatest dimension is present. Five additional small lymph nodes, the largest measuring 0.3 cm in greatest dimension, are present.

Cassettes #1 and 2: Deepest invasion by tumor and deep margin, 2 frags, RSS.
Cassettes #3 and 4: Tumor and adjacent mucosa, 2 frags, RSS.
Cassette #5: Proximal margin, en face, cardia, 1 frag, RSS.
Cassette #6: Distal margin, en face, duodenum, 1 frag, RSS.
Cassette #7: Fundus, 1 frag, RSS.
Cassette #8: Antrum, 1 frag, RSS.
Cassette #9: Large lymph node, 2 frags, ESS.
Cassettes #10 and 11: Five lymph nodes, 5 frags, ESS.

Pathologic prognostic/diagnostic features sign-out checklist for stomach carcinomas

Specimen type*
Incisional biopsy, excisional biopsy, partial gastrectomy, total gastrectomy, other.

Tumor site*
Cardia (<2 or 2 cm distal to GE junction), fundus (anterior or posterior wall), body (anterior or posterior wall, greater or lesser curvature), antrum/pylorus (anterior or posterior wall, greater or lesser curvature).
If the carcinoma involves the GE junction, the anatomic location of the center of the tumor and the proportion of the tumor in the esophagus and stomach should be given to aid in determining if the carcinoma is gastric or esophageal.

Histologic type*
Adenocarcinoma (intestinal or diffuse type), papillary adenocarcinoma, tubular adenocarcinoma, signet ring cell carcinoma (>50% signet ring cells), mucinous adenocarcinoma (>50% mucinous), carcinoma in situ (or high grade/severe dysplasia), other rare types.

Histologic grade
Well, moderate, poor, undifferentiated (Box 19-3 and Table 19-5).

Extent of invasion*
In situ (Tis), invasion into lamina propria (T1a) or submucosa (T1b), muscularis propria (T2a) or subserosa (T2b), penetration of visceral peritoneum (T3), invasion of adjacent structures or organs (T4).

Regional lymph nodes*
Number of positive nodes: metastasis in 1 to 6 nodes (N1), metastasis in 7 to 15 nodes (N2), metastasis in more than 15 nodes (N3).
Total number of nodes examined. At least 15 lymph nodes should be examined.

Tumor configuration (Box 19-4)
Exophytic (polypoid), infiltrative, ulcerating, ulcerating and infiltrative, diffusely infiltrative (linitis plastica).

Tumor size*

Greatest dimension.

Lymphatic (small vessel) invasion

Present or absent.

Venous (large vessel) invasion

Present or absent.

Perineural invasion

Present or absent.

Margins*

Proximal, distal, radial (omental), distance from closest margin, invasive or in situ carcinoma or adenoma.

Nonlesional mucosa

Chronic gastritis, *H. pylori*, intestinal metaplasia, dysplasia, atrophic gastritis, polyps (types, size).

Post-treatment changes

Location and extent of residual tumor.

This checklist incorporates information from the ADASP (see www.panix.com/~adasp) and the CAP Cancer Committee protocols for reporting on cancer specimens (see www.cap.org/). The asterisked elements are considered to be scientifically validated or regularly used data elements that must be present in reports of cancer-directed surgical resection specimens from ACS CoC-approved cancer programs. The specific details of reporting the elements may vary among institutions.

Box 19-3 Gastric adenocarcinoma: CAP recommended grading system

Grade 1	Well differentiated (>95% of tumor composed of glands)
Grade 2	Moderately differentiated (50–95% of tumor composed of glands)
Grade 3	Poorly differentiated (<49% of tumor composed of glands)
Grade 4	Undifferentiated (cannot be determined to be squamous or adenocarcinoma)

Tubular carcinomas are not usually graded but would correspond to grade 1.
Signet ring cell carcinomas are not typically graded but would correspond to grade 3.
Small cell carcinomas and undifferentiated carcinomas are not typically graded but would correspond to grade 4.

Box 19-4 Gross configuration of gastric carcinomas

Borrmann type I	Polypoid
Borrmann type II	Ulcerating
Borrmann type III	Ulcerating and infiltrating
Borrmann type IV	Diffusely infiltrating (linitis plastica)

Types I and II have been shown to have a better prognosis than types III and IV in some (but not all) studies.

Classification of gastric carcinomas according to the Japanese Research Society for Gastric Carcinoma, Lewin KJ, Appelman HD. Tumors of the esophagus and stomach, Fascicle 18, Third Series. AFIP, Washington, DC., 1995.

Table 19-4 AJCC (6th edition) classification of stomach carcinomas

Tumor	TX	Primary tumor cannot be assessed
	T0	No evidence of primary tumor
	Tis	Carcinoma in situ: intraepithelial tumor without invasion of the lamina propria
	T1	Tumor invades lamina propria or submucosa
	T1a[a]	Tumor invades lamina propria (mucosa)
	T1b[a]	Tumor invades submucosa
	T2	Tumor invades muscularis propria or the subserosa (this includes tumors that invade into the gastrocolic or gastrohepatic ligaments or into the greater or lesser omentum without perforation of the visceral peritoneum)
	T2a	Tumor invades muscularis propria
	T2b	Tumor invades subserosa
	T3	Tumor penetrates the serosa (visceral peritoneum) without invasion of adjacent structures
	T4	Tumor invades adjacent structures (e.g., spleen, transverse colon, liver, diaphragm, pancreas, abdominal wall, adrenal gland, kidney, small intestine, and retroperitoneum)
Regional lymph nodes	NX	Regional lymph node(s) cannot be assessed
	N0	No regional lymph node metastasis
	N1	Metastasis in 1 to 6 regional lymph node(s)
	N2	Metastasis in 7 to 15 regional lymph nodes.
	N3	Metastasis in more than 15 regional lymph nodes

Regional lymph nodes are perigastric lymph nodes(s) found along the greater or lesser curvatures and the nodes located along the left gastric, common hepatic, splenic, or celiac arteries, or in the greater or lesser omentum. Involvement of other intra-abdominal lymph nodes, such as the hepatoduodenal, retropancreatic, mesenteric, and para-aortic, is classified as distant metastasis.

Distant metastasis	MX	Distant metastasis cannot be assessed
	M0	No distant metastasis
	M1	Distant metastasis

[a] These subcategories are not yet part of the AJCC staging system. The T1 subcategories differ in the incidence of lymph node metastases.
The AJCC classification applies only to carcinomas, and should not be used for carcinoid tumors, lymphomas, or sarcomas.

Table 19-5 Grading system for gastric adenocarcinoma[2]

FEATURE	WELL (1)	MODERATE (2)	POOR (3)	UNDIFFERENTIATED (4)
Gland formation	Well developed	Less well developed, cribriform or acinar patterns	Poor gland formation, loss of cell cohesion, small clusters of cells	No gland formation, solid sheets of cells
Stroma	Desmoplasia present but less pronounced	Desmoplasia present but less pronounced	Desmoplastic	Desmoplastic
Cell types	Well differentiated, specialized types may be present	Some differentiation	Minimal differentiation. Most signet ring cell carcinomas belong in this group	No differentiation

■ SMALL INTESTINE

The small intestine is subject to immunologic disease (e.g., sprue or Crohn disease), infectious disease (e.g., *Giardia*, *Cryptosporidium*, or rarely *Isospora*), ischemia, and neoplasms (carcinoids, lymphomas, ampullary adenomas, adenocarcinomas, and leiomyosarcomas).

Relevant clinical history (in addition to age and gender)

See Table 19-6.

Table 19-6 Relevant clinical history (in addition to age and gender)	
HISTORY RELEVANT TO ALL SPECIMENS	HISTORY RELEVANT TO SMALL BOWEL SPECIMENS
Organ/tissue resected or biopsied	Celiac disease (or other cause of malabsorption)
Purpose of the procedure	Inherited polyposis syndromes (including familial adenomatous polyposis, hereditary non-polyposis colon cancer, and Peutz–Jeghers syndrome, see "Hereditary Tumor Syndromes" Table 17-36)
Gross appearance of the organ/tissue/lesion sampled	
Any unusual features of the clinical presentation	
Any unusual features of the gross appearance	Crohn disease
Prior surgery/biopsies—results	
Prior malignancy	
Prior treatment (radiation therapy, chemotherapy, drug use that can change the histologic appearance of tissues)	
Compromised immune system	

Biopsy

Biopsies are usually performed to evaluate patients with malabsorption and less commonly for neoplasms.

Processing the specimen

1. Specimens submitted in formalin can be processed like other small biopsies (see Chapter 13).
2. Some specimens may be submitted in Hollendes, possibly a better fixative for histologic detail. The biopsies are on mesh to preserve orientation. The biopsies must fix in Hollendes for 2 to 4 hours.
3. Each biopsy with the attached mesh is wrapped together in lens paper. Submit each biopsy in a separate cassette in order for each one to be oriented by the histotechnologist. Tissue fixed in Hollendes must be washed in water for at least 3 hours up to overnight. Transfer to formalin and submit after washing.

Special studies

Systemic mastocytosis

Rarely, biopsies are received in saline for evaluation of systemic mastocytosis. These specimens are submitted for EM plastic-embedded thick sections and toluidine blue staining to look for mast cells (mast cells degranulate in formalin fixative) (see Table 7-32).

Resection

The small bowel is usually resected as part of a larger resection (Whipple, right colectomy), for inflammatory bowel disease (e.g., Crohn disease), or for ischemic bowel (e.g., due to a volvulus). Resection for primary tumors is unusual. Although carcinoid is the most common neoplasm, lymphoma, adenomas, adenocarcinoma, and gastrointestinal stromal tumor are occasionally seen.

Resections for tumors can be processed in the same manner as colon resections. If the resection is for Crohn disease, follow the guidelines for examination of the specimen and microscopic sections in the "Colon" section, below.

If the small intestine has been resected due to ischemia, sample the margins, the ischemic portion, and vessels found in the mesentery to look for vascular lesions such as atherosclerosis, thrombi, or vasculitis.

Pathologic prognostic/diagnostic features sign-out checklist for small intestine tumors

Specimen type*
Polypectomy, segmental resection, Whipple procedure, other organs included.

Tumor site*
Segment of small intestine, if known (duodenum, jejunum, ileum).

Tumor configuration
Exophytic (polypoid), infiltrative, ulcerating.

Tumor size*
Size of greatest dimension (and in 3 dimensions).

Histologic type*
Carcinoid, adenoma, adenocarcinoma, signet ring cell carcinoma (>50% signet ring cells), mucinous adenocarcinoma (>50% mucinous), squamous cell carcinoma, all others rare.

Histologic grade* (Box 19-5)
Carcinomas: well, moderately, poorly, undifferentiated (similar to stomach and colorectal carcinomas).

Extent of invasion*
In situ (Tis), invasion into lamina propria or submucosa (T1), invasion into muscularis propria (T2), invasion through muscularis propria into subserosa or the nonperitonealized perimuscular tissue with extension of 2 cm or less (T3), perforation of the visceral peritoneum, invasion into retroperitoneal soft tissue (specify distance in cm) or directly invades other organs or structures (T4).

Regional lymph nodes*
Number of positive nodes and total number of nodes, with locations specified when possible.

Distant metastases*
Absent (M0) or present (M1).

Lymphatic invasion
Present or absent, intramural or extramural.

Perineural invasion
Present or absent.

Margins*
Proximal, distal, serosal, distance to margin, radial (circumferential) margin for retroperitoneal carcinomas, specify invasive or in situ carcinoma or adenoma.
Pancreatic and bile duct margins for Whipple resections.

Nontumorous bowel

Crohn disease, celiac disease, polyps, epithelial dysplasia, ulcers, strictures

If polyps are present, specify type, sessile or pedunculated, presence or absence of high-grade dysplasia or adenocarcinoma.

Staging information

Note that AJCC staging (Table 19-7) is slightly different from staging for colonic carcinomas.

This checklist incorporates information from the ADASP (see www.panix.com/~adasp) and the CAP Cancer Committee protocols for reporting on cancer specimens (see www.cap.org/). The asterisked elements are considered to be scientifically validated or regularly used data elements that must be present in reports of cancer-directed surgical resection specimens from ACS CoC-approved cancer programs. The specific details of reporting the elements may vary among institutions.

Box 19-5 Histologic grade of small intestine carcinomas

Grade 1	Well differentiated (>95% of tumor composed of glands) with <5% of solid or cord-like growth patterns
Grade 2	Moderately differentiated (50–95% of tumor composed of glands) with 5% to 50% solid or cord-like growth patterns
Grade 3	Poorly differentiated (<50% of tumor composed of glands) with >50% of solid or cord-like growth patterns
Grade 4	Undifferentiated carcinoma and small cell carcinoma

Table 19-7 AJCC (6th edition) classification for small intestine carcinomas

Tumor	TX	Primary tumor cannot be assessed
	T0	No evidence of primary tumor
	Tis	Carcinoma in situ
	T1	Tumor invades lamina propria or submucosa
	T2	Tumor invades the muscularis propria
	T3	Tumor invades through the muscularis propria into the subserosa or into the non-peritonealized perimuscular tissue (mesentery or retroperitoneum) with extension 2 cm or less. The non-peritonealized perimuscular tissue is, for jejunum and ileum, part of the mesentery and, for duodenum in areas where serosa is lacking, part of the retroperitoneum
	T4	Tumor perforates the visceral peritoneum, or directly invades other organs or structures (includes other loops of small intestine, mesentery, or retroperitoneum more than 2 cm, and abdominal wall by way of serosa; for duodenum only, invasion of pancreas)
Regional lymph nodes	NX	Regional lymph nodes cannot be assessed
	N0	No regional lymph node metastasis
	N1	Regional lymph node metastasis
Metastasis	MX	Distant metastasis cannot be assessed
	M0	No distant metastasis
	M1	Distant metastasis

Note: This classification is not used for carcinoma arising at the ileocecal valve, carcinomas arising in Meckel's diverticulum, carcinomas arising in the ampulla of Vater, carcinoid tumors, sarcomas, or lymphomas.

■ MECKEL'S DIVERTICULUM

Meckel's diverticulum is persistence of a portion of the vitelline duct and is always present on the antimesenteric border of the small bowel. This is a "true" congenital diverticulum that has a complete muscular wall (unlike the acquired sigmoid diverticula of diverticulosis or the esophageal Zenker's diverticulum: both lack complete muscular walls). Ectopic tissue (gastric, pancreatic) may be found within the diverticulum. Often a diverticulum is removed because the ectopic gastric mucosa produces acid and causes ulceration; rarely, a diverticulum causes intussusception or is involved by tumor.

Processing the specimen

1. Orient the specimen. The specimen usually consists of a segmental resection of the ileum with a small outpouching from the wall (it often is the size and shape of an appendix). Record the dimensions of the ileum (length and circumference) and diverticulum (length and diameter). Examine the ileal mucosa for ulceration, erosion, or inflammation (sometimes seen with production of acid by ectopic gastric mucosa).
2. The diverticulum can be processed like an appendix. Cut off the tip and submit one of the longitudinal sections. Submit a second cassette with cross-sections of the middle portion. Look carefully for heterogeneous areas. Ectopic gastric mucosa or pancreatic parenchyma is often found.

   Submit the two margins of the ileum and representative sections of any lesions present.

■ COLON

The most common surgical diseases of the colon are neoplasms (almost all adenocarcinomas or adenomatous polyps), inflammatory bowel disease (both ulcerative colitis and Crohn disease), diverticulosis, and rarely hemorrhage from ectatic blood vessels.

Relevant clinical history (in addition to age and gender)

See Table 19-8.

Table 19-8 Relevant clinical history (in addition to age and gender)	
HISTORY RELEVANT TO ALL SPECIMENS	HISTORY RELEVANT TO COLON SPECIMENS
Organ/tissue resected or biopsied	Inflammatory bowel disease (type, history of dysplasia)
Purpose of the procedure	Inherited polyposis syndromes (including familial adenomatous polyposis, hereditary non-polyposis colon cancer, and Peutz–Jeghers syndrome, see "Hereditary Tumor Syndromes" Table 17-36)
Gross appearance of the organ/tissue/lesion sampled	
Any unusual features of the clinical presentation	→ pedunculated polyp or ulcerated mass
Any unusual features of the gross appearance	Colonic bleeding
Prior surgery/biopsies—results	
Prior malignancy	
Prior treatment (radiation therapy, chemotherapy, drug use that can change the histologic appearance of tissues)	
Compromised immune system	

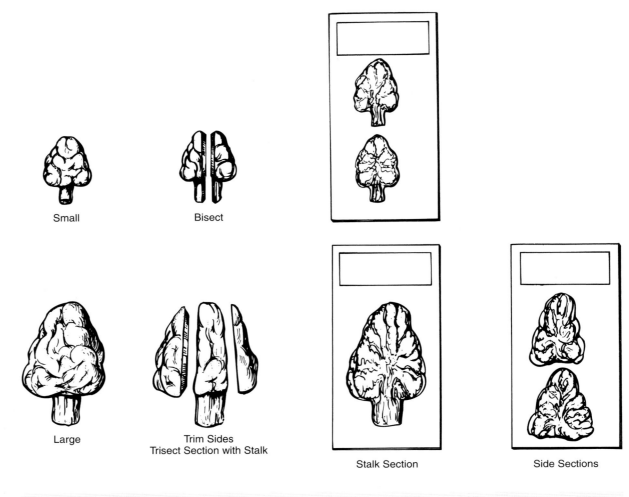

Figure 19-3 Polypectomies.

Biopsies

Most biopsies can be processed as described in Chapter 13.

Small or large pedunculated polyps can be removed during colonoscopy. "Hot" polypectomies are polyps removed with a cauterizing wire: the presence of a cautery artifact may allow identification of the surgical margin.

Processing the specimen: Polyps (Fig. 19-3)

1. Describe size, color, surface configuration (polypoid or villiform), and the base of the polyp (sessile, stalk: include length and width). Often the stalks (consisting of normal mucosa pulled out by the polyp) retract into the base and are difficult to see.
2. Always ink the base, if possible. The presence of cautery artifact is also a helpful landmark for the location of the margin.

   Small polyps. Bisect the polyp along the vertical plane of the stalk to reveal the surgical margin and submit both halves in one cassette. Order three levels on this section if the polyp is over 1 cm in size.

   Large polyps. If the head of the polyp is too wide to fit in a cassette, trim the sides away from the stalk. Submit the sections of the stalk in a designated cassette and order three levels. The peripheral fragments not containing the stalk are submitted in a separate cassette and can be examined in one level.

Special studies

Hirschsprung disease

Children with constipation may undergo endoscopic or open biopsy. Normal bowel has nerve fibers and ganglion cells in the submucosa and muscularis propria with thin nerve fibers extending to the muscularis mucosa. In Hirschsprung disease, ganglion cells are absent from the submucosal (and myenteric) plexuses. Frozen tissue may be used for acetylcholinesterase reactions to demonstrate coarse, irregular nerve fibers that extend from the muscularis propria to the lamina propria. Similar findings can be seen with neurofibromatosis, Crohn disease, and neuronal dysplasia (see Table 7–36).

Identification of colon segments

Large resections of colon are often submitted as specimens with nonspecific labels such as "colon" or misleading labels such as "sigmoid" when the specimen is actually recto-sigmoid. It is important to identify all the anatomical subdivisions of the resected bowel. This is especially important in distinguishing rectal from sigmoid carcinomas as they have different natural histories, prognostic features, and treatment. Use Figures 19-4, 19-5, Table 19-9 and the following descriptions to identify specimens. Isolated portions of the ascending, descending, and sigmoid colon cannot be distinguished by morphologic features.

Typical specimens

Rectosigmoid

To preserve the anal sphincter only a limited amount of rectum can be resected. The tumor is usually very close to the distal end of the specimen, as no more colon can be resected in this

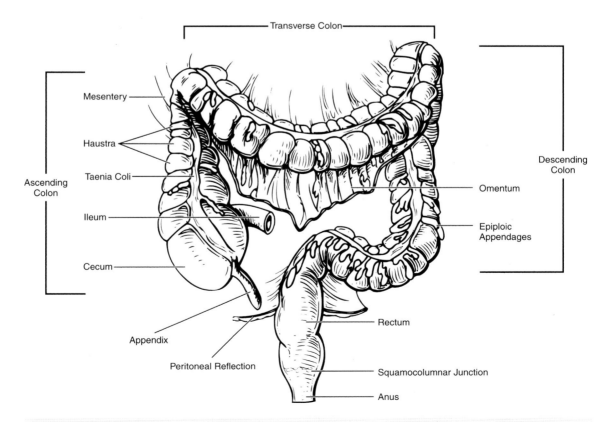

Figure 19-4 Gross anatomy of the colon.

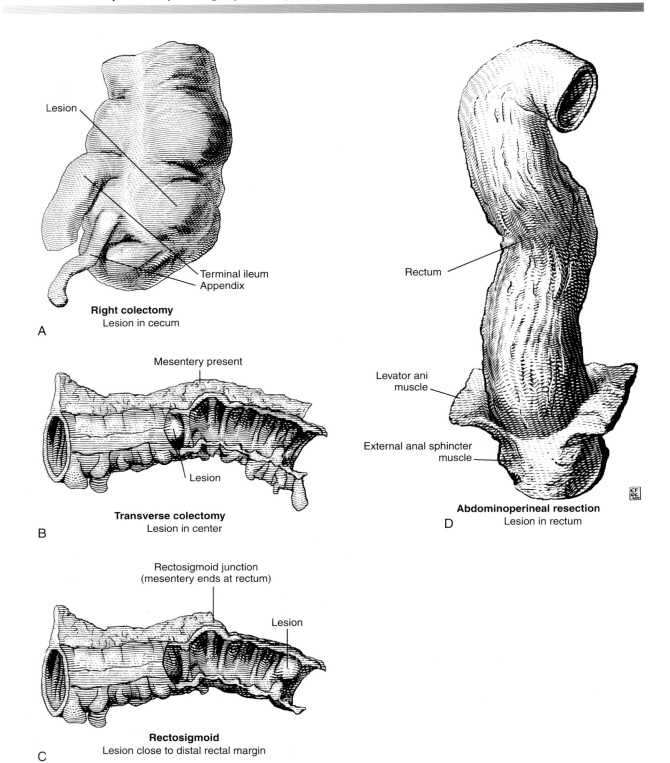

Right colectomy
Lesion in cecum

Lesion
Terminal ileum
Appendix

A

Transverse colectomy
Lesion in center

Mesentery present
Lesion

B

Rectosigmoid
Lesion close to distal rectal margin

Rectosigmoid junction
(mesentery ends at rectum)
Lesion

C

Abdominoperineal resection
Lesion in rectum

Rectum
Levator ani
muscle
External anal sphincter
muscle

D

Figure 19-5 Common colon resections.

Table 19-9 Gross features of colon segments

COLON SEGMENTS	SEROSA	TAENIAE COLI	EPIPLOIC APPENDAGES	MESENTERY	OMENTUM
Ileum	Present	Absent	Absent	Present	Absent
Appendix	Present	Present	Present or absent	Present	Absent
Cecum	Present	Present	Absent	Absent	Absent
Ascending colon	Present	Present	Present	Present or absent	Absent
Transverse colon	Present	Present	Present	Present	Present
Descending colon	Present	Present	Present	Present or absent	Absent
Sigmoid	Present	Present	Present	Present	Absent
Rectum	Absent	Absent	Absent	Absent	Absent
Anus	Absent	Absent	Absent	Absent	Absent

Taeniae coli: Three longitudinal bands of muscle.
Haustra: Sacculation of wall due to taeniae coli.
Epiploic appendages: Pouches of peritoneum filled with fat.

area without removing the anal sphincter. The transition from the sigmoid to the rectum is marked by the fusion of the longitudinal taeniae coli of the sigmoid to form the complete outer longitudinal muscle sheath of the rectum. However, it is easier to mark the transition to the rectum by identifying the end of the mesentery and the peritoneal serosal surface. Specifically, the rectum is covered by peritoneum on its anterior and lateral sides in the upper third, only the anterior aspect in the middle third, and has no peritoneal covering over the lower third. The point at which the peritoneal covering no longer completely surrounds the bowel segment is the rectosigmoid junction. In the gross description and in the final report, state the location of the tumor within the specimen (i.e., "sigmoid," "rectal," or "rectosigmoid junction").

The distance to the distal, usually closest, margin is important to document. Immediate examination after excision (before the colon contracts) is optimal. The length of this margin may be used to decide whether post-surgical radiation therapy is required.

Right colectomy

This specimen consists of terminal ileum (which may be very short, only 1 to 2 cm, but is invariably present), cecum (has a wider lumen than the remainder of the colon), appendix (may have been removed by previous surgery), and a variable length of ascending colon. The ileo-cecal valve is used as a landmark for measurement of the lengths of the ileum and colon. The proximal portion of the ascending colon may be retroperitoneal; the distal portion is on a mesentery. The transverse colon has a mesentery and is usually not included in the resection.

Transverse colon

This is the only portion of the colon with omentum. The omentum is sometimes submitted separately. The transverse colon is entirely intraperitoneal (i.e., surrounded by visceral peritoneum/serosa).

Abdominoperineal (A-P) resection

The specimen consists of perianal skin, anus, and rectum, and may include sigmoid. This procedure is used to resect tumors of the low rectum and anal tumors located at or near the anal sphincter.

The anus is a complex structure, usually 3 to 4 cm in length, demarcated by the proximal and distal margins of the internal sphincter muscle.[3] The luminal surface is marked proximally by longitudinal folds (the rectal columns) that interface with distal folds (the anal columns) at the zone of transition from colonic to anal mucosa (the pectinate or dentate line). Anal papillae are raised projections of anal mucosa that extend upward on the rectal columns. Between the rectal columns are depressions termed rectal sinuses. The anal columns are linked circumferentially at the dentate line by transverse plicae, known as anal or semilunar valves, which delineate the anal crypts. Although prominent in young persons, they may be indistinct or absent in adults.

There are many different definitions of what constitutes the anal canal. The surgical definition is most widely accepted and is used by the AJCC. It is based on clinically identifiable landmarks that are difficult to define in surgical specimens. The start of the anal canal is defined as the point where the rectum enters the puborectalis sling at the apex of the anal sphincter complex, which can be palpated clinically as the anorectal ring. By this definition, the upper portion of the anal canal is lined by 1 to 2 cm of rectal-type glandular mucosa and transitional (cloacogenic) mucosa (if present) at the dentate line (anal transition zone) and the lower portion by the non-keratinized squamous epithelium that extends to the perianal hair-bearing skin. On the anal papillae, the squamous and columnar mucosa interface directly.

Bowel rings

Separate specimens of small rings of colon, sometimes on a plastic rod, may be received. These are the products of the stapler that creates the surgical anastomosis. These rings represent the true margins of the specimen. Examine them for lesions and submit representative sections. Make sure that the submitted tissue does not contain staples or suture material.

Total colectomy with ileo-anal pull-through reconstruction

The technique is performed for ulcerative colitis or familial adenomatous polyposis. The specimen includes terminal ileum to rectum and a second specimen designated "rectal mucosa." The subdivisions of the total colectomy specimen (ileum, cecum, colon, and rectum) are identified and described as above. To perform the pull-through, the surgeon dissects the rectal mucosa off the internal anal sphincter along the plane of the submucosa, generating an unoriented and traumatized collar of rectal tissue that is submitted as a separate specimen. The muscularis propria (i.e., the "sphincter") is not removed. One representative section of this latter specimen is submitted.

Rectal resection

Small tumors of the rectum may be resected transanally without removing an entire circumferential segment in order to preserve the sphincter. The specimens are usually small and consist of an ovoid fragment of mucosa, submucosa, and superficial muscularis propria consisting almost entirely of tumor with a 1 to 2 mm rim of uninvolved mucosa around the tumor. The normal mucosa may curl under and may be difficult to see. Careful orientation, inking, fixation, and evaluation of all margins by taking perpendicular sections is very important to evaluate the completeness of the excision.

Processing resection specimens

See sections below for specific instructions depending on the underlying disease process.

1. Identify and record the components of the colon present. Palpate the specimen to identify the location of mass lesions. If no mass lesion is present, open the specimen along the antimesenteric border using blunt scissors. If a mass lesion is present, cut through an area of uninvolved mucosa and wall.

   For some specimens, primarily those with diverticular disease, inflation of the bowel segment with formalin is advantageous, followed by further dissection (see "Diverticulosis," below).

   Clean the lumen using saline. Record the dimensions of each of the components of the specimen (length and circumference) including length of mesentery and size of omentum if present. If a mass lesion or stricture is present, document any dilatation of the lumen proximal to the lesion. Record the bowel wall thickness and any variation in thickness (e.g., tumor, stricture, or muscular hypertrophy associated with diverticulosis).

2. Identify and describe any lesions (see Gross differential diagnosis). The distance of lesions (especially invasive carcinomas) from margins is noted.

   Bowel segments may contract as much as 40% within 10 to 20 minutes of resection,[4] therefore margins are best measured as soon as possible after excision. The distal margin of rectal carcinomas is typically short (due to the desire to avoid resecting the anal sphincter) and the length of this margin may indicate the need for postoperative radiation therapy (e.g., if the margin is <2 cm in length).

3. **Tumor cases.** Identify all lymph nodes present.[5,6] The fat can be stripped off the colon and placed in Bouin's. *However*, leave the fat at the deep margin of tumors intact and do not strip the fat in cases of diverticulosis (this maneuver will also remove the base of the diverticula). Soft tissue nodules in continuity with the main tumor mass must be described as such and submitted in designated cassettes. If there is no histologic evidence of residual lymph node, such nodules are usually best interpreted as direct spread of tumor. Well-circumscribed soft tissue nodules with a smooth outer contour that are separate from the main tumor mass are classified as nodal metastasis, even in the absence of definitive nodal architecture.

   The number of lymph nodes present will depend on the length of the specimen. At least 20 should be present in an entire colectomy. In segmental resections, at least 12 (the minimum number considered necessary for accurate staging) are usually present. The minimum number of nodes that should be found is controversial. If fewer than 12 are identified, post-fix in Bouin's and look again and/or submit any areas that grossly may represent nodes. Lymph nodes in these specimens tend to be small (<0.5 cm) even when involved by metastatic disease.

   There may be prognostic significance if metastases are present in proximal or distal lymph nodes with respect to the tumor. If the specimen can be oriented (e.g., right colectomy, rectosigmoid colectomy, obstructing tumors with obvious proximal dilatation of the bowel lumen, or as oriented by surgeon), lymph nodes can be examined as separate groups. Strip the fat as above but keep proximal and distal soft tissue in separate containers of Bouin's. Identify lymph nodes in cassettes as "distal" or "proximal."

   Non-tumor cases. Abnormal lymph nodes (enlarged, hard) must be diligently sought and submitted for examination. Occasionally, a tumor is first discovered by finding unsuspected lymph node metastases. However, it is not necessary to extensively search for and document at least 12 nodes. Only one block of the largest nodes found may be submitted. If carcinoma is found to be present after microscopic examination, however, all nodes should be retrieved and submitted.

4. Pin the colon out on a paraffin block. Float it upside down in formalin overnight.

5. Submit sections including representative sections of all components present (e.g., ileum, appendix, ascending colon, sigmoid, rectum) and all lesions (including polyps) present. Submit at least one representative block from grossly uninvolved colon mucosa (this can also serve as a margin if grossly normal). Submit sections of margins that are within 5 cm

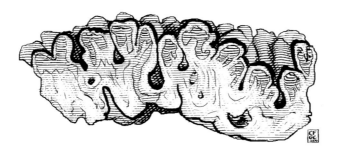

Figure 19-6 Cross-section of bowel showing diverticulosis.

of the carcinoma. Grossly normal margins that are more than 5 cm from the carcinoma need not be submitted. Submit all lymph nodes (see above).

Gross differential diagnosis

Diverticulosis (Fig. 19-6)

Diverticulosis of the descending colon and sigmoid is a common disease. The colon is resected after multiple episodes of diverticulitis. The muscularis propria becomes markedly hypertrophied (presumably due to long-term straining at stool), resulting in a thickened bowel wall and a narrowed lumen. The increased intraluminal pressure causes herniation of mucosa through weak points in the muscularis propria adjacent to the penetrating vasculature on either side of each taenia coli. These are false diverticula because they lack a complete muscular coat. True diverticula (e.g., Meckel's diverticulum or a solitary cecal diverticulum) have a complete muscle coat and are thought to be congenital in origin.

The best demonstration of diverticula requires the intact specimen to be inflated with formalin. Close off the ends with hemostats or twine and fix overnight. Open along the antimesenteric side or hemisect. The fat should not be stripped from the specimen, as this will also remove the diverticula.

A metal probe can be used to find the ostia of the diverticula. Count the number of diverticula or estimate the number if there are many. Sections of diverticula can be obtained by cutting in the plane of the probe. Sample areas of interdiverticular mucosa (2 to 3 sections) to look for superimposed diverticulosis-associated colitis, inflammatory bowel disease, or ischemia.

If the history is of diverticulitis or there is gross evidence of perforation (induration of pericolonic fat, a serosal exudate, hemorrhage, pericolonic necrosis), the perforated diverticulum should be identified. Probe the diverticula in the most inflamed area and cut cross-sections. A perforated diverticulum shows effacement of the mucosa associated with necrosis and hemorrhage in the surrounding soft tissue. If the wall of the diverticulum can be seen, then it is not perforated and it is just an adjacent diverticulum surrounded by the inflammation. Submit sections of all diverticula that appear to be inflamed. In a case of peritonitis, lack of a documented site of perforation can constitute a medical emergency because the site of perforation is presumably still within the patient.

> *Linguistic note*
>
> *The plural form of diverticulum is diverticula, not diverticuli or diverticulae as is commonly believed (look it up in the dictionary!).*

Solitary cecal diverticulum

Patients usually present with symptoms of acute appendicitis. However, at surgery the appendix appears normal and a pericecal abscess is found. Often a right colectomy is performed. A solitary cecal diverticulum is thought to be congenital in origin (it is a true diverticulum with a complete muscular wall), is usually located within a few centimeters of the ileo-cecal valve, and has a broad orifice (as opposed to the narrow orifices of diverticulosis).

Vascular ectasia (angiodysplasia)

Vascular ectasia is a degenerative acquired lesion of older adults (>60 years) and usually presents as bleeding from the cecum or ascending colon. Clinical arteriography may reveal bleeding from an area of ectatic vessels and embolization is sometimes attempted. The lesion consists of multiple small (5 to 10 mm) areas of ectatic thin-walled vessels in the submucosa and mucosa that rupture and bleed. The pathogenesis is thought to be obstruction of veins passing through the muscularis propria due to high wall tension in the right colon (Laplace's law predicts the highest wall tension in the area of greatest bowel diameter).

The specimen is usually unrevealing grossly because bleeding has usually been controlled at the time of surgery. There may be small petechial hemorrhages or areas of congestion; commonly, there are no mucosal lesions. The area most often affected is near the cecum and the first 10 cm of ascending colon. Take sections of any mucosal lesions. If no lesion is visible, look on the outer surface of the specimen for the major vessels tied off with sutures. If sections near these vessels are examined, large dilated vessels traversing the muscularis propria are sometimes identified.

Alternative methods have been developed to demonstrate these lesions.[7,8]

Inflammatory bowel disease (Fig. 19-7, Table 19-10)

Segments of bowel may be removed in Crohn disease because of complications (e.g., strictures, fistulas) or a total colectomy may be performed for long-standing ulcerative colitis (UC) due to the increased risk of carcinoma.

Ulcerative colitis and Crohn disease can be distinguished in resected segments of bowel by their gross features (Table 19-10). Typically, segments of large or small bowel involved by Crohn disease do not lie flat when opened due to the transmural inflammation and thickening of the bowel wall. Mesenteric fat also surrounds a greater portion of the bowel circumference ("creeping substitution"). In contrast, since UC involves only the mucosa, the bowel flattens out once opened, similar to normal non-inflamed bowel.

The pattern of mucosal involvement is an important feature to distinguish UC (which has continuous involvement) from colonic Crohn disease (which can have discontinuous involvement). Sequential sections are taken every 10 cm (including both normal and abnormal appearing mucosa) to determine if the involvement is continuous or patchy. Additional sections of any raised, polypoid areas, or areas of flat mucosa with velvety, villiform, or granular areas are taken as these gross findings may indicate areas of dysplasia or early carcinoma. A mass lesion (mass, plaque-like region, polyp, or group of polyps) associated with microscopic dysplasia is associated with an increased risk of carcinoma (dysplasia-associated lesion or mass, DALM). These lesions are described as to whether they resemble an adenoma (which can possibly be treated with local excision) or do not resemble an adenoma (e.g., broad-based, irregular, associated with a stricture—may be best treated with colectomy).

Gross mucosal disease (aphthous ulcers) at or near (within 1 cm) of the surgical margins of resections for Crohn disease is very useful in determining the likelihood of recurrence after surgery. Microscopic involvement alone (e.g., a single crypt abscess) does not predict recurrence. Gross ulcers present at or near the margins predict a 100% probability of recurrence. Grossly non-ulcerated margins have a 50% risk of recurrence. However, the amount of normal tissue required for adequate margins is controversial.

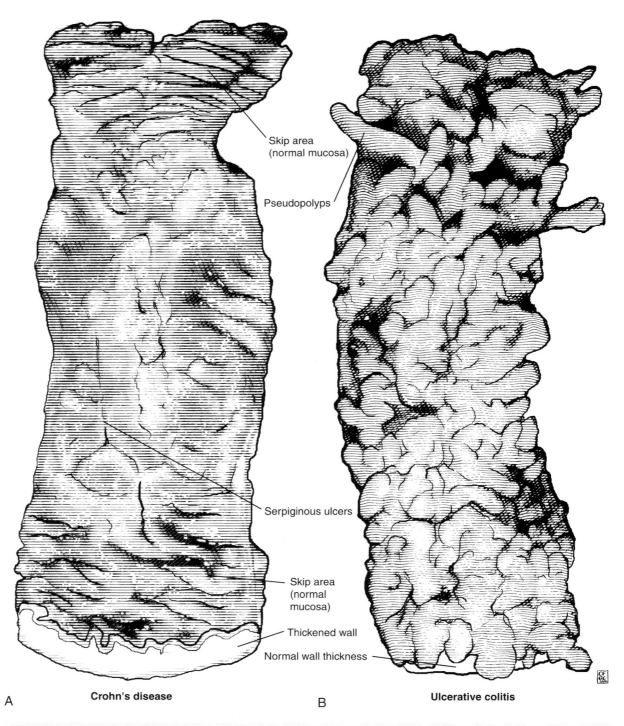

Skip area
(normal mucosa)

Pseudopolyps

Serpiginous ulcers

Skip area
(normal
mucosa)

Thickened wall

Normal wall thickness

A   **Crohn's disease**   B   **Ulcerative colitis**

Figure 19-7 Inflammatory bowel disease.

Table 19-10 Gross features of inflammatory bowel disease in colonic resections

GROSS FEATURE	ULCERATIVE COLITIS	CROHN DISEASE
Distribution	Starts in rectum and spreads proximally. Discontinuous cecal/appendiceal involvement is rarely present (~10%)	Focal involvement with skip lesions; right > left
Depth of inflammation	Mucosal and submucosal	Mucosal, submucosal, or transmural
Mucosal lesions	Irregular geographic ulcers. Adjacent mucosa is hyperemic with an inflammatory exudate. The mucosa may become atrophic	Linear serpiginous ulcers connected by transverse ulcers ("cobblestoning"[a]). The adjacent mucosa is relatively normal in appearance
Pseudopolyps	May be present May have mucosal bridges	May be present May have mucosal bridges
Bowel wall	Not involved or may be fibrotic in late stages	May be relatively normal or thickened and edematous
Creeping substitution[b]	Absent	Often present
Strictures	Usually absent	Occasionally present
Internal fistulas	Usually absent	May be present
Fissuring	Usually absent	Common, but may be absent.
Ileal involvement	Present in <10% of patients ("backwash ileitis" of distal 2–3 cm), with mild superficial active mucosal inflammation only	Present in 50% of patients, often stenotic
Rectal involvement	Present in all patients, but may appear minimal due to prior enema therapy	Present in 15% of patients
Anal involvement	Present in 5–10% of patients, may have a perianal fistula	Present in 75% of patients; fissures, fistulas, and ulcerations are common
Carcinoma	Increased risk	Increased risk

[a] The use of the term "cobblestone appearance" should be avoided because this term is imprecise and is used to describe different findings by clinicians, radiologists, and pathologists. Depending on the way it is used, it may be associated either with Crohn disease or with UC. Be descriptive in the gross dictation. If linear and transverse ulcers are present, describe them as such. If pseudopolyp formation is present (i.e., islands of normal mucosa surrounded by ulcerated areas) describe this accordingly.
[b] Extension of fat onto antimesenteric surface.

Resections for UC are always "complete," i.e., all colonic mucosa is removed leaving the proximal margin in the small intestine. A section from the ileal mucosal margin, designated "proximal mucosal margin," is submitted.

Specimen integrity is better preserved if longitudinal, rather than transverse, sections are taken. Good perpendicular sections of the wall are taken after fixation to help determine wall thickness. The appendix is sampled if present.

Lymph nodes must be searched for and carefully evaluated because of the increased risk of carcinoma associated with inflammatory bowel disease. These cancers can occur in young patients and may be difficult to detect by biopsy due to the extensive inflammatory changes in the mucosa.

Polyposis syndromes

Affected patients may have tens to thousands of colonic polyps. Total colectomy is performed to prevent the development of colon carcinoma. The specimen is carefully examined to look for any lesion suspicious for invasion. All polyps greater than 1 cm in size are sampled. Representative samples from smaller polyps are taken as one section per quadrant (four sections for a total colectomy). Lymph nodes are identified and abnormal nodes submitted for histologic examination.

Tumors (Fig. 19-8)

The description includes:

- **Size.**
- **Appearance.** The typical colonic adenocarcinoma is firm, tan/pink, and has raised serpentine borders with an ulcerated center. Mucinous tumors may produce lakes of gelatinous mucin within the tumor mass or bowel wall.
- **Anatomic depth of invasion** (e.g., into or through the muscularis propria).
- **Location.** If the specimen includes sigmoid colon and rectum, describe the location of the carcinoma with respect to the mesentery (i.e., sigmoid, junction of sigmoid and rectum, or rectal).
- **Distance from margins** including deep or serosal margin. The radial margin represents the adventitial (i.e., non-peritonealized) soft tissue margin closest to the deepest penetration of tumor. This margin is significant for rectal carcinomas and for colon carcinomas penetrating into the mesentery. This margin is not significant for colon carcinomas invading into adipose tissue on the antimesenteric side of the bowel unless the carcinoma penetrates the visceral peritoneum. For segments of colon that are completely surrounded by a peritonealized (serosal) surface (e.g., transverse colon), the only circumferential/radial margin is the mesenteric resection margin.
- **Distance from anatomical landmarks** such as ileo-cecal valve, rectosigmoid junction, squamo-columnar junction).
- **Percent of circumference** occupied by tumor and minimal luminal diameter at the site of the tumor (if the lesion is obstructing, describe the dilation of the proximal colon).
- **Presence or absence of perforation.** There may be induration of surrounding fat, a purulent exudate, and adhesions to other serosal surfaces.

While the specimen is fresh, ink the radial margin at the site of the tumor. The remainder of the fat can be stripped and placed in Bouin's to aid in searching for lymph nodes. It may be useful to separate proximal from distal lymph nodes (see above).

Primary carcinomas versus metastatic carcinomas to the colon

The epicenter of a primary tumor is usually in the mucosa and submucosa and the intraluminal component predominates. Sections from the edge of a primary tumor often reveal continuity with the remainder of the mucosa and association with a preexisting adenoma. The epicenter of metastatic tumors is usually in pericolonic fat (because the tumor originates in a focus of lymphatic spread). The tumor may then invade through the muscularis propria and erode through the overlying mucosa. Metastatic carcinomas usually appear to be erupting upwards from below and may ulcerate the mucosal surface without an exophytic component. Findings consistent with a preexisting polyp are not present, although carcinomas can sometimes grow for a distance along the surface.

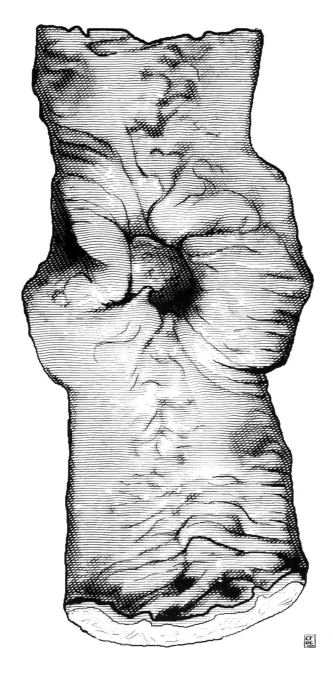

Figure 19-8 Gross appearance of colon carcinoma.

Recurrent colon carcinoma

Carcinomas occasionally recur at a prior colonic resection site. The mucosa heals without scarring and the anastomosis is not grossly evident on the surface. However, surgical staples may be present and the history will support the location of the carcinoma at the prior surgical site.

Melanosis coli

The colonic mucosa is dark brown in color due to the accumulation of pigment in lamina propria histiocytes. The right colon is involved more frequently than the left. This finding is secondary to chronic laxative ingestion and is generally an incidental finding.

Microscopic sections

Tumor

Four or fewer of the tumor including relationship to adjacent mucosa (in situ changes may reveal a preexisting adenoma or exclude metastasis from another site), deepest extent of invasion, and any involvement of contiguous organs.

Other lesions

Representative of all other lesions (e.g., polyps).

Diverticula

One representative section. If resection was for diverticulitis, submit one section of the perforated diverticulum.

Inflammatory bowel

Sequential sections, every 10 cm, including all unusual, raised, or polypoid disease lesions and areas of grossly normal appearing mucosa.

Lymph nodes

All lymph nodes from tumor cases. Submit nodes so that the total number of positive nodes can be determined (e.g. by inking with different colors). If proximal and distal nodes have been separated, submit in separate identified cassettes. See Chapter 27. If cancer is not present, submit all abnormal lymph nodes.

Surgical margins

Proximal and distal margins and the deep margin or serosal surface. The margins may be taken en face if the tumor is far from the margin. If the tumor is close to the margin, the section is taken perpendicular to the margin and through the tumor (if possible). If the tumor is ≥5 cm from the margin, sections need not be submitted if the mucosal surface appears normal.

Normal structures

Any normal components that have not been sampled in the sections already: for example, in a right colectomy the margins are usually a sample of normal colon and ileum but also submit a section of the appendix.

Sample dictation for tumors

Received fresh, labeled with the patient's name and unit number and "colon," is a 35 cm in length segment of rectosigmoid colon which is 6 cm in circumference at the sigmoid margin and 3 cm in circumference at the rectal margin. A 6 cm in length mesentery is present along the 32 proximal cm of the colon and is absent from the distal 3 cm. There is a 2.5 × 3 × 2 cm tan/pink centrally ulcerated tumor with serpiginous borders arising 1 cm distal to the rectosigmoid junction. The tumor invades into, but not through, the muscularis propria. The tumor spares only 0.5 cm of the colon circumference and the lumen is narrowed to approximately 0.5 cm in diameter. The proximal colon is markedly dilated. The tumor is 1 cm from the distal margin and 32 cm from the proximal margin. The remainder of the mucosal surface is unremarkable. Ten firm lymph nodes are present in the pericolonic soft tissue, the largest measuring 0.6 cm in greatest dimension.

Cassettes #1 and 2: Tumor at area of deepest invasion and deep margin, 2 frags, ESS.
Cassette #3: Tumor and adjacent mucosa, 1 frag, RSS.
Cassette #4: Distal margin and tumor, perpendicular, 1 frag, RSS.
Cassette #5–9: Lymph nodes, two per cassette, 10 frags, ESS.

Sample dictation for diverticulitis

The specimen is received fresh, labeled with the patient's name and unit number, in two parts.
The first part, labeled "colon," consists of a segment of colon (12 cm in length by 3 cm in circumference

with one stapled margin and one open margin). The bowel wall is markedly thickened and there are 5 diverticula. The tip of one diverticulum is perforated and is surrounded by a green yellow purulent exudate which also covers the adjacent serosal surface. There is a 0.4 cm pedunculated polyp which is 4 cm from the closest margin (stapled). Three lymph nodes are found in the pericolonic fat.

Cassette #1: Area of perforation, 1 frag, RSS.
Cassette #2: Non-perforated diverticulum, 1 frag, RSS.
Cassette #3: Polyp, 2 frags, ESS.
Cassette #4: Three lymph nodes (inked black, blue, and green), 5 frags, ESS.

The second part, labeled "rings," consists of two ring-shaped sections of colonic mucosa with tan/brown normal-appearing mucosa. One ring is attached to a 5-cm green plastic rod.

Cassette #5: Representative mucosa from both rings, 2 frags, RSS.

Sample dictation for inflammatory bowel disease

The specimen is received in two parts, labeled with the patient's name and unit number.
The first part, labeled "total colectomy," consists of a total colectomy specimen extending from the terminal ileum (4 cm in length by 4 cm in circumference), cecum with appendix (appendix 5 cm in length by 0.8 cm in diameter), and colon (100 cm in length × 5 cm circumference). The mucosal surface over the distal 50 cm is dusky red and has multiple ulcers and pseudopolyp formation. No gross skip lesions are seen. The remainder of the proximal mucosa is tan/brown and unremarkable. The bowel wall is thin and the distribution of the adipose tissue is normal. The ulcerations extend to the distal margin. Twenty lymph nodes are found in the pericolic fat, the largest measuring 0.8 cm in size.

Cassettes #1–10: Sequential sections of colon from distal to proximal, every 10 cm, 10 frags, RSS.
Cassette #11: Terminal ileum, margin, 1 frag, RSS.
Cassette #12: Appendix, 2 frags, RSS.
Cassette #13: Two largest lymph nodes (one inked in black), 4 frags, ESS.
Cassettes #14–19: Three lymph nodes per cassette, 18 frags, ESS.

The second part, labeled "rectum," consists of a mucosal segment measuring 10 cm in length by 4 cm in circumference. The mucosal surface is brown/red and irregular with effacement of the normal mucosal surface. The mucosal changes extend throughout the length of the specimen. No muscularis propria is present.

Cassette #20: Representative sections from one end, 2 frags, RSS.
Cassette #21: Representative sections from opposite end, 2 frags, RSS.

Pathologic prognostic/diagnostic features sign-out checklist for colon and rectal carcinomas

Specimen type*
Right colectomy (include structures present with lengths: terminal ileum, colon, and appendix), segmental resection (length of colon), left hemicolectomy (length of colon), low anterior resection (length of sigmoid and rectum), abdominal perineal resection (length of colon and anus), subtotal colectomy (length of colon), total proctocolectomy (length of terminal ileum, colon, appendix, and rectum).

Tumor site*
Ileocecal valve, cecum, ascending colon, hepatic flexure, transverse colon, splenic flexure, descending colon, sigmoid, rectum.

Tumor configuration
Exophytic (pedunculated or sessile), endophytic (ulcerative), diffusely infiltrative (linitis plastica).

Tumor size*
Greatest dimension (cm), or three dimensions.

Mesorectum
Complete, near complete, incomplete: evaluates the completion of resection of rectal tumors (Box 19-6).

Histologic type*
Adenoma, adenocarcinoma, signet ring cell carcinoma (>50% signet ring cells), mucinous (colloid) adenocarcinoma (>50% mucinous), undifferentiated (no gland formation), "medullary" (solid growth of uniform cells with prominent lymphocytic response: strongly associated with microsatellite instability, may be sporadic or occur in association with the hereditary nonpolyposis colon cancer syndrome, HNPCC, Box 19-7), small cell (neuroendocrine undifferentiated), squamous cell carcinoma, all others rare.

Histologic grade*
Low grade (well to moderately differentiated) or high grade (poorly differentiated to undifferentiated) (Boxes 19-8, 19-9).

Extent of invasion*
Carcinoma in situ (including invasion into lamina propria) (Tis), invasion into submucosa (T1), invasion into muscularis propria (T2), invasion through muscularis propria into the subserosa, or into non-peritonealized pericolic or perirectal tissues (T3), direct invasion of other organs or structures and/or perforates visceral peritoneum (T4). A measurement of the depth of invasion is sometimes used for rectal carcinomas.

The distance of invasion into the subserosa may be prognostic for T3 carcinomas (T3a/b: invasion 0.5 cm or less beyond the muscularis propria; T3c/d: invasion >0.5 cm beyond the muscularis propria). Extension of carcinoma within lymphatics or blood vessels is not included in determining the depth of invasion.

Invasion into another segment of the colorectum by way of the serosa or mesocolon is classified as T4. Invasion into another segment of colorectum by extent along the bowel wall (e.g., a cecal carcinoma extending into the ileum) would not be sufficient for classification as T4.

Perforation of visceral peritoneum has been classified[9]:

1. A mesothelial inflammatory and/or hyperplastic reaction with tumor close to, but not at, the serosal surface.
2. Tumor present at the serosal surface with inflammatory reaction, mesothelial hyperplasia, and/or erosion/ulceration.
3. Free tumor cells on the serosal surface (in the peritoneum) with underlying ulceration of the visceral peritoneum.

All three types of peritoneal involvement have been associated with decreased survival. CAP recommends that T4b include at least types 2 and 3. Free perforation of a colorectal carcinoma into the peritoneal cavity is classified as T4.

Regional lymph nodes*
Number of positive nodes, number of nodes examined, presence of extracapsular invasion, specify location or "apical" if designated by surgeon.

All nodes should be examined (preferably at least 12). If fewer than 12 nodes are found, additional techniques to identify lymph nodes and additional tissue sampling should be considered.

Rounded tumor nodules in pericolonic/perirectal fat without histologic evidence of residual lymph node tissue are classified as lymph node metastases. If the nodule is irregular, it is classified as "discontinuous extramural extension."

Distant metastasis*
Present, absent, cannot be assessed.

Margins*

Proximal, distal, serosal, circumferential (radial) margin (for rectal carcinomas), mesenteric, distance to margin. Anastomotic recurrences are rare if the distance is more than 5 cm. A distal margin less than 2 cm for a rectal carcinoma may be an indication for radiation therapy.

The distance of a rectal carcinoma from the radial margin may be important for rectal carcinomas. Margins should be evaluated for adenomatous changes, carcinoma in situ, and invasive carcinoma.

Colon segments contract after excision. Distances to margins are best determined while the specimen is fresh, immediately after excision.

The distance of a carcinoma from a non-peritonealized surface (the radial or circumferential margin) predicts local recurrence if positive or less than 0.1 cm. This includes carcinoma within a lymph node close to this margin. This margin should be considered negative if more than 0.1 cm.

Perforation of bowel wall

Present or absent, related to tumor or other process.

Lymphatic (small vessel) invasion*

Present or absent, intramural or extramural.

Venous invasion

Should be in a definite muscular vein: absent, intramural, or extramural.

Perineural invasion

Present or absent. This feature is also used to classify borders (Box 19-10).

Tumor border configuration

Not assessed, pushing type (expansile, uniformly smooth), or irregular (infiltrative, streaming dissection), mixed (Box 19-10).

Crohn-like lymphoid reaction

None, low grade (3 to 15 lymphocytes per 40× HPF), high grade (>15 lymphocytes per 40× HPF)

Tumor-infiltrating lymphocytes

None, low grade (3 to 15 lymphocytes per 40× HPF), high grade (>15 lymphocytes per 40× HPF). Intratumoral lymphocytic infiltrates are associated with microsatellite instability and medullary histology.

Nontumorous bowel

Inflammatory bowel disease (with or without dysplasia), hyperplastic polyps, adenomas, serrated adenomas, diverticular disease, ulcers, strictures.

Treatment effect

Present or absent.

Note specific location of acellular mucin pools in wall and margins.

Post-chemotherapy inflammatory changes: fibrosis, obliterative vasculopathy, telangiectasia, cellular atypia, active inflammation, ulceration.

This checklist incorporates information from the ADASP (see www.panix.com/~adasp) and the CAP Cancer Committee protocols for reporting on cancer specimens (see www.cap.org/). The asterisked elements are considered to be scientifically validated or regularly used data elements that must be present in reports of cancer-directed surgical resection specimens from ACS CoC-approved cancer programs. The specific details of reporting the elements may vary among institutions.

The AJCC classification is given in Table 19-11.

Box 19-6 Evaluation of the mesorectal envelope

Complete excision of the rectum and surrounding tissues decreases the risk of local recurrence. The extent of resection can be determined by gross evaluation of the non-peritonealized surface of the specimen. The entire specimen is scored according to the worst area.

Incomplete

- Little bulk to the mesorectum
- Defects in the mesorectum down to the muscularis propria
- After transverse sectioning, the circumferential margin appears very irregular

Nearly complete

- Moderate bulk to the mesorectum
- Irregularity of the mesorectal surface with defects >0.5 cm, but none extending to the muscularis propria
- No areas of visibility of the muscularis propria except at the insertion site of the levator ani muscles

Complete

- Intact bulky mesorectum with a smooth surface
- Only minor irregularities of the mesorectal surface
- No surface defects >0.5 cm in depth
- No coning towards the distal margin of the specimen
- After transverse sectioning the circumferential margin appears smooth

Box 19-7 Hereditary non-polyposis colorectal cancer (HNPCC)

HNPCC is an autosomal dominant disorder caused by mutations in DNA repair genes, present in 0.1% of the population. There is 80% penetrance. HNPCC accounts for 1% to 5% of all colon carcinomas.

Clinical

- Young age (mean age 42 years compared to 65 for sporadic tumors), women > men
- Right-sided carcinomas more common than left
- Multiple synchronous or metachronous tumors are common
- Extracolonic carcinomas: endometrium, stomach, small bowel, urothelium, kidney, ovary, skin
- Better prognosis than sporadic carcinomas (fewer regional or distant metastases)
- Better response to anti-metabolic chemotherapy than to alkylating agents
- 95% due to germline mutations in two genes involved in mismatch DNA repair: *hMSH2* (human mutS homolog 2) and *hMLH1* (human mutL homolog 1). Other mutations are in *hPMS1, hPMS2, hMSH6*, as well as others. These mutations result in microsatellite instability (MSI).

Pathologic

- Large bulky tumors with pushing borders
- Prominent lymphocytic infiltrate (Crohn like)
- Poorly differentiated carcinomas with necrosis, mucin production, or signet ring cell features
- Diploid DNA content
- Lack of *hMSH2* and *hMLH1* can be confirmed by immunohistochemistry: PCR assays can also be used to detect microsatellite instability. Pathologic features may vary with the mutation present.

Approximately 10% to 20% of sporadic tumors have inactivation of the same genes by methylation of the promoter (most commonly in *hMLH1*). These carcinomas also have similar clinical, histologic, and prognostic features and can be identified by immunohistochemistry or PCR assays.

Box 19-8 Grading system for adenocarcinomas of no special type[11,12]

Well differentiated	Complex or simple tubules, easily discerned nuclear polarity, and uniformly sized nuclei
Moderately differentiated	Complex, simple, or slightly irregular tubules, nuclear polarity just discerned or lost
Poorly differentiated	Highly irregular glands or an absence of glandular differentiation with loss of nuclear polarity

Box 19-9 AJCC grade

GX   Grade cannot be assessed

G1   Well differentiated (>95% gland forming)

G2   Moderately differentiated (50–95% gland forming)

G3   Poorly differentiated (≤50% gland forming)

G4   Undifferentiated

The AJCC recommends using a two-tiered system:

Low grade (well and moderately differentiated carcinomas): >50% gland formation

High grade (poorly differentiated and undifferentiated carcinomas): <50% gland formation; includes signet ring cell carcinomas, small cell carcinomas, and undifferentiated carcinomas. Signet ring cell carcinomas in association with MSI-H may not have the same prognosis as those not associated with MSI-H.

Some authors suggest that G4 lesions be reported separately as they may have a worse prognosis than G3 carcinomas.

Box 19-10 Diagnostic criteria for an infiltrative border of colorectal carcinoma[13,14]

Naked eye examination of a microscopic slide of the tumor border

Inability to define limits of invasive border of tumor and/or

Inability to resolve host tissue from malignant tissue

Microscopic examination of the tumor border

"Streaming dissection" of muscularis propria (dissection of tumor through the full thickness of the muscularis propria without stromal response) and/or

Dissection of mesenteric adipose tissue by small glands or irregular clusters of cords of cells and/or 'perineural invasion'

Table 19-11 AJCC (6th edition) classification of colon and rectal carcinomas

Tumor	TX	Primary tumor cannot be assessed
	T0	No evidence of primary tumor
	Tis	Carcinoma in situ: intraepithelial or invasion of lamina propria
	T1	Tumor invades submucosa
	T2	Tumor invades muscularis propria
	T3	Tumor invades through the muscularis propria into the subserosa or into non-peritonealized pericolic or perirectal tissues *Optional subclassification of T3[a]:* T3a Minimal invasion: less than 0.1 cm beyond the border of the muscularis propria T3b Slight invasion: 0.1 to 0.5 cm beyond the border of the muscularis propria T3c Moderate invasion: >0.5 to 1.5 cm beyond the border of the muscularis propria T3d Extensive invasion: >1.5 cm beyond the border of the muscularis propria
	T4	Tumor directly invades other organs (including other segments of bowel) or structures and/or perforates visceral peritoneum
	T4a	Tumor directly invades other organs or structures
	T4b	Tumor penetrates the visceral peritoneum. This includes tumors with a mesothelial inflammatory and/or hyperplastic reaction with tumor close to, but not at, the serosal surface, tumor present at the serosal surface with inflammatory reaction, mesothelial hyperplasia, and/or erosion/ulceration, and free tumor cells on the serosal surface (in the peritoneum) with underlying ulceration of the visceral peritoneum
Regional lymph nodes	NX	Regional lymph nodes cannot be assessed
	N0	No regional lymph node metastasis
	N1	Metastasis in one to three regional lymph nodes
	N2	Metastasis in four or more regional lymph nodes

Note: Tumor nodules in perirectal and pericolic fat or in adjacent mesentery without histologic evidence of residual lymph node tissue are classified as regional lymph node metastases if they have the form and smooth contour of a lymph node. If the nodule has an irregular contour, it should be classified as V1 (microscopic venous involvement) or V2 (grossly evident involvement). Multiple metastatic foci seen microscopically only in the pericolic fat should be considered lymph node metastases. It is desirable to obtain at least 12 lymph nodes for staging. Regional lymph nodes for the anatomic subsites of the colon and rectum are as follows:

Cecum: anterior cecal, posterior cecal, ileocolic, right colic
Ascending colon: ileocolic, right colic, middle colic
Hepatic flexure: middle colic, right colic
Transverse colon: middle colic
Splenic flexure: middle colic, left colic, inferior mesenteric
Descending colon: left colic, inferior mesenteric, sigmoid
Sigmoid colon: inferior mesenteric, superior rectal sigmoidal, sigmoid mesenteric
Rectosigmoid: perirectal, left colic, sigmoid mesenteric, sigmoidal, inferior mesenteric, superior rectal, middle rectal
Rectum: perirectal, sigmoid mesenteric, inferior mesenteric, lateral sacral, presacral, internal iliac, sacral promontory, superior rectal, middle rectal, inferior rectal
Metastases to non-regional lymph nodes (e.g. external iliac, para-aortic) should be classified as distant metastases (M1).
Micrometastases found only after immunoperoxidase studies or by PCR should be classified as N0 with an explanation

Metastasis	MX	Distant metastasis cannot be assessed
	M0	No distant metastasis
	M1	Distant metastasis

Seeding of abdominal organs is considered M1

Lymphatic and vessel invasion does not change the T category. These findings are coded separately:

Lymphatic vessel invasion (L)	LX	Lymphatic vessel invasion cannot be assessed
	L0	No lymphatic vessel invasion
	L1	Lymphatic vessel invasion

Table 19-11 AJCC (6th edition) classification of colon and rectal carcinomas—cont'd

Venous invasion (V)	VX	Venous invasion cannot be assessed
	V0	No venous invasion
	V1	Microscopic venous invasion
	V2	Macroscopic venous invasion

[a] The T3 subclassification is not currently part of the AJCC 6th edition cancer staging but may have prognostic significance, especially if invasion is greater than 0.5 cm.
This staging system should not be used for appendiceal carcinomas or carcinoid tumors.
This list also incorporates recommendations for reporting from the AJCC.[10]

Table 19-12 AJCC (6th edition) classification of anal carcinomas[a]

Tumor	TX	Primary tumor cannot be assessed
	T0	No evidence of primary tumor
	Tis	Carcinoma in situ:
		Intraepithelial
		Invasion of lamina propria
		Invasion of muscularis mucosae
	T1	Tumor ≤2 cm in greatest dimension
	T2	Tumor >2 cm but ≤5 cm in greatest dimension
	T3	Tumor >5 cm in greatest dimension
	T4	Tumor of any size with invasion of adjacent organ(s): e.g., vagina, urethra, bladder (involvement of sphincter muscles alone is not classified as T4).
Regional lymph nodes	NX	Regional lymph nodes cannot be assessed
	N0	No regional lymph node metastasis
	N1	Metastasis in perirectal lymph nodes
	N2	Metastasis in unilateral internal iliac and/or inguinal lymph nodes
	N3	Metastasis in perirectal and inguinal lymph nodes and/or bilateral internal iliac and/or inguinal lymph nodes
		Regional lymph nodes include perirectal (anorectal, perirectal, and lateral sacral), internal iliac (hypogastric), and inguinal (superficial and deep). All other lymph node groups are considered distant metastasis.
Metastasis	MX	Distant metastasis cannot be assessed
	M0	No distant metastasis
	M1	Distant metastasis

[a] Carcinomas arising at the junction of the hair-bearing skin and mucous membrane of the anal canal are staged as skin cancers.

Box 19-11 Histologic grade of anal adenocarcinomas

Grade X	Grade cannot be assessed
Grade 1	Well differentiated (>95% of tumor composed of glands)
Grade 2	Moderately differentiated (50–95% of tumor composed of glands)
Grade 3	Poorly differentiated (<49% of tumor composed of glands)
Grade 4	Undifferentiated

Small cell carcinomas and tumors with no differentiation or minimal differentiation that is only present in rare small foci (classified as WHO undifferentiated carcinomas) are categorized as grade 4.

Pathologic prognostic/diagnostic features sign-out checklist for anal carcinomas

Specimen type*
Abdominoperineal resection (length of bowel segment, length of anus), transanal disk excision (intact, fragmented—the number of fragments may be given).

Tumor site*
Rectum, anal canal, relationship to squamo-columnar junction, anterior wall.

Tumor size*
Greatest dimension (T1 ≤2 cm; T2 >2 but ≤5 cm; T3 >5 cm), three dimensions.

Tumor configuration
Polypoid, exophytic, infiltrative, ulcerating, other.

Histologic type*
Squamous cell carcinoma, adenocarcinoma, mucinous adenocarcinoma, small cell carcinoma, other rare types.

Histologic grade*
Well, moderately, poorly differentiated, or undifferentiated (Box 19-11).

Extent of invasion*
In situ, invasion into lamina propria or submucosa, muscularis propria or subserosa, invasion into perineal soft tissue, invasion of adjacent structures or organs. A measurement of the depth of invasion is sometimes used as a prognostic factor for rectal carcinomas.

Regional lymph nodes*
Present or absent, number of nodes examined, number with metastases, location, size, presence of extracapsular invasion, specify location or "apical" if designated by surgeon.
Carcinomas of the anal canal usually metastasize to the anorectal and perirectal nodes.
Carcinomas of the anal margin metastasize to superficial inguinal nodes.

Distant metastasis*
Absent, present.

Margins*
Uninvolved (distance to closest margin), involved.
Specify proximal, distal, distance to margin, radial (circumferential) margin.
Specify if it is carcinoma in situ or invasive carcinoma at the margin.

Perineural invasion
Absent, present.

Venous/lymphatic (large/small vessel) invasion
Absent, present (intramural or extramural)

Other findings
Condyloma acuminatum, Paget disease, dysplasia, Crohn disease.

This checklist incorporates information from the ADASP (see www.panix.com/~adasp) and the CAP Cancer Committee protocols for reporting on cancer specimens (see www.cap.org/). The asterisked elements are considered to be scientifically validated or regularly used data elements that must be present in reports of cancer-directed surgical resection specimens from ACS CoC-approved cancer programs. The specific details of reporting the elements may vary among institutions.

■ APPENDIX

Appendices are generally removed due to acute appendicitis, occasionally "incidentally" during operations for other reasons, and as part of a right colectomy.

Processing the specimen

1. Record dimensions (length, diameter including range), color (tan/pink, gray/green), external surface (edematous, fibrinous exudate, hyperemia, purulence, perforations, hemorrhagic—may be seen in endometriosis).

   If the mesoappendix is present, record dimensions, color, appearance (edema, fibrinous exudate, purulence).

2. Make a longitudinal section of the tip, just long enough to fit into a cassette. The serosal side may be inked to orient the tip for embedding. The remainder of the appendix is sectioned at 3-mm intervals (Fig. 19-9).

3. Record the thickness of the wall, the diameter of the lumen (dilated, fibrosed, constricted), the condition of the mucosa (glistening, ulcerated, hyperemic), and the contents of the lumen:
   - Fecalith
   - Foreign body (e.g., seeds, gallstone calculus)
   - Purulence or blood (acute appendicitis)
   - Parasites (*Oxyuris vermicularis*)
   - Mucin—may be associated with a mucocele or a mucinous neoplasm (check for mucinous implants on serosa)
   - Fibrous obliteration.

4. Submit one longitudinal section of the tip and two transverse sections (one near the resection margin and one near the tip), including any abnormalities seen (perforations, ulcerations, serositis).

   If there is mucin accumulation in the lumen (i.e., a possible cystadenoma or cystadenocarcinoma) or an area suspicious for tumor, submit the entire appendix and submit the resection margin in a separate cassette.

   If the appendectomy was performed for appendicitis, and the appendix is grossly normal, the entire specimen must be submitted.

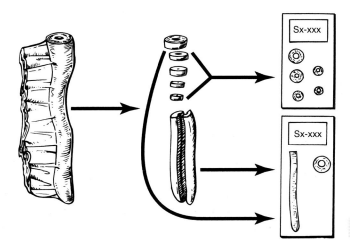

Figure 19-9 Appendectomies.

Gross differential diagnosis

Appendicitis is usually apparent as a purulent exudate on the serosal surface of the appendix, often with a gross perforation. More subtle cases may appear edematous or may not be grossly apparent. Surgeons may be incorrect in up to 7% of cases of acute appendicitis (both false positive and false negative clinical diagnoses). Thus, histologic confirmation is useful for clinical management after appendectomy.

Neuroendocrine tumors (e.g., carcinoid, tubular or goblet cell carcinoid, crypt cell carcinoma) are usually found at the tip of the appendix. Carcinoids are found incidentally in 1 to 6 specimens out of 1000 appendectomies and are the most common appendiceal tumor. Small tumors are often difficult or impossible to see grossly because of their infiltrative growth pattern in the submucosa. The normal architecture may be effaced. Large tumors may be firm, yellow to white, well circumscribed but not encapsulated, and are usually found near the tip.

Endometriosis is not an uncommon finding in the appendix. Often the muscularis propria appears to be markedly hypertrophied and areas of focal hemorrhage may be present.

Mucocele is seen as diffuse globular enlargement of the appendix which is filled with mucus. Mucinous cystadenomas and mucinous cystadenocarcinomas have this same appearance.

Adenocarcinoma of the appendix is rare and has the same gross appearance as a colonic adenocarcinoma. The AJCC staging system does not apply to appendiceal carcinomas. Some tumors may perforate and present as acute appendicitis. These cases may be difficult to distinguish from inflammation grossly.

A cecal diverticulum (thought to be of congenital origin) may present clinically as appendicitis. Intraoperatively, the surgeon finds a pericecal abscess with a normal appendix and a right colectomy is performed. Search for the diverticulum in the proximal cecum with a metal probe: the probe will enter the abscess cavity from the mucosal surface.

Specific infections, such as tuberculosis and *Yersinia*, are rarely causes of appendiceal inflammation but may be more common in patients from outside the US. The gross appearance may be unremarkable or the same as for acute appendicitis.

Sample dictation

Received fresh, labeled with the patient's name and unit number and "appendix," is a 5 cm in length × 0.9 cm in diameter appendix with attached mesoappendix (5 × 1 × 0.8 cm). There is a 0.3 cm in diameter perforation of the appendiceal wall, 1.5 cm from the tip. The serosal surface is dull and covered with purulent material. The mesoappendix is edematous, tan/brown, and has areas of focal hemorrhage. The mucosal surface is red/brown and ulcerated. There is a 0.5 × 0.5 × 0.5 cm brown friable fecalith in the lumen of the proximal appendix.

Cassette #1: longitudinal section of tip and proximal margin, 2 frags, RSS.
Cassette #2: cross-sections, including area of perforation, 4 frags, RSS.

■ HEMORRHOIDS

Hemorrhoids are dilated veins of the hemorrhoidal plexus resected due to recurrent bleeding and pain. The specimen consists of a local resection of anal mucosa and submucosa. Squamous cell carcinomas, condylomata, tuberculosis, and nonspecific granulomas can sometimes be found incidentally in the adjacent anal tissue. Occasionally a fibroepithelial polyp clinically mimics a hemorrhoid.

Processing the specimen

1. Record the number of fragments and size of each one. Examine the anal mucosa carefully for any lesions. Serially section each fragment. Dilated vascular spaces with or without thrombosis can sometimes be seen grossly.
2. Submit one cassette of representative tissue. Submit additional cassettes to document any lesions seen.

■ LIVER

The liver is involved by a wide variety of non-neoplastic and, less commonly, neoplastic diseases. See Chapter 27 for processing of liver biopsies performed for staging of Hodgkin's disease. Biopsies may be performed to evaluate a liver prior to transplantation, see Chapter 6, Operating Room Consultations for more information.

Relevant clinical history (in addition to age and gender)

See Table 19-13.

Table 19-13 Relevant clinical history	
HISTORY RELEVANT TO ALL SPECIMENS	HISTORY RELEVANT TO LIVER SPECIMENS
Organ/tissue resected or biopsied	Viral hepatitis (A, B, or C)
Purpose of the procedure	Hemochromatosis
Gross appearance of the organ/tissue/lesion sampled	Cirrhosis
Any unusual features of the clinical presentation	Bile duct disease (e.g., liver fluke infection, obstruction, jaundice)
Any unusual features of the gross appearance	Liver function tests, serum AFP
Prior surgery/biopsies—results	Family history of liver tumors
Prior malignancy	Pregnancy
Prior treatment (radiation therapy, chemotherapy, drug use that can change the histologic appearance of tissues)	→ Drug use that can alter the histologic appearance of the liver
Compromised immune system	

Needle biopsy

Needle biopsies are commonly used to assess liver diseases affecting hepatic function and are also used to evaluate liver masses (primary tumors or metastases). Scoring systems are available for chronic hepatitis[15,16] (Table 19-14).

Processing the specimen

1. Describe the specimen including color (tan/brown, white probably indicates capsular tissue or tumor), length, diameter, and whether the specimen appears fragmented (may indicate a cirrhotic liver).

Table 19-14 A system for grading and staging of liver specimens with chronic viral hepatitis[16]

SCORE	GRADE OF NECROINFLAMMATORY ACTIVITY		STAGE OF FIBROSIS/CIRRHOSIS
	PORTAL ACTIVITY	*LOBULAR ACTIVITY*	
0	No portal inflammation	None	No fibrosis
1	Portal inflammation only, no/minimal piecemeal necrosis	Minimal inflammation, no necrosis	Enlarged fibrotic portal tracts
2	Mild piecemeal necrosis (some or all portal tracts)	Focal hepatocyte necrosis	Periportal or portal to portal septa; no bridging
3	Moderate piecemeal necrosis (all portal tracts)	Moderate, with multifocal necrosis	Bridging fibrosis with architectural distortion, no obvious cirrhosis
4	Severe piecemeal necrosis	Severe with prominent diffuse necrosis (may be bridging)	Cirrhosis

Grade refers to the extent of current inflammation and can increase or decrease over time. The most severe degree of portal or lobular injury is graded.
Stage refers to the degree of fibrosis and is usually progressive over time; fibrosis may regress during antiviral therapy.

2. Wrap in lens paper and submit in entirety. Trichrome, reticulin, and iron stains are often used in the evaluation.

Special studies

Hemochromatosis (iron). Iron stains show increased iron within hepatocytes. Fixed or unfixed tissue biopsies may be used for quantitative iron assessment by a specialty laboratory.

Wilson's disease (copper). Quantitative copper measurements may require that the specimen be acquired and handled with special equipment to avoid contamination of the specimen with trace metals. The specialty laboratory should be contacted before processing such a specimen. Special stains for copper (rhodanine stain) or copper associated protein (orcein stain) can be used to visualize the abnormal copper stores within hepatocytes. These stains may also be positive in other diseases, such as chronic biliary disorders.

Acute fatty liver of pregnancy, Reye's syndrome, etc. These diseases require the demonstration of microvesicular fat, which is removed by routine processing. Oil red O stains may be performed on frozen tissue sections that have been air dried (do not fix in methanol). EM can also be used. These patients are acutely ill and a timely diagnosis is clinically useful, so a frozen section is generally preferable to EM studies.

α_1-Antitrypsin deficiency. PAS-positive, diastase-resistant, eosinophilic hyaline globules can be seen in periportal hepatocytes in routinely fixed tissues.

Lymphoma. Evaluation of the disease process using a cytologic preparation may be helpful before allocating tissue. If lymphoma is suspected, a portion of the tissue may be fixed in B5. The entire specimen should not be fixed in B5 because nonlymphoid markers may not be optimally preserved (e.g., keratins). If a portion is frozen, histologic sections of the frozen tissue should always be examined.

Lobectomy

Hepatocellular carcinomas may be treated with surgery but cholangiocarcinomas are rarely resectable. More commonly, resections are performed for adenomas and focal nodular hyperplasia. An individual metastasis from colon carcinoma also may be resected.

Processing the specimen

1. Weigh and measure the specimen. Identify the cut surgical margins and the capsular surface. Assess the overall appearance of the resected liver (e.g., normal homogeneous parenchyma with a smooth capsule versus the nodular and fibrotic appearance of a cirrhotic liver). Identify the vascular pedicle.
2. Section the specimen thinly at 0.5 cm to look for lesions.
3. Describe the size, location (with respect to the liver capsule and with respect to the surgical margins), color, and other gross features (central scar, hemorrhage, nodularity, bulging on cut section).
4. Describe the remainder of the liver parenchyma including color, presence of nodules (give range of sizes), congestion, and fibrosis. Describe the appearance of the capsule: normal = thin smooth and glistening; abnormal = thickened, nodular, adhesions, etc.

   Examine the major portal vein and hepatic vein structures for gross evidence of vascular invasion.
5. Take sections to demonstrate the lesion, nearby vasculature, cauterized margins, vascular margins, and uninvolved liver.

Gross differential diagnosis (Fig. 19-10)

Focal nodular hyperplasia (FNH). FNH usually takes the form of a solitary (but 20% are multiple) gray/white unencapsulated nodule that may be located beneath the liver capsule. Most are less than 5 cm. On cut section there is a very characteristic white depressed area of fibrosis with broad strands radiating out in a stellate configuration and prominent nodularity of the intervening parenchyma. The surrounding liver is most commonly normal in appearance. An elastic stain on a section from the central scarred area helps to delineate the abnormal vasculature.

Adenoma. An adenoma is usually a solitary well-encapsulated mass with a homogeneous parenchyma that has a slightly different color from the adjacent normal parenchyma (yellow to tan/brown). Some can be quite large (up to 30 cm). Usually located beneath the liver capsule and some are pedunculated. Hemorrhage and necrosis are common. Look carefully for gross vascular invasion or pale areas that would suggest a well-differentiated carcinoma. The surrounding liver is usually normal in appearance. Most occur in young women and are related to oral contraceptive use.

Hepatocellular carcinoma may consist of multiple nodules or a large infiltrating mass. Tumors are usually white/yellow with areas of punctate hemorrhage and necrosis, although bile-producing tumors may be green. The surrounding liver parenchyma is often cirrhotic. Look for a "nodule within a nodule." This may represent an incipient carcinoma arising in a benign hyperplastic nodule.

Fibrolamellar carcinoma is an unusual variant but may be more likely to be resected because it has a better prognosis. It usually presents as a single large mass that may have a capsule in a liver that is non-cirrhotic. The mass appears to be composed of smaller nodules (reminiscent of FNH).

Cholangiocarcinoma. These carcinomas are often unresectable at presentation, so excisional specimens are very uncommon. Intrahepatic tumors are gray/white hard irregular masses.

Extrahepatic tumors may be nodular or flat and usually invade the wall of the bile duct. Klatskin (hilar) tumors originate at the hepatic duct junction and spread along the biliary tree. The liver may be green due to bile duct obstruction. The intrahepatic bile duct and distal extrahepatic bile duct margins must be evaluated.

Metastatic carcinoma is usually of colonic origin if resected. The tumor often appears as a circumscribed necrotic mass with a central depression beneath the surface of the liver. Multiple lesions may be present. The surrounding liver is usually normal in appearance. Margins are evaluated.

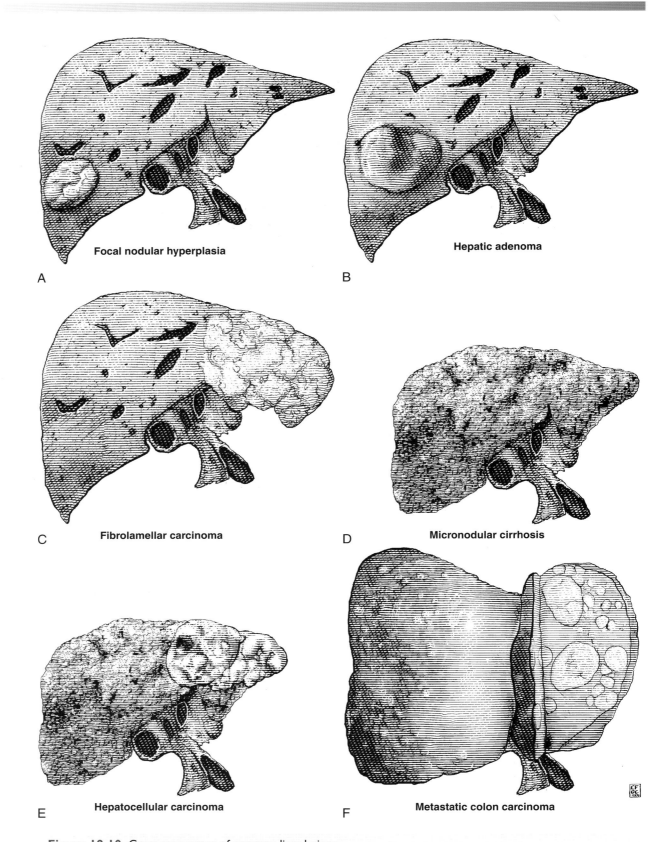

Focal nodular hyperplasia

A

Hepatic adenoma

B

Fibrolamellar carcinoma

C

Micronodular cirrhosis

D

Hepatocellular carcinoma

E

Metastatic colon carcinoma

F

Figure 19-10 Gross appearance of common liver lesions.

Pediatric tumors. Children are subject to a wider variety of liver lesions including hepatoblastoma, infantile hemangioendothelioma, mesenchymal hamartoma, and undifferentiated "embryonal" sarcoma, as well as lesions also found in adults.[17] At least one section per centimeter of greatest dimension of the tumor should be examined, including all areas of differing appearance. Some tumors may have been treated prior to resection with chemotherapy or embolization. Special studies are not needed for the diagnosis of these tumors. However, since these tumors are rare, tissue should be saved for EM, frozen, and submitted for cytogenetic analysis if feasible.

Hepatoblastoma. Essentially only occurs in infants. The tumor can be large (up to 25 cm) and is variegated in appearance with cysts, necrosis, and hemorrhage. The surrounding liver appears normal.

Mesenchymal hamartoma. Presents in the first 2 years of life as a large circumscribed mass comprised of multiple cystic spaces filled with clear fluid. Solid areas may be fibrous and white, myxoid, or resemble normal liver.

Embryonal (undifferentiated) sarcoma. Most common between the ages of 6 and 10. The tumors are circumscribed and soft with a variegated solid and cystic appearance. Necrosis and hemorrhage may be present.

Bile duct hamartomas (Meyenburg complexes). These are usually multiple small (<0.5 cm) well-circumscribed nodules on the surface of the liver. They are most commonly biopsied during laparotomy to exclude metastatic carcinoma.

Bile duct adenomas. These are solitary lesions, usually less than 1 cm in size, located below the capsule. Like bile duct hamartomas, they are most commonly biopsied during laparotomy to exclude carcinoma.

Microscopic sections

Tumor
Four cassettes, including relationship to liver capsule, capsule of tumor, relationship to other anatomic landmarks (e.g., large vessels).

Margins
Representative sections of all margins at the closest approach of the tumor. Take vascular margins if they can be identified.

Uninvolved liver
Two cassettes of uninvolved liver parenchyma. Order reticulin, iron, and trichrome stains on one of the cassettes if diffuse liver disease is suspected clinically or grossly.

Pathologic prognostic/diagnostic features sign-out checklist for liver tumors

Specimen type*
Lobectomy (right or left), segmentectomy (medial, left lateral), explanted liver.

Focality*
Solitary (location), multiple (locations).

Tumor size*
Size of greatest dimension (additional dimensions optional).

Histologic type*
Hepatocellular carcinoma, cholangiocarcinoma, fibrolamellar hepatocellular carcinoma, metastatic carcinoma, bile duct cystadenocarcinoma, other rare types. The WHO classification is recommended.

Histologic grade*
Well, moderately, poorly differentiated, undifferentiated, or grades I to IV (Table 19-15, Box 19-12).

Extent of invasion*

Solitary tumor with no vascular invasion (T1), solitary tumor with vascular invasion or multiple tumors, none more than 5 cm (T2), multiple tumors more than 5 cm or tumor involving a major branch of the portal or hepatic veins (T3), tumors with direct invasion of adjacent organs other than the gallbladder or perforation of visceral peritoneum (T4).

Regional lymph nodes*

Absent (N0), present (N1), number of nodes examined, number with metastases.

Distant metastasis*

Absent (M0), present (M1).

Margins*

Not involved or involved (distance from closest margin), bile duct margin (only for cholangiocarcinoma), invasive or in situ.

Tumor necrosis

Present or absent (minimal, moderate, or extensive).

Venous (large vessel) invasion

Absent or present. Portal vein or hepatic vein invasion is an important prognostic factor. Identify the vessel involved, if possible.

Lymphatic invasion

Absent or present.

Perineural invasion

Absent or present.

Nonlesional liver

Cirrhosis/fibrosis, hepatitis (type and activity), steatosis, macroregenerative nodule, hepatocellular dysplasia (large cell dysplasia, small cell dysplasia), ductal dysplasia, iron overload.

This checklist incorporates information from the CAP Cancer Committee protocols for reporting on cancer specimens. The asterisked elements are considered to be scientifically validated or regularly used data elements that must be present in reports from ACS CoC-approved cancer programs. For this purpose, the protocol applies to primary carcinomas of the liver, but not hepatoblastoma. The specific reporting of some data elements may vary among institutions. This checklist also incorporates recommendations from the ADASP (see www.panix.com/~adasp/).

Box 19-12 Grading system for cholangiocarcinomas	
Grade 1	Well differentiated (>95% of tumor composed of glands)
Grade 2	Moderately differentiated (50–95% of tumor composed of glands)
Grade 3	Poorly differentiated (5–49% of tumor composed of glands)
Grade 4	Undifferentiated (<5% to tumor composed of glands)

Table 19-15 Grading of hepatocellular carcinomas (Edmondson and Steiner System)[18]

	CYTOPLASM	NUCLEI	N/C RATIO	COHESION	CELL FUNCTION	ARCHITECTURE
Grade I	Granular and acidophilic	Slightly abnormal	Normal	Normal	Bile frequent	Normal
Grade II	Granular and acidophilic with sharp and clear-cut borders	Larger and more hyper-chromatic	Higher	Normal	Bile frequent	Frequent acini
Grade III	Not as granular and acidophilic	Larger and more hyper-chromatic than grade II	Higher, tumor giant cells may be present	Some intra-vascular single cells	Bile less frequent	Breakup or distortion of the trabecular pattern
Grade IV	Variable, often scanty, with fewer granules	Intensely hyper-chromatic	Very high	Lack of cohesiveness	Rare acini with bile	Trabeculae difficult to find, spindle cells may be present

Table 19-16 AJCC (6th edition) classification of liver tumors

Tumor	TX	Primary tumor cannot be assessed
	T0	No evidence of primary tumor
	T1	Solitary tumor without vascular invasion
	T2	Solitary tumor with vascular invasion or multiple tumors none more than 5 cm
	T3	Multiple tumors more than 5 cm or tumor involving a major branch of the portal or hepatic vein(s)
	T4	Tumor(s) with direct invasion of adjacent organs other than the gallbladder or with perforation of the visceral peritoneum
		Vascular invasion includes either gross or histologic involvement of vessels
Regional nodes	NX	Regional lymph nodes cannot be assessed
	N0	No regional lymph node metastasis
	N1	Regional lymph node metastasis
		A regional lymphadenectomy usually includes three or more lymph nodes. Regional lymph nodes include hilar, hepatoduodenal ligament, and caval lymph nodes. Inferior phrenic or other lymph nodes distal to the hilar, hepatoduodenal ligament, and caval lymph nodes are classified as distant metastases
Distant metastasis	MX	Distant metastasis cannot be assessed
	M0	No distant metastasis
	M1	Distant metastasis

Note: This classification does not include sarcomas or metastatic tumors. It does include hepatomas or hepatocellular carcinomas, intrahepatic bile duct carcinomas or cholangiocarcinomas, bile duct cystadenocarcinomas, and mixed types.

Grade I	Best reserved for those areas in grade II hepatocellular carcinomas where the difference between the tumor cells and hyperplastic liver cells is so minor that a diagnosis of carcinoma rests upon the demonstration of more aggressive growths in other parts of the neoplasm.
Grade II	Cells show a marked resemblance to normal hepatic cells. Nuclei are larger and more hyperchromatic than normal cells but the cytoplasm is abundant and acidophilic. The cell borders are often sharp and clear cut. Acini are frequent with lumina varying in size from tiny canaliculi to large thyroid-like spaces. The lumina are often filled with bile or protein precipitate.
Grade III	Nuclei are usually larger and more hyperchromatic than grade II cells. The nuclei occupy a relatively greater proportion of the cell (high N:C ratio). Cytoplasm is granular and acidophilic, but less so than in grade II tumors. Acini are less frequent and not as often filled with bile or protein precipitate. More single cells were seen in the intravascular growths than in grade II. Tumor giant cells are the most numerous in this group.
Grade IV	Nuclei are intensely hyperchromatic and occupy a high percentage of the cell volume. Cytoplasm is variable in amount, often scanty and contains fewer granules. The growth pattern is medullary in character, trabeculae difficult to find, and cell masses seem to lie loosely without cohesion in vascular channels. Only rare acini are seen. Spindle cell areas are present in some tumors. Short plump cell forms, resembling "oat cell" carcinoma of the lung, are seen in some.

This system is sometimes simplified to a three grade system with grades I and II equivalent to grade I, grade III equivalent to grade II, and grade IV equivalent to grade III. This modification should be stated if used.

■ GALLBLADDER

Gallbladders are commonly removed for chronic cholecystitis with cholelithiasis. Tumors are uncommon, and are usually associated with gallstones. Carcinoma may also be associated with an anomalous choledochopancreatic junction or with chronic inflammatory bowel disease.

Laparoscopic cholecystectomies are frequently performed procedures. It is sometimes necessary for the surgeon to fragment the gallstones within the intact gallbladder with forceps prior to removing it through the small laparotomy incision. This can lead to a rather tattered appearance of the specimen. Gallbladders are occasionally torn during this procedure, spilling the contents into the abdominal cavity. Note should be made of whether the specimen is intact or whether perforations and tears are present. The peritoneal cavity is not well visualized in a laparoscopic procedure as it would be in a routine cholecystectomy. Therefore, be alert to serosal implants or inflammation that could indicate clinically unsuspected disease outside of the gallbladder.

Processing the specimen

1. Describe the serosal appearance.
   - Normal: smooth and glistening.
   - Adhesions and/or portion of attached liver: normally found at the attachment of the gallbladder to the liver capsule.
   - Inflammation: dull and irregular, subserosal fibrosis, fat necrosis (very firm yellow hemorrhagic soft tissue, may indicate pancreatitis), fibrinous or purulent exudates.
   - Tumor implants: firm tan/white nodules.
   - Necrosis: blue-black discoloration (gangrene) associated with possible perforation.

- Porcelain gallbladder: the wall may be markedly thickened in chronic cholecystitis. If there is extensive calcification the gallbladder may take on the appearance of "porcelain" (shiny hard and white).
- Intact or with perforations and tears or previously opened.
  Look for lymph nodes, most commonly present near the cystic duct.

2. Open the gallbladder longitudinally, starting away from the cystic duct. The cystic duct is tortuous and need not be opened completely. Record the length, circumference and wall thickness. Describe the mucosa.

Normal. Tan/green and velvety with a honeycomb pattern, thin pliable wall.

Cholesterolosis ("strawberry gallbladder"). Speckled yellow mucosa due to aggregates of foamy histiocytes in the mucosa. This finding has no definite clinical significance.

Inflammation. Ulcerated, friable, flattened and white (atrophy), wall thickened and fibrotic or edematous. Acute acalculous cholecystitis (i.e., without gallstones) is a life-threatening disease of severely ill or debilitated patients. Often transmural (gangrenous) necrosis is present which may be apparent on examination of the serosa. The wall may be very thin and friable or markedly thickened by edema.

Polyps. Usually small and papillary, uncommon.

Carcinoma is rare and usually appears as a solid white mass infiltrating the wall or as an exophytic soft fronded intraluminal tumor. Papillary carcinomas may have a more favorable prognosis. However, infiltrating tumor may be obscured by superimposed inflammation and be occult grossly. The wall may be slightly thickened with effacement of the normal tissue planes. If present, describe and document invasion through the wall (including serosa and adjacent liver if present), and submit the cystic duct as a margin.

3. Record the number (estimate if there are many, do not just state "several" or "many"), size in aggregate and range of sizes, color, quality, and shape (ovoid or faceted—if faceted there must have been multiple stones) of any gallstones present.

- Cholesterol calculi: green/yellow/black, hard and crystalline.
- Pigment calculi: black, soft and crumbly.

Note if there are stones lodged in the isthmus or cystic duct.

If stones were fragmented during laparoscopy, the stones may appear to be "gravel" within the bile. Note if the luminal contents include bile (viscous green/black fluid) or clear watery mucin (suggests total obstruction resulting in hydrops or mucocele).

Gallstones are sometimes requested for return to the patient (see Chapter 2, "Returning specimens to patients"). In these cases place them in a sealed container, labeled with the patient's name. Do not release a container filled with liquid formalin—the fixative is a biohazard. If the stones were placed in formalin, they can be rinsed in water and then placed in an empty container. If chemical analysis is requested, see below.

4. Submit one cassette of gallbladder with sections demonstrating cross-sections of the fundus, neck with serosa, and cystic duct. If a cystic duct lymph node is present, a representative section should be submitted as well. Submit additional sections of gross lesions.

Gross differential diagnosis

Adenocarcinomas. These tumors are rare (6 to 15 per 1000 cholecystectomies) and many may be grossly inapparent. Most have an infiltrating pattern and appear as a diffuse homogeneous thickening of the wall that effaces the normal texture. Approximately one third of tumors are exophytic and grow into the lumen as a mass as well as invading the wall. In most cases, gallstones and fibrosis are also present. Porcelain gallbladder is associated with an increased risk of carcinoma.

Metastatic carcinomas. Metastatic carcinoma (usually to the serosal surface) is found in 1 to 5 cases per 1000. Rarely, a removed lymph node adjacent to the cystic duct will reveal metastatic carcinoma or a lymphoma.

Acute calculous or acalculous cholecystitis. The gallbladder is enlarged and firm and bright red, green black, or violaceous. The lumen may be filled with cloudy hemorrhagic or purulent fluid. The wall may be markedly thickened and edematous. In gangrenous cholecystitis the entire gland is necrotic with multiple perforations. The serosal surface is often covered with a fibrinous or purulent exudate.

Chronic cholecystitis. The wall may be thickened and fibrotic. The mucosa is usually preserved. Serosal adhesions may be present. If the wall is thickened with multiple calcifications it may give the appearance of a porcelain gallbladder. Xanthogranulomatous cholecystitis has the appearance of a small shrunken nodular gallbladder that can be mistaken for a malignancy.

Mucoceles can be mistaken for mucinous carcinomas. Muciphages may resemble signet ring cells in the wall. However, these cells are not immunoreactive for cytokeratin.

Infections. Gallbladders from patients with AIDS may show CMV, *Cryptosporidium* sp., or MAI. Rarely, parasites may be found.

Microscopic sections

Grossly normal
Three sections (1 from fundus, 1 from body, and 1 from neck).
If carcinoma in situ or invasive carcinoma is found, additional sections should be submitted.

Tumors
Most lesions can be submitted in entirety including the deepest extent of invasion and relationship to attached liver (if present).
If a gross lesion is present, submit the cystic duct separately.

Lymph node
If a lymph node is present, submit in its entirety.

Sample dictation

Received fresh, labeled with the patient's name and unit number and "gallbladder," is a 6 × 4 × 0.5 cm (wall thickness) gallbladder with a green/tan velvety mucosa with focal ulcerations (largest 0.5 × 0.3 cm). The wall is slightly thickened but pliable and the serosal surface is smooth and glistening. Within the gallbladder are green/black bile and approximately 20 hard yellow crystalline faceted gallstones (in aggregate 4 × 3 × 2 cm; largest 1.5 cm). One of the gallstones is lodged within the cystic duct.

Cassette: Sections of wall and cystic duct, 6 frags, RSS.

Pathologic prognostic/diagnostic features sign-out checklist for gallbladder carcinomas

Specimen type*
Laparoscopic or open cholecystectomy, resection of other organs, including adjacent liver tissue.

Tumor site*
Fundus, body, neck, indeterminate.

Tumor size*
Size of greatest dimension (additional dimensions optional).

Histologic type*
Carcinoma in situ, adenocarcinoma, papillary adenocarcinoma, adenocarcinoma—intestinal type, adenocarcinoma—gastric type, mucinous adenocarcinoma (>50% mucinous), adenosquamous carcinoma, small cell carcinoma, other rare types. The WHO classification is recommended.

Configuration
Exophytic (fungating/polypoid), endophytic (ulcerating), or diffusely infiltrating.
Papillary carcinomas (usually polypoid) have a favorable prognosis.

Histologic grade*
Well, moderately, poorly differentiated, undifferentiated (Table 19-17).
Papillary adenocarcinoma and clear cell adenocarcinoma are usually not graded.

Extent of invasion*
In situ (Tis), invasion into lamina propria (T1a), invasion into muscle layer (T1b), invasion into perimuscular connective tissue (no extension beyond serosa or into liver) (T2), perforates serosa (visceral peritoneum) and/or directly invades liver and/or adjacent organ or structure, such as the stomach, duodenum, colon, or pancreas, omentum, or extrahepatic bile ducts (T3), tumor invades the main portal vein or hepatic artery or invades multiple extrahepatic organs or structures (T4).

Regional lymph nodes*
No regional lymph node metastasis (N0), regional lymph node metastasis (N1).
Number of nodes examined, number of nodes involved.

Distant metastasis*
Absent (M0), present (M1).

Margins*
Involved or not involved (distance from nearest margin), involved by invasive carcinoma or in situ carcinoma: cystic duct, liver parenchymal margin.

Venous/lymphatic (large/small vessel) invasion
Absent, present, indeterminate.

Perineural invasion
Absent, present, indeterminate.

Gallstones
Absent, present. If absent, the carcinoma may be associated with anatomic abnormalities (e.g., an anomalous choledochopancreatic junction) or inflammatory bowel disease.

Other findings
Acute cholecystitis, chronic cholecystitis, metaplasia (squamous, pyloric gland, intestinal), chronic inflammatory changes, dysplasia/adenoma.

This checklist incorporates information from the ADASP (see panix.com/~adasp/) and the CAP Cancer Committee protocols for reporting on cancer specimens. The asterisked elements are considered to be scientifically validated or regularly used data elements that must be present in reports from ACS CoC-approved cancer programs, although the details of reporting each element may vary among institutions. For this purpose, this protocol applies to carcinomas, including those with endocrine differentiation, but excludes carcinoid tumors.
The AJCC classification is given in Table 19-18.

Table 19-17 Grading system for gallbladder adenocarcinomas		
Grade 1	Well differentiated	>95% of tumor composed of glands
Grade 2	Moderately differentiated	50–95% of tumor composed of glands
Grade 3	Poorly differentiated	<49% of tumor composed of glands (includes signet ring cell carcinomas)
Grade 4	Undifferentiated	Small cell carcinomas, undifferentiated carcinomas

Papillary carcinomas and clear cell carcinomas are usually not graded.

Table 19-18 AJCC Classification of gallbladder tumors

Tumor	TX	Primary tumor cannot be assessed
	T0	No evidence of primary tumor
	Tis	Carcinoma in situ
	T1	Tumor invades lamina propria or muscle layer
	T1a	Tumor invades lamina propria
	T1b	Tumor invades muscle layer
	T2	Tumor invades perimuscular connective tissue; no extension beyond serosa or into liver
	T3	Tumor perforates the serosa (visceral peritoneum) and/or directly invades the liver and/or one other adjacent organ or structure, such as the stomach, duodenum, colon, or pancreas, omentum or extrahepatic bile ducts
	T4	Tumor invades main portal vein or hepatic artery or invades multiple extrahepatic organs or structures
Regional nodes	NX	Regional lymph nodes cannot be assessed
	N0	No regional lymph node metastasis
	N1	Metastasis in regional lymph nodes: hilar (i.e., in the hepatoduodenal ligament, along the inferior vena cava, hepatic artery, portal vein, and hepatic pedicle), peripancreatic (only the head), periduodenal, periportal, celiac, and superior mesenteric.
Distant metastasis	MX	Distant metastasis cannot be assessed
	M0	No distant metastasis
	M1	Distant metastasis (includes lymph nodes in peripancreatic nodes along the body and tail)

Note: This classification does not include carcinoid tumors or sarcomas. Tumors of the extrahepatic bile ducts have a separate AJCC classification system.

Chemical analysis of gallstones

Rarely, there may be a request from a clinician for chemical analysis of gallstones to determine their cholesterol content. This is an expensive test and is only ordered by special request. In these cases the gallstones are placed in a separate dry sterile container and sent to a specialty laboratory.

■ PANCREAS

The pancreas is most frequently biopsied or resected because of tumors or severe debilitating chronic pancreatitis.

Relevant clinical history (in addition to age and gender)

See Table 19-19.

Biopsy

Pancreatic biopsies may be obtained transabdominally (usually fine needle biopsies), via ERCP (often brushings), or may be intraoperative needle or incisional biopsies. Small biopsies are processed as described in Chapter 13. Frozen sections of pancreatic biopsies can be very difficult to interpret (see chapter 6).

Table 19-19 Relevant clinical history (in addition to age and gender)

HISTORY RELEVANT TO ALL SPECIMENS	HISTORY RELEVANT FOR PANCREATIC SPECIMENS
Organ/tissue resected or biopsied	Diabetes mellitus
Purpose of the procedure	Pancreatitis
Gross appearance of the organ/tissue/lesion sampled	Jaundice
Any unusual features of the clinical presentation	Zollinger–Ellison syndrome
Any unusual features of the gross appearance	Family or personal history of tumors or hyperplasia of other endocrine organs (i.e., MEN syndromes)
Prior surgery/biopsies—results	
Prior malignancy	
Prior treatment (radiation therapy, chemotherapy, drug use that can change the histologic appearance of tissues)	
Compromised immune system	

Pancreatic resections

Pancreatic adenocarcinomas of the body or tail usually present late (because they do not cause obstruction) with extension into peripancreatic tissue or metastases and are rarely resectable. Resectable tumors of this region are more likely to be tumors of the ampullary region (presenting with obstruction), endocrine tumors, or unusual non-endocrine tumors (e.g., cystic lesions such as cystadenoma or cystadenocarcinoma). Benign conditions (e.g., pancreatic pseudocyst) or chronic pancreatitis are resected less frequently.

Examination of the lymph nodes as separate groups is important for staging and prognosis.[19]

Approximately half of small ampullary and duodenal carcinomas will have metastases at surgery. These tumors commonly metastasize to a single location (most often the posterior or inferior lymph node groups) and often to a single lymph node.

In contrast, most tumors of the head of the pancreas metastasize to multiple lymph node groups and often to multiple lymph nodes within the group. The most common sites are posterior, superior, and inferior nodal groups.

Metastases to gastric or splenic nodes are rare, probably due to the lack of lymphatic connections between these nodes and the pancreas. Therefore, metastases to these nodes indicate either a very aggressive tumor or a second primary site.

Distal pancreatectomy

The specimen usually consists of distal pancreas and attached spleen (Fig. 19-11) but may also include transverse colon or stomach.

Processing the specimen

1. Orient the specimen (anterior, posterior, superior, inferior). Identify the pancreatic resection margin and the main pancreatic duct. Photographs are taken of the entire specimen and cross-sections when appropriate. Record the outer appearance including color (tan/yellow, white), consistency (firm, hard), texture (finely nodular, fibrous bands, architecture obscured by dense white infiltrate), noting if there are areas grossly suspicious for tumor.

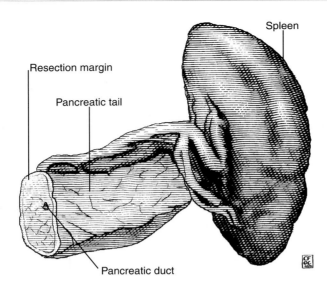

Figure 19-11 Distal pancreatectomy.

Ink the soft tissue margins around the pancreas. The proximal (pancreatic) resection margin may be taken en face or perpendicular, depending on the distance of the tumor from the margin.

2. Serially section through the pancreas, perpendicular to the long axis. Describe any lesions including size, location (body or tail), color, borders (encapsulated, infiltrating), relationship to margins (pancreatic, anterior, retroperitoneal, superior, inferior).

3. Separate the spleen if not directly involved by tumor. Section thinly, looking for lesions (see Chapter 27, "Spleen"). Evaluate the splenic vein (if present) for thrombosis or tumor.

4. Fix the entire specimen in formalin overnight. Take microscopic sections the following day. Cystic lesions are carefully sectioned and sections of any thickened walls or solid areas taken. Most should have the entire wall submitted. Take perpendicular sections of the closest approach of tumor to soft tissue margins (posterior, anterior, superior, and inferior) and place in labeled cassettes.

After the tumor and margins have been sampled, the soft tissue is examined carefully for lymph nodes. These are of great importance for prognosis (curative versus palliative resection) and diagnosis (malignant versus benign endocrine tumors). The peripancreatic nodes are described and submitted separately from the splenic nodes. These are all regional nodes for tumors in the body and tail. The adipose tissue may be carefully sectioned while attached to the specimen, or the adipose tissue can be removed and fixed in Bouin's overnight. Nodes adjacent to other structures (stomach, transverse colon) are submitted separately because these are not considered regional nodes.

Microscopic sections

Tumor
Submit at least one cassette per cm of tumor including borders and relationship to uninvolved pancreas. Cystic lesions are usually completely submitted unless more than 5 cm. In these cases one section per cm is taken including the most irregular and nodular areas.

Margins
Proximal pancreatic margin (usually the most important): submit en face. This section should include the pancreatic duct.
Soft tissue margins (perpendicular) around pancreas to evaluate invasion into soft tissue and/or retroperitoneum.

Pancreatic duct
The duct margin is sampled in the en face margin section.

Other structures
One section of spleen (if no lesions). Representative sections of any other structures.

Lymph nodes
Submit each lymph node. Describe as separate groups peripancreatic, splenic, and any other sites.

Received fresh, labeled with the patient's name and unit number and "pancreas," is the pancreatic tail (7 × 4 × 3 cm) and attached spleen (10 × 5 × 4 cm; 150 g). Within the pancreas there is a 5 × 4 × 3 cm well-circumscribed fleshy homogeneous yellow/tan tumor mass. The tumor is 2 cm from the pancreatic resection margin, which is uninvolved. The outer margins of the specimen consist of yellow/white adipose tissue varying in thickness from 0.5 to 2.0 cm. The margins are grossly uninvolved by tumor. The remainder of the pancreatic parenchyma is yellow/tan and grossly unremarkable. The spleen has a dark red/brown homogeneous parenchyma with slight prominence of the white pulp. Two lymph nodes are present in the perihilar soft tissue, the largest measuring 0.5 cm in greatest dimension. Two additional lymph nodes are present in the posterior and inferior soft tissue surrounding the distal pancreas, the largest measuring 0.4 cm in greatest dimension. A frozen section was performed on the pancreatic resection margin (en face). Tumor is saved for EM and snap freezing. The margins are inked and taken perpendicular to the specimen except as noted. Photographs are taken.

Cassette #1: Pancreatic resection margin, en face, FSR, 1 frag, ESS.
Cassette #2: Tumor and anterior margin, 1 frag, RSS.
Cassette #3: Tumor and superior margin, 1 frag, RSS.
Cassette #4: Tumor and posterior margin, 1 frag, RSS.
Cassette #5: Tumor and inferior margin, 1 frag, RSS.
Cassette #6: Tumor and adjacent pancreas, 1 frag, RSS.
Cassette #7: Spleen, 1 frag, RSS.
Cassette #8: Perihilar lymph nodes, 2 frags, ESS.
Cassette #9: Inferior lymph node, 2 frags, ESS.
Cassette #10: Posterior lymph node, 2 frags, ESS.

Whipple procedure (partial gastrectomy, duodenectomy, partial pancreatectomy)

A Whipple procedure is performed for resection of tumors in the head of the pancreas or in the ampullary or periampullary region.

The specimen usually consists of distal stomach (although the pylorus may be spared), duodenum, head of pancreas, and common bile duct remnant (Fig. 19-12). The gallbladder is usually submitted as a separate specimen. The specimen is dissected carefully to determine the site of origin of the tumor (e.g., duodenal, ampullary, periampullary, bile duct, pancreatic duct, head of pancreas). Anatomic orientation must be maintained at all times.

Processing the specimen

1. While the specimen is unfixed and pliable, open the stomach along the greater curvature, across the anterior wall of the pylorus, and down the outer curvature of the duodenum. The distal portion of the duodenal mucosa usually looks dusky because the blood supply to this portion is ligated earlier in the operation. Record the dimensions of the stomach (proximal to distal, greater curvature and lesser curvature, circumference, wall thickness), duodenum (length and circumference), pancreatic head (three dimensions), common bile duct (length and diameter), and margins (stapled versus open, length, diameter).

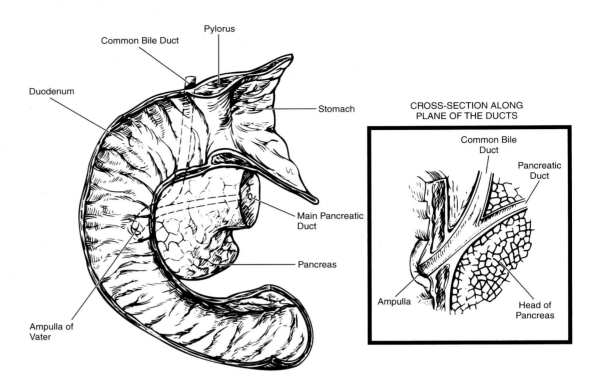

Figure 19-12 Whipple procedure.

Clean the mucosa with saline and look for mucosal lesions, especially around the ampulla. A probe in the common bile duct extending to the ampulla is helpful for orientation.

Identify the distal pancreatic resection margin. It will be the only pancreatic tissue visible (the remainder being surrounded by a thin rim of soft tissue). Take two or more en face sections including the pancreatic duct if visible (more if suspicious for involvement by tumor) and place in labeled cassettes.

Alternatively (particularly if the tumor appears close to the distal margin), this margin may be taken perpendicular to the resection margin after further dissection (see below).

Identify the uncinate process of the pancreas, which extends inferiorly from the pancreatic head. The posterior surface of this portion of the pancreas is not peritonealized as it lies directly on the superior mesenteric vessels for a distance of approximately 3 to 4 cm. This pancreatic margin is sometimes specifically designated by the surgeon, but is critical in all cases, since it represents a true surgical margin. Carcinomas may be closest to this margin as the surgeon must preserve the mesenteric vessels and he or she is limited in the amount of surrounding tissue that can be taken.

2. Identify the common bile duct as it exits the pancreas and passes behind the proximal duodenum. The duct is often markedly dilated because the tumor has usually caused obstruction. Remove the proximal bile duct margin en face and place in a separate cassette. Gently place a probe in the duct and advance it until it exits through the ampulla of Vater. It is usually possible to do this even if the duct is functionally obstructed. This must be done while the specimen is fresh and pliable. Ink the soft tissue and uncinate process margins of the pancreas, excluding the distal resection margin (to be able to identify it for orientation).

Identify the main pancreatic duct. This may be difficult and may require two or three serial sections starting at the pancreatic margin to look for the duct as it enlarges proximally. If the duct is found, gently place a probe in it and advance the probe to the ampulla if possible.

If a probe cannot be advanced through the bile duct or the pancreatic duct into the ampulla, find the ampulla starting at the mucosal surface. It is usually more distal than it seems it should be and may have the appearance of an edematous fold of mucosa. Note whether the duodenal mucosa appears grossly normal or abnormal in this region.

In approximately 8% of individuals the main pancreatic duct from the body and tail empties via the accessory duct of Santorini into an accessory papilla, usually located proximal to the ampulla of Vater. The uncinate head only drains into the ampulla. Thus, there may be no communication between the main ampulla and the main pancreatic duct.

3. Make a section along the plane of both pancreatic duct and bile duct probes or along the probe in the common bile duct. This bisects the ampulla and gives the best demonstration of the relationship of the tumor to the ampulla, duodenal mucosa, common bile duct, pancreatic duct, and pancreatic parenchyma. If two parallel cuts are made on either side of this cut, the resulting sections are usually very photogenic and demonstrate the tumor relationships well. An alternative method involves cutting along the main pancreatic duct in the transverse (i.e., anterior to posterior) plane. This method illustrates the relationship of the tumor to the posterior margin and preserves the uncinate process in the inferior half of the specimen.

   Describe the tumor including size, color, consistency, cysts, relationship to anatomic sites, distance from margins, and obstruction of ducts.

   The tumor may be grossly subtle but is best identified as a lesion that partially effaces or blurs the normal lobular architecture of the pancreatic parenchyma, usually without gross scarring.

   Describe the remainder of the pancreatic parenchyma including color, fibrosis, nodularity, fat necrosis, cysts, ducts (?dilated), calculi. Describe any anatomic variations of the merger of the common bile duct and pancreatic duct.

   Only at this point is the specimen is fixed overnight (pinning out the stomach and duodenum) before taking additional sections.

4. Lymph node involvement is the most important prognostic indicator. Carefully section through the surrounding soft tissue to look for lymph nodes. The location of each lymph node found is recorded (i.e., anterior, inferior, posterior, superior pancreas, pyloric, stomach, distal duodenal, and splenic) as this information is used in staging. Although little adipose tissue is present, several lymph nodes are always present. Commonly, a lymph node is present near the common bile duct. Some lymph nodes may be submitted by the surgeon as separate specimens.

5. If other specimens are submitted (commonly the gallbladder or spleen), they are examined as described in the separate sections. However, special attention is paid to looking for tumor involvement as well as identifying additional lymph nodes.

Gross differential diagnosis (Fig. 19-13)

Adenocarcinoma may be difficult to define grossly. The tumor may be an infiltrating white mass that effaces the normal architecture and can resemble a chronically inflamed fibrotic pancreas. The distal common bile duct or pancreatic duct is frequently invaded at the head of the pancreas with obstruction and proximal dilatation of the duct. Carcinomas involving the ampulla typically present earlier with symptoms and are frequently small in size. In larger carcinomas, invasion into the retroperitoneum is common.

Endocrine tumors tend to be well circumscribed with a capsule and occur within the tail. They may be fleshy, yellow, and homogeneous in appearance. Necrosis, cysts, and hemorrhage may be present. Save tissue for EM and snap freezing.

Solid-pseudopapillary tumor is usually a well-circumscribed large mass arising anywhere in the pancreas, comprised of single or multiple cystic spaces. Central necrosis is common. The inner wall must be sectioned extensively to look for solid areas. This tumor is most common in young women and carries a relatively good prognosis.

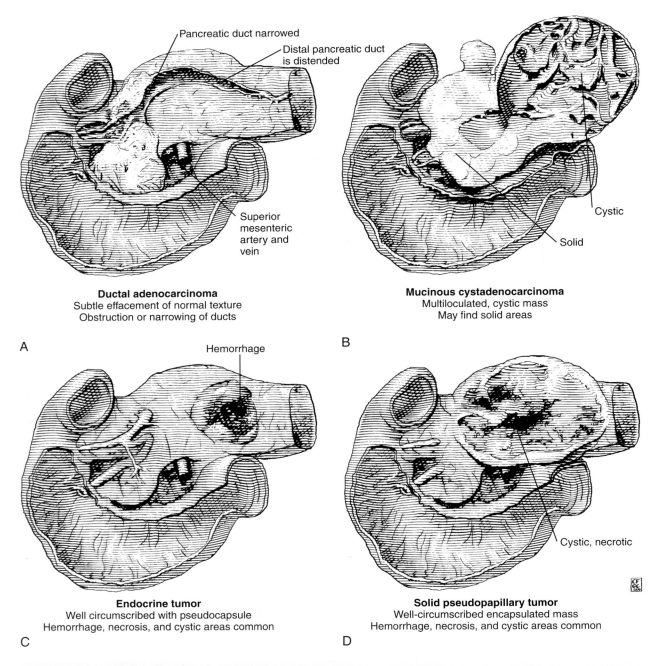

Figure 19-13 Differential diagnosis of pancreatic tumors.

Mucinous cystic tumors of the pancreas (cystadenoma and cystadenocarcinoma) can be found anywhere in the pancreas, but more commonly occur in the body or tail. The tumors are comprised of mucin-containing cystic spaces, usually thin-walled. Look for solid areas or thickened walls with papillary excrescences; these areas are more likely to contain invasive tumor.

Serous cystic neoplasms are more uniform in appearance and are virtually always benign. These tumors only occasionally communicate with the normal ductal system. The tumors consist of a circumscribed area of small cysts separated by thin septa and may have a central stellate scar.

Intraductal papillary mucinous neoplasms are grossly similar to mucinous cystic tumors in that they are comprised of mucin-containing spaces. However, these tumors are usually in continuity with the main pancreatic duct and are more common in the head region.

Acinar cell carcinoma occurs anywhere in the pancreas and consists of multiple soft well-circumscribed red/brown nodules separated by fibrous septa. Occasionally tumors can consist of multiple cysts.

Pancreatoblastoma is the most common pancreatic tumor of childhood. The large soft encapsulated mass can occur at any site in the pancreas.

Chronic pancreatitis can result in a very hard, scarred pancreas that is difficult to distinguish from an invasive carcinoma. Calculi may be present within the pancreatic duct and pseudocysts may form in peripancreatic soft tissue.

Pseudocysts are usually associated with pancreatitis and arise due to digestion of tissues by pancreatic enzymes. The cystic cavity is generally extrapancreatic but attached by fibrotic tissue. A portion of the adjacent stomach may be included with the specimen. The cyst may be filled with blood and necrotic material.

Microscopic sections

Tumor
Up to six blocks including relationship to pancreas, ducts, ampulla, duodenal mucosa, and surrounding soft tissue.

Margins
Pancreatic resection margin (either perpendicular or en face, soft tissue around pancreas, common bile duct, stomach, duodenum. Only the posterior retroperitoneal soft tissue and the posterior (non-peritonealized) surface of the uncinate process are true margins, being in continuity with the patient. The remaining soft tissue "margins" evaluate tumor invasion outside of the pancreas and are taken perpendicular to the tumor.

Uninvolved pancreas
One to two cassettes including normal and abnormal appearing areas.

Ampulla
One cassette (if not previously submitted).

Lymph nodes
Submit all lymph nodes as separate groups.
Regional lymph nodes include the following:

- Superior pancreatic nodes: superior to the head and body of the pancreas
- Anterior pancreatic nodes: anterior pancreaticoduodenal, pyloric, and proximal mesenteric
- Inferior pancreatic nodes: inferior to the head and body of the pancreas
- Posterior pancreatic nodes: posterior pancreaticoduodenal, common bile duct or pericholedochal, and proximal mesenteric
- Retroperitoneal nodes
- Lateral aortic nodes
- Hepatic artery nodes
- Superior mesenteric nodes
- Infrapyloric nodes (tumors of the head only)
- Subpyloric nodes (tumors of the head only)
- Celiac nodes (tumors of the head only)
- Pancreaticolienal nodes (tumors of the body and tail only)
- Splenic nodes: hilum of spleen and tail of the pancreas (tumors of the body and tail only).

Involvement of other nodal groups is considered distant metastasis.

Sample dictation

Received fresh, labeled with the patient's name and unit number and "Whipple," is the stomach (20 cm in length × 15 cm in circumference × 0.5 cm wall thickness), duodenum (30 cm in length × 4 cm in circumference) and pancreatic head (5 × 4 × 4 cm (length)). There is a tan/white 3 × 2 × 2 cm diffusely infiltrating tumor mass in the head of the pancreas which surrounds the main pancreatic duct and the common bile duct at their junction. The bile duct is patent but dilated to 0.7 cm in diameter. The pancreatic duct is obstructed by the tumor mass. The tumor is 1 cm from the ampulla of Vater and does not grossly involve the duodenal muscularis or mucosa. The tumor is 2 cm from the distal pancreatic resection margin which is grossly free of tumor. The lateral margins are comprised of yellow/white adipose tissue ranging in thickness from 1 to 3 cm and are grossly free of tumor. The remainder of the pancreatic parenchyma is firm and nodular. The cystic duct remnant is 2 cm in length by 0.7 cm in diameter. There is an adjacent 1.1 cm fleshy lymph node. The gastric mucosa is unremarkable. Two lymph nodes are present in the perigastric soft tissue (0.5 and 0.3 cm). The distal 20 cm of the duodenal mucosa has a dusky red/brown color. Three periduodenal lymph nodes are found, the largest measuring 0.6 cm. Three lymph nodes are found adjacent to the pancreas (one anterior and two inferior), the largest measuring 0.9 cm. The margins are inked. Photographs are taken.

Cassettes #1 and 2: Pancreatic resection margin, en face, 2 frags, ESS.
Cassettes #3 and 4: Tumor and common bile duct, 2 frags, RSS.
Cassettes #5 and 6: Tumor and pancreatic duct, 2 frags, RSS.
Cassettes #7 and 8: Tumor and pancreatic parenchyma, 2 frags, RSS.
Cassette #9: Anterior margin, perpendicular, 1 frag, RSS.
Cassette #10: Superior margin, perpendicular, 1 frag, RSS.
Cassette #11: Posterior margin, perpendicular, 1 frag, RSS.
Cassette #12: Inferior margin, perpendicular, 1 frag, RSS.
Cassette #13: Gastric resection margin, en face, 1 frag, RSS.
Cassette #14: Duodenal resection margin, en face, 1 frag, RSS.
Cassette #15: Common bile duct margin, en face, 1 frag, RSS.
Cassette #16: Uninvolved pancreas, 2 frags, RSS.
Cassette #17: Ampulla, 1 frag, RSS.
Cassette #18: Common bile duct lymph node, 2 frags, ESS.
Cassette #19: Two perigastric lymph nodes, 2 frags, ESS.
Cassette #20: Three periduodenal lymph nodes, 3 frags, ESS.
Cassette #21: One anterior pancreatic node, 2 frags, ESS.
Cassette #22: Two inferior pancreatic nodes, 2 frags, ESS.

Pathologic prognostic/diagnostic features sign-out checklist for pancreatic tumors

Specimen type*
Pancreatoduodenectomy (Whipple procedure), distal pancreatectomy, other organs included (spleen, gallbladder).

Tumor site*
Ampulla, periampullary, head of pancreas (to the right of the left border of the superior mesenteric vein including the uncinate process), body of pancreas (between the left border of the superior mesenteric vein and the left border of the aorta), tail of pancreas (between the left border of the aorta and the hilum of the spleen). Clinical information may be necessary to identify the location of some tumors.

Tumor focality*
For endocrine tumors: unifocal, multifocal.

Tumor configuration
Infiltrative, circumscribed (solid or cystic, partially or entirely circumscribed).

Tumor size*

Greatest dimension. For exocrine tumors, ≤2 cm, >2 cm is used for staging (other dimensions optional). For endocrine tumors, tumors ≥2.5 cm are correlated with aggressive biologic behavior (tumors <2.5 cm are almost always benign, tumors >10 cm are highly likely to be malignant).

Histologic type*

Pancreas: Infiltrating ductal adenocarcinoma, mucinous noncystic carcinoma, signet ring cell carcinoma (>50% signet ring cells), adenosquamous carcinoma, undifferentiated (anaplastic) carcinoma, acinar cell carcinoma, serous cystadenoma, mucinous cystic neoplasm, mucinous cystadenocarcinoma, intraductal papillary mucinous neoplasm (without or with invasion) (Box 19-13, Table 19-20), solid pseudopapillary tumor, pancreatic endocrine tumor (Tables 19-21, 19-22), mixed tumors, others.

Ampulla: Papillary adenocarcinoma, intestinal adenocarcinoma, mucinous adenocarcinoma, signet ring cell carcinoma (>50% signet ring cells), carcinoid, others.

Functional type

If endocrine tumor, correlation with clinical syndrome and/or elevated serum levels of hormone product.

Histologic grade*

Well, moderately, poorly differentiated, undifferentiated (Box 19-14).

Extent of invasion*

Carcinoma in situ (Tis), limited to pancreas, less than or equal to 2 cm (T1), limited to pancreas, greater than 2 cm (T2), extension beyond pancreas but without involvement of the celiac axis or the superior mesenteric artery (T3), involvement of the celiac axis or the superior mesenteric artery (T4).

Invasion of duodenum, ampulla of Vater, common bile duct, peripancreatic tissues, stomach, spleen, colon, large vessels (portal vein, mesenteric vessels, common hepatic artery), mesentery, omentum.

Ampullary tumors: confined to duodenal wall; invasion ≤2 cm into pancreas; invasion >2 cm into pancreas; invasion into adjacent organs.

Intraductal papillary mucinous neoplasms are grossly visible, usually clinically detected, noninvasive neoplasms arising from the pancreatic ducts. The involved ducts are usually dilated and the lesions are usually larger than 1 cm.

Intraductal lesions

Papillary hyperplasia, carcinoma in situ.

Venous/lymphatic (large/small) vessel invasion

Absent, present, indeterminate.

Perineural invasion

Absent, present.

Mitotic activity

Absent, present (≤4 mitoses/HPF), present >4 mitoses/HPF)

Margins*

Invasive carcinoma or in situ dysplasia or carcinoma:

Involved or not involved (distance from closest margin), including common bile duct margin, pancreatic parenchymal margin including pancreatic duct margin, uncinate process margin (non-peritonealized surface of the uncinate process), posterior (retroperitoneal) pancreas, duodenum, stomach, peripancreatic soft tissue margins (anterior, inferior, posterior, superior).

Type of ductal epithelium at parenchymal margin (normal, mucinous metaplasia, dysplasia). The PanIN classification scheme should be used (Box 19-15, Table 19-23).

Regional lymph nodes*

Metastases present or absent, number of metastases, number of nodes examined.

Regional versus distant

Note: The definition of regional nodes depends on the location of the tumor.

- Gastric lymph nodes: distant for all.
- Pyloric lymph nodes: regional for head, distant for body and tail.
- Peripancreatic lymph nodes: regional for all. Divide into superior, inferior, anterior, and posterior groups.
- Splenic lymph nodes: regional for body and tail, distant for head.

Distant metastasis*
Absent or present.

Nonlesional pancreas
Chronic pancreatitis, acute pancreatitis, fibrosis, pancreatic intraepithelial neoplasia, intraductal pancreatic mucinous tumor, islet cell hyperplasia, adenomatosis.

Stomach and duodenum
Gastritis (chemical or *H. pylori*), duodenitis, peptic ulcer disease, ampullitis.

This checklist incorporates information from the ADASP (see www.panix.com/~adasp) and the CAP Cancer Committee protocols for reporting on cancer specimens (see www.cap.org/). The asterisked elements are considered to be scientifically validated or regularly used data elements that must be present in reports of cancer-directed surgical resection specimens from ACS CoC-approved cancer programs. The specific details of reporting the elements may vary among institutions.

Box 19-13 Grading system for infiltrating ductal carcinomas of the pancreas[21]

Grade I — Well differentiated (>95% of tumor composed of glands)
Grade II — Moderately differentiated (50–95% of tumor composed of glands)
Grade III — Poorly differentiated (5–49% of tumor composed of glands)
Grade IV — Undifferentiated (<5% of tumor composed of glands)

Table 19-20 Classification of intraductal papillary mucinous neoplasms

	ARCHITECTURE	CELLULAR DIFFERENTIATION	DYSPLASIA	MITOSES
IPMN adenoma	Papillary	Tall columnar Mucin-containing	Slight or none	Absent
IPMN borderline	Papillary; pseudo-papillary structures may be present	Tall columnar Mucin-containing	Moderate	Usually absent
Intraductal papillary mucinous carcinoma	Papillary or micropapillary. Cribriform growth and budding of small clusters of cells into the lumen may be present	Cellular pleomorphism Diminished or absent mucin	Severe (carcinoma in situ) Loss of polarity Nuclear pleomorphism Nuclear enlargement	May be present, may be suprabasal or luminal

Intraductal papillary mucinous neoplasms are grossly visible, usually clinically detected, noninvasive neoplasms arising from the pancreatic ducts. The involved ducts are usually dilated and the lesions are usually larger than 1 cm.

Box 19-14 Grading system for nonpapillary carcinomas of the ampulla of Vater

Grade I	Well differentiated (>95% of tumor composed of glands)
Grade II	Moderately differentiated (50–95% of tumor composed of glands)
Grade III	Poorly differentiated (less than 49% of tumor composed of glands)
Grade IV	Undifferentiated carcinomas and small cell carcinoma (high-grade neuroendocrine carcinomas in the WHO classification

Table 19-21 Classification of pancreatic endocrine tumors

TUMOR TYPE	CLINICAL SYMPTOMS
Pancreatic endocrine tumor, functional	
Insulinoma (insulin-secreting)	Hypoglycemia, neuropsychiatric disorders
Glucagonoma (glucagon-secreting)	Diabetes, skin rash (necrolytic migratory erythema), stomatitis
Gastrinoma (gastrin-secreting)	Abdominal pain, ulcer disease, diarrhea, gastrointestinal bleeding
Somatostatinoma (somatostatin-secreting)	Diabetes, steatorrhea, achlorhydria
PPoma (pancreatic polypeptide-secreting)	Clinically silent, elevated serum PP levels
VIPoma (vasoactive intestinal polypeptide secreting, Verner–Morrison tumors)	Watery diarrhea, hypokalemia, achlorhydria
Adrenocorticotropic hormone secreting	Cushing's syndrome: central obesity, muscle weakness, glucose intolerance, hypertension
Carcinoid tumor (serotonin-producing)	Carcinoid syndrome: flushing, diarrhea
Pancreatic endocrine tumor, non-functional	
Pancreatic endocrine tumor, nonsecretory	
Mixed ductal-endocrine carcinoma	
Mixed acinar-endocrine carcinoma	

High mitotic activity (>4 per 10 HPF, 80% malignant), a high degree of pleomorphism, and tumor necrosis correlate with malignant potential. Larger tumor size ($\geq$2.5 cm) correlates with local invasion, vascular invasion, and metastasis.

Table 19-22 WHO Classification of endocrine tumors of the pancreas

	WELL DIFFERENTIATED ENDOCRINE TUMOR	WELL DIFFERENTIATED ENDOCRINE CARCINOMA	POORLY DIFFERENTIATED ENDOCRINE CARCINOMA OR SMALL CELL CARCINOMA
Growth pattern	Small solid nests, trabeculae, gyriform cords, or pseudoglandular structures	Solid nests and sheets, trabeculae, gyriform cords, or pseudo-glandular structures	Large, ill-defined solid aggregates or diffuse sheets of cells
Cytologic features	No or minimal atypia	Mild to moderate atypia, hyperchromatic nuclei, fairly prominent nucleoli	Highly atypical, small to intermediate sized cells with high N:C ratio, poorly granular or agranular cytoplasm
Local extent	Usually circumscribed, can be ill defined, confined to pancreas	May invade local structures	Usually invades locally
Size	<2 cm	Most >3 cm	Any size
Necrosis	Absent	Usually absent	Often present
Lymphovascular or perineural invasion	Absent	Often present	Usually prominent
Mitoses (per 10 HPF)	≤2	2–10	>10
Ki-67 (% of cells)	≤2%	>5%	>15%
P53			Frequently present
Metastases	Absent	May be present (regional lymph nodes or liver)	Often present (liver and extra-abdominal sites)

Mixed exocrine–endocrine carcinomas are tumors with an admixture of the two components; the biologic behavior is determined by that of the exocrine component.

Table 19-23 Classification of pancreatic intraepithelial neoplasia (PanIN)[20,22,23]

	ARCHITECTURE	CYTOLOGY	MITOSES	NECROSIS
Normal	Flat	Flattened or cuboidal, nonmucinous	Absent	Absent
PanIN-1a[a]	Flat	Tall columnar cells Orientation to basal membrane Basally located nuclei Abundant supra-nuclear mucin Nuclei small, round to oval	Absent	Absent
PanIN-1B	Papillary, micro-papillary, or basally pseudostratified	Same as PanIN-1a	Absent	Absent
PanIN-2	Most are papillary but some may be flat. Cribriform growth would be unusual	Some nuclear abnormalities are present: Loss of polarity Nuclear crowding Enlarged nuclei Pseudostratification Hyperchromatism	Rare. If present, they are not abnormal and are non-luminal (not apical)	Absent or very rare
PanIN-3[b]	Usually papillary or micropapillary, rarely flat. Cribriform growth with the appearance of budding off of small clusters of epithelial cells into the lumen, may be present	Marked nuclear abnormalities are present: Loss of polarity Nuclear crowding Enlarged nuclei Irregular nuclei Hyperchromasia Prominent (macro) nuclei Dystrophic goblet cells[c]	Mitoses may be present and may be abnormal	May be present

Pancreatic intraepithelial neoplasia is a microscopic flat or papillary noninvasive neoplasm arising in pancreatic ducts. The involved ducts are generally not dilated or are less than 0.5 cm in size. These lesions are usually not detected clinically or on gross examination but are often found in pancreatic parenchyma surrounding ductal adenocarcinomas.
[a] This category can also be called PanIN/L-1A (lesion) to acknowledge that not all cases may be neoplastic.
[b] For tumor staging, PanIN-3 is equivalent to carcinoma in situ and is classified as Tis.
[c] Dystrophic goblet cells have nuclei oriented toward the lumen and mucinous cytoplasm oriented toward the basement membrane.

Table 19-24 AJCC (6th edition) classification of exocrine pancreatic tumors

Tumor	TX	Primary tumor cannot be assessed
	T0	No evidence of primary tumor
	Tis	In situ carcinoma
	T1	Tumor limited to the pancreas 2 cm or less in greatest dimension
	T2	Tumor limited to the pancreas more than 2 cm in greatest dimension
	T3	Tumor extends beyond the pancreas but without involvement of the celiac axis or the superior mesenteric artery
	T4	Tumor involves the celiac axis or the superior mesenteric artery (unresectable primary tumor)
Regional nodes	NX	Regional lymph nodes cannot be assessed
	N0	No regional lymph node metastasis
	N1	Regional lymph node metastasis
	N1a	Metastasis to one regional lymph node
	N1b	Metastasis to multiple regional lymph nodes
		Note: 10 or more regional lymph nodes are optimally assessed
Distant metastasis	MX	Distant metastasis cannot be assessed
	M0	No distant metastasis
	M1	Distant metastasis (includes direct invasion into the liver, peritoneal seeding, or positive peritoneal cytology on fluid)

Note: This staging system is not used for endocrine cell tumors.

Pathologic prognostic/diagnostic features sign-out checklist for carcinomas of the ampulla of Vater

Specimen type*
Pancreatoduodenectomy (Whipple procedure), ampullectomy.

Tumor site*
Intra-ampullary, periampullary, junction of ampullary and duodenal mucosa, not specified.

Tumor size*
Greatest dimension (tumors <2.5 cm have a 65% 5-year survival rate whereas tumors >2.5 cm have a 20% 5-year survival rate).

Tumor type*
Papillary adenocarcinoma, adenocarcinoma—intestinal type, adenocarcinoma—gastric type, mucinous adenocarcinoma, clear cell adenocarcinoma, signet ring cell carcinoma (>50% signet ring cells), adenosquamous carcinoma, others.

Tumor grade*
Well, moderate, poorly differentiated, undifferentiated (Box 19-16).

Extent of invasion*
Carcinoma in situ, tumor limited to ampulla of Vater or sphincter of Oddi, invasion of muscle of the sphincter of Oddi, invasion of duodenal wall, invasion into pancreas, invasion into peripancreatic soft tissue or other adjacent organs or structures.

Intraductal lesions
Papillary hyperplasia, carcinoma in situ.

Lymphovascular invasion
Present or absent.

Perineural invasion
Present or absent.

Margins*

Involved or not involved, pancreatic margins, duodenal margins, distance to closest margin including common bile duct and pancreatic duct.

Nodal status*

Regional lymph nodes include nodes superior, inferior, and posterior to the head and body of pancreas, pyloric nodes, proximal mesenteric nodes, hepatic artery nodes, common bile duct nodes, infrapyloric nodes, subpyloric nodes, celiac nodes, superior mesenteric nodes, retroperitoneal nodes, and lateral aortic nodes.

Distant metastasis*

All other nodal groups are considered distant metastatic sites, present or absent.

Nonlesional pancreas

Chronic pancreatitis, metaplasia, pancreatic intraepithelial neoplasia, acute pancreatitis, fibrosis, islet cell hyperplasia.

This protocol includes primary carcinomas of the ampulla, including those with focal neuroendocrine differentiation, but is not designed for carcinoid tumors, GISTs, or lymphomas. This checklist incorporates information from the ADASP (see www.panix.com/~adasp/) and the CAP Cancer Committee protocols for reporting on cancer specimens (see www.cap.org/). The asterisked elements are considered to be scientifically validated or regularly used data elements that must be present in reports of cancer-directed surgical resection specimens from ACS CoC-approved cancer programs. The specific details of reporting the elements may vary among institutions.

The AJCC classification is given in Table 19-25.

Table 19-25 AJCC (6th edition) classification of tumors of the ampulla of Vater

Tumor	TX	Primary tumor cannot be assessed
	T0	No evidence of primary tumor
	Tis	Carcinoma in situ
	T1	Tumor limited to the ampulla of Vater or sphincter of Oddi
	T2	Tumor invades duodenal wall
	T3	Tumor invades into the pancreas
	T4	Tumor invades peripancreatic soft tissues and/or into other adjacent organs or structures
Regional nodes	NX	Regional lymph nodes cannot be assessed
	N0	No regional lymph node metastasis
	N1	Regional lymph node metastasis
		Note: Regional lymph nodes are the same as regional lymph nodes for tumors of the head of the pancreas. Optimal evaluation will include at least 10 lymph nodes
Distant metastasis	MX	Distant metastasis cannot be assessed
	M0	No distant metastasis
	M1	Distant metastasis

Note: This staging system is not used for carcinoid tumors or other neuroendocrine tumors.

REFERENCES

1. Lee RG, et al. Protocol for the examination of specimens removed from patients with esophageal carcinoma: A basis for checklists. Arch Pathol Lab Med 121:925-929, 1997.

2. Lewin KJ, Appelman HD. Tumors of the Esophagus and Stomach, Fascicle 18, Third Series. AFIP, Washington, D.C., 1995, p. 293.

3. Fenger C. Histology of the anal canal. Am J Surg Pathol 12:41-55, 1988.

4. Goldstein JS, Somon A, Sacksner J. Disparate surgical margin lengths of colorectal resection specimens between in vivo and in vitro measurements. The effects of surgical resection and formalin fixation on organ shrinkage. Am J Clin Pathol 111:349-351, 1999.

5. Goldstein NS. Lymph node recoveries from 2427 pT3 colorectal resection specimens spanning 45 years: recommendations for a minimum number of recovered lymph nodes based on predictive probabilities. Am J Surg Pathol 26:179-189, 2002.

6. Sanchez-Maldonado W, Rodriquez-Bigas MA, Weber TK, Penetrante RB, Petrelli NJ. Utility of mapping lymph nodes cleared from rectal adenocarcinoma specimens. Surg Oncol 5:123-126, 1996.

7. Angiodysplasia of colon revisited: Pathologic demonstration without the use of intravascular injection technique. Hum Pathol 23:37-40, 1992. *A description of an alternative method for processing these specimens. The specimen is fixed inflated for 3 hours. The mucosa is carefully removed and passed through ethanol. Dilated vessels in the mucosa are visualized grossly using transillumination.*

8. Mitsudo SM, et al. Vascular ectasias of the right colon in the elderly: A distinct pathologic entity. Hum Pathol 10:585, 1979.

9. Shepherd N, Baxter K, Love S. The prognostic importance of peritoneal involvement in colonic cancer: a prospective evaluation. Gastroenterology 112:1096-1102, 1997.

10. Compton C, Fenoglio-Preiser CM, Pettigrew N, Fielding LP. American Joint Committee on Cancer Prognostic Factors Consensus Conference, Colorectal Working Group. Cancer 88:1739-1757, 2000.

11. Jass JR, Sobin LH. Histological typing of intestinal tumors, 2nd edn. World Health Organization. New York, NY, Springer-Verlag, 1989.

12. Jass JR, et al. The grading of rectal cancer: Historical perspectives and a multivariate analysis of 447 cases. Histopathology 10:437-459, 1986.

13. Jass J, Ajioka Y, Allen JP, et al. Assessment of invasive growth pattern and lymphocytic infiltration in colorectal cancer. Histopathology 28:543-548, 1996.

14. Jass JR. Lymphocytic infiltration and survival in rectal cancer. J Clin Pathol 39:585-589, 1986.

15. Hytiroglou P, Thung SN, Gerber MA. Histological classification and quantitation of the severity of chronic hepatitis: keep it simple! Semin Liver Dis 15:414-421, 1995.

16. Scheuer PJ. Classification of chronic viral hepatitis: a need for reassessment. J Hepatol 13:372-374, 1991.

17. Stocker JT. An approach to handling pediatric liver tumors. Am J Clin Pathol 109 (Suppl 1):S67-S72, 1998.

18. Edmondson HA, Steiner PE. Primary carcinoma of the liver, a study of 100 cases among 48,900 necroscopies. Cancer 7:462-503, 1954.

19. Cubilla AL, et al. Lymph node involvement of the head of the pancreas area. Cancer 41:880-887, 1978.

20. Hruban RH, Takaori K, Klimstra DS, et al. An illustrated consensus on the classification of pancreatic intraepithelial neoplasia and intraductal papillary mucinous neoplasms. Am J Surg Pathol 28:977-987, 2004.

21. Recommendations for reporting resected pancreatic neoplasms. HDASP Mod Pathol 11:500-504, 1998.

22. Hruban RH, Adsay VN, Albores-Saavedra J, et al. Pancreatic intraepithelial neoplasia: a new nomenclature and classification system for pancreatic duct lesions. Am J Surg Pathol 25:579-586, 2001.

23. Klein WM, Hruban RH, Klein-Szanto AJP, Wilenz RE. Direct correlation between proliferative activity and dysplasia in pancreatic intraepithelial neoplasia (PanIN): additional evidence for a recently proposed model of progression. Mod Pathol 15:441-447, 2002.

Genitourinary specimens

20

Genitourinary specimens include those from the kidney, ureters, bladder, prostate, and testis. The kidney may be biopsied as part of the evaluation of renal function. Otherwise, genitourinary specimens are generally biopsied or excised for neoplastic disease.

■ KIDNEY

Needle or wedge biopsies

Renal biopsies are usually performed to evaluate glomerular function in patients with renal dysfunction. Resectable masses are rarely biopsied because of the virtually diagnostic appearance of tumors on CT scan and the need for resection for treatment. Unresectable tumors are usually diagnosed by fine needle aspiration (FNA). Occasionally, biopsies are performed on kidneys with tumors that will be treated with cryotherapy or before a kidney is used for transplantation (Chapter 6).

Relevant clinical history

See Table 20-1.

Table 20-1 Relevant clinical history	
HISTORY RELEVANT TO ALL SPECIMENS	HISTORY RELEVANT TO KIDNEY SPECIMENS
Organ/tissue resected or biopsied	Results of urine analysis
Purpose of the procedure	Renal function tests (BUN and creatinine)
Gross appearance of the organ/tissue/lesion sampled	Systemic diseases (e.g., lupus erythematosus, scleroderma, diabetes mellitus, anti-phospholipid syndrome, myeloma, hemoglobinopathies, vasculitis, HUS)
Any unusual features of the clinical presentation	
Any unusual features of the gross appearance	
Prior surgery/biopsies—results	Results of serology (e.g., ANCA, ANA, C3, C4, cryoglobulins, hepatitis C)
Prior malignancy	
Prior treatment (radiation therapy, chemotherapy, chemotherapeutic agents) appearance of tissues)	Drug use (analgesics, penicillamine, hydralazine, chemotherapeutic agents)
Compromised immune system	Organ transplantation (native versus transplant kidney)
	Infection (e.g., hepatitis)
	Pregnancy

Processing the specimen

1. The specimen is often examined for adequacy by stereo-microscopy in the ultrasound suite during the procedure. Additional cores of tissue may be requested when the sample does not contain sufficient cortex.
2. Representative samples are fixed in formalin. Additional tissue is saved for electron microscopy and immunofluorescence microscopy.
3. Special stains are usually evaluated on all renal biopsies (e.g., PAS, trichrome, Jones silver methenamine).

Nephrectomy

Nephrectomy is commonly performed for tumor (usually renal cell carcinoma [RCC], rarely urothelial [transitional] cell carcinoma [TCC] of the renal pelvis) or to remove a nonfunctioning graft. Native nonfunctioning kidneys are also sometimes removed. Partial nephrectomy is increasingly used to resect tumor if the other kidney is absent or nonfunctioning or if the primary tumor is small (e.g., a tumor found incidentally on CT scan or ultrasound).

Transplant nephrectomy

Renal grafts are transplanted to the pelvis with a short vascular pedicle connected to the inguinal vessels. The specimen usually consists simply of the kidney, without surrounding soft tissue, and vessels cut flush with the hilum. Transplant failure may be caused by preexisting disease in the allograft, vascular insufficiency (e.g., thrombosis or plaque), rejection, or recurrence of the patient's original renal disease.

Processing the specimen

1. Weigh (normal is 125 to 170 g for males and 115 to 155 g for females) and record the measurements of the kidney. Record the length and diameter of any vessels at the hilum. Look for patency of vessels (thrombosis, intimal proliferation, atherosclerotic plaques).
2. Describe the renal parenchyma including color (tan/red, gray/green), thickness of cortex, shape of calyces and papillae (normal, blunted), state of pelvis and ureter, vessels, infarcts (size and location), hemorrhage, and necrosis.
3. Submit four cassettes including cortex and medulla, hilar vessels, and focal lesions and request a PAS stain on one block.

   If the transplant has failed six months or more after transplantation, or if there is significant proteinuria, and recurrence of the patient's original disease is suspected, always save cortex for EM and immunofluorescence microscopy.

Native kidney nephrectomy

Nonfunctioning kidneys may be removed because of hypertension refractory to medical therapy, persistent pyelonephritis, severe renal protein loss, polycystic kidneys, or in patients with bilateral renal tumors. A native kidney may also be removed to provide a native ureter for the allograft.

Acquired cystic kidney disease (ACKD) occurs in over 30% of patients with end stage renal disease and the incidence increases over time. Papillary hyperplasia is commonly present in the walls of the cysts and is thought to be a precursor lesion for carcinomas. Adenomas are frequently found in this population (approximately 25%) and are typically multiple and bilateral.

Renal cell carcinomas develop in 5% to 10% of patients, and 70% to 80% of these patients have ACKD. Although many carcinomas are small and incidental, some do metastasize, resulting in an overall 5-year survival rate of 35%. The relative proportion of papillary renal cell carcinomas is increased in this group. The incidence of urothelial carcinomas is increased in patients with analgesic-related renal failure.

The cortex is examined as for a diagnostic renal biopsy to identify the etiology of the renal failure.

Processing the specimen

1. Weigh (normal is 125 to 170 g for males and 115 to 155 g for females) and record the measurements of the kidney. Record the length and diameter of any vessels at the hilum. Look for patency of vessels (thrombosis, intimal proliferation, atherosclerotic plaques).

2. Describe the renal parenchyma including color (tan/red, gray/green), thickness of cortex, shape of calyces and papillae (normal, blunted), state of pelvis and ureter, vessels, infarcts (size and location), hemorrhage, and necrosis. The number and size of cysts are recorded.

    The entire kidney is thinly sectioned and examined for solid lesions. The lining of cysts is examined for any areas of thickening or irregularities.

    Fresh normal cortical tissue may be saved for immunofluorescence (Zeus medium) and fixed for EM if these studies might be requested.

3. Submit four cassettes including cortex and medulla and hilar vessels.

    PAS, silver methenamine, and AFOG stains on the best block of normal cortex may be helpful for evaluation in some cases.

    Additional cassettes are submitted to document any solid or cystic area suspicious for carcinoma.

Laparoscopic nephrectomy with morcellation

Laparoscopic surgery offers numerous advantages for patients. However, before tissues and organs can be removed through a small skin incision they must be morcellated (i.e., reduced to small fragments) and this procedure introduces new challenges to pathologists. The procedure has been used for the removal of adrenal glands, kidneys, spleens, and prostate glands.

It may not be possible to determine the size, status of margins, and renal vein involvement for such specimens. However, this information can be determined from imaging studies, and the decreased morbidity to the patient from a laparoscopic procedure may outweigh the loss of specific pathologic confirmation. A method to allow inking of margins prior to morcellation has been described.[1] If gross tumor, vessels, and/or ureter are apparent, these specific structures can be selected for microscopic examination.

Pathologic examination is more problematic if there is a small mass and a prior diagnosis has not been made. In most cases, fragments containing tumor are grossly identifiable. A model has been described to estimate the amount of tissue that would need to be examined in order to find a tumor of a given size in a specimen of a certain size with 95% certainty if gross tumor cannot be identified.[2] For example, to find a 4.5 cm tumor in a normal-sized kidney, approximately 11 cassettes of tissue would need to be examined. However, it could take over 100 cassettes to find a 1 cm tumor. Cytology washings from the retrieval bag can also provide a diagnosis in the majority of patients.[3]

Radical nephrectomy

A radical nephrectomy consists of the kidney, most of the ureter, renal vein and artery, perinephric fat, and surrounding Gerota's fascia. An adrenal gland may or may not be present.

Processing the specimen

1. Weigh the entire specimen and record its dimensions. Examine the hilum carefully and identify the ureter, renal vein, and renal artery. The vessels will usually be tied off with sutures.

Tumor involvement of the renal vein is usually obvious and has the appearance of a smoothly surfaced projection of tumor extending out from the hilum. There may be a "plug" of tumor in the lumen, or the tumor may invade into the vessel wall. It is useful to determine whether vessel invasion was seen on preoperative radiologic studies in order to specifically document this finding.

Take cross-sections of the margins (vein, artery, and ureter) and place in a labeled cassette.

Palpate the hilar region for any lymph nodes and save in a labeled cassette. Typically lymph nodes are not found.

2. Inspect the outer portion of the specimen. The kidney is surrounded by perirenal fat. Surrounding this fat, the kidney, and the adrenal gland is the renal fascia (Gerota's fascia).

If there are areas suspicious for tumor at the margin (which is rarely seen as most tumors are limited to the renal parenchyma), ink these areas selectively.

The kidney is then bivalved with a single longitudinal cut.

If the section starts at the hilum, place a probe in the ureter. Cut along the probe to bisect the ureter and extend the cut to divide the kidney. This method facilitates the complete evaluation of the urothelium in cases of urothelial (transitional) cell carcinoma.

Alternatively, start at the side of the kidney opposite the hilum and bivalve the kidney, but do not cut completely through the hilum.

Describe all lesions including size, number (both RCC and TCC may be multifocal), location (with respect to the upper and lower pole, cortex, pelvis), distance from margins (Gerota's fascia, vascular, ureteral), involvement of calyceal or pelvic mucosa (open completely with scissors), gross invasion of capsule or into perirenal soft tissue, involvement of adjacent structures (renal vein, adrenal). Make additional cuts as necessary to assess the parenchyma. Photograph any gross lesion.

Describe the uninvolved renal parenchyma including color, thickness of the cortex, corticomedullary junction (well defined, effaced), shape of the papillae (blunted, necrotic), calyces, renal pelvis (dilation, petechiae, mucosa), presence of calculi, and types of cysts (simple cysts are usually benign; complex cysts may represent tumor). Note any tan/yellow or white nodules in the cortex that might represent a cortical "adenoma" or additional foci of tumor.

3. Fix the entire specimen in formalin overnight. Large tumors are partially sectioned and gauze is used to wick formalin around the sections.

4. The following day, sections of the tumor, margins, and kidney are taken. The adrenal gland is identified at the upper pole. It is usually, but not always, present. Free the gland from the surrounding fat and describe, including color, size, and nodularity (see Chapter 11). Section it carefully looking for evidence of tumor metastasis (nodules). If abnormal, weigh the gland and/or focal lesions.

5. Carefully section through the remainder of the fat looking for lymph nodes. Most nodes will be near the renal hilum.

6. A portion of rib is usually submitted with the nephrectomy specimen. See Chapter 14 for instructions on processing.

Gross differential diagnosis (Fig. 20-1)

Renal cell carcinoma. The most common type of carcinoma—clear cell (conventional)—is usually golden yellow to red, spongy to firm, and occurs in discrete nodules with pushing borders. Blood lakes are typical. Necrosis may be present. The tumor may appear brown if the cytoplasm is granular. Cysts may be absent or quite prominent. Most RCC arise in the upper pole. The tumor may bulge out beyond the contour of the renal capsule, but rarely invades into adipose tissue. RCC arising in acquired cystic disease may be quite subtle and have the appearance of an irregular area or papillary projection within a cyst.

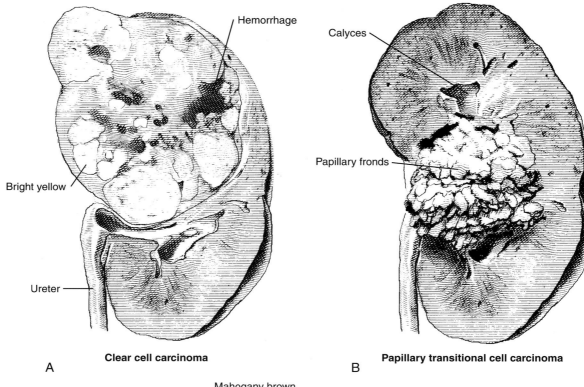

A   **Clear cell carcinoma**

B   **Papillary transitional cell carcinoma**

C   **Oncocytoma**

Figure 20-1 Renal lesions.

- **Papillary carcinomas** are brown (due to hemosiderin), very soft and friable, and may appear to be necrotic (although they usually are not).
- **Chromophobe carcinomas** are usually well circumscribed and tan/brown in color with possible focal necrosis or hemorrhage.
- **Granular cell renal carcinoma** is brown and typically has an invasive border. Hemorrhage and necrosis are usually present.
- **Collecting duct carcinomas** occur in the renal medulla and have a hard gray/white appearance. The borders are typically irregular and necrosis is frequent.
- Tumors of other types with **sarcomatoid features** are gray/white firm to fleshy masses. Hemorrhage and necrosis are common.

Cytogenetic studies can be helpful to distinguish the different types of RCC (see Table 7-33). EM can be helpful to distinguish chromophobe carcinomas from oncocytomas (see Table 7-32).

Urothelial (transitional) cell carcinoma is usually a tan/pink friable mass with a minute villous architecture. There may be a rather small base, compared to the size of the tumor, attached to the renal pelvic urothelium. However, some tumors have a broad base and involve the majority of the urothelium of the renal pelvis.

Renal cortical adenomas are usually well circumscribed, unencapsulated gray or yellow tumors present below the renal capsule. They are typically an incidental finding and are less than 2 cm in size. They are sometimes associated with long-term hemodialysis or chronic pyelonephritis.

Metanephric adenomas are also well circumscribed but can range in size from 1 to 15 cm. The color is fleshy tan/yellow and hemorrhage or necrosis may be present.

Oncocytomas are usually deep red/brown, soft, and well circumscribed, without areas of necrosis, and located in the cortex. Central "scarring" is present in approximately half of cases, especially in larger tumors.

Pediatric tumors. The types of renal tumors occurring in children are quite different from those occurring in adults and include nephroblastoma (Wilms tumor), clear cell sarcoma, rhabdoid tumor, mesoblastic nephroma, lymphoma, neural tumors, renal cell carcinoma, and angiomyolipoma. The specimens may be processed as above but additional sections should be taken to document the relationship of the tumor to the normal kidney and to evaluate possible capsular invasion. Since these tumors tend to be more heterogeneous in appearance, at least one section per cm of greatest tumor dimension should be taken, including all areas of differing appearance. Tissue should also be taken for special studies (Box 20-1).

- **Nephroblastoma (Wilms tumor)** is a well-circumscribed lobulated mass with a gray to pink variegated appearance. Extensive necrosis and hemorrhage are common. If there are multiple nodules, each should be sampled. Cysts may be present. The tumor may invade into the renal vein, ureter, or adipose tissue. Characteristic cytogenetic changes are present (see Table 7-33).

The weight of the kidney may be used as an eligibility factor for clinical protocols and must be accurately determined.

At least one section per cm of tumor should be taken, as tumors can be quite heterogeneous. Most sections should be taken from the periphery to evaluate the relationship to the capsule, the normal kidney, and possible vascular involvement.

More than one third of cases are associated with nephrogenic rests (Table 20-2). These appear as grossly pale areas. The presence of nephrogenic rests is associated with the probability of a syndrome and involvement of the contralateral kidney. Renal lobes are more easily seen in the kidneys of infants and children.

Nephroblastomatosis is defined as multiple or diffusely distributed rests.

The renal sinus (the hilum of the kidney occupied by the renal pelvis, hilar vessels, and fat) should be well sampled as tumors often involve vessels at this point. The renal cortex lacks a capsule at this point. The tumor often involves the renal vein as a tumor

Box 20-1 Special studies in pediatric renal tumors[4,5]

Snap-frozen tissue

The National Wilms Tumor Study Protocols (www.nwstg.org) require snap-frozen tissue from all pediatric renal tumors and adjacent normal tissue (preferably 1 g or a minimum of 100 mg in two or more vials along with a separate portion of normal kidney in at least one vial). Nephrogenic rests may also be frozen. Adjacent tissue should be sampled for formalin fixation for histologic correlation.

Electron microscopy

EM may occasionally be of use.

Touch preparations

Fixed in 95% alcohol. Can be used for some studies (e.g., FISH) if other tissue is not available.

Flow cytometry

In some cases flow cytometric analysis of ploidy, S-phase fraction, or surface markers (i.e., for lymphomas) may be requested.

Cytogenetics

Can be useful for prognosis and classification as these tumors have charascteristic changes— neuroblastoma (N-*myc* amplification, 1p deletion), peripheral primitive neuroectodermal tumor— characteristic t(11,22), cellular mesoblastic nephroma—t(12;15), malignant rhabdoid tumor—22q11.2 deletion, or Wilms tumor—11p13 deletion.

Table 20-2 Types of nephrogenic rest[a]

FEATURE	PERILOBAR REST	INTRALOBAR REST
Site in renal lobe	Periphery (including subcortical)	Random; cortex, medulla, sinus
Margins	Clearly demarcated	Poorly demarcated
Relation to nephrons	No nephrons within rest	Dispersed between nephrons
Composition	Blastemal or tubular; stroma scanty or sclerotic	Tubules, blastema, cysts; stroma usually predominates
Number	Usually numerous	Often single
Associations	Beckwith–Wiedemann syndrome, Perlman syndrome, and hemihypertrophy	WAGR syndrome and Denys–Drash syndrome

[a] Modified from Sternberg's Diagnostic Surgical Pathology, 2004.

thrombus. The vein may retract around a tumor thrombus. This should not be interpreted as a positive margin if the thrombus is not transected.

- **Clear cell sarcoma** is usually a large and well-circumscribed gray/white mass with pushing borders into the adjacent renal parenchyma.[6] Focal necrosis and hemorrhage may be present. Characteristic cytogenetic changes are present (see Table 7-33).
- **Rhabdoid tumor.** Most are well defined and fleshy in appearance with frequent necrosis and hemorrhage. The renal pelvis is usually involved. Characteristic cytogenetic changes are present (see Table 7-33).
- **Congenital mesoblastic nephroma** is an irregular gray/white to tan mass, often of large size. Few cases are associated with cysts, necrosis, or hemorrhage. These tumors can involve the renal vein and the vessels at the hilum and this is an important prognostic factor. This

area should be thoroughly sampled. Characteristic cytogenetic changes are present (see Table 7-33).

There are two main types:

1. Classic CMN (24% of cases) corresponds to infantile fibromatosis.
2. Cellular CMN (66% of cases) corresponds to infantile fibrosarcoma and has a t(12;15). Most relapses are of this type.

   Mixed CMN (10%) has features of both histologic types.

- **Lymphoma.** A well-defined homogenous gray to white mass involving the cortex or medulla.

Cystic kidney disease. Genetic (presenting at birth or as an adult), sporadic, and acquired (due to long-term hemodialysis) forms occur. The location and size of the cysts vary among the different types of cystic renal disease (Table 20-3). The increased risk of RCC in acquired cystic disease mandates that all cysts be carefully examined for mural nodules or papillary projections.

Xanthogranulomatous pyelonephritis. There are single or multiple golden yellow nodules in and around the pelvis and calyces. The nodules may rarely be found in the renal capsule or in adjacent fat. The gross appearance can mimic a renal cell carcinoma.

Angiomyolipoma. This tumor is usually well circumscribed. The radiologic appearance is often diagnostic. The tumors are variegated due to the mixture of adipose tissue (yellow) and smooth muscle (gray/white). The smooth muscle cells are positive for HMB-45 and other melanoma markers. The vascular component is often associated with hemorrhage. The tumor may be confined to the kidney or extend through the capsule. Rare cases may involve the renal vein or regional lymph nodes. The gross appearance can closely mimic a RCC. Approximately half the cases are associated with tuberous sclerosis: these patients more commonly have

Table 20-3 Cystic kidney disease

DISEASE	KIDNEY SIZE	LOCATION OF CYSTS	SIZE OF CYSTS	CLINICAL CORRELATIONS
Infantile polycystic kidney disease	Massively enlarged	Cortex and medulla, radially arranged and oriented perpendicular to renal capsule	Small	Usually fatal at birth
Medullary sponge kidney	Normal	Arise in collecting ducts and found in medullary pyramids and renal papillae	Small, <0.5 cm	Rarely progress to renal failure, associated with urolithiasis
Medullary cystic kidney disease/ Familial nephrolithiasis	Small, contracted, granular surface	Corticomedullary junction	Small, <2 cm	Usually present in childhood with renal failure
Adult polycystic kidney disease	Normal to marked increase	Cortex and medulla	Small to very large (several cm)	Approximately half progress to renal failure in adulthood
Acquired cystic disease	Small	Cortex	Variable—small to very large	Occurs after long-term hemodialysis. There is an increased risk of RCC

multiple and bilateral tumors. These tumors can rarely be associated with RCC, therefore adequate sampling of non-fatty areas is necessary to evaluate this possibility.

Microscopic sections

Tumor
Three to four cassettes including portions of tumor with varying appearance, relationship to adjacent uninvolved tissue, invasion of adjacent structures. If involvement of the renal vein is known or suspected, representative sections of the vein should be submitted.

Margins
Radial margin in perirenal fat, vascular margins, and ureter margin (these latter three sections can be submitted in the same cassette).

Other lesions
Cysts, infarcts, adenomas, etc. One section of each.

Normal kidney
At least one cassette of uninvolved kidney. If an underlying disease is suspected that could affect the other kidney, tissue for EM or immunofluorescence and special stains may be indicated.

Adrenal
At least one cassette demonstrating normal adrenal. Additional cassettes to demonstrate lesions.

Lymph nodes
Submit all lymph nodes found.

Sample dictation

Received fresh, labeled with the patient's name, unit number, and "kidney," is a 333-g left radical nephrectomy specimen including kidney (12 × 8 × 5.5 cm) and left adrenal gland (3.8 × 1.8 × 0.7 cm) and surrounding perirenal fat measuring in thickness from 2 to 3 cm. Extending from the renal pelvis is a ureter (1 cm in length by 0.3 cm in diameter), renal vein (2.5 cm in length by 1 cm in diameter), and renal artery (1 cm in diameter by 0.4 cm in diameter). In the upper pole is a circumscribed golden yellow tumor mass with areas of hemorrhage (5 × 5 × 3 cm). The tumor protrudes into the renal vein for a distance of 3.2 cm but is not present at the vein margin. The tumor pushes against the renal capsule but does not appear to penetrate the capsule or invade into the perirenal fat. The remainder of the renal cortex is tan/brown with a well-defined cortical medullary junction. The pelvis and calyces are covered by smooth glistening mucosa. The adrenal gland consists of normal medulla and cortex without focal lesions. The adipose tissue is thinly sectioned and no lymph nodes are found.

Cassette #1: Tumor and capsule and perirenal fat, 1 frag, RSS.
Cassette #2: Tumor and adjacent normal kidney, 1 frag, RSS.
Cassette #3: Tumor and renal vein, 1 frag, RSS.
Cassette #4: Renal vein margin, 1 frag, ESS.
Cassette #5: Renal artery and ureter margins, 2 frags, ESS.
Cassette #6: Normal kidney, 1 frag, RSS.
Cassette #7: Representative sections of adrenal, 2 frags, RSS.

Partial nephrectomy

A partial nephrectomy is performed for a radiologically indeterminate mass, tumor in a solitary kidney (the contralateral nephrectomy may have been performed for prior tumor), or underlying disease expected to affect renal function (e.g., diabetes). Process as above with the following exceptions:

1. Examine the cut surface of the kidney for areas suspicious for tumor. Ink this margin. Often, the surgeon will indicate the resection margin using a surgical suture. Because orientation and evaluation of this margin is very important, contact the surgeon for orientation if necessary. Serially section through the specimen. Describe the distance of the tumor from the cut renal resection margin.
2. No major vessel nor the ureter will be present.
3. Take multiple sections demonstrating the relationship of the tumor to the renal resection margin as well as to the deep (perirenal fat) margin.

Pathologic prognostic/diagnostic features sign-out checklist for renal tumors

Specimen type*
Partial nephrectomy, radical nephrectomy.

Laterality*
Right, left.

Tumor site
Upper pole, middle, lower pole, hilum, medulla, cortex.

Focality*
Unifocal, multifocal.

Tumor size*
Greatest dimension (4 cm and 7 cm are used for staging); if multiple tumors, give the size of the largest tumor.

Macroscopic extent of tumor*
RCC:
Limited to kidney, extension into perinephric tissues, extension beyond Gerota's fascia, extension into adrenal, extension into major veins.
TCC:
Into or through renal pelvis into parenchyma or invades into peripelvic fat.
Ureter:
Involvement of lamina propria, muscularis propria, periureteric soft tissue.

Histologic type*
Clear cell (conventional) renal cell carcinoma, papillary renal cell carcinoma, chromophobe renal cell carcinoma, collecting duct carcinoma, urothelial (transitional) cell carcinoma, oncocytoma, Wilms tumor, others.

Histologic grade*
RCC:
Fuhrman nuclear grade (Table 20-4).
TCC:
Various systems (see "Grading of bladder urothelial neoplasms," Table 20-9).

Adrenal gland*
Not present, uninvolved by tumor, direct invasion (T3a), metastasis (M1).

Margins*
Involved or not involved, renal vein, ureter, perinephric fat, Gerota's fascial margin, renal parenchyma (for partial nephrectomies), renal capsular margin (for partial nephrectomies).

Regional lymph nodes*
Metastases present or absent, number of involved nodes, number of nodes examined, size of largest metastasis, extracapsular invasion.

Distant metastases*
Present or absent.

Lymphatic (small vessel) invasion
Present or absent.

Venous (large vessel) invasion
Present or absent.

Nonlesional kidney
Glomerular disease, interstitial disease, cysts, adenomas, inflammation.
For Wilms tumor—nephrogenic rests (intralobar or perilobar).

This checklist incorporates information from the ADASP (see www.panix.com/~adasp) and the CAP Cancer Committee protocols for reporting on cancer specimens (see www.cap.org/). The asterisked elements are considered to be scientifically validated or regularly used data elements that must be present in reports of cancer-directed surgical resection specimens from ACS CoC-approved cancer programs. The specific details of reporting the elements may vary among institutions.

There is a separate checklist for resections of pediatric Wilms tumor (see Reporting on Cancer Specimens at www.cap.org).

Table 20-4 Fuhrman nuclear grading system for renal cell carcinomas[7]

	NUCLEI	NUCLEOLI
Grade I	Round, uniform, measure 10 μm	Inconspicuous or absent
Grade II	Slightly irregular, measure 15 μm	Small
Grade III	Very irregular, measure 20 μm	Prominent, large
Grade IV	Bizarre multilobated, chromatin clumping, ≥20 μm	Prominent

Table 20-5 AJCC (6th edition) classification for renal cell carcinomas

Tumor	TX	Primary tumor cannot be assessed
	T0	No evidence of primary tumor
	T1	Tumor 7 cm or less limited to the kidney
	T1a	Tumor 4 cm or less limited to the kidney
	T1b	Tumor more than 4 cm but less than 7 cm limited to the kidney
	T2	Tumor more than 7 cm in greatest dimension limited to the kidney
	T3	Tumor extends into major veins or invades the adrenal gland or perinephric tissues, but not beyond Gerota's fascia
	T3a	Tumor directly invades the adrenal gland or perirenal and/or renal sinus fat but not beyond Gerota's fascia
	T3b	Tumor grossly extends into the renal vein or its segmental (muscle-containing) branches, or vena cava below the diaphragm
	T3c	Tumor grossly extends into the vena cava above the diaphragm or invades the wall of the vena cava
	T4	Tumor invades beyond Gerota's fascia
Regional nodes	NX	Regional lymph nodes cannot be assessed
	N0	No regional lymph node metastasis
	N1	Metastasis in a single regional lymph node
	N2	Metastases in more than one regional lymph node
		Note: Regional lymph nodes include renal hilar, paracaval, aortic, and retroperitoneal. Laterality does not affect the N classification. If a lymph node dissection is performed, usually at least 8 would be included
Distant metastasis	MX	Distant metastasis cannot be assessed
	M0	No distant metastasis
	M1	Distant metastasis

Note: Sarcomas and adenomas are not included in this classification.
There is a separate staging system for pediatric Wilms tumors (see reference 4 or "Wilms Tumor" protocol in Reporting on Cancer Specimens at www.cap.org).

Table 20-6 AJCC (6th edition) classification for tumors of the renal pelvis and ureter		
Tumor	TX	Primary tumor cannot be assessed
	T0	No evidence of primary tumor
	Ta	Papillary noninvasive carcinoma
	Tis	Carcinoma in situ
	T1	Tumor invades subepithelial connective tissue
	T2	Tumor invades the muscularis
	T3	(For renal pelvis only) Tumor invades beyond muscularis into peripelvic fat or the renal parenchyma
	T3	(For ureter only) Tumor invades beyond muscularis into periureteric fat
	T4	Tumor invades adjacent organs, or through the kidney into perinephric fat
Regional nodes	NX	Regional lymph nodes cannot be assessed
	N0	No regional lymph node metastasis
	N1	Metastasis in a single lymph node, ≤2 cm
	N2	Metastasis in a single lymph node > 2 cm but ≤5 cm or in multiple lymph nodes ≤5 cm
	N3	Metastasis in a lymph node >5 cm
		Note: Regional lymph nodes for the renal pelvis are renal hilar, paracaval, aortic, and retroperitoneal. Regional lymph nodes for the ureter are renal hilar, iliac, paracaval, peri-ureteral, and pelvic. Laterality does not affect N classification
Distant metastasis	MX	Cannot be assessed
	M0	No distant metastasis
	M1	Distant metastasis

■ BLADDER

Urothelial (transitional) cell carcinoma is the most common tumor of the bladder. Other tumors at this site are rare (e.g., squamous cell carcinoma, adenocarcinoma).

The bladder muscularis mucosae is poorly defined (not unlike the gallbladder) and incomplete. Therefore the term "submucosa" is not used. Invasion is reported as being into the lamina propria or deeper into the muscularis propria.

Relevant clinical history (in addition to age and gender)

See Table 20-7.

Biopsy

Bladder biopsies are processed as small biopsies (see Chapter 13). Transurethral resections of bladder tumors (TURBT) sometimes result in specimens grossly recognizable as papillary tumors. Orient if possible; however, the specimens generally cannot be oriented.

Order two levels on each small biopsy. Order one level on grossly recognizable tumor specimens.

Fresh tissue for DNA ploidy can be submitted by clinician request. Only submit portions of biopsies that are clearly tumor by gross examination (but do not submit solid areas that may represent muscle invasion) or one of a set of paired biopsies specifically taken for the purpose of flow cytometry (see Chapter 7).

Pathologic prognostic/diagnostic features sign-out checklist for bladder tumor biopsies

Histologic type
Urothelial (transitional) cell, squamous cell, adenocarcinoma.

Grade
WHO 2003 grading system (see Table 20-9).

Depth of invasion
Not invasive, superficial, into muscularis propria.

Muscularis propria
Present or absent.

This list incorporates the recommendations of Gephardt and Baker.[8]

Table 20-7 Relevant clinical history	
HISTORY RELEVANT TO ALL SPECIMENS	HISTORY RELEVANT TO BLADDER SPECIMENS
Organ/tissue resected or biopsied	Renal or bladder stones
Purpose of the procedure	Recent urinary tract infections
Gross appearance of the organ/tissue/lesion sampled	Recent urinary tract procedures
Any unusual features of the clinical presentation	Obstruction
Any unusual features of the gross appearance	Infections
Prior surgery/biopsies—results	
Prior malignancy	Hereditary non-polyposis colon cancer (HNPCC syndrome—can be associated with carcinomas of the ureter
Prior treatment (radiation therapy, chemotherapy, drug use that can change the histologic appearance of tissues)	Systemic or intravesical chemotherapy, immunotherapy with BCG, or radiation
	Analgesic nephropathy, with papillary necrosis—may increase the risk of renal pelvic tumors
Compromised immune system	

Radical or partial cystectomy

The bladder is usually resected because of biopsy-proven invasive urothelial (transitional) cell carcinoma. Rarely, the bladder is removed because of prostatic carcinoma invasive into the bladder or because of synchronous bladder and prostatic primary tumors. It is not uncommon to have the majority of the tumor removed by biopsy (TURBT) and have only minimal, or no, tumor present in the cystectomy specimen. It is also common to find an incidental (clinically occult) prostate carcinoma.

Processing the specimen

1. Record outer dimension of the bladder and length and diameter of attached ureters.
   Males: The prostate is attached (Fig. 20-2). Record outer dimensions, seminal vesicles (dimensions), vasa deferentia (length and diameter).
   Females: The anterior vaginal wall is attached. Describe size (length, width, depth), color (usually white), and any lesions.
   Record the outer appearance of the specimen (i.e., is any gross tumor present at the resection margin). Usually the margin consists of unremarkable adipose tissue. Palpate (but do not remove) this tissue, looking for grossly involved lymph nodes. Usually lymph nodes will not be found.

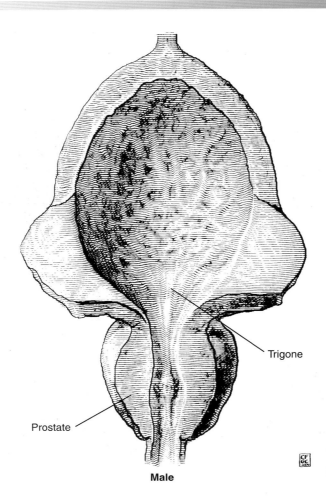

Trigone

Prostate

Male

Figure 20-2 Cystectomy.

2. Ink the prostate (if present) and any suspicious areas of the external bladder.

    Bladders that arrive intact are inflated with formalin through the urethra and allowed to fix in an expanded state overnight. It is very difficult to examine a contracted and highly folded bladder mucosa for small or multicentric tumors.

    Hold the bladder neck upright with a hemostat. Fill the lumen with formalin. When the bladder is full, the urethra can be plugged with a large cotton swab.

    If the bladder has already been opened, the specimen is pinned out on a paraffin board for fixation overnight.

3. Before opening the bladder, determine the location of the tumor by looking up prior biopsy specimens or radiology reports. Avoid cutting through the tumor when opening the bladder.

    If the location is unknown, or if it is in the usual location near the trigone, open the bladder anteriorly through the urethra and extend the incision to the dome. A probe placed in the urethra is helpful to guide the knife.

4. Locate the site of the tumor. Avoid touching the mucosal surface because it is very delicate and is easily denuded. In some cases the luminal tumor is very small, or only a shallow ulceration from a prior biopsy may be present.

    Ink the deep margin at the site of the tumor. Make parallel sections through the tumor.

    Record the tumor's size, configuration (papillary, sessile, ulcerated, fungating, flat or plaque-like), color, consistency (firm, soft), depth of penetration of wall (submucosa, into or through muscularis propria, into perivesical soft tissue), location (dome, anterior, posterior, lateral wall, trigone), and relationship to ureteral orifices (obstructing, extending into ureter).

    Submit up to four sections of tumor (more if the tumor is very large) including junction with uninvolved mucosa, deepest extension through wall, and deep margin.

5. Describe the remainder of the bladder mucosa (smooth and glistening, hemorrhagic, edematous). If there are any abnormal areas describe location and appearance.

   Submit representative sections of anterior wall, posterior wall, lateral wall, dome, and any abnormal areas.

6. The true ureteral margins are usually submitted separately and have often been examined by frozen section. Additional margins from the specimen do not need to be submitted.

   The entire length of the ureter is examined for additional foci of tumor. Take multiple cross-sections or open longitudinally. Submit any suspicious lesions.

7. **Males:** The prostate can be processed similar to radical prostatectomies (see sections on prostatectomies, below, for details). The prostate is sectioned through the posterior surface in serial sections perpendicular to the prostatic urethra. Describe color (white, yellow), consistency (firm, hard), any areas of necrosis or hemorrhage, and texture (nodular or effaced). The most common location of tumors is along the posterior wall. If no gross lesion is present, submit four sections from the posterior right lobe and four sections from the posterior left lobe. If lesions are present, submit enough sections to document them as well as representative sections from the uninvolved prostate.

   The bladder base is not a margin and is not submitted. However, if gross tumor is present take a section to document invasion into prostate.

   The urethral margin (also the apex of the prostate) is best sampled with a perpendicular section through the urethra to try to assess urethral mucosa which may be retracted and not seen in an en face apical margin.

   Section the seminal vesicles perpendicular to the long axis. Submit one section of each at the junction with the prostate.

   Females: Submit one representative section of the vaginal mucosa and any gross lesions.

8. After all microscopic sections have been taken, the perivesical soft tissue is carefully sectioned to look for lymph nodes. These nodes are found in only a small percentage of cases and more often in females than in males.

Microscopic sections

Tumor
Up to four cassettes including junction with normal mucosa, deepest point of invasion, deep margin.

Bladder mucosa
Up to six cassettes of representative sections of anterior wall, posterior wall, right and left lateral walls, if no gross tumor is present. If gross tumor is present, additional representative mucosa need not be sampled in that area.

Ureters
Need not be submitted if margins have been evaluated in separate specimens.
Up to four cassettes including left and right specimen margins, and all lesions.

Prostate
Four cassettes of posterior right lobe and four cassettes of posterior left lobe.

Urethral margin
One perpendicular section.

Seminal vesicles
Two cassettes documenting left seminal vesicle and right seminal vesicle.

Anterior vaginal wall
One cassette documenting normal mucosa and any lesions present.

Lymph nodes
All lymph nodes present in perivesical soft tissue.

Sample dictation

Received fresh, labeled "Bladder," is a radical cystectomy specimen containing bladder (15 × 10 × 5 cm), prostate (5 × 4.5 × 4 cm), and right (7 cm in length × 0.8 cm in diameter) and left (6 cm in length × 0.8 cm in diameter) ureters. There is a soft tan/pink papillary tumor (3.0 × 2.0 × 1.5 cm) located at the base of the posterior wall. The tumor extends into, but not through, the muscularis propria, and is 1.5 cm from the deep margin.

There is a second soft tan/pink papillary tumor (1.2 × 0.8 × 0.7 cm) located in the dome of the bladder which is confined to the mucosal surface. This tumor is 8 cm from the previously described tumor.

The remainder of the bladder mucosa is edematous and congested, however, no other gross lesions are noted.

The right ureter is unremarkable. In the left ureter there is an area of mucosal irregularity (0.3 × 0.3 cm) which is 3 cm from the unremarkable surgical margin.

The prostate consists of diffusely firm white parenchyma with a whorled appearance. The right seminal vesicle (3 × 1.5 × 0.5 cm), left seminal vesicle (2.5 × 1.8 × 0.6 cm), right vas deferens (0.8 cm in length × 0.5 cm in diameter), and left vas deferens (0.6 cm in length × 0.6 cm in diameter) are unremarkable. Three fleshy tan lymph nodes are present in the perivesical soft tissue, the largest measuring 0.5 cm in greatest dimension.

Cassettes #1 and 2: deepest extent of invasion of large tumor including deep margin, 2 frags, ESS.
Cassettes #3 and 4: large tumor and adjacent mucosa, 2 frags, RSS.
Cassettes #5 and 6: small tumor including deep margin, 2 frags, ESS.
Cassette #7: anterior wall, 1 frag, RSS.
Cassette #8: right lateral wall, 1 frag, RSS.
Cassette #9: posterior wall, between the two tumors, 1 frag, RSS.
Cassette #10: left lateral wall, 1 frag, RSS.
Cassette #11: right ureter margin, 1 frag, ESS.
Cassette #12: left ureter margin, 1 frag, ESS.
Cassette #13: suspicious area in left ureter, 3 frags, ESS.
Cassette #14: right seminal vesicle, 2 frags, RSS.
Cassette #15: left seminal vesicle, 2 frags, RSS.
Cassette #16: urethral margin of prostate, perpendicular, 1 frag, RSS.
Cassette #17–20: right lobe, 4 frags, RSS.
Cassette #21–24: left lobe, 4 frags, RSS.
Cassette #25: three lymph nodes, 3 frags, ESS.

Pathologic prognostic/diagnostic features sign-out checklist for bladder tumors

Specimen type*
Partial cystectomy, total cystectomy, radical cystectomy, radical cystoprostatectomy, anterior exenteration.

Tumor site
Trigone, right lateral wall, left lateral wall, anterior wall, posterior wall, dome, not specified.
Tumors at the dome or anterior surface of the bladder have a worse prognosis than those at the base. Most tumors occur near the trigone.

Tumor size*
Greatest dimension (additional dimensions optional).

Histologic type*
Urothelial (transitional cell) carcinoma (papillary, noninvasive, microinvasive [≤0.2 cm], or invasive or nonpapillary), rarely adenocarcinoma or squamous cell carcinoma, other rare types.

Histologic grade*

Three and four grade systems: specify the system used (see "Grading of bladder urothelial neoplasms," below). The WHO system is recommended (Table 20-9).

Tumor configuration

Papillary, solid/nodule, flat, ulcerated, indeterminate.

Extent of invasion*

Noninvasive papillary carcinoma (pTa), flat carcinoma in situ (pTis), tumor invades subepithelial connective tissue (lamina propria) (T1), tumor invades superficial muscle (inner half—pT2a), tumor invades deep muscle (pT2b), tumor invades perivesical tissue microscopically (pT3a), tumor invades perivesical tissue (an extravesicular mass is present) (pT3b), tumor invades prostate, uterus, or vagina (pT4a), tumor invades pelvic wall or abdominal wall (pT4b). See also Box 20-2.

Also specify if the carcinoma invades rectum, seminal vesicle, or ureter. Carcinoma in situ may involve the prostatic urethra, ducts, and acini.

Distinguish invasion of muscularis mucosae from invasion of muscularis propria.

Extent of invasion: focal or extensive; depth in mm; by level—above, at, or below muscularis mucosae. The depth of invasion in muscularis propria should not be staged in TURBT specimens. Adipose tissue is sometimes present in the lamina propria and muscularis propria and involvement does not necessarily indicate extravesicular invasion.

Multiple tumors

Multiple tumors are common and if present predict a greater likelihood of tumor at other sites (ureter, renal pelvis) and recurrence; pagetoid spread of carcinoma in situ in urethral mucosa.

Venous/lymphatic (large/small) vessel invasion

Absent, present, indeterminate.

Associated with increased recurrence rate.

Margins*

Uninvolved or involved, distance from closest margin, invasive carcinoma or in situ carcinoma.

Ureteral, urethral, soft tissue, invasion through to peritoneal surface.

Regional lymph nodes*

Absent (N0), present in one node, ≤2 cm in size (N1), present in one node >2 cm but ≤5 cm, or multiple nodes, none >5 cm (N2), or present in a lymph node >5 cm (N3).

Number of nodes examined, number with metastases, size of metastasis (≤2, >2, ≤5, >5 cm), single versus multiple. Pelvic nodes are usually submitted separately. Nodes in the perivesical fat are also reported.

Distant metastasis*

Absent (M0), present (M1).

Associated epithelial lesions*

None, urothelial (transitional cell) papilloma, urothelial (transitional cell) papilloma, inverted type, papillary urothelial (transitional cell) neoplasm, low malignant potential.

Nonlesional tissue

Urothelial dysplasia (low-grade intra-urothelial neoplasia), inflammation/regenerative changes, cystitis cystica glandularis, keratinizing squamous metaplasia, intestinal metaplasia, granulomatous cystitis, ulceration, therapy-related changes,

Specify whether or not muscularis propria is present.

Prostate

Normal, hyperplasia, PIN, carcinoma (report as for prostatectomies), invasion by bladder carcinoma.

Vaginal wall
Normal, lesions.

Flow cytometry
In some studies aneuploidy has been associated with prognosis.

This checklist incorporates information from the ADASP (see www.panix.com/~adasp) and the CAP Cancer Committee protocols for reporting on cancer specimens (see www.cap.org/). The asterisked elements are considered to be scientifically validated or regularly used data elements that must be present in reports of cancer-directed surgical resection specimens from ACS CoC-approved cancer programs. The specific details of reporting the elements may vary among institutions.

Box 20-2 The Marshall modification of the Jewett and Strong system for staging bladder carcinomas[9]

Stage 0	No tumor in specimen or carcinoma in situ, or papillary tumor
Stage A	Invasion into the lamina propria
Stage B1	Invasion into superficial muscle
Stage B2	Invasion into deep muscle
Stage C	Invasion into perivesical tissue
Stage D1	Invasion into contiguous organs or tissues or metastases to regional lymph nodes
Stage D2	Metastases to distant sites

Table 20-8 AJCC (6th edition) or WHO (2003) classification for bladder carcinomas

Tumor	TX	Primary tumor cannot be assessed
	T0	No evidence of primary tumor
	Ta	Papillary noninvasive carcinoma
	Tis	Carcinoma in situ: "flat tumor"
	T1	Tumor invades subepithelial connective tissue
	T2	Tumor invades muscle
	T2a	Tumor invades superficial muscle (inner half)
	T2b	Tumor invades deep muscle (outer half)
	T3	Tumor invades perivesical tissue
	T3a	Microscopically
	T3b	Macroscopically (extravesicular mass)
	T4	Tumor invades any of the following: prostate uterus, vagina, pelvic wall, abdominal wall
	T4a	Tumor invades prostate, uterus, or vagina
	T4b	Tumor invades pelvic wall or abdominal wall
		The suffix (m) should be added to the appropriate T category to indicate multiple tumors. The suffix (is) may be added to any T to indicate the presence of associated carcinoma in situ
Regional nodes	NX	Regional lymph nodes cannot be assessed
	N0	No regional lymph node metastasis
	N1	Metastasis in a single lymph node, ≤2 cm
	N2	Metastasis in a single lymph node >2 cm but ≤5 cm or to multiple lymph nodes ≤5 cm
	N3	Metastasis to a lymph node >5 cm
		Note: Regional lymph nodes are those within the true pelvis
Distant metastasis	MX	Distant metastasis cannot be assessed
	M0	No distant metastasis
	M1	Distant metastasis

Grading of bladder urothelial (transitional cell) neoplasms

Numerous grading systems for bladder tumors have been proposed over the years. However, by consensus, the new WHO 2003 system[10] (Table 20-9) has been accepted as the best current working model. Revisions are expected with the advent of new molecular diagnostic tests.

The grading systems shown in Box 20-3 and Table 20-10 were used in the past.

Table 20-9 WHO/International Society of Urological Pathology Consensus Classification of urothelial (transitional cell) neoplasms of the urinary bladder (WHO 2003)[10]

	ARCHITECTURE		CYTOLOGY					
	PAPILLAE	ORGANIZATION OF CELLS	NUCLEAR SIZE	NUCLEAR SHAPE	NUCLEAR CHROMATIN	NUCLEOLI	MITOSES	UMBRELLA CELLS
Papilloma	Delicate	Identical to normal	Identical to normal	Identical to normal	Fine	Absent	Absent	Uniformly present
PUNLUMP[a]	Delicate, occasionally fused	Polarity identical to normal; any thickness, cohesive	May be uniformly enlarged	Elongated, round-oval, uniform	Fine	Absent to inconspicuous	Rare, basal	Present
Low-grade papillary carcinoma	Fused, branching, delicate	Predominantly ordered, yet minimal crowding and minimal loss of polarity; any thickness; cohesive	Enlarged with variation in size	Round-oval; slight variation in shape and contour	Mild variation within and between cells	Usually inconspicuous[b]	Occasional at any level	Usually present
High-grade papillary carcinoma[c]	Fused, branching, delicate	Predominantly ordered with frequent loss of polarity; any thickness; often discohesive	Enlarged with variation in size	Moderate-marked pleomorphism	Moderate-marked variation both within and between cells with hyperchromasia	Multiple prominent nucleoli may be present	Usually frequent, at any level	May be absent

[a] Papillary urothelial neoplasm of low malignant potential. It is suggested that this diagnosis be accompanied by the following note: "Patients with these tumors are at risk of developing new bladder tumors ("recurrence"), usually of a similar histology. However, occasionally these subsequent lesions manifest as urothelial carcinoma, such that follow-up of the patient is warranted."
[b] If present, small and regular and not accompanied by other features of high-grade carcinoma.
[c] The degree of nuclear anaplasia may be included in a note.

Definitions

Urothelial papilloma. Exophytic urothelial papilloma composed of a delicate fibrovascular core covered by urothelium indistinguishable from that of the normal urothelium.

Inverted papilloma. Benign urothelial tumor that has an inverted growth pattern with normal to minimal cytologic atypia of the neoplastic cells.

Papillary urothelial neoplasm of low malignant potential (PUNLMP; former WHO Grade 1). A papillary urothelial tumor that resembles the exophytic urothelial papilloma, but shows increased cellular proliferation exceeding the thickness of normal urothelium.

Noninvasive low-grade papillary urothelial carcinoma (former WHO Grade 2). A neoplasm of urothelium lining papillary fronds that shows an orderly appearance, but easily recognizable variations in architecture and cytologic features.

Noninvasive high-grade papillary urothelial carcinoma (former WHO Grade 3). A neoplasm of urothelium lining papillary fronds that shows a predominant pattern of disorder with moderate to marked architectural and cytologic atypia.

Urothelial carcinoma in situ. A nonpapillary (i.e., flat) lesion in which the surface epithelium cells are cytologically malignant.

Box 20-3 WHO grading system[11]

Papilloma	Benign tumors
Grade 1	Tumors with the least degree of cellular anaplasia compatible with a diagnosis of malignancy
Grade 2	Tumors with degrees of anaplasia intermediate between Grades 1 and 3
Grade 3	Tumors with the most severe degrees of cellular anaplasia

Table 20-10 Grading system based on WHO system[12]

	PAPILLOMA	TCC-I	TCC-II	TCC-III
Hyperplasia (>7 layers)	None	Variable	Variable	Prominent
Superficial cell layer	Preserved	Preserved	Variable	Absent
"Clear" cytoplasm	Present	Often absent	Often absent	Absent, vacuoles common
Pleomorphism	None	Slight	Variable	Prominent
Nuclear polarization	Normal	Slightly abnormal	Abnormal	Absent
Nuclear crowding	None	Slight	Moderate	Moderate
Chromatin	Normal	Fine-regular	Fine-regular	Coarse, usually irregular
Mitoses	Rare	Uncommon	Common	Prominent

■ URETER

Ureters are rarely removed intentionally except as part of a radical cystectomy, radical nephrectomies for urothelial (transitional) cell carcinoma, or if there is a tumor present in the ureter. Almost all tumors of the ureter are transitional cell carcinomas and are sometimes associated with HNPCC. The uretero-pelvic junction is sometimes resected to relieve obstruction (see "Uretero-pelvic junction," below).

Processing the specimen

1. Record the length and diameter (range if it varies). Palpate the specimen and determine whether a lesion is present. The proximal and distal margins are taken as thin cross-sections at either end of the specimen.
2. Carefully open the ureter longitudinally with a small pair of scissors and avoid cutting into any lesions. Examine the mucosal surface for lesions. Urothelial (transitional) cell carcinoma usually looks like a soft tan/pink papillary mass on a stalk.
3. If a lesion is present, photograph the specimen. Ink the deep margin. Pin out on a paraffin board and fix overnight.
4. Section through the tumor looking for the deepest extent of invasion. If soft tissue is attached, look for lymph nodes.

Microscopic sections

Tumor
Up to four cassettes including greatest depth of invasion into the wall of the ureter and deep margin.

Margins
Proximal and distal mucosal margins.

Ureter
Submit at least one cassette of uninvolved ureter to look for additional lesions.

Lymph nodes
Submit all lymph nodes.

Pathologic prognostic/diagnostic features sign-out checklist for ureteral tumors

Specimen type*
Ureterectomy, nephroureterectomy.

Laterality*
Right, left, not specified.

Tumor size*
Greatest dimension (additional dimensions optional).

Histologic type*
Urothelial (transitional cell) carcinoma (papillary or nonpapillary), rarely adenocarcinoma or squamous cell carcinoma. The WHO classification is recommended.

Histologic grade*
Use the bladder tumor grading systems.

Extent of invasion*
Papillary noninvasive carcinoma (pTa), carcinoma in situ (Tis), tumor invades subepithelial connective tissue (lamina propria) (pT1), tumor invades the muscularis (pT2), tumor invades beyond muscularis into periureteric fat (pT3), tumor invades adjacent organs (pT4).

Tumor configuration

Papillary, solid/nodule, ulcerated, flat.

Associated epithelial lesions*

None, urothelial (transitional cell) papilloma, urothelial (transitional cell) papilloma, inverted type, papillary urothelial (transitional cell) neoplasm, low malignant potential.

Multiple tumors

Multiple tumors are common and if present predict a greater likelihood of tumor at other sites (ureter, renal pelvis) and recurrence; pagetoid spread of carcinoma in situ in urethral mucosa.

Venous/lymphatic (large/small) vessel invasion

Absent, present, indeterminate.

Associated with increased recurrence rate.

Margins*

Uninvolved, involved, invasive or in situ carcinoma, distance to closest margin.

Ureteral, soft tissue.

Regional lymph nodes*

Absent (N0), present in one node, ≤2 cm in size (N1), present in one node >2 cm but ≤5 cm, or multiple nodes, none >5 cm (N2), or present in a lymph node >5 cm (N3).

Number of nodes examined, number with metastases, size of metastasis. Pelvic nodes are usually submitted separately.

Distant metastasis*

Absent (M0), present (M1).

Additional findings

Urothelial carcinoma in situ, urothelial dysplasia (low-grade intra-urothelial neoplasia), inflammation/regenerative changes, cystitis cystica glandularis, keratinizing squamous metaplasia, intestinal metaplasia, granulomatous cystitis, ulceration, therapy-related changes,

This checklist incorporates information from the ADASP (see www.panix.com/~adasp/) and the CAP Cancer Committee protocols for reporting on cancer specimens (see www.cap.org/). The asterisked elements are considered to be scientifically validated or regularly used data elements that must be present in reports of cancer-directed surgical resection specimens from ACS CoC-approved cancer programs. The specific details of reporting the elements may vary among institutions.

For the AJCC classification of tumors of the renal pelvis and ureter, see Table 20-6.

Uretero-pelvic junction

Primary causes of uretero-pelvic junction obstruction are usually congenital in origin and may consist of muscular bundle disarray or absence, increased collagen deposition, or abnormal anatomic location of the renal pelvis. The diagnosis of these lesions is histologically problematic, does not affect the treatment or prognosis of the patient, and should not be attempted except on a research basis.

In adults, secondary causes of obstruction such as papillary urothelial (transitional) cell carcinoma or external compression by metastatic carcinoma, as well as lesions unrelated to the obstruction such as urothelial dysplasia, must be excluded.

Processing the specimen

1. The specimen may be funnel shaped if unopened. Describe the length, diameter at both ends, thickness of wall, and presence and size of any strictures. Open the specimen along the long axis.

   If the specimen has been opened, it may look like a triangular fragment of mucosa. Describe the dimensions including the wall thickness.

2. Carefully examine the surface of the mucosa for lesions or irregularities in texture. Examine the outer surface for mass lesions or fibrosis.

3. Take sections along the long axis. Submit multiple sections in one cassette.

■ CALCULI (KIDNEY AND BLADDER)

Kidney and bladder calculi are submitted for chemical analysis.

- Phosphate stones: gray to gray/white and may be hard or soft.
- Urate stones: yellow or brown, hard, and round to oval.
- Cystine stones: yellow, hard, smooth, with a waxy appearance.
- Oxalate stones: hard and may be either multilobated or spiculated.
- If bleeding has occurred the stones may be black or dark brown.

The specimen is described including number, color, shape (round, multilobated, spiculated), consistency (soft, hard), and dimensions (in aggregate and range of sizes). *Do not place in fixative!* The unfixed specimen may be sent to a commercial laboratory for chemical analysis.

■ PROSTATE

The prostate is biopsied to evaluate nodules or to investigate an increased serum prostate-specific antigen (PSA). Transurethral resection of the prostate (TURP) is performed to relieve urinary obstruction, generally for benign disease. However, tumor may be found incidentally. The prostate is resected for tumor (radical prostatectomy) or, less commonly, for benign hyperplasia (suprapubic prostatectomy).

Relevant clinical history (in addition to age)

See Table 20-11.

Needle biopsy[13-15]

Biopsies are usually thin, obtained using a "biopty gun," and processed as described in Chapter 13. Three levels are needed to detect significant lesions. In cases of focal glandular atypia found in the first three slides, an additional level was diagnostic of prostatic carcinoma in 4% of cases.[13]

It may be helpful to request intervening unstained slides between the H&E levels. If a difficult to classify glandular lesion is present, these slides can be used for immunoperoxidase studies.

Pathologic prognostic/diagnostic features sign-out checklist for prostate carcinoma diagnosed on needle biopsy

Tumor volume

Number of cores involved/total number of cores present, percent of involvement of each core.

Grade of tumor

All tumors are given a Gleason grade and score (see below).

Perineural invasion

Present or absent.

Table 20-11 Relevant clinical history	
HISTORY RELEVANT TO ALL SPECIMENS	HISTORY RELEVANT FOR PROSTATE SPECIMENS
Organ/tissue resected or biopsied	PSA level
Purpose of the procedure	Results of prior biopsies
Gross appearance of the organ/tissue/lesion sampled	
Any unusual features of the clinical presentation	
Any unusual features of the gross appearance	
Prior surgery/biopsies—results	
Prior malignancy	
Prior treatment (radiation therapy, chemotherapy, drug use that can change the histologic appearance of tissues)	→ radiation or hormone treatment
Compromised immune system	

Transurethral resection of prostate (TURP)[16-23]

In a TURP procedure, multiple fragments are curetted from the central transitional zone of the prostate in order to relieve obstruction. TURPs are performed less commonly than in the past due to advances in the nonsurgical therapy of prostatic enlargement. The intent is not to diagnose cancer, as the majority of carcinomas (approximately 75%) arise in the unsampled peripheral zone.

Nevertheless, carcinoma is found in 7% to 8% of TURPs with limited sampling and 14% to 19% if the entire specimen is examined. The likelihood of finding cancer is 6.4% if preoperative PSA and digital rectal examination are negative, 11.9% to 15% if either is positive, and 43.9% if both are positive.[16] The majority (70% to 80%) are T1a (involving 5% or less of tissue) carcinomas and the remainder T1b (involving >5% of tissue).

The criteria for "clinically significant" prostate cancer have included extent, grade, and age of the patient, but there is no universally accepted definition. A quarter to a third of incidentally found prostate carcinomas will progress if followed for 10 years, but the selection of patients for treatment remains controversial.

Because the likelihood of finding incidental carcinoma varies according to how much tissue is examined, and the amount of tissue from a TURP may be quite large, studies have been undertaken to determine how much sampling is necessary.[17-22] In some studies, limited sampling has been effective in detecting all carcinomas defined to be clinically important: for example, examination of 6 g of chips found all stage A2 carcinomas.[17] Examination of 12 g revealed 90% of the incidental carcinomas, including all of the clinically significant cancers (i.e., excluding small, well-differentiated stage A1 cancers). However, in other studies, 6% to 7% of the incidental cancers were high grade and could have been missed if the entire specimen had not been examined.[18,19]

CAP recommends examining specimens weighing 12 g or less in their entirety (see www.cap.org). For larger specimens, the first 12 g should be submitted (in 6 to 8 cassettes—in general 1 to 2 g of tissue will fit in one cassette), with one more cassette for each additional 5 g of tissue. If an unsuspected carcinoma is found involving <5% of tissue, the remaining tissue is generally submitted for examination.

If firm, yellow or yellow-orange chips are present, they should be submitted, as these chips are more likely to contain carcinoma.[20]

Additional recommendations in the literature have been to submit the entire specimen in the following situations:

- Patients under 60 years of age (small, low-grade carcinomas may be more likely to become clinically significant in this group)
- Patients with elevated PSA (may have centrally located carcinomas).

Each institution may develop its own policy for the extent of examination.

Processing the specimen

1. Weigh the specimen. The easiest method is to weigh the entire container (without fixative) and subtract the weight of the container. Record the dimensions in aggregate. Describe the fragments including color (gray/tan is normal, yellow suggests tumor), consistency (rubbery is normal, hard suggests tumor), and all areas with a different appearance (e.g., necrosis, hemorrhage).

    Note: The yellow or yellow-orange color seen in association with carcinoma is best seen in unfixed tissue.

2. Submit the entire specimen if possible, up to 12 blocks. For larger specimens, the institutional protocol should be followed (see discussion above).

    If carcinoma is present on the initial slides, and involves less than 5% of tissue, all the remaining tissue is generally submitted.

3. Since carcinomas tend to be near the capsule, and the clinician may take smaller slices to avoid going through the capsule, smaller fragments may be more likely to contain carcinoma.

4. For cases with one to two cassettes, order two levels.

    For cases with three or more cassettes, order one level.

The proportion of prostatic tissue involved by tumor (≤5% or >5%) is reported. The number of chips with tumor and the total number of chips may also be reported.

Suprapubic prostatectomy or retropubic simple prostatectomy for benign prostatic hyperplasia

Prostatectomy is performed rather than a TURP if the prostate is very enlarged or if there are other contraindications for transurethral surgery (e.g., urethral disease, bladder diverticula). The specimen usually looks like a large apple with a wedge cut out of one side, but may be in two or more fragments. There are usually no orienting features. The entire prostate is not removed so margins are irrelevant.

As for TURP specimens, there is no consensus on the appropriate amount of sampling. From 4% to 13% of cases will reveal unsuspected carcinoma. A minimum of one cassette for each 5 g of tissue has been suggested. CAP recommends submitting 8 cassettes. If an unsuspected carcinoma is found, and it involves less than 5% of tissue, additional blocks should be submitted.

Processing the specimen

1. Weigh the entire specimen and record aggregate dimensions. Serially section the specimen at 3 to 4 mm. If the urethra can be identified (usually it cannot) make the sections perpendicular to it.

2. Describe the parenchyma including color (white/tan, yellow, gray), consistency (firm, hard, soft, indurated), and areas of necrosis or hemorrhage. Carcinomas may be yellower and firmer than hyperplastic nodules.

3. Submit at least eight cassettes from different areas including (if recognizable) urethra, right and left lobes, and capsule and any area suspicious for tumor.

The percentage of tissue involved by carcinoma is reported. If a dominant nodule can be identified, the size should be given.

Radical prostatectomy

Radical prostatectomy is performed after carcinoma has been documented. Numerous protocols for submitting tissue have been proposed ranging from submission of the entire specimen in whole mount specimens to limited sampling using standard slides.[23,24] The method used should be designed to evaluate the extent of carcinoma, grade, stage, and margin status.

Processing the specimen

1. Weigh the entire specimen and record the outer dimensions including prostate and seminal vesicles. Orient the specimen (Fig. 20-3) to identify right and left, anterior and posterior, superior and inferior. It may be helpful to place a probe through the urethra. Note any unusual appearance to the prostatic capsule, which is normally relatively smooth (irregular areas may indicate tumor invasion or incomplete surgical excision).

2. Ink the right and left halves of the specimen different colors, including the soft tissue around the seminal vesicles and ductus deferentia.

3. Amputate each seminal vesicle and submit the basal section of each one at the junction with the prostate. Carcinomas may penetrate the prostatic capsule at the base and invade through adipose tissue and into the seminal vesicle in this area.

4. The bladder neck base margin (also referred to as the proximal urethral margin) surrounds the prostatic urethra nearest the seminal vesicles on the superior surface. This margin is cut perpendicular to the urethra as thin (0.7 cm) shave margin. Tissue slice is cut perpendicular to the initial cut and submitted on edge. The right and left sides are submitted separately.

   The apex (also referred to as the distal urethral margin) is cut perpendicular to the urethra as a thin (0.7 cm) shave margin. Tissue slice is cut perpendicular to the initial cut and submitted on edge. The right and left sides are submitted separately.

5. Section the remaining prostate at 5 mm intervals using cuts perpendicular to the urethral axis. Alternate sections are quartered and submitted from base to apex. Each cassette should be coded as to the slice number (e.g. "1," "3," "5"), right versus left, and anterior versus posterior.

   Examine each slice for the presence of gross lesions (see below). Note the location of any lesions (anterior/posterior, right/left, superior/inferior), color, extension to capsule or other structures, and their size. However, many tumors are small (due to the effects of screening) and are not detectable grossly.

   Describe the remainder of the parenchyma including color, consistency, and nodularity. If a gross lesion is present, a photograph should be taken.

Gross differential diagnosis

Adenocarcinoma

Prostate carcinoma is the most difficult malignancy to detect grossly because of the underlying firmness of the normal or hyperplastic gland, the small size of many tumors, and the tendency of many tumors to infiltrate into and around normal tissue or to grow in a nodular pattern mimicking normal parenchyma.

The majority of carcinomas (approximately 75%) are located in the posterior peripheral zone. It is helpful to look for smooth solid areas with effacement of the normal spongy or cystic appearance or an area where the capsule appears to be effaced. Asymmetry of the right and left posterior lobes may indicate the location of a tumor. Tumors may have a slightly different color (sometimes yellow) but often do not. Palpation may be helpful in fresh tissues (carcinomas may be firm or gritty and less spongy than normal tissue), but is not helpful after

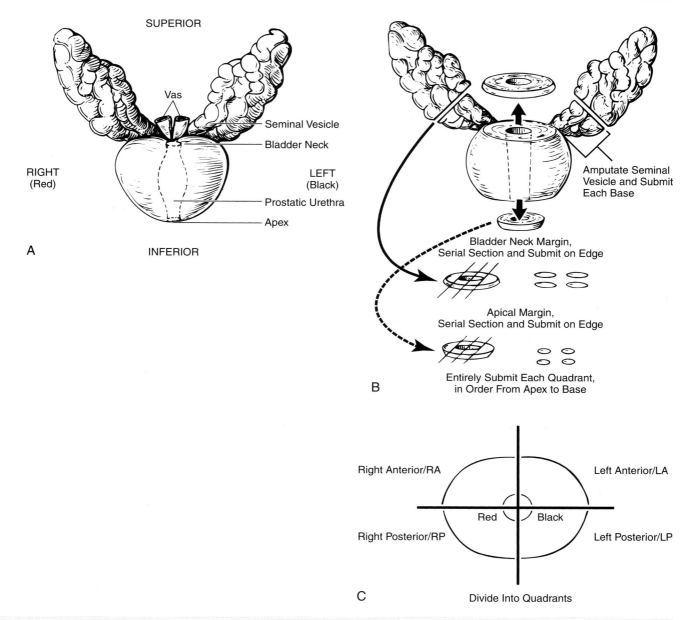

Figure 20-3 Radical prostatectomy. **A**, Orientation; **B**, margins and seminal vesicles; **C**, quadrants.

fixation. Even experienced pathologists cannot identify at least 50% of prostate carcinomas grossly.

Historical data may be helpful. Prior biopsy reports may indicate location (i.e., right versus left). Lesions diagnosed by needle biopsy and/or as a palpable mass are most likely located in the posterior portion of the gland. Lesions diagnosed by TURP specimens are often located centrally or anteriorly.

Nodular hyperplasia (benign prostatic hypertrophy or hyperplasia)

The gland is diffusely enlarged due to centrally located nodules of variable size. The nodules may be soft and tan/pink and exude prostatic fluid or be firm and gray with a whorled appearance. The nodules often encroach laterally on the prostatic urethra. The peripheral zone may appear compressed.

Microscopic sections

Lesions
Make sure all sections can be identified as either the right lobe or the left lobe (right inked red, left inked black, and designate in cassette code). Submit lesions in their entirety.

Grossly normal prostate
Submit alternate sections.

Margins
Submit bladder neck margin and apical margin (see Fig. 20-3).

Seminal vesicle
Submit one section from the base of each vesicle.

Sample dictation

Received fresh, labeled with the patient's name and unit number and "prostate," is a 52-g radical prostatectomy specimen that measures 6 cm right to left, 5.5 cm anterior to posterior, and 4.7 cm superior to inferior. The right seminal vesicle measures 1.5 × 0.8 × 0.4 cm and the left seminal vesicle measures 1.7 × 0.6 × 0.4 cm. The right side of the prostate is inked in red, the left side in black. The external surface of the prostate is smooth. There are multiple nodules grossly consistent with benign prostatic hyperplasia located centrally, the largest of which measures 1 × 1 × 0.5 cm. There is a 0.9 × 0.5 × 0.5 cm gray/yellow mass in the right posterior lobe which may represent tumor that does not extend across the midline. This lesion is within 0.1 cm of the posterior margin, but is not grossly present at the margins. The prostate is sectioned into 5 slices. Alternate slices are submitted completely for histologic examination.

Cassette #1: Right seminal vesicle, RSS, 1 frag.
Cassette #2: Left seminal vesicle, RSS, 1 frag.
Cassette #3: Right proximal urethral margin RPUM, ESS, 5 frags.
Cassette #4: Left proximal urethral margin LPUM, ESS, 6 frags.
Cassette #5: Right digital urethral margin RDUM, ESS, 1 frag.
Cassette #6: Left digital urethral margin LDUM, ESS, 1 frag.
Cassette #7: 1 Right anterior, ESS, 1 frag.
Cassette #8: 1 Left anterior, ESS, 1 frag.
Cassette #9: 1 Right posterior, ESS, 1 frag.
Cassette #10: 1 Left posterior, ESS, 1 frag.
Cassette #11: 3 Right anterior, ESS, 1 frag.
Cassette #12: 3 Left anterior, ESS, 1 frag.
Cassette #13: 3 Right posterior, ESS, 1 frag.
Cassette #14: 3 Left posterior, ESS, 1 frag.
Cassette #15: 5 Right anterior, ESS, 1 frag.
Cassette #16: 5 Left anterior, ESS, 1 frag.
Cassette #17, 5 Right posterior, ESS, 1 frag.
Cassette #18: 5 Left posterior, ESS, 1 frag.

Pathologic prognostic/diagnostic features sign-out checklist for prostate tumors

Specimen type*
Needle biopsy, TURP, suprapubic or retropubic prostatectomy (subtotal prostatectomy), radical prostatectomy.

Histologic type*
Adenocarcinoma (acinar type), prostatic duct adenocarcinoma, mucinous (colloid) adenocarcinoma, signet ring cell carcinoma, others.

Tumor quantitation
Needle biopsy:
Size or percentage of core involved, number of cores involved.
TURP or suprapubic prostatectomies:
Number of foci of carcinoma, number of chips involved, percentage chips involved by carcinoma.
Radical prostatectomy:
Various methods are used, some requiring submission of the entire gland and image analysis.[25] The greatest dimension of tumor on the glass slides can be used to predict tumor volume.[26,27]

Proportion (%) of prostate involved by tumor.
Tumor size (dominant nodule, if present), in cm.
Number of tissue blocks with tumor.

Histologic grade*
All tumors are given a Gleason grade and score (see below).
If three patterns are present, record the most predominant and second most common patterns; the tertiary pattern should be recorded if higher than the first two patterns.

Extent of invasion*
Incidental finding in ≤5% of tissue (T1a), incidental finding in >5% of tissue, identified by needle biopsy (T1c), unilateral, involving one half of one lobe or less (T2a), unilateral involving more than one half of one lobe (T2b), involving both lobes (T2c), extension beyond the prostate (T3a), extension beyond prostate and into seminal vesicle (T3b), invasion of the bladder neck, external sphincter, rectum, levator muscles, and/or pelvic wall (T4).

Regional lymph nodes*
Present or absent, number of involved nodes, number of nodes examined.

Distant metastases*
Absent (M0), non-regional lymph nodes (M1a), bone (M1b), other sites (M1c).

Margins*
Absent or present, location—apical (the most inferior portion of the prostate), bladder neck, anterior, lateral, posterolateral (neurovascular bundle), posterior, other.
Unifocal or multifocal, extent (focal or extensive, number of blocks, linear mm, etc.).
Positive margins are defined as ink on tumor cells. Close margins (without ink on tumor cells) are reported as negative. A margin may be positive without the presence of extraprostatic invasion.

Extraprostatic extension*
Absent or present.
Unifocal or multifocal (extensive): The extent of extraprostatic invasion is of prognostic value. Extraprostatic invasion may be defined as "focal" (≤1 HPF on ≤2 slides) or "nonfocal" (any degree of invasion more than focal).
Defined as tumor beyond the confines of the prostatic gland:

Tumor abutting on or admixed with fat.

Tumor involving perineural spaces in neurovascular bundles beyond the prostate.
Tumor beyond the confines of the normal glandular prostate (anterior prostate and bladder neck).
However, a T4 designation usually requires gross involvement of the bladder neck.

Skeletal muscle is present at the apex. Carcinoma in skeletal muscle at this site does not constitute extraprostatic extension.
The prostatic capsule is ill defined and incomplete. Carcinomas typically extend along the periphery of the posterior lobes. Only unequivocal extraprostatic extension into adjacent adipose tissue should be diagnosed as extraprostatic extension.

Seminal vesicle invasion*

Absent or present, or no seminal vesicle present.
Invasion must be into the muscular wall of the vesicle (invasion into the adventitia but not the wall does not qualify as invasion into the seminal vesicle).

Perineural invasion

Absent or present, within or outside the capsule. Perineural invasion is a common finding and there is not a universal consensus as to its significance within the capsule. On needle biopsies, some studies have shown an association with an increased risk of capsular penetration.

Venous (large vessel) invasion
Absent or present.

Lymphatic (small vessel) invasion
Absent or present.

Prostatic intraepithelial neoplasia (PIN)
Present or absent. Only high-grade PIN is reported. If present on a needle biopsy, it signifies an increased probability for invasive carcinoma on subsequent biopsies.

Table 20-12 AJCC (6th edition) classification of prostate tumors

Tumor	TX	Primary tumor cannot be assessed
	T0	No evidence of primary tumor
	T1	Clinically inapparent tumor not palpable nor visible by imaging
	T1a	Tumor incidental histologic finding in 5% or less of tissue resected
	T1b	Tumor incidental histologic finding in >5% of tissue resected
	T1c	Tumor identified by needle biopsy (e.g., because of elevated PSA) Includes tumors found in both lobes by needle biopsy
	pT2	Tumor confined within the prostate
	pT2a	Tumor involves one half of one lobe or less
	pT2b	Tumor involves more than one half of one lobe but not both lobes
	PTc	Tumor involves both lobes
	pT3	Tumor extends through the prostate capsule
	pT3a	Extracapsular extension (unilateral or bilateral)
	pT3b	Tumor invades seminal vesicle(s)
	pT4	Tumor invades into the bladder or rectum
Regional lymph nodes	NX	Regional lymph nodes cannot be assessed
	N0	No regional lymph node metastases
	N1	Metastasis in regional lymph node or nodes
Metastasis	MX	Distant metastasis cannot be assessed
	M0	No distant metastasis
	M1	Distant metastasis
	M1a	Non-regional lymph node(s)
	M1b	Bone(s)
	M1c	Other site(s) with or without bone disease

Note: This classification system does not apply to sarcomas or urothelial (transitional) cell carcinomas. Urothelial (transitional) cell carcinomas of the prostate should be classified as urethral tumors.

Nonlesional prostate

Benign prostatic hyperplasia, atypical adenomatous hyperplasia, inflammation.

This checklist incorporates information from the ADASP (see www.panix.com/~adasp) and the CAP Cancer Committee protocols for reporting on cancer specimens (see www.cap.org/). The asterisked elements are considered to be scientifically validated or regularly used data elements that must be present in reports of cancer-directed surgical resection specimens from ACS CoC-approved cancer programs. The specific details of reporting the elements may vary among institutions.

Gleason grading of prostatic adenocarcinomas[28] (Box 20-4; Fig. 20-4)

The two predominant patterns are graded from 1 to 5 and added together to derive a Gleason's score. If there is only one pattern, the same grade is duplicated. The score and the grade should be reported with the predominant grade listed first: e.g., Gleason score 7 (3+4) or Gleason score 7 (4+3).

Box 20-4 Gleason score	
2–4	Well differentiated
5–6	Moderately differentiated
7	Moderately poorly differentiated
8–10	Poorly differentiated

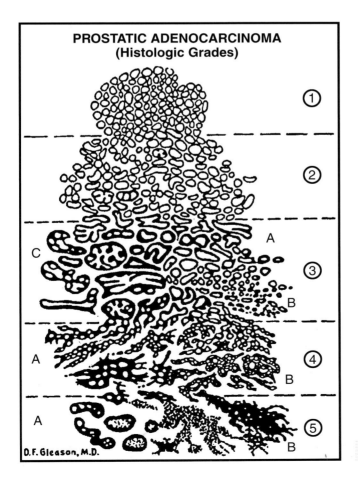

Figure 20-4 Gleason grade.

In core needle biopsies, when more than two patterns are present, and the highest grade is not the predominant or second most common grade, the predominant pattern and the highest grade are used to derive a score. For example, if 70% of the carcinoma is grade 3, 20% grade 2, and 10% grade 4, this would be reported as Gleason score 7 (3+4).

If more than one tumor of different grade is found in a prostatectomy specimen, the grade of each should be reported.

In current practice, Gleason grade 1 carcinomas are vanishingly rare and grade 2 carcinomas are uncommon.

Grade description

1. Simple round glands, close-packed in rounded masses with well-defined edges
2. Simple rounded glands, loosely packed in vague, rounded masses with loosely defined edges
3A. Medium-sized single glands of irregular shape and irregular spacing with ill-defined infiltrating edges
3B. Very similar to 3A, but small to very small glands, which must not form significant chains or cords
3C. Papillary and cribriform epithelium in smooth, rounded cylinders and masses; no necrosis
4A. Small, medium, or large glands fused into cords, chains, or ragged infiltrating masses
4B. Very similar to 4A, but with many large clear cells, sometimes resembling "hypernephroma"
5A. Papillary and cribriform epithelium in smooth, rounded masses, more solid than 3C and with central necrosis
5B. Anaplastic adenocarcinoma in ragged sheets

■ TESTIS

Biopsies are usually performed for the evaluation of infertility. Unilateral orchiectomies are performed to resect tumors (almost all germ cell tumors). Retroperitoneal lymph node dissections for testicular carcinoma require special evaluation (see below). Bilateral orchiectomies are sometimes performed for the treatment of prostate carcinoma.

Relevant clinical history

See Table 20-13.

Biopsy for infertility

Bouin's is the preferred fixative. The yellow/tan tubules of the testicular parenchyma can be identified grossly. The entire specimen is submitted. Order 2 H&E, trichrome, elastic stain, and PAS to aid in the evaluation of basement membranes.

In lesions in which some spermatogenesis is seen (categories 3 and 4 in Box 20-5, rarely 5), count the spermatids in selected (10 to 20) tubules and derive an average spermatid per tubular cross-section count. Count all small, elongated, compact oval nuclei (these cells have no tails yet). Then use Figure 20-5 to calculate the predicted sperm count and report this number as well. 100×10^6 sperm/mL is considered a normal count.

Unilateral orchiectomy for tumor

Germ cell tumors are the most common tumors of the testis. They are readily locally controlled but often metastasize.

Processing the specimen

1. Weigh the specimen and record the dimensions of the testis (three dimensions), epididymis (three dimensions), and spermatic cord (length and diameter).

2. The tunica vaginalis is a closed peritoneal sac surrounding the front and sides of the testis and extends upwards over the spermatic cord. Open the sac along the anterior border.

   The testis is surrounded by the thick white tunica albuginea. The epididymis is posterior and in continuity with the spermatic cord. Bisect the testis parallel to, and through, the epididymis. Additional cuts can be made parallel to this plane.

   Describe any lesions including size, color, consistency, variegation (it is very important to sample all areas with a different gross appearance), hemorrhage, and necrosis. Determine whether tumor extends through the tunica albuginea or into the epididymis. Invasion most commonly occurs at the junction of the testis and the epididymis.

   Describe the remainder of the testicular parenchyma including color (tan/yellow) and consistency (stringy). The normal seminiferous tubules can be demonstrated grossly by gently teasing them out with a forceps.

3. Remove the proximal resection margin of the spermatic cord and place in a labeled cassette. **Note:** The vas deferens often retracts. Try to find the end of the vas by looking for a thin, firm, white, tubular structure.

Table 20-13 Relevant clinical history

HISTORY RELEVANT TO ALL SPECIMENS	HISTORY RELEVANT TO TESTICULAR SPECIMENS
Organ/tissue resected or biopsied	Cryptorchidism (with or without prior orchiopexy)
Purpose of the procedure	Retroperitoneal or para-aortic lymphadenectomy
Gross appearance of the organ/tissue/lesion sampled	Prior contralateral testicular tumor
Any unusual features of the clinical presentation	
Any unusual features of the gross appearance	
Prior surgery/biopsies—results	Serum levels of alpha-fetoprotein (AFP) and human chorionic gonadotropin (β-hCG)
Prior malignancy	
Prior treatment (radiation therapy, chemotherapy, drug use that can change the histologic appearance of tissues)	Gynecomastia (more frequently associated with sex cord/stromal tumors than with germ cell tumors)
Compromised immune system	Intersex syndrome (e.g., ambiguous genitalia or feminization)

Box 20-5 Histologic patterns in testicular biopsies

1. Normal
2. Prepubertal
3. Sloughing
4. Hypospermatogenesis
5. Spermatogenic arrest
6. Sertoli only
7. Hyalinized

QUANTITATIVE TESTICLE BIOPSY AND SPERM COUNT

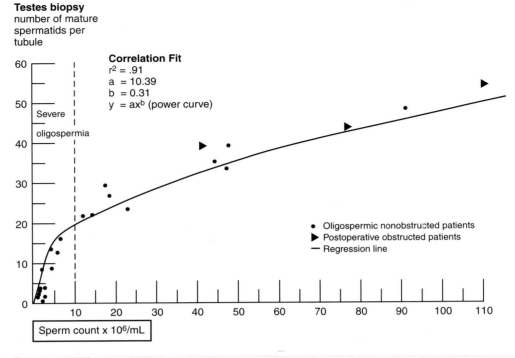

Figure 20-5 Correlation between the number of mature spermatids per tubule and the sperm counts. (From Silber SJ, Rodriguez-Rigau LJ. Quantitative analysis of testicle biopsy: determination of partial obstruction and prediction of sperm count after surgery for obstruction. Fertil Steril 36:480-485, 1981.)

Section through the remainder of the cord looking for gross evidence of tumor spread.
4. Take sections of all lesions, including all areas of different gross appearance, and relationship to tunica vaginalis and epididymis. Take one section of uninvolved testis.

Gross differential diagnosis

Seminomas are usually solid homogeneous light yellow to tan fleshy nodules which often have sharply circumscribed areas of necrosis. Cystic areas or hemorrhage are unusual and may indicate that another type of germ cell tumor is present. Some patients have elevated serum hCG (10% to 25%) due to the presence of syncytiotrophoblast cells. AFP is usually normal.

Embryonal carcinomas are firm with a more heterogeneous gray/white coloration and may have areas of hemorrhage and necrosis.

Choriocarcinomas are often small, gray/white, and usually very hemorrhagic and necrotic. Almost all patients will have elevated serum hCG.

Teratomas are usually cystic or multiloculated and often have grossly evident cartilaginous differentiation. Fat and bone may be present. Immature teratomas may grossly resemble brain tissue.

Endodermal sinus tumors (yolk sac) are rarely seen in a pure form in adults and are usually not evident grossly if a minor component. Pure tumors in children under 2 years of age may have a soft gelatinous microcystic appearance and be pale tan or yellow. Larger tumors may be focally necrotic. Almost all patients will have elevated serum AFP.

Regressed germ cell tumors may consist of a small fibrous scar or area of calcification. If a patient has a known metastatic germ cell tumor, and a gross lesion cannot be found, the entire testis should be examined histologically.

Leydig cell tumors are well circumscribed or lobulated and yellow, tan, or brown. Hemorrhage and necrosis are uncommon.

Sertoli cell tumors are gray/white, firm, and circumscribed.

Lymphomas are rare, usually seen in older males, and usually part of more generalized involvement (i.e., not solely present in testis). The testis is diffusely enlarged by homogeneous fleshy gray/creamy white tissue that may be multinodular. Approximately half the cases also involve epididymis or spermatic cord. Tissue is taken for hematopathologic studies (see Chapter 27).

Acute and chronic leukemia frequently involve the testes. The tumors may closely resemble a seminoma with a creamy yellow to white homogeneous appearance. The testis is a frequent site of relapse after treatment of acute leukemia.

Pediatric germ cell tumors. These tumors are more commonly endodermal sinus tumors or teratomas and the behavior may be different from that observed in adults.[29] Cytogenetic studies may be useful as the genetic changes have been reported to be different from those observed in adults and may predict different behavior. Tissue for EM and snap freezing is not used routinely for diagnosis but may be saved for possible studies in unusual cases.

Microscopic sections

Tumor
Four to 10 cassettes demonstrating all types of gross appearances including all hemorrhagic and necrotic areas. In general, at least one cassette per 1 cm of greatest dimension should be examined. Include sections demonstrating relationship to tunica vaginalis and near the base of the epididymis (this is the most common site to find tumor invasion outside the testis).
If serum β-hCG is increased in the absence of Leydig cell hyperplasia or choriocarcinoma, take more samples to look for choriocarcinoma.
If serum alpha-fetoprotein is increased and yolk sac carcinoma is not seen, take more samples to look for possible yolk sac carcinoma.

Testis
One cassette of uninvolved testis and epididymis.

Spermatic cord
Resection margin, representative sections from center of cord, representative sections from peri-testicular cord.

Sample dictation

Received, labeled with the patient's name and unit number and "right testis," is a 30-g orchiectomy specimen including testis (4.5 × 4 × 4 cm), epididymis (1 × 1 × 0.5), and spermatic cord (9 cm in length × 1.5 cm in diameter). There is a 3 × 2 × 2 cm tan/white firm circumscribed mass with focal areas of hemorrhage and necrosis and small (0.2 cm) cystic spaces within the testis. The tumor does not grossly extend into the tunica albuginea or into the epididymis. The remainder of the testicular parenchyma is brown/tan with grossly normal tubules present. The spermatic cord consists of vas deferens, arteries, and veins, and is grossly unremarkable.

Cassettes #1 and 2: Tumor with homogeneous appearance, 3 frags, RSS.
Cassettes #3 and 4: Tumor with necrosis and hemorrhage, 3 frags, RSS.
Cassettes #5 and 6: Tumor with small cystic areas, 2 frags, RSS.
Cassette #7: Tumor and tunica vaginalis, 1 frag, RSS.
Cassette #8: Tumor and epididymis, 1 frag, RSS.
Cassette #9: Uninvolved adjacent testis, 1 frag, RSS.
Cassette #10: Spermatic cord, resection margin, 1 frag, ESS.
Cassette #11: Spermatic cord, mid section, 1 frag, RSS.
Cassette #12: Spermatic cord, peri-testicular, 1 frag, RSS.

Pathologic prognostic/diagnostic features sign-out checklist for testicular tumors

Serum hormone levels
Unknown, normal, alpha-fetoprotein (AFP) elevation, beta-subunit of human chorionic gonadotropin (β-hCG) elevation, lactate dehydrogenase (LDH) elevation.
If the serum markers are elevated and a histologic correlate is not found (i.e., yolk sac for AFP or choriocarcinoma or Leydig cell hyperplasia for β-hCG) additional tumor sampling may be helpful.

Laterality*
Right, left, both.

Focality*
Unifocal, multifocal.

Tumor size*
Greatest dimension of main tumor (additional dimensions). Seminomas >4 cm in size have an increased risk of recurrence.

Histologic type*
Seminoma (classic type or with syncytiotrophoblastic cells), teratoma, embryonal carcinoma, choriocarcinoma, endodermal sinus (yolk sac) tumor, intratubular germ cell neoplasia, sex cord stromal tumors, others. Include the presence of syncytiotrophoblasts.
Many tumors are of mixed types. The proportion of each type is given.

Extent of invasion*
Intratubular germ cell neoplasia (Tis), limited to testis (including rete testis and epididymis) without vascular/lymphatic invasion (tumor may invade tunica albuginea but not tunica vaginalis) (T1), tumor with vascular/lymphatic invasion or extension through tunica albuginea with involvement of tunica vaginalis (T2), tumor invades spermatic cord (T3), tumor invades scrotum (T4).
Rete testis involvement (extension of tumor into testicular mediastinum without necessarily involving tubular lumens) is associated with increased risk for recurrence for seminoma.[30] Involvement of parenchyma beyond the area of the main tumor mass may also be of prognostic importance for seminoma.

Direct extension of invasive tumor*
Rete testis, epididymis, perihilar fat, spermatic cord, tunica vaginalis, scrotal wall.

Regional lymph nodes*
Absent or present, number of involved nodes (number of nodes examined), size of metastasis (<2 cm, <5 cm, <10 cm), presence of extranodal invasion.

Distant metastasis*
Absent (M0), non-regional lymph nodes or pulmonary metastases (M1a), other sites (M1b), specific site if known.

Venous/lymphatic (large/small vessel) invasion
Present or absent.

Nonlesional testis
Intratubular germ cell neoplasia, atrophy, fibrosis, hemosiderin-laden macrophages and intratubular calcifications (possibly regressed tumor), spermatogenesis present or absent, Leydig cell hyperplasia, Sertoli cells, abnormal testicular development (e.g., due to dysgenesis or androgen insensitivity syndrome).

Margins*
Spermatic cord, parietal layer of tunica vaginalis, scrotal skin.

This checklist incorporates information from the ADASP (see www.panix.com/~adasp/) and the CAP Cancer Committee protocols for reporting on cancer specimens (see www.cap.org/). The asterisked

Box 20-6 Modified Royal Marsden staging system for seminoma[31]

Stage I	Tumor confined to the testis
Stage II	Infradiaphragmatic nodal involvement
IIA	greatest dimension of involved nodes <2 cm
IIB	greatest dimension of involved nodes ≥2 cm but <5 cm
IIC	greatest dimension of involved nodes ≥5 cm but <10 cm
IID	greatest dimension of involved nodes ≥10 cm
Stage III	Supraclavicular or mediastinal involvement
Stage IV	Extranodal metastasis

Some studies suggest this staging system provides more prognostic information than the AJCC system.

elements are considered to be scientifically validated or regularly used data elements that must be present in reports of cancer-directed surgical resection specimens from ACS CoC-approved cancer programs. The specific details of reporting the elements may vary among institutions.

■ RETROPERITONEAL LYMPH NODE DISSECTION FOR TESTICULAR CARCINOMA

Retroperitoneal lymph node dissection is often performed following chemotherapy, so much of the tissue may be hemorrhagic, cystic, and/or necrotic. In such cases, it is especially important to take many sections to document the presence or absence of *viable* residual high-grade tumor (embryonal carcinoma, endodermal sinus tumor, or choriocarcinoma). Otherwise, follow the directions for non-hematopathology lymph nodes. The size of the largest lymph node metastasis (or confluent area of tumor involvement) and number of involved lymph nodes is recorded.

Pathologic prognostic/diagnostic features sign-out checklist for retroperitoneal lymphadenectomy for testicular tumors

Pre-lymphadenectomy treatment
None, chemotherapy, radiation therapy.

Serum hormone levels
Unknown, normal, AFP, β-hCG, LDH.
If the serum markers are elevated and a histologic correlate is not found (i.e., yolk sac for AFP or choriocarcinoma or Leydig cell hyperplasia for β-hCG) additional tumor sampling may be helpful.

Specimen site(s)
Nodal groups

Number of nodal groups present
Give number.

Size of largest metastasis*
Greatest dimension.

Viability of tumor*
No tumor present, nonviable tumor present, viable tumor present.

Histologic type*
Same as for testicular tumors.

Regional lymph nodes
Number of nodes with metastases, number of nodes examined, size of largest metastatic deposit.

Non-regional lymph node metastasis*
Absent, present.

This checklist incorporates information from the ADASP (see www.panix.com/~adasp/) and the CAP Cancer Committee protocols for reporting on cancer specimens (see www.cap.org/). The asterisked elements are considered to be scientifically validated or regularly used data elements that must be present in reports of cancer-directed surgical resection specimens from ACS CoC-approved cancer programs. The specific details of reporting the elements may vary among institutions.

■ BILATERAL SIMPLE ORCHIECTOMY: NON-TUMOR

Bilateral orchiectomy is sometimes performed for the treatment of prostate cancer. A unilateral simple orchiectomy may be performed for torsion.

Table 20-14 AJCC (6th edition) classification of testicular tumors

Tumor	pTX	Primary tumor cannot be assessed
	pT0	No evidence of primary tumor (e.g., histologic scar in testis)
	pTis	Intratubular germ cell neoplasia (carcinoma in situ)
	pT1	Tumor limited to the testis and epididymis without vascular/lymphatic invasion; tumor may invade into the tunica albuginea but not the tunica vaginalis
	pT2	Tumor limited to the testis and epididymis with vascular/lymphatic invasion, or tumor extending through the tunica albuginea with involvement of the tunica vaginalis
	pT3	Tumor invades the spermatic cord with or without vascular/lymphatic invasion
	pT4	Tumor invades the scrotum with or without vascular/lymphatic invasion
Regional lymph nodes	pNX	Regional lymph nodes cannot be assessed
	pN0	No regional lymph node metastasis
	pN1	Metastasis with a lymph node mass, ≤ 2 cm in greatest dimension and ≤ 5 nodes positive, none $> \leq 2$ cm.
	pN2	Metastasis with a lymph node mass, > 2 but ≤ 5 cm in greatest dimension; or more than 5 nodes positive, none > 5 cm; or evidence of extranodal extension of tumor
	pN3	Metastasis with a lymph node mass > 5 cm in greatest dimension
		Note: Regional lymph nodes include interaortocaval, para-aortic (peri-aortic), paracaval, preaortic, precaval, retroaortic, and retrocaval. Intrapelvic, external iliac, and inguinal nodes are considered regional only after scrotal or inguinal surgery prior to the presentation of the testis tumor. Laterality does not affect N classification

Serum tumor markers (S)	SX	Not available or not performed		
	S0:	Normal		

	LDH	hCG (mIu/mL)		AFP (ng/mL)
S1	$<1.5 \times$ nL and	<5000	and	<1000
S2	$1.5–10 \times$ nL or	$5000–50,000$	or	$1000–10,000$
S3	$>10 \times$ nL or	$>50,000$	or	$>10,000$

Metastasis	MX	Distant metastasis cannot be assessed
	M0	No distant metastasis
	M1	Distant metastasis
	M1a	Non-regional nodal or pulmonary metastasis
	M1b	Distant metastasis other than to non-regional lymph nodes and lungs

Processing the specimen

1. Weigh each testis and record the measurements of the testis and spermatic cord (length and diameter), if present.
2. Make a single incision through the testis. If focal lesions are present, follow the protocol above for tumors. If no lesion is present, describe the parenchyma (soft, yellow/tan) and look for the presence of tubules and capsule (smooth white).
3. Submit one representative section of each testis.

REFERENCES

1. Meng MV, Koppie TM, Duh Q-Y, Stoller ML. Novel method of assessing surgical margin status in laparoscopic specimens. Urology 58:677-682, 2001.
2. Meng MV, Koppie TM, Stoller ML. Pathologic sampling of laparoscopically morcellated kidneys: a mathematical model. J Endourol 17:229-233, 2003.
3. Meng MV, Miller TR, Stoller ML. Cytology of morcellated renal specimens: significance in diagnosis and dissemination. J Urol 169:45-48, 2003.
4. Qualman SJ, et al. Protocol for the examination of specimens from patients (children and young adults) with Wilms tumor (nephroblastoma) or other renal tumors of childhood, Arch Pathol Lab Med 127:1280-1289, 2003.
5. Zuppan CW. Handling and evaluation of pediatric renal tumors. Am J Clin Pathol 109 (Suppl 1):S31-S37, 1998.
6. Argani P, et al. Clear cell sarcoma of the kidney: a review of 351 cases from the National Wilms Tumor Study Group Pathology Center. Am J Surg Pathol 24:4-18, 2000.
7. Fuhrman SA, et al. Prognostic significance of morphologic parameters in renal cell carcinoma. Am J Surg Pathol 6:655, 1982.
8. Gephardt GN, Baker PB. Interinstitutional comparison of bladder carcinoma surgical pathology report adequacy. A College of American Pathologists Q-probes study of 7234 bladder biopsies and curettings in 268 institutions. Arch Pathol Lab Med 119:681-685, 1995.
9. Murphy WM, et al. Tumors of the kidneys, bladder and related urinary structures. Atlas of Tumor Pathology, 3rd series, Fascicle 4. Armed Forces Institute of Pathology, Washington, DC, 1994, p. 199.
10. Epstein JI, Amin MB, Reuter VR, Mostofi FK, and the Bladder Consensus Conference Committee. The World Health Organization/International Society of Urological Pathology Consensus Classification of Urothelial (Transitional Cell) Neoplasms of the Urinary Bladder. Am J Surg Pathol 22:1435-1448, 1998.
11. Mostofi FK, et al. Histological typing of urinary bladder tumours. International Histological Classification of Tumours, No. 10. WHO, Geneva, 1973.
12. Jordon AM, et al. Transitional cell neoplasms of the urinary bladder: Can potential be predicted from histologic grading? Cancer 60:2766-2774, 1987.
13. Reyes AO, Humphrey PA. Diagnostic effect of complete histologic sampling of prostate needle biopsy specimens, Am J Clin Pathol 109:416-422, 1998.
14. Renshaw AA. Adequate tissue sampling of prostate core needle biopsies. Am J Clin Pathol 107:26-29, 1997.
15. Rubin MA, Bismar TA, Curtis S, Montie JE. Prostate needle biopsy reporting. How are the surgical members of the Society of Urologic Oncology using pathology reports to guide treatment of prostate cancer patients? Am J Surg Pathol 28:946-952, 2004.
16. Zigeuner RE, Lipsky K, Riedler I, et al. Did the rate of incidental prostate cancer change in the era of PSA testing? A retrospective study of 1127 patients. Urology 62:451-455, 2003.
17. Murphy WM, Dean PJ, Brasfield JA, Tatum L. Incidental carcinoma of the prostate. How much sampling is adequate? Am J Surg Pathol 10:170-174, 1986.
18. Moore GH, Lawshe B, Murphy J. Diagnosis of adenocarcinoma in transurethral resectates of the prostate gland. Am J Surg Pathol 10:165-169, 1986.
19. Newman AJ, Graham MA, Carlton CE, et al. Incidental carcinoma of the prostate at the time of transurethral resection: Importance of evaluating every chip. J Urol 128:948-950, 1982.
20. Geddy PM, Reid IN. Selective sampling of yellow prostate chips: a specific method for detecting prostatic adenocarcinoma. Urol Int 56:33-35, 1996.
21. Graham SD Jr, Bostwick DG, Hoisaeter A, et al. Report of the Committee on Staging and Pathology. Cancer 70 (1 suppl):359-361, 1992.
22. Harden P, Parkinson MC. Macroscopic examination of prostatic specimens. J Clin Pathol 48:693-700, 1995.
23. Humphrey PA, Walther PJ. Adenocarcinoma of the prostate. I. Tissue sampling considerations. Am J Clin Pathol 99:746-759, 1993.

24. Bova GS, Fox WM, Epstein JI. Methods of radical prostatectomy specimen processing: A novel technique for harvesting fresh prostate cancer tissue and review of processing techniques. Mod Pathol 6:201-207, 1993.

25. Humphrey PA, Vollmer RT. Percentage carcinoma as a measure of prostatic tumor size in radical prostatectomy tissues. Mod Pathol 10:326-333, 1997.

26. Renshaw AA, Chang H, D'Amico AV. Estimation of tumor volume in radical prostatectomy specimen in routine clinical practice. Am J Clin Pathol 107:704-708, 1997.

27. Renshaw AA, Richie JP, Loughlin KR, Jiroutek M, Chung A, D'Amico AV. The greatest dimension of prostate carcinoma is a simple, inexpensive predictor of prostate specific antigen failure in radical prostatectomy specimens. Cancer 83:748-752, 1998.

28. Gleason DF. Histologic grading of prostate cancer: A perspective. Hum Pathol 23:273-279, 1992.

29. Hawkins EP. Germ cell tumors. Am J Clin Pathol 109 (Suppl 1):S82-S88, 1998.

30. Warde P, et al. Prognostic factors for relapse in stage I seminoma managed by surveillance: a pooled analysis. J Clin Oncol 20:4448-4452, 2002.

31. Thomas G, Jones W, VanOosterom A, Kawai T. Consensus statement on the investigation and management of testicular seminoma 1989. Prog Clin Biol Res 357:285-294, 1990.

Gross examination

21

Certain specimens do not need to be submitted for histologic examination. These specimens include inanimate objects that cannot be examined under the microscope and tissue specimens that do not yield useful diagnostic information.

Each hospital must develop guidelines and policies to determine which types of specimens need not be examined histologically. The following factors should be considered:

- The likelihood of a clinically significant finding
- The need for documentation of surgical procedures for quality assurance
- Educational value for doctors in training
- Potential medicolegal issues.

In accordance with JCAHO guidelines, such decisions are made by consensus of the hospital staff and are put in writing. All clinicians should be informed as to the types of specimens that are not examined routinely in order that a specific request can be made in those cases in which microscopic examination is indicated.

A Q-Probes study by CAP revealed that 87.1% of institutions had written policies concerning specimens to be examined by gross examination only.[1] Only four tissue specimens were exempt from submission to the pathology department in more than 50% of institutions:

1. Placentas from routine uncomplicated pregnancies that were grossly normal
2. Foreskins from the circumcision of newborn children
3. Lens cataracts
4. Teeth.

Five types of tissue specimens were exempt from microscopic examination (i.e. only examined grossly) in more than 50% of institutions:

1. Calculi (renal, ureteral, bladder)
2. Teeth
3. Lens cataracts
4. Cartilage and bone from septorhinoplasty
5. Toenails and fingernails.

Thus, most institutions continue to examine most specimens grossly and microscopically.

Inanimate objects generally not examined microscopically

- Orthopedic hardware (see Chapter 28)
- Foreign bodies (see Chapter 28)
- Bullets (see Chapter 28)
- Gallstones (see Chapter 19)
- Bladder stones (usually sent for chemical analysis, see Chapter 20)
- Silicone implants (see Chapter 15)
- Vascular grafts may be submitted for histologic examination (see Chapter 16)

Tissue specimens generally not examined microscopically
• Teeth
• Skin from plastic surgery reconstruction if the surgeon does not request examination, no lesions are present, and there is no history of malignancy
• Skin with cicatrix (if there is no history of malignancy)
• Rib (as part of a resection if there is no history of malignancy and no gross lesions)
• Nasal septum (if part of a plastic surgery procedure or for chronic sinusitis)
• Stapes (removed to treat otosclerosis)
• Tonsils from children with hyperplasia but without gross lesions
• Foreskins from newborns
• Saphenous vein harvest for CABG
• Placentas from routine pregnancies
• Fetuses from therapeutic abortions (if there is no clinical indication for examination)
• Fingernails and toenails (if there is no clinical indication for examination)
• Lens (if removed for cataract)
• Pannus or bowel resections for treatment of obesity if grossly normal

Other specimens

It has been suggested that some specimens (specifically gallbladders, tonsils in adults, appendices, bone from orthopedic procedures, and hernia sacs) need not be examined, as the diagnostic yield is small. In sufficiently large studies, the incidence of clinically important unsuspected diagnoses in this group of specimens is approximately 1 to 10 per 1000 specimens. Thus, it is an economic decision as to whether it is of value to examine all of these specimens histologically. In a cost-benefit analysis, it was concluded that at least 1 of every 2000 specimens would need to show a clinically significant diagnosis to justify histologic examination.[2]

Studies have clearly shown that specimens that generally have a low diagnostic yield have a much higher yield of important diagnoses if certain features are present. These include:

• Specimens taken because of a "non-routine" clinical presentation (e.g., asymmetric tonsils).
• Grossly abnormal findings noted by the surgeon.
• Grossly abnormal findings noted by the pathologist.
• Specimens from patients with a history of malignancy.
• Specimens from patients in whom an infectious process is suspected.
• Specimens from patients who are known to be immunocompromised or who are at higher risk for unusual infections (e.g., because of organ transplant, corticosteroid therapy, chemotherapy, chronic ambulatory peritoneal dialysis, diabetes mellitus, antibiotic therapy, antifungal therapy, assisted ventilation, extensive burns, implanted monitoring devices or catheters, or chronic sinusitis).

Thus, if a decision is made to not examine some types of "routine" specimens, it is important that none of the above applies. The absence of clinical history provided by the submitting physician can never be interpreted to mean that no relevant clinical history exists. Figure 21-1 is an example of a requisition form that could be required from a submitting physician for specimens that need to be examined microscopically.

If the answers to the above questions are all "yes" and the tissue appears grossly unremarkable, then the specimen may not be examined microscopically.

If any of the answers are "no" or unknown, or if the tissue appears to be abnormal in appearance, or at the discretion of the pathologist, the tissue may be examined microscopically.

Request for pathologic examination.

Yes   **No**

☐   ☐   Is this a "routine" specimen (i.e., with the typical clinical presentation for this procedure)?

If no, explain: _____

☐   ☐   Did the tissue appear typical for a routine specimen?

If no, explain: _____

☐   ☐   Is the patient free of known malignances?

If no, explain: _____

☐   ☐   Does the patient lack conditions that could place him or her at higher risk for unusual infections or other diseases, such as immunocompromise (e.g., HIV), organ transplant, corticosteroid therapy, chemotherapy, chronic ambulatory peritoneal dialysis, diabetes mellitus, antibiotic therapy, antifungal therapy, assisted ventilation, extensive burns, implanted monitoring devices or catheters, or chronic sinusitis?

If no, explain: _____

☐   ☐   Is only a gross examination of tissue requested?

If no, explain: _____

Figure 21-1 Request for pathologic examination.

REFERENCES

1. Zarbo RJ, Nakhleh RE. Surgical pathology specimens for gross examination only and exempt from submission. A College of American Pathologists Q-Probes study of current policies in 413 institutions. Arch Pathol Lab Med 123:133-139, 1999.

2. Raab SS. The cost-effectiveness of routine histologic examination. Am J Clin Pathol 110:391-396, 1998).

Gynecologic and perinatal pathology

22

■ UTERUS

Relevant clinical history (in addition to age and gender)

See Table 22-1.

Table 22-1 Relevant clinical history	
HISTORY RELEVANT TO ALL SPECIMENS	HISTORY RELEVANT TO UTERINE SPECIMENS
Organ/tissue resected or biopsied	Date of last menstrual period or if postmenopausal
Purpose of the procedure	Current or recent pregnancy
Gross appearance of the organ/tissue/lesion sampled	Use of exogenous hormones (type and duration) or hormonal treatment (e.g., tamoxifen)
Any unusual features of the clinical presentation	Family history of breast or ovarian carcinoma
Any unusual features of the gross appearance	Abnormal bleeding
Prior surgery/biopsies—results	
Prior malignancy	
Prior treatment (radiation therapy, chemotherapy, drug use that can change the histologic appearance of tissues)	
Compromised immune system	

Endometrial biopsies or curettings

The endometrium is biopsied to evaluate abnormal bleeding in post-menopausal women, to monitor patients at high risk for endometrial carcinoma (e.g., women taking tamoxifen), and to evaluate infertility.

For patients with trophoblastic disease, the history would include the week of pregnancy, passage of tissue, prior history of hydatidiform mole, and human chorionic gonadotropin (hCG) level.

Processing the specimen

The entire specimen is submitted. For women younger than 45 years, one level is examined (usually luteal phase defect, increased bleeding due to suspected polyps, endometritis); for women of 45 years or more, or for women with a history or clinical question of hyperplasia or carcinoma, three levels are examined.

Table 22-2 Endometrial dating (Noyes Criteria)

Proliferative endometrium (PE)	Round or tubular glands, pseudostratified nuclei, no cytoplasmic vacuolization, apical *mitoses, no vacuoles*
Day 16 endometrium	Like PE, tubular glands with mitoses, but with *scattered basal cytoplasmic vacuoles*
	These changes can be caused by estrogen alone and are not diagnostic of ovulation
Secretory endometrium	
Day 17	Tubular glands with very regular, even subnuclear vacuoles ("*piano keys*"). A few mitoses may be present
Day 18	*Increased glandular complexity* (infolding) and intraglandular secretions, persistent cytoplasmic vacuoles
Day 19	Like Day 18 with only *scattered* cytoplasmic vacuoles. There are increased intraluminal secretions. No mitoses are present
Day 20	Like Day 19 *without* cytoplasmic vacuoles. Secretions peak
Day 21–22	Like Day 20 with *maximal stromal edema; no decidual change* On Day 22 the nuclei appear "naked"
Day 23	Decidual change *cuffing around arterioles*
Day 24	Decidual change expanding *from gland-to-gland,* but not going to surface
Day 25	A *thin* layer of decidual change underneath the surface
Day 26	A *thick* layer of decidual change underneath the surface
Day 27	"Inflammatory cells" (*stromal granulocytes*) in decidua; *scattered karyorrhexis* in glandular epithelium
Day 28 (menstrual endometrium, ME)	Hemorrhagic stroma (falling apart), prominent glandular karyorrhexis, and balls of necrotic stroma ("blue balls") surrounded by eosinophilic ("reparative") epithelium

As a general rule of thumb, pathology residents are always one day off the correct day.
Modified from Noyes RW, Hertig AT, Rock J. Dating the endometrial biopsy. Fertil Steril 1:3-25, 1950.

Hysterectomy and salpingo-oophorectomy

The type of hysterectomy (total or radical) and the disease (benign or malignant) determine the method of processing the specimen. Specimens fall into three categories:

1. Total hysterectomies for benign conditions (e.g., prolapse or fibroids)
2. Total hysterectomies for malignant conditions (e.g., endometrial carcinoma)
3. Radical hysterectomies for malignant conditions (e.g., cervical carcinoma) that include vaginal cuff, parametrium, and regional lymph nodes.

Gravid hysterectomies are rarely performed. These specimens are unusual and may have medicolegal implications.

Orientation of hysterectomies (Fig. 22-1)

Proceeding anterior to posterior are the round ligament, the fallopian tube, the ovary, and finally the ovarian ligament.

The peritoneal reflection is lower on the posterior surface and often comes to a point. It is higher and blunter on the anterior surface where the bladder has been dissected away.

If a specimen cannot be oriented, designate the two sides "A" and "B" when submitting sections.

Processing the specimen: Total hysterectomy for benign conditions

1. Weigh the specimen.
   Orient the specimen as to anterior and posterior.
   Examine the serosal surface for adhesions, endometriosis, tumor implants, or inflammation and describe.

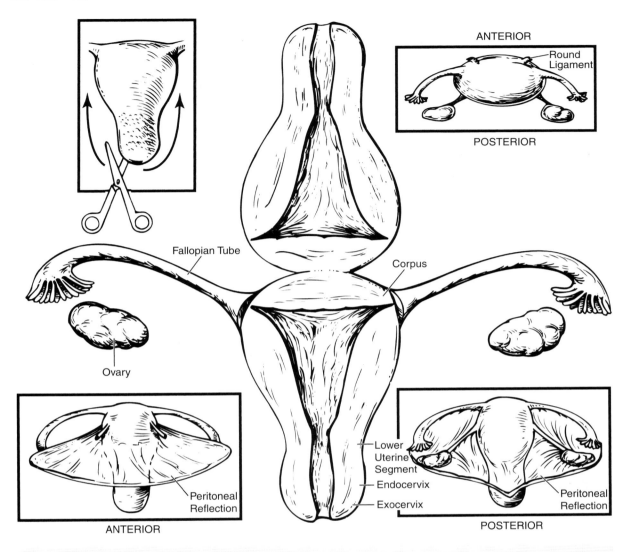

Figure 22-1 Total abdominal hysterectomy: orientation.

Record the overall dimensions of the uterus (three dimensions), tubes (length and diameter), and ovaries (three dimensions).

Record the dimensions of the exocervix and the size (greatest dimension, size of os) and shape (slit-like, round) of the os. Describe the appearance (smooth, white, glistening) and any lesions of the cervix (ulcerated, irregular, granular).

2. Open the uterus along the lateral margins from the external os to the cornu with scissors. Never use a scalpel. It is useful to use a probe within the os to guide the scissors. Make transverse incisions through the entire mucosa to, but not through, the serosa. Do not abrade the mucosa or wash with water.

Describe the endometrial cavity and lining including size (cornu to cornu, fundus to endocervical canal), distortion (by leiomyomas), color (tan, hemorrhagic), thickness, and any lesions. If lesions are present describe location (anterior or posterior), size, color, consistency, and depth of invasion into myometrium.

Describe the endocervix including size (length and width), color, normal herringbone pattern, and any lesions.

Describe the myometrium including average thickness, normal trabeculated pattern, or adenomyosis (coarse trabeculations or cystic hemorrhagic areas). If leiomyomata are present describe number, size (or range in size if many), location (subserosal, mural, submucosal, anterior or posterior), color, presence of hemorrhage or necrosis or variation in pattern.

Describe each fallopian tube (see separate section).

Serially section along short axis and describe each ovary (see "ovary" page 435).

Remove the adnexa and weigh the uterus.

3. Hysterectomies for benign disease can have sections taken from unfixed tissue. The remainder of the specimen is stored in the refrigerator. However, if a neoplastic process is known or suspected, follow the next protocol.

Microscopic sections

Cervix
Anterior and posterior cervix taken to include both exocervix and endocervix and the transformation zone.

Lower uterine segment (LUS)
One transmural section from the posterior side.

Endometrium and myometrium
Two transmural endometrial sections from anterior and posterior walls; if the myometrium is very thick, include only a portion of wall. Sample any lesions (e.g., polyps). If leiomyomas are present, section through each one and examine grossly. Take up to three representative sections total. More sections are taken if there are areas of necrosis, hemorrhage, or unusual appearance.

If the hysterectomy is supracervical, take a section perpendicular to the resection margin to determine at what level (endocervix or lower uterine segment) the resection was performed. If all endometrium is not removed, the patient may be at risk for developing carcinoma and decisions concerning hormonal treatment could be affected.

Serosa
If serosa is not included in the sections of endometrium, submit a separate section.

Fallopian tubes
Sample proximal, mid, and distal (fimbriae) segments and submit right and left in separate cassettes.

Ovary
Serially section the ovaries transversely to the long axis and submit one representative section from each ovary including the capsule. This section can be submitted with the fallopian tube in the same cassette.

Sample dictation

Received fresh, labeled with the patient's name and unit number and "TAH-BSO," is a 350-g specimen including an unopened uterus (10 × 6.5 × 4.0 cm), right fallopian tube (5 cm in length × 0.7 cm in diameter), right ovary (3.5 × 2.0 × 0.9 cm), left fallopian tube (4.3 cm in length × 0.7 cm in diameter), and left ovary (3.8 × 2.4 × 1.0 cm). The exocervix (3.0 × 2.8 cm) is covered by smooth glistening white mucosa. The external os is circular and measures 0.7 cm in diameter. The endocervical canal (2.7 cm in length) has a tan herringbone mucosa. The endometrial cavity (6.5 cm from cornu to cornu, 5.0 cm in length) has a tan/pink hemorrhagic endometrium (0.5 cm in average thickness). The myometrium measures 1.5 cm in maximum thickness and contains two subserosal leiomyomata (1.2 and 0.8 cm in greatest dimension) that have a white/tan whorled appearance without hemorrhage or necrosis. The serosa is dull and there are multiple fine adhesions.

The fallopian tubes are patent and have fimbriated ends. The left tube has a 0.3 cm in greatest dimension thin-walled paratubal cyst filled with clear fluid.

The right ovary has a smooth white surface and a single smooth-walled cortical cyst (0.3 cm in greatest dimension). The left ovary has multiple fine adhesions on the outer surface and a golden yellow corpus luteum is present with a hemorrhagic center. Multiple corpora albicantia are present in both ovaries.

Cassette #1: Anterior cervix, 1 frag, RSS.
Cassette #2: Posterior cervix, 1 frag, RSS.
Cassette #3: Lower uterine segment, 1 frag, RSS.
Cassette #4: Anterior endometrium, 1 frag, RSS.
Cassette #5: Posterior endometrium, 1 frag, RSS.
Cassette #6: Serosa including adhesions, 3 frags, RSS.
Cassette #7: Right fallopian tube and ovary with cyst, 4 frags, RSS.
Cassette #8: Left fallopian tube with cyst and left ovary with corpus luteum and adhesions, 4 frags, RSS.

Processing the specimen: Total hysterectomy for endometrial tumors (Fig. 22-2)

1. Weigh the specimen and orient as before. Examine the serosal surface carefully for adhesions, serosal implants, or direct invasion by tumor. The vaginal reflection at the cervix should be examined for tumor implants.

    Ink the serosal surface and the vaginal margin. Do not ink surfaces exposed by cutting into the specimen.

    State in the description whether the specimen was received intact or was previously opened.
2. Open with scissors along the lateral margins from external os to cornu. Avoid cutting through areas suspicious for involvement by tumor. Try to make clean cuts when opening the uterus so that true surgical margins and serosal surface will be apparent. Do not abrade the mucosa or wash with water.
3. Make serial transverse incisions from the mucosal surface to, but not through, the serosal surface at approximately 0.5 cm intervals. Leave all tissues attached in order to maintain orientation.
4. Describe as above but include any irregularities or piling up of the mucosal surface, location of lesions (e.g., anterior versus posterior), the portion of the endometrial surface involved, and gross invasion (depth). Gross invasion is appreciated as an effacement of the normal myometrial texture but may be difficult to appreciate grossly.
5. Pin to a paraffin board and fix overnight in formalin.
6. Sections are taken the following day. Search for all parametrial lymph nodes and note their location. Usually nodes are not found.

Microscopic sections

Tumor
Transmural sections demonstrating depth of invasion to the inked margin. In most cases four anterior and four posterior sections are adequate. If the tumor is in the LUS or near the cervix the entire vaginal margin (inked) is divided into quadrants and submitted and extra slides of the LUS are also submitted.

Note: The edges of transmural sections are trimmed to remove areas of myometrium without overlying endometrium (see Fig. 22-2).

Cervix
Anterior and posterior cervix taken to include both exocervix and endocervix and the transformation zone.

Lower uterine segment
Two transmural sections from the posterior and anterior sides. See "Tumor," above, if the tumor is near the LUS.

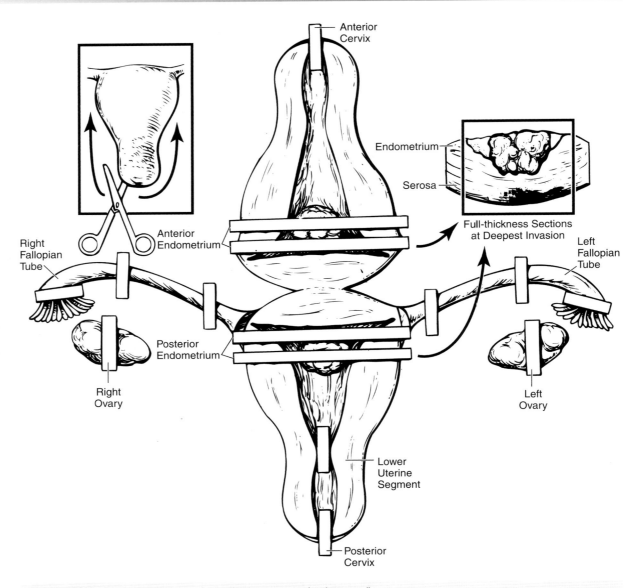

Figure 22-2 Total hysterectomy for malignant tumors (endometrial).

Fallopian tubes
Sample proximal, mid, and distal (fimbriae) segments and submit right and left in separate cassettes.

Ovary
Submit the entire ovaries (sections taken transverse to the longitudinal axis) including capsule.

Serosa
If serosa is not included in the sections of endometrium, submit a separate section.

Parametrium
Submit any parametrial nodules or lymph nodes.

Other lesions
Submit sections of any other lesions (e.g., polyps, leiomyomata).

Received fresh, labeled with the patient's name and unit number and "Hysterectomy," is a 400-g specimen including an unopened uterus (11 × 7 × 5.2 cm), right fallopian tube (4.5 cm in length × 0.7 cm in diameter), right ovary (3.0 × 2.0 × 1.0 cm), left fallopian tube (5.1 cm in length × 0.7 cm in diameter), and left ovary (3.5 × 3.2 × 0.9 cm). The exocervix (3.0 × 3.0 cm) is covered by smooth glistening white mucosa. The external os is circular and measures 0.6 cm in diameter. The endocervical canal (3.1 cm in length) has a tan herringbone mucosa. The endometrial cavity (7.1 cm from cornu to cornu, 6.0 cm in length) has a tan/pink hemorrhagic endometrial lining. There is a 2 × 2 cm mass of heaped up pink/gray mucosa on the posterior wall. There appears to be invasion of the underlying mucosa to a depth of one third of the myometrium. A representative section was used for frozen section. The mass is located 3 cm from the lower uterine segment. The myometrium measures 2.1 cm in maximum thickness. The serosa is shiny and glistening without adhesions.
The fallopian tubes are patent and have fimbriated ends.
The right ovary has a smooth white outer surface and multiple corpora albicantia. The left ovary has a smooth white outer surface and a single smooth-walled simple cyst (0.8 cm in greatest dimension).
One lymph node (0.6 cm) is located within parametrial soft tissue.

Cassette #1: Frozen section remnant, 1 frag, ESS.
Cassettes #2–5: Posterior wall of uterus including deepest extent of invasion, 4 frags, RSS.
Cassettes #6–9: Anterior wall of uterus including areas suspicious for tumor involvement, 4 frags, RSS.
Cassette #10: Anterior cervix, 1 frag, RSS.
Cassette #11: Posterior cervix, 1 frag, RSS.
Cassette #12: Lower uterine segment, posterior, 1 frag, RSS.
Cassette #13: Lower uterine segment, anterior, 1 frag, RSS.
Cassette #14: Left fallopian tube, 3 frags, RSS.
Cassette #15: Left ovary, 4 frags, ESS.
Cassette #16: Right fallopian tube, 3 frags, RSS.
Cassette #17: Right ovary, 5 frags, ESS.
Cassette #18: Lymph node, 2 frags, ESS.

Processing the specimen: Radical hysterectomy for cervical carcinoma (Fig. 22-3)

1. Weigh the specimen and orient as described previously.

   Examine the serosal surface for adhesions, serosal tumor nodules, or direct invasion by tumor.

   Ink the uterine and cervical serosal surface and the vaginal cuff margin. Do not spill ink onto the exocervix. If tumor extends directly into parametrium, ink this area also. Do not ink surfaces exposed by cutting into the specimen.

   State in the description if the specimen was received intact or was previously opened.

2. Amputate the cervix with the vaginal cuff. Open the anterior surface (12 o'clock). Pin onto corkboard and fix in formalin overnight.

   Open the uterine corpus with scissors along the lateral margins from external os to cornu. Avoid cutting through areas suspicious for involvement by tumor. Try to make clean cuts when opening the uterus so that true surgical margins and serosal surface will be apparent. Do not abrade the mucosa or wash with water.

3. Make serial transverse incisions from the mucosal surface to, but not through, the serosal surface at approximately 0.5 cm intervals. Leave all tissues attached in order to maintain orientation.

4. Describe as for a non-tumor hysterectomy but include location of lesions (e.g., anterior versus posterior, involvement of exocervix, endocervix, and/or LUS), distance from

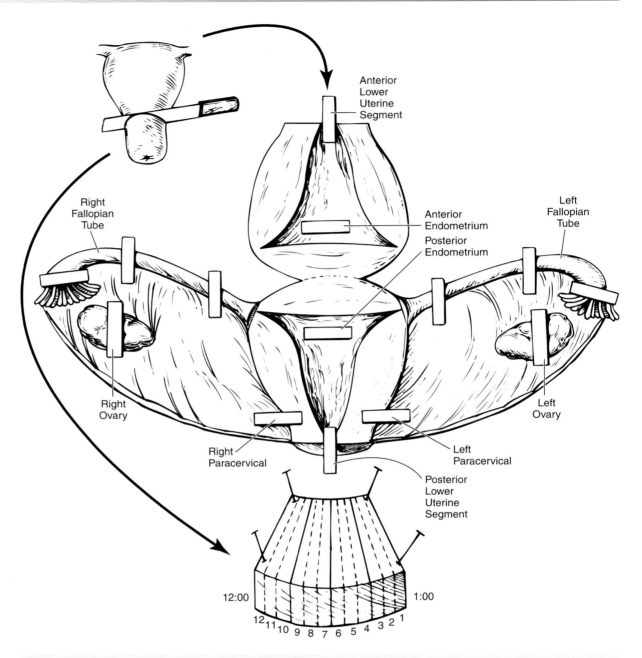

Figure 22-3 Radical hysterectomy for malignant tumors (cervical carcinoma).

margins, and gross invasion (depth). Pin to a paraffin board and fix overnight in formalin.

5. Carefully search for parametrial lymph nodes and note their location, side, and number. Lymph nodes are often also submitted as separate specimens.

Microscopic sections

Tumor (cervix)

Submit the entire cervix by clock positions (as described for "Cone biopsies," page 448). The vaginal margin can be left on the cervix and included with these sections if small. If this margin is large, representative sections can be submitted using clock positions. If tumor is close to or involves the vaginal margin, the entire margin should be submitted as clock positions.

If the tumor extends beyond the cervix, sample these areas (e.g., parametrium and adjacent uterine serosa).

Lower uterine segment
Two transmural sections from the posterior and anterior sides. See "Tumor," above, if the tumor is near the LUS.

Endometrium
Two sections (anterior and posterior).

Fallopian tubes
Sample proximal, mid, and distal (fimbriae) segments and submit right and left in separate cassettes.

Ovary
Submit one representative section from each ovary (taken transverse to the longitudinal axis) including capsule. This section can be submitted with the fallopian tube in the same cassette.

Serosa
If serosa is not included in the sections of endometrium, submit a separate section.

Parametrium
Submit any parametrial nodules or lymph nodes. Note number, location, and side. If no gross tumor is present in this location, submit two representative sections.

Other lesions
Submit sections of any other lesions (e.g., polyps, leiomyomata).

Sample dictation

Received fresh, labeled with the patient's name and unit number and "Radical Hysterectomy," is a 420-g specimen including an unopened uterus (9.0 × 5.5 × 5.0 cm) with attached cervix and vaginal cuff, right fallopian tube (4.5 cm in length × 0.7 cm in diameter), right ovary (3.8 × 1.8 × 1.2 cm), left fallopian tube (5.0 cm in length × 0.7 cm in diameter), and left ovary (4.2 × 3.0 × 1.2 cm). There is a white/tan centrally ulcerated mass (1.5 × 1.0 × 0.5 cm) located on the posterior surface of the exocervix (3.0 × 2.8 cm). The mass appears to invade to a depth of 0.5 cm but is grossly 0.8 cm from the outer surface. The mass extends into the endocervical canal but not to the lower uterine segment. The mass is 4 cm from the vaginal cuff margin. The external os is distorted by the mass and is 0.2 cm in diameter. The endocervical canal (3.1 cm in length) has a tan herringbone mucosa. The endometrial cavity (6.3 cm from cornu to cornu, 4.8 cm in length) has a tan/pink hemorrhagic endometrium (0.3 cm in average thickness). The myometrium measures 1.2 cm in maximum thickness and contains one submucosal leiomyoma (2.5 cm in greatest dimension) that has a white/tan whorled appearance without hemorrhage or necrosis. The serosa is glistening with an adhesion on the posterior surface.
The fallopian tubes are patent and have fimbriated ends.
The right ovary has a smooth white surface and multiple corpora albicantia. The left ovary has multiple corpora albicantia and a golden yellow corpus luteum.
Three lymph nodes are located in the right parametrial soft tissue. The largest node measures 1.2 cm and is grossly white and firm. Two lymph nodes are located in the left parametrial soft tissue. Both are tan and the largest measures 0.8 cm in greatest dimension.

Cassettes #1–4: Posterior cervix including mass, 4 o'clock to 7 o'clock, 4 frags, ESS.
Cassette #5–12: Remainder of cervix, 8 o'clock to 3 o'clock, 8 frags, ESS.
Cassette #13–16: Vaginal cuff margin, sections at 12, 3, 6, and 9 o'clock, 4 frags, RSS.
Cassette #17: Lower uterine segment, posterior, closest to mass, 1 frag, RSS.
Cassette #18: Lower uterine segment, anterior, 1 frag, RSS.
Cassette #19: Anterior endometrium, 1 frag, RSS.
Cassette #20: Posterior endometrium, 1 frag, RSS.
Cassette #21: Right fallopian tube and right ovary, 4 frags, RSS.

Cassette #22: Left fallopian tube and left ovary, 4 frags, RSS.
Cassette #23: Leiomyoma, 2 frags, RSS.
Cassette #24: Largest right lymph node, 2 frags, ESS.
Cassette #25: Two additional right lymph nodes (inked blue and black), 4 frags, ESS.
Cassette #26: Two left lymph nodes (inked blue and black), 4 frags, ESS.

Special studies

Hormone receptors, DNA content, proliferative fraction, and oncogene expression have been studied on a research basis. There are no routinely indicated special studies of endometrial lesions for clinical decision making.

Gross differential diagnosis of endometrial and myometrial lesions

Leiomyomata. These tumors are firm, whorled, white to tan nodules present within myometrium, bulging into the endometrial lumen or protruding into the peritoneal cavity. Cystic degeneration and softening may be seen in the center of large leiomyomata. Hemorrhage and necrosis should not be seen. Their location may be:

- Subserosal: immediately below the serosa; some are pedunculated and can appear to be periuterine masses.
- Intramural: within the myometrium.
- Submucosal: immediately below the endometrium.

Leiomyosarcoma. These are usually larger and softer than leiomyomas and more commonly solitary. The color may be gray/yellow rather than white. Areas of hemorrhage and necrosis may be present. Invasion into the surrounding myometrium may be present. However, some are grossly indistinguishable from leiomyomas. Malignant lesions generally have complex karyotypes as compared to leiomyomas.

Stromal sarcomas may be well circumscribed or diffusely infiltrative as single or multiple masses. Lymphovascular invasion can often be seen as "worm-like" masses within the myometrium. Approximately one third invade into adjacent tissues. Necrosis and hemorrhage are common.

Adenomyosis results from benign glands embedded within myometrium. The myometrium appears thickened with coarse trabeculations. Pinpoint hemorrhage may be present.

Endometrial polyps are usually large, broad-based, finger-like projections from the endometrial wall. The center is comprised of fibrous stroma and the surface is covered by endometrium.

Endometrial carcinoma. The endometrial lining may be heaped up, but a yellow friable appearance is more characteristic of carcinomas. This may be best appreciated on cross-section. Invasive carcinomas may efface the normal myometrial texture. This finding may be subtle or obscured by adenomyosis.

Malignant mixed mesodermal tumor (carcinosarcoma) usually takes the form of a very large friable mass completely filling the endometrial cavity and extending through the cervical os. The myometrium is typically deeply invaded. Foci of bone or cartilage may be present.

Adenomatoid tumor is a poorly circumscribed soft mass within the myometrium, near the serosal surface. Large tumors may extend into the endometrium.

Gestational trophoblastic tumors. Complete or partial hydatidiform moles are usually received as products of conception and are grossly recognized by the numerous dilated grape-like vesicles. Fetal parts may be present in partial hydatidiform moles. Hysterectomy is rarely performed in the case of an invasive mole, which grossly looks like a hemorrhagic mass adherent to the wall of the uterus.

Gestational choriocarcinoma can arise from placental tissues from either a normal or abnormal pregnancy. It is a soft, fleshy, yellow-white tumor, often with large areas of necrosis and usually with extensive hemorrhage. The tumor invades into the myometrium and may extend out into the serosa. There is a separate AJCC staging system for these tumors.

Pathologic diagnostic/prognostic features sign-out checklist for endometrial carcinomas

Specimen type*
Hysterectomy, radical hysterectomy (including parametria), pelvic exenteration.

Other organs present*
None, ovary (right and/or left), fallopian tube (right and/or left), urinary bladder, vagina, rectum.

Tumor site
Location (if known).

Histologic type*
Endometrioid carcinoma (and subtypes), mucinous adenocarcinoma, serous adenocarcinoma, clear cell adenocarcinoma, squamous cell carcinoma, undifferentiated carcinoma, other rare types. The WHO classification is recommended.

Tumor size*
Greatest dimension (additional margins are optional).
Extent of surface area involved (<4 cm versus >4 cm) is correlated with higher stage disease.

Histologic grade*
Different grading systems are used for different tumor types (see page 431).

Myometrial invasion*
Given as percentage of myometrium involved (<50%, ≥50%) and depth of invasion measured in millimeters. Also give thickness of myometrium in this area. See also Box 22-1.

Extent of invasion*
Carcinoma in situ (pTis), tumor limited to endometrium (pT1a), tumor invades less than one half of the myometrium (pT1b), tumor invades one half or more of the myometrium (pT1c), tumor invades the endocervical glands of the cervix (pT2a), tumor invades cervical stroma (pT2b), tumor involves serosa, parametria, and/or adnexa (direct extension or metastasis) and/or cancer cells are present in ascites or peritoneal washings (pT3a), tumor involves vagina (direct extension or metastasis), rectal or bladder wall (without mucosal involvement), or pelvic wall(s) (frozen pelvis) (pT3b), tumor invades bladder mucosa and/or bowel mucosa (pT4).

Venous/lymphatic (large/small vessel) invasion*
Absent, present, indeterminate.

Involvement of other structures
Involvement of fallopian tube, ovary, serosa of uterus, endocervix, vagina, peritoneum, bladder mucosa, colon or rectal mucosa, etc.

Regional lymph nodes*
Absent (N0), present (N1).
Number of nodes examined, number involved.

Distant metastasis*
Absent (M0), present (M1).

Cytology
Ascites or peritoneal washings: Positive or negative for malignant cells.

Other findings
Endometrial intraepithelial neoplasia (EIN), atrophy, polyps.

Margins*

Uninvolved, involved, distance of invasive carcinoma from the margin.
Cervical margin, serosal margin.

This checklist incorporates information from the ADASP (see www.panix.com/~adasp) and the CAP Cancer Committee protocols for reporting on cancer specimens (see www.cap.org/). The asterisked elements are considered to be scientifically validated or regularly used data elements that must be present in reports of cancer-directed surgical resection specimens from ACS CoC-approved cancer programs. The specific details of reporting the elements may vary among institutions.

The AJCC classification is given in Table 22-3.

Box 22-1 Criteria defining stromal invasion of endometrial carcinomas[1]

One of the following should be present:
1. Irregular infiltration of glands associated with an altered fibroblastic stroma (desmoplastic response)
2. Confluent glandular pattern (cribriform growth)
3. Extensive papillary growth pattern (at least 0.42 cm in diameter)

Pathologic diagnostic/prognostic features sign-out checklist for gestational trophoblastic malignancies

Specimen type*
Dilatation and curettage, hysterectomy, radical hysterectomy, pelvic exenteration.

Other organs involved by tumor*
None, specify organ, direct extension or separate metastasis.

Tumor site*
Location (if known).

Fetal tissue*
Absent, present (specify type).

Fetal anomalies*
Cannot be determined, absent, present (specify type).

Histologic type*
Hydatidiform mole (complete, partial, or invasive), choriocarcinoma, placental site trophoblastic tumor, epithelioid trophoblastic tumor, malignant trophoblastic tumor, type cannot be determined.

Tumor size*
Greatest dimension (additional margins are optional).

Extent of invasion*
Tumor limited to uterus (pT1), tumor extends outside uterus but is limited to the genital structures (adnexa, vagina, broad ligament) (pT2).
Myometrial invasion: Present (% of thickness), absent.
Serosal surface: Involved, not involved.

Venous/lymphatic (large/small vessel) invasion*
Absent, present, indeterminate.

Distant metastasis*
Absent (M0), tumor extends to the lungs with or without genital tract involvement (M1a), tumor involves other metastatic sites (M1b).

Margins
Uninvolved, involved, distance to nearest margin.

Additional findings
Implantation site, leiomyoma, adenomyosis.

This checklist incorporates information from the ADASP (see www.panix.com/~adasp) and the CAP Cancer Committee protocols for reporting on cancer specimens (see www.cap.org/). The asterisked elements are considered to be scientifically validated or regularly used data elements that must be present in reports of cancer-directed surgical resection specimens from ACS CoC-approved cancer programs. The specific details of reporting the elements may vary among institutions.

The AJCC classification is given in Table 22-4.

Grading of gynecologic tumors

In serous and clear cell adenocarcinomas, nuclear grading takes precedence. Most are high grade. Rare serous tumors with a solid growth pattern in small nests with a high degree of nuclear maturation and psammoma bodies are assigned grade 1.

There is no universally accepted system for mucinous carcinomas. Architectural and nuclear features are evaluated.

Table 22-3 AJCC and FIGO (6th edition) classification of endometrial carcinomas

AJCC (TNM)	FIGO	DEFINITION
Primary tumor		
TX	—	Primary tumor cannot be assessed
T0	—	No evidence of primary tumor
Tis	—	Carcinoma in situ
T1	I	Tumor confined to the corpus uteri
T1a	IA	Tumor limited to the endometrium
T1b	IB	Tumor invades up to or less than one half of the myometrium
T1c	IC	Tumor invades more than one half of the myometrium
T2	II	Tumor invades cervix but does not extend beyond the uterus
T2a	IIA	Endocervical glandular involvement only
T2b	IIB	Cervical stromal invasion
T3	III	Local and/or regional spread as specified in T3a, b, and/or N1 and FIGO IIIA, B, and C below
T3a	IIIA	Tumor involves serosa and/or adnexa (direct extension or metastasis) and/or cancer cells in ascites or peritoneal washings
T3b	IIIB	Vaginal involvement (direct extension or metastasis)
N1	IIIC	Metastasis to the pelvic and/or para-aortic lymph nodes
T4	IVA	Tumor invades bladder mucosa and/or bowel mucosa (bullous edema is not sufficient to classify a tumor as T4)
M1	IVB	Distant metastasis (excluding metastasis to vagina, pelvic serosa, or adnexa; including metastasis to intra-abdominal lymph nodes other than para-aortic, and/or inguinal lymph nodes)
Regional lymph nodes		
NX	—	Regional lymph nodes cannot be assessed
N0	—	No regional lymph node metastasis
N1	—	Regional lymph node metastasis
Distant metastasis		
MX	—	Distant metastasis cannot be assessed
M0	—	No distant metastasis
M1	IVB	Distant metastasis (excludes peritoneal metastasis)

Table 22-4 AJCC and FIGO (6th edition) classification of gestational trophoblastic tumors

AJCC (TNM)	FIGO	DEFINITION
Tx		Primary tumor cannot be assessed
T0		No evidence of primary tumor
T1	I	Tumor confined to uterus
T2	II	Tumor extends to other genital structures (ovary, tube, vagina, broad ligaments) by metastasis or direct extension
	IIA	With low-risk prognostic score (see Table 22-5)
	IIB	With high-risk prognostic score

Distant metastasis

MX		Metastasis cannot be assessed
M0		No distant metastasis
M1		Distant metastasis
M1a	III	Lung metastasis
	IIIA	With low-risk prognostic score
	IIIB	With high-risk prognostic score
M1b	IV	All other distant metastasis
	IVA	With low-risk prognostic score
	IVB	With high-risk prognostic score

Table 22-5 Gestational trophoblastic neoplasia: Prognostic score

PROGNOSTIC FACTOR	0	1	2	3
Age	<40	≥40		
Antecedent pregnancy	Hydatidiform mole	Abortion	Term pregnancy	
Months from index pregnancy	<4	4–<7	7–12	>12
Pretreatment serum hCG (U/mL)	$<10^3$	$10^3-<10^4$	$10^4-<10^5$	$\geq10^5$
Largest tumor size including uterus	<3 cm	3–<5 cm	≥5 cm	
Sites of metastasis	Lung	Spleen, kidney	Gastrointestinal tract	Liver, brain
Number of metastases		1–4	5–8	>8
Previous failed chemotherapy			Single drug	Two or more drugs

Risk categories

Low risk	7 or less (add "A" to FIGO stage)
High risk	8 or more (add "B" to FIGO stage)

This classification is used for invasive hydatidiform mole, choriocarcinoma, placental site trophoblastic tumors, and epithelioid trophoblastic tumors.

Adenocarcinomas with squamous differentiation are graded according to the nuclear grade of the glandular component.

Urothelial (transitional) cell and squamous cell carcinomas are graded using nuclear grade.

Immature teratomas are graded by the quantity of embryonal elements, almost always neuroectodermal.

Granulosa cell tumors are not graded.

FIGO grading of endometrial carcinomas

Architectural grade (endometrioid carcinomas)

- Well differentiated (G1): 5% or less solid growth (excluding squamous or morular growth patterns)
- Moderately differentiated (G2): 6–50% solid growth (nonsquamous or nonmorular growth pattern)
- Poorly differentiated (G3): >50% solid growth (nonsquamous or nonmorular growth pattern)

Notable nuclear atypia (grade 3 nuclear atypia), inappropriate for the architectural grade, raises the grade of a grade 1 or grade 2 tumor by 1 grade.

Nuclear grade (clear cell, squamous, and serous carcinomas)

1. Uniform nuclei (round to oval), small nucleoli, even chromatin, usually in a single row or moderately stratified, rare mitoses.
2. Variable size and shape of nuclei, larger nucleoli, more mitoses.
3. Enlarged pleomorphic nuclei, prominent nucleoli, coarse chromatin, frequent mitoses.

Sample reports

Hysterectomies should be reported in a standardized format:

Example of a hysterectomy report with benign findings

SPECIMEN LABELED "UTERUS, TUBES, AND OVARIES"

Cervix
Squamous metaplasia

Endometrium
Proliferative endometrium

Myometrium
Leiomyomata, intramural, submucosal (largest 5.0 cm)

Serosa
Adhesions

Right fallopian tube
No significant pathologic change

Right ovary
Recent corpus luteum
Cystic follicle

Left fallopian tube
Peritubal adhesions

Left ovary
Cortical inclusion cysts

Example of a hysterectomy report with an endometrial carcinoma

SPECIMEN LABELED "UTERUS, TUBES, AND OVARIES"

Cervix
Squamous metaplasia

Endomyometrium
Endometrial adenocarcinoma, endometrioid type, grade 1 (of 3).
● The tumor invades through 30% of the myometrial thickness.
● Capillary/lymphatic space invasion is *not* seen.
Leiomyomata, subserosal (largest 3.0 cm)

Serosa
No significant pathologic change

Right fallopian tube
No significant pathologic change

Right ovary
Recent corpus luteum
Cystic follicle

Left fallopian tube
Peritubal adhesions

Left ovary
Cortical inclusion cysts

Example of a report with a cervical carcinoma

SPECIMEN LABELED "UTERUS, TUBES, AND OVARIES"

Cervix
SQUAMOUS CELL CARCINOMA, moderately differentiated.
● The tumor is 6.0 cm in length by 5.0 cm in greatest depth.
● Capillary/lymphatic space invasion is present.
Squamous intraepithelial lesion, high grade (CIN 2/3).
Margins are free of intraepithelial and invasive neoplasia.

Endometrium
Proliferative endometrium

Myometrium
Adenomyosis

Serosa
No significant pathologic change

Right fallopian tube
No significant pathologic change

Right ovary
Recent corpus luteum
Cystic follicle

Left fallopian tube
Peritubal adhesions

Left ovary
Cortical inclusion cysts

Example of a report with an ovarian carcinoma

SPECIMEN LABELED "UTERUS, TUBES, AND OVARIES"

Cervix
Squamous metaplasia

Endometrium
Atrophy

Myometrium
Adenomyosis

Serosa
No significant pathologic change

Right fallopian tube
No significant pathologic change

Right ovary
PAPILLARY SEROUS ADENOCARCINOMA, moderately differentiated (20 cm).
The tumor is located within a cyst and does not involve the ovarian surface.

Left fallopian tube
Peritubal adhesions

Left ovary
Cortical inclusion cysts

Omentum
No significant pathologic change

Pelvic lymph nodes
No tumor seen in three (3) of three lymph nodes

■ OVARY

Ovaries are removed for evaluation of a mass or as part of a larger resection (Fig. 22-4). Occasionally biopsies are performed for incidental mass lesions (e.g., a corpus luteum of pregnancy during a cesarean section) or for treatment (e.g., Stein–Leventhal syndrome).

Neoplasms generally have one of the three following appearances:

1. **Simple cyst:** thin-walled, without solid areas. These cysts are almost always benign. Most are follicular cysts (cystic follicles), corpus luteum cysts, or cystadenomas (epithelium-lined cysts).
2. **Complex cyst** with or without a solid component. Such a cyst may be nonneoplastic (e.g., an endometriotic or "chocolate" cyst), a benign neoplasm (dermoid), a borderline tumor, or a malignant tumor.

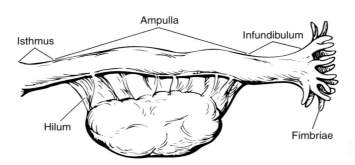

Figure 22-4 Ovary and fallopian tube.

3. **Solid tumors.** These may be benign fibromas, Brenner tumors, granulosa cell tumors, or malignant carcinomas.

Relevant clinical history (in addition to age)

See Table 22-6.

Table 22-6 Relevant clinical history	
HISTORY RELEVANT TO ALL SPECIMENS	HISTORY RELEVANT TO OVARIAN SPECIMENS
Organ/tissue resected or biopsied	Pregnancy
Purpose of the procedure	Abnormal uterine bleeding
Gross appearance of the organ/tissue/lesion sampled	Personal or family history or ovarian or breast carcinoma
Any unusual features of the clinical presentation	Stein–Leventhal syndrome
Any unusual features of the gross appearance	
Prior surgery/biopsies—results	
Prior malignancy	
Prior treatment (radiation therapy, chemotherapy, drug use that can change the histologic appearance of tissues)	
Compromised immune system	

Processing the specimen: Incidental ovaries or prophylactic oophorectomies

1. Record the overall dimensions of the ovary and describe the outer surface including color (white), surface (smooth or convoluted, adhesions, papillary projections), simple cysts (thin-walled without a solid component).

   Avoid rubbing or abrading the outer surface in order to preserve the delicate (and very fragile) epithelial lining.

2. If any abnormality is present (e.g., cysts, papillary projections), ink the outer surface.

   Serially section the ovary, parallel to the short axis.

   Describe the ovary including color and presence of corpus luteum and corpora albicantia. If cysts are present, describe number, size, unilocular versus multilocular, lining (smooth, irregular, papillary projections, velvety as in endometriotic cyst), thickness of wall, contents (fluid versus keratinaceous material and hair as in mature teratoma, serous versus mucinous, hemorrhagic), calcified areas or bone. If it is a large cyst, try to identify remaining ovary as a focal thickening of the wall.

3. The usual unremarkable ovary with only small simple cysts can be sampled with one section demonstrating any features noted above.

If the ovary was removed as a prophylactic procedure in a woman with a family history of ovarian carcinoma, the entire specimen (ovary and fallopian tube) is examined histologically.

Large thin-walled cysts can be rolled into a "jelly roll" and fixed in formalin overnight. Submit transverse sections of the roll. Try to submit a section of the residual ovary.

If there is any suspicion of malignancy (e.g., mucinous cyst, complex cyst, papillary projections, solid areas), additional sections must be taken to document these areas and any extension into adjacent tissues (see "ovary with complex cyst," "ovary with solid tumor").

Received fresh, labeled with the patient's name and unit number and "right ovary," is an ovary (3.0 × 2.5 × 1.0 cm) with a smooth white convoluted surface and multiple corpora albicantia. There is a smooth-walled 0.6 cm superficial intact cyst.

Cassette #1: Representative cross-section including cyst, 1 frag, RSS.

Processing the specimen: Ovary with simple cyst

1. Record the overall dimensions of the ovary and describe the outer surface including color (white), surface (smooth or convoluted, adhesions, papillary projections), and simple (thin-walled without a solid component) cysts. Papillations or a "nubby" appearance on the surface of the ovary could indicate either invasion of a tumor through the capsule or a serosal implant.

Avoid rubbing or abrading the outer surface in order to preserve the surface epithelial lining.

2. Ink the outer surface including all areas of irregularity.

Ovarian cysts are opened with great care as the cyst fluid may be under pressure. Wear goggles and appropriate clothing protection. Open in a pan or on sufficient numbers of surgical drapes to absorb all the fluid. Very large cysts may need to be opened in a sink. Make a small initial incision inferiorly (away from the face of the prosector) to allow the fluid to drain slowly.

Try to identify remaining ovarian tissue. It can sometimes be seen as a thickened portion of the wall, readily visible on transillumination. Do not abrade the lining by excessive handling.

Describe the cyst including size, inner surface (smooth or with papillary areas or solid areas, velvety texture as in endometriotic cysts), wall thickness, contents (blood, serous fluid, mucinous fluid, keratinaceous and sebaceous material and hair as in mature teratoma), and solid areas (color, texture, extension to serosal surface). If the fallopian tube is included, describe its relationship to the cyst. Describe the remaining ovary including color, corpus luteum, and corpora albicantia.

3. Large thin-walled cysts can be rolled into a "jelly roll" and fixed in formalin overnight. Submit transverse sections of the roll. Submit a section of the residual ovary.

If there is any suspicion of malignancy (e.g., mucinous cyst, complex cyst, papillary projections, solid areas), additional sections must be taken to document these areas and any extension into adjacent tissues. At least one cassette per cm of greatest dimension of the cyst must be taken if the cyst is mucinous (malignant features can be focal in this type of neoplasm).

Submit a section with fallopian tube, if present.

Received fresh, labeled with the patient's name and unit number and "left ovary," is an intact 10 × 8 × 8 cm thin-walled (0.3 cm) white/tan unilocular cyst with smooth inner and outer surfaces. A 1 × 1 × 0.8 cm area of white fibrotic tissue is present, possibly representing residual ovarian tissue. No corpora albicantia are seen. The cyst is filled with clear non-viscous fluid.

Cassette #1: Transverse sections of cyst wall, 2 frags, RSS.

Cassette #2: Possible residual ovarian tissue, 1 frag, RSS.

Processing the specimen: Ovary with complex cyst

1. Record the overall dimensions of the ovary and describe the outer surface including color (white), surface (smooth or convoluted, adhesions, papillary projections), and simple (thin-walled without a solid component) cysts. Carefully examine the surface for invasion or adhesion to adjacent structures.

    Avoid rubbing or abrading the outer surface in order to preserve the surface epithelial lining.

2. Ink the outer surface in all irregular areas. Open *all* cysts and examine carefully for papillary or solid components. See the section above for precautions on opening cysts with fluid under pressure.

    Try to identify remaining ovarian tissue. It can sometimes be seen as a thickened portion of the wall, readily visible on transillumination. Do not abrade the lining by excessive handling.

    Describe the cystic spaces including number, size, inner surface (smooth or with papillary areas or solid areas, velvety texture as in endometriotic cysts), wall thickness, contents (blood, serous fluid, mucinous fluid, keratinaceous and sebaceous material and hair as in mature teratoma), and solid areas (color, texture, extension to serosal surface). If the fallopian tube is included, describe its relationship to the cyst. Describe the remaining ovary including color, corpus luteum, and corpora albicantia.

3. Fix the specimen in formalin overnight. One cassette per cm of largest cyst diameter should be submitted if there is any suspicion of malignancy. Include solid or papillary areas within the wall and areas of gross invasion. Submit a section of the residual ovary.

    Submit a section with fallopian tube, if present.

Received fresh, labeled with the patient's name and unit number and "left ovary," is an intact 18 × 15 × 10 cm multilocular tan/white cyst. Most of the cyst wall is thin (0.2 cm) but focal areas of thickening are present measuring up to 0.8 cm. The outer surface is smooth. Within the inner surface of the cysts there are multiple minute papillary areas (all less than 0.4 cm in height). A representative frozen section was taken of one of these areas. A 1 × 0.8 cm area of residual ovarian tissue is present with a single corpus albicans. The cysts are filled with thick yellow viscous fluid.

Cassette #1: Frozen-section remnant, papillary area, 1 frag, ESS.

Cassettes #2–19: Representative sections of cyst including papillary areas and areas of thickened wall, 18 frags, RSS.

Cassette #20: Residual ovarian tissue, 1 frag, RSS.

Processing the specimen: Ovary with solid tumor

1. Record the overall dimensions of the ovary and describe the outer surface including:
- Color: usually white
- Surface: smooth or convoluted, adhesions, papillary projections
- Presence of simple cysts: thin-walled cysts without a solid component.

Carefully examine the surface for invasion or adhesion to adjacent structures.

Avoid rubbing or abrading the outer surface in order to preserve the surface epithelial lining.

2. Ink the outer surface. Serially section through the tumor. Describe size, surface, color, relationship to surface and adjacent ovary (i.e., margins), the presence of a cystic component (describe as above), and texture upon cutting.

3. Fix the specimen in formalin overnight. One cassette per cm of largest tumor diameter should be submitted if there is any suspicion of malignancy. Include at least one section to demonstrate the relationship of the tumor to adjacent ovary and peritoneal surface. Include all areas of gross invasion. Submit a section of the residual ovary.

Submit a section with fallopian tube, if present. Sample any structures adherent to the ovary (e.g., fat or muscle).

Sample dictation

Received fresh, labeled with the patient's name and unit number and "left ovary," is a 12 × 10 × 7 cm lobulated mass attached to the fallopian tube (5 cm in length × 0.8 cm in diameter with a fimbriated end). The mass has multiple small cysts of variable size (0.3 to 2 cm) filled with hemorrhagic viscous fluid occupying approximately half the area. The remaining portion of the mass is firm and solid with a mottled appearance ranging from dark red/brown to yellow. The outer surface is irregular with multiple shaggy adhesions. Definite residual ovarian tissue is not identified. The mass does not grossly involve the grossly unremarkable fallopian tube. During an intraoperative consultation a representative frozen section of a solid area was taken.

Cassette #1: Frozen-section remnant, solid area, 1 frag, ESS.
Cassettes #2–7: Representative sections of cystic areas of mass, 6 frags, RSS.
Cassettes #8–10: Representative sections of solid areas of mass, 3 frags, RSS.
Cassette #11 and 12: Mass and relationship to surface, 2 frags, RSS.
Cassette #13: Mass and fallopian tube and additional section of fallopian tube, 2 frags, RSS.
Cassette #14: Possible residual ovarian tissue, 1 frag, RSS.

Processing the specimen: Omental biopsies for staging ovarian malignancies

Carcinomas. If there is a grossly evident metastatic focus, one section is sufficient to document it. If the omentum is grossly negative, take 5 to 10 sections (or the entire specimen if possible) to evaluate for microscopic metastases.

Borderline tumors or immature teratomas. Multiple sections of grossly evident metastases are taken to evaluate invasive versus noninvasive implants (borderline tumors) and maturity of implants (teratomas). If the omentum is grossly negative, take 5 to 10 sections (or the entire specimen if possible) to evaluate for microscopic metastases.

Special studies

Ovarian carcinoma

Special studies—including hormone receptor analysis, DNA analysis, and genetic studies—are under investigation but none is routinely used for clinical decision making.

Steroid-producing tumors

It may be helpful to save frozen tissue of solid yellow tumors for oil red O stains. However, such stains are rarely necessary.

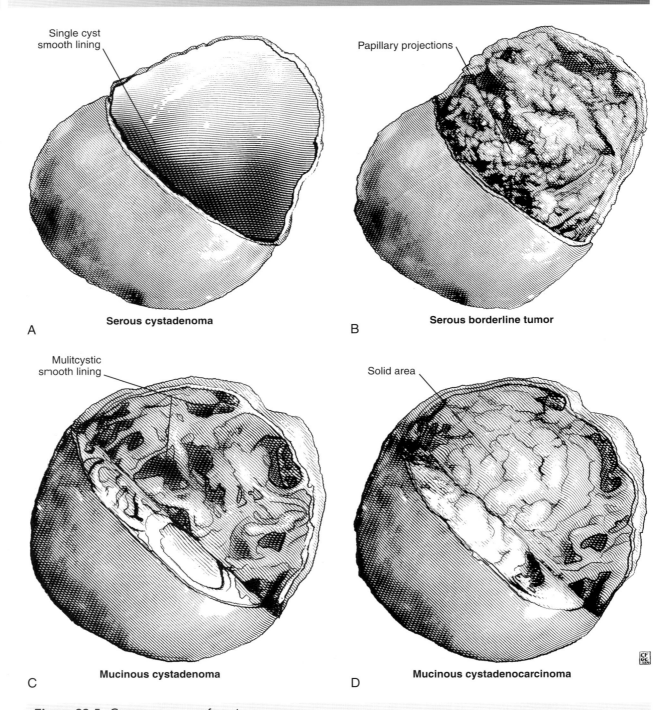

Single cyst
smooth lining

Serous cystadenoma

A

Papillary projections

Serous borderline tumor

B

Mulitcystic
smooth lining

Mucinous cystadenoma

C

Solid area

Mucinous cystadenocarcinoma

D

Figure 22-5 Gross appearance of ovarian tumors.

Gross differential diagnosis of ovarian lesions (Fig. 22-5)

Follicular cysts. Small (<2 cm) unilocular smooth-surfaced cysts filled with clear serous fluid.

Corpus luteum is a yellow/orange 1.5 to 2.0 cm ovoid structure with convoluted borders and a hemorrhagic center. The corpus luteum associated with pregnancy is larger (it may occupy half the area of the ovary), brighter yellow, and has a cystic center.

Corpora albicantia. A corpus luteum regresses to become a corpus albicans. Corpora albicantia are small fibrotic well-circumscribed white structures with convoluted borders that are usually multiple in both ovaries.

Polycystic ovaries (Stein–Leventhal syndrome). Both ovaries are generally enlarged (to 2 to 5 times normal) with a thick superficial cortex and multiple superficial small smooth-walled cysts measuring less than 1 cm in size. Corpora lutea or albicantia are absent.

Brenner tumor. This is usually a small (<2 cm) well-circumscribed white/tan or yellow solid fibrous tumor. Cysts may be present. In 25% of cases, there will be a second tumor (most are mucinous cystadenomas).

Teratomas (dermoid cysts) are unilocular (less commonly multilocular) cysts containing hair and cheesy sebaceous material. Ten to 15% are bilateral. A nodule of tissue projects into the cyst cavity (Rokitansky's protuberance) and often contains bone or teeth. Immature teratomas are more likely to be solid, may resemble brain tissue (gray and fleshy), and may have foci of necrosis. These tumors are more likely to spontaneously rupture. The immature elements may be intermingled with mature areas. Struma ovarii is red/brown and has small colloid-filled cysts (with brown or green/brown fluid) that correspond to thyroid tissue.

Endometriotic (chocolate) cyst ("endometrioma"). The cyst has a dark red or brown ("chocolate") shaggy lining containing coagulated blood. The term "powder burn" is used to describe ecchymotic or brown areas of involvement. The surface is usually covered by dense fibrous adhesions. Solid areas or thickened plaque-like areas may represent malignancy arising within the cyst (most commonly endometrioid carcinoma or clear cell carcinoma).

Mucinous neoplasms. These tumors tend to be large and consist of multiple cysts of varying size and shape. The cysts are filled with viscous gelatinous fluid. Approximately 10% are malignant, and 10% to 15% are borderline. Benign lesions have thin delicate cyst walls and smooth inner linings. Malignant tumors often have solid areas of growth and may have areas of necrosis. Borderline tumors may have subtle areas of papillary projections from the inner cyst wall. Surface involvement is less common than that seen in serous tumors. Mucinous tumors may exhibit histologic variation within the tumor, thus extensive sampling is necessary to exclude malignancy. Approximately 5% of cystadenomas and 20% of carcinomas are bilateral.

Serous neoplasms. One to several cysts filled with watery clear fluid are generally present. Benign lesions have thin walls and smooth cyst linings. Approximately 20% to 25% are malignant and 5% to 10% are borderline. Malignant lesions have areas of solid and/or papillary growth with possible areas of necrosis. Invasion into adjacent structures may be present. Borderline lesions usually have numerous small soft friable papillary projections. Surface involvement may be present. Twenty five to 30% are bilateral and 30% have extraovarian implants.

Endometrioid neoplasms. There is usually a mixture of solid and cystic areas. Most are malignant. The cysts may be filled with bloody or mucinous fluid. Approximately 15% to 20% are associated with endometriosis and 40% are bilateral.

Clear cell carcinomas. These tumors may be solid or have cystic areas. There may be white/tan papillary projections into the lumens. Some arise in endometriotic cysts and may look like fleshy nodules in the wall of the cyst.

Metastatic carcinomas are most commonly from primaries in the breast, stomach, colon, biliary tract, and pancreas. Bilaterality is common, but some primary ovarian neoplasms can also be bilateral. The tumor may have a homogeneous appearance and may look like a fibroma or involve the ovary as multiple nodules. The classic Krukenberg tumor is a signet ring cell carcinoma (usually from stomach but also arising in other sites) metastatic to the ovary.

Fibroma has a circumscribed hard, chalky-white whorled appearance and is usually 5 to 6 cm in size. Calcifications may be present. More than 90% are bilateral. Fibrosarcomas are rare and are usually softer, with areas of hemorrhage and necrosis.

Thecoma is a lobulated solid yellow tumor, often large in size (10 cm). Most are unilateral. Foci of calcification, cysts, hemorrhage, and necrosis may be present. Endometrial hyperplasia may be present due to tumor secretion of estrogen.

Granulosa cell tumor. Most granulosa cell tumors are unilateral and large (12 cm). The tumor is circumscribed, soft, and yellow to gray. Hemorrhagic cysts or necrosis may be present. Endometrial hyperplasia may be present due to tumor secretion of estrogen. Five per cent are bilateral.

Pseudomyxoma peritonei. The tumor may involve one or both ovaries and mimic a primary mucinous ovarian tumor. However, most cases arise from the appendix. The appendix should also be carefully examined during surgery.

Microscopic sections

Ovary
Normal/incidental:
One section.
Prophylactic for family history of ovarian carcinoma:
Submit entire ovary and fallopian tube.
Simple cysts:
One section of wall, one section of residual ovary.
Complex cysts:
One section per cm of greatest dimension including all thickened or papillary areas and relationship to surface, one section of residual ovary.
Solid masses:
One section per cm of greatest dimension including relationship to surface, one section of residual ovary.

Fallopian tube
One section demonstrating relationship to ovary.

Soft tissue
Sections of any abnormal areas of adjacent soft tissue (e.g., suspicion of tumor implant) or any lymph nodes found in soft tissue.

Omentum
Multiple sections (5 to 10) including all gross lesions as well as grossly normal-appearing adipose tissue. Some metastases are not grossly apparent.

Pathologic diagnostic/prognostic features sign-out checklist for ovarian carcinomas

Specimen type*
Oophorectomy (right or left), salpingo-oophorectomy (right or left), subtotal oophorectomy (right or left), removal of tumor in fragments, hysterectomy with salpingo-oophorectomy, omentectomy.

Tumor site*
Ovary (right or left), parenchymal growth, growth on surface, uninvolved.

Specimen integrity*
Intact, ruptured, fragmented. List separately for right and left ovary.

Tumor size*
Greatest dimension (additional dimensions optional).

Histologic type*
Serous carcinoma, mucinous carcinoma, endometrioid carcinoma, clear cell carcinomas, transitional carcinoma, squamous carcinoma, undifferentiated carcinomas, borderline carcinomas, granulosa cell tumor, germ cell tumor. The WHO classification is recommended.

Histologic grade*

Well, moderately, poorly differentiated.

Endometrioid:

Use grading system for endometrial carcinomas (see Box 22-2).

Serous, clear cell, transitional, squamous:

Use nuclear grading system (see Box 22-2).

Immature teratoma:

See Table 22-7.

Involvement of other organs/tissues

One ovary, both ovaries, omentum, uterus, fallopian tube, serosa of uterus, peritoneum, etc.

Extent of invasion*

Tumor limited to ovaries, involvement of capsule, presence or absence on ovarian surface, presence or absence in ascites or peritoneal washings, extension and/or implants on uterus and/or tubes, microscopic or macroscopic peritoneal metastases.

Superficial tumors (<0.5 cm invasion into ovary) may be primary peritoneal carcinomas or metastases. Tumors at the hilum are more commonly metastatic carcinomas.

Ovarian capsule

Intact or ruptured, relationship of rupture to carcinoma (i.e., is the malignancy at the site of the rupture).

Regional lymph nodes*

Absent (N0), present (N1). Number of nodes examined, number with metastases.

Distant metastasis*

Absent (M0), present (M1). Specify site, if known.

Implants (for borderline tumors)*

Non-invasive (epithelial) implants: Not present, present, site.

Non-invasive (desmoplastic) implants: Not present, present, site.

Invasive implants:

Not present, present, site.

Size of peritoneal metastases (<2 cm or >2 cm).

Venous/lymphatic (large/small vessel) invasion

Absent, present, indeterminate. This finding has not been clearly linked to prognosis. It is more commonly seen in tumors metastatic to the ovary.

Cytology

Ascitic fluid or peritoneal washings: Positive or negative for malignant cells

Other findings

Endometriosis (ovarian or extraovarian), endosalpingiosis, ovarian or tubal cysts, etc.

This checklist incorporates information from the ADASP (see www.panix.com/~adasp) and the CAP Cancer Committee protocols for reporting on cancer specimens (see www.cap.org/). The asterisked elements are considered to be scientifically validated or regularly used data elements that must be present in reports of cancer-directed surgical resection specimens from ACS CoC-approved cancer programs. The specific details of reporting the elements may vary among institutions.

The AJCC classification is presented in Table 22-8.

Table 22-7 Immature teratoma: Grade	
Grade I	Rare foci of immature neural tissue occupying <1 low-power field per slide
Grade II	Moderate amounts of immature neural tissue occupying >1 but <4 low-power fields per slide
Grade III	Large quantities of immature neural tissue occupying ≥4 low-power fields per slide

Other germ cell tumors are not routinely graded.

■ FALLOPIAN TUBE

Fallopian tubes are most commonly received as part of a TAH-BSO specimen but may be submitted after tubal ligation (small cross-sections), in cases of ectopic pregnancy, or very rarely for tumors.

Some women present with a sudden discharge of clear fluid from the vagina accompanied by abdominal pain and reduction of an abdominal mass.

Processing the specimen

1. Describe the size (length and diameter), and the presence or absence of a fimbriated end. Check for patency with a probe. A plastic ring may be present if there has been a tubal ligation.
2. Describe the serosal surface (normal is smooth and glistening) including adhesions, paratubal cysts, purulent or fibrinous exudates, and ruptures.
3. Make cross-sections across the tube. Note any luminal contents (purulent exudate, hemorrhage, placental or fetal tissue or membranes, see below).
4. Submit three sections in one cassette including the fimbriated end, midportion, and cornual portion of the tube. Additional cassettes can be used to document any gross lesions.
5. If the procedure was a tubal ligation, instruct the histology laboratory to embed the specimen as cross-sections. A complete cross-section of the tube is necessary to document that a sterilizing procedure was performed.

Special studies

Tubal pregnancies

Tissue may be sent for karyotyping if requested.

Gross differential diagnosis of fallopian tube lesions

Tubal cysts. Commonly seen are benign inclusion cysts. These are 0.1 to 0.2 cm unilocular smooth- surfaced cysts located beneath the serosal surface.

Tubal pregnancies. The tube is dilated and darkened due to blood within the lumen. An embryo or villi may be identifiable within the hemorrhagic area. The outer surface may be ruptured. Peritubal adhesions may be present, indicating prior salpingitis.

Tubal carcinomas. Malignancies are very uncommon. The tube may appear enlarged (resembling a sausage) and filled with a papillary or solid growth. More commonly the tube is secondarily involved by invasion by an ovarian or endometrial carcinoma. Careful gross examination and sectioning may be necessary to distinguish these two processes.

Tubes in women exposed to diethylstilbestrol (DES). Abnormalities, such as hypoplasia, may be present.

Table 22-8 AJCC and FIGO (6th edition) classification of ovarian carcinomas

AJCC (TNM)	FIGO	DEFINITION
Primary tumor		
TX	—	Primary tumor cannot be assessed
T0	—	No evidence of primary tumor
T1	I	Tumor limited to ovaries (one or both)
T1a	IA	Tumor limited to one ovary; capsule intact, no tumor on ovarian surface, no malignant cells in ascites or peritoneal washings
T1b	IB	Tumor limited to both ovaries; capsules intact, no tumor on ovarian surface, no malignant cells in ascites or peritoneal washings
T1c	IC	Tumor limited to one or both ovaries with any of the following: capsule ruptured, tumor on ovarian surface, malignant cells in ascites or peritoneal washings
T2	II	Tumor involves one or both ovaries with pelvic extension
T2a	IIA	Extension and/or implants on the uterus and/or tube(s); no malignant cells in ascites or peritoneal washings
T2b	IIB	Extension to other pelvic tissues; no malignant cells in ascites or peritoneal washings
T2c	IIC	Pelvic extension (2a or 2b) with malignant cells in ascites or peritoneal washings
T3 and/or N1	III	Tumor involves one or both ovaries with microscopically confirmed peritoneal metastasis outside the pelvis and/or regional lymph node metastasis. This would include metastasis to the liver capsule
T3a	IIIA	Microscopic peritoneal metastasis beyond the pelvis
T3b	IIIB	Macroscopic peritoneal metastasis beyond the pelvis 2 cm or less in greatest dimension
T3c and/or N1	IIIC	Peritoneal metastasis beyond the pelvis more than 2 cm in the greatest dimension and/or regional lymph node metastasis
M1	IV	Distant metastasis (excludes peritoneal metastasis). This would include liver parenchymal metastasis or positive pleural fluid cytology
Regional lymph nodes		
NX	—	Regional lymph nodes cannot be assessed
N0	—	No regional lymph node metastasis
N1	—	Regional lymph node metastasis
Distant metastasis		
MX	—	Presence of distant metastasis cannot be assessed
M0	—	No distant metastasis
M1	IV	Distant metastasis (excludes peritoneal metastasis)

Microscopic sections

Incidental tube
One cassette including fimbriated end, midportion, and cornual portion.

Ectopic pregnancy
Representative sections of hemorrhagic areas and grossly evident placental or embryonic tissue.

Carcinomas
One section per cm of tumor including relationship to surface, relationship to ovary, and representative section of uninvolved mucosa.

Table 22-9 AJCC and FIGO (6th edition) classification of fallopian tube tumors

AJCC (TNM)	FIGO		DEFINITION
Primary tumor			
TX	—		Primary tumor cannot be assessed
T0	—		No evidence of primary tumor
Tis	0		Carcinoma in situ (limited to tubal mucosa = epithelium)
TI	I		Tumor limited to the fallopian tube(s)
T1a		IA	Tumor limited to one tube, without penetrating the serosal surface; no ascites
T1b		IB	Tumor limited to both tubes, without penetrating the serosal surface; no ascites
T1c		IC	Tumor limited to one or both tubes with extension onto or through the tubal serosa, or with malignant cells in ascites or peritoneal washings
T2	II		Tumor involves one or both fallopian tubes with pelvic extension
T2a		IIA	Extension and/or metastasis to the uterus and/or ovaries
T2b		IIB	Extension to other pelvic structures
T2c		IIC	Pelvic extension with malignant cells in ascites or peritoneal washings
T3 and/or N1	III		Tumor involves one or both fallopian tubes, with peritoneal implants outside the pelvis and/or positive regional lymph nodes. This would include metastasis to the liver capsule
T3a		IIIA	Microscopic peritoneal metastasis outside the pelvis
T3b		IIIB	Macroscopic peritoneal metastasis beyond the pelvis 2 cm or less in greatest dimension
T3c and/or N1		IIIC	Peritoneal metastasis more than 2 cm in greatest dimension and/or regional lymph node metastasis
M1	IV		Distant metastasis (excludes peritoneal metastasis). This would include liver parenchymal metastasis or positive pleural fluid cytology
Regional lymph nodes			
NX	—		Regional lymph nodes cannot be assessed
N0	—		No regional lymph node metastasis
N1	—		Regional lymph node metastasis
Distant metastasis			
MX	—		Distant metastasis cannot be assessed
M0	—		No distant metastasis
M1	IV		Distant metastasis (excludes peritoneal metastasis)

Pathologic diagnostic/prognostic features sign-out checklist for fallopian tube carcinoma

Specimen type*
Salpingectomy (right or left), salpingo-oophorectomy (right or left), hysterectomy with salpingo-oophorectomy.

Primary tumor site*
Fallopian tube (right or left).
Relationship to ovary: not fused or fused.
Status of fimbriated end: open or closed.
The closure of the fimbriated end may be associated with a more favorable prognosis.

Specimen integrity*
Intact, ruptured, fragmented, other (specify).

Tumor location*
Fimbria(e), ampulla, infundibular portion, isthmus (all that apply).

Tumor size*
Greatest dimension (additional dimensions optional).

Other organs*
None, specify identity of organs.

Histologic type*
Carcinoma in situ, serous carcinoma, mucinous carcinoma, endometrioid carcinoma, clear cell carcinoma, other rare types.

Histologic grade*
Use the grading system for endometrial carcinomas (see Box 22-2).

Extent of invasion*
Carcinoma in situ (limited to fallopian tube/s) (pTis), tumor limited to one tube without penetrating the serosal surface and without ascites (pT1a), tumor limited to both tubes without penetrating the serosal surface and without ascites (pT1b), tumor limited to one or both tubes with extension into or through the tubal serosa or with malignant cells in ascites or peritoneal washings (pT1c), tumor involves one or both tubes with pelvic extension and/or metastasis to the uterus and/or ovaries (pT2a), extension to other pelvic structures (pT2b), pelvic extension with malignant cells in ascites or peritoneal washings (pT2c), tumor involves one or both tubes with microscopic peritoneal metastasis beyond pelvis (pT3a), macroscopic peritoneal metastasis beyond the pelvis ≤2 cm in size (pT3b), peritoneal metastasis beyond the pelvis >2 cm in size and/or regional lymph node metastasis (pT3c).

Summary of organs/tissues involved by tumor
Fallopian tube only, ovary, broad ligament, uterus, pelvic peritoneum, omentum, abdominal peritoneum, bowel serosa.

Venous/lymphatic (large/small vessel) invasion*
Absent, present, indeterminate.

Cytology
Ascites or peritoneal washings: positive or negative for malignancy.

Other tubal findings
Hyperplasia, in situ carcinoma, dysplasia, salpingitis isthmica nodosa, chronic salpingitis, mucosal metaplasia.
Severe salpingitis (e.g., tuberculous salpingitis) can be associated with pseudocarcinomatous changes. Carcinoma is rarely associated with salpingitis.
Endometriosis can be associated with endometrioid carcinoma of the tube.

Other findings
Endometriosis, endosalpingiosis.

Regional lymph nodes*
Absent (N0), present (N1).
Number of nodes examined, number with metastases
Note: Endosalpingiosis or mullerian inclusions are common findings in lymph nodes. These should be reported but distinguished from metastases.

Distant metastasis*
Absent (M0), present (M1).

This checklist incorporates information from the ADASP (see www.panix.com/~adasp/) and the CAP Cancer Committee protocols for reporting on cancer specimens (see www.cap.org/). The asterisked elements are considered to be scientifically validated or regularly used data elements that must be present in reports of cancer-directed surgical resection specimens from ACS CoC-approved cancer programs. The specific details of reporting the elements may vary among institutions.

■ CERVIX

The cervix is one of the tissues most frequently sampled due to the high incidence of dysplasia and carcinoma. Cervical biopsies and cone biopsies are frequent surgical procedures to evaluate or treat cervical lesions.

Relevant clinical history (in addition to age)

See Table 22-10.

Table 22-10 Relevant clinical history	
HISTORY RELEVANT TO ALL SPECIMENS	HISTORY RELEVANT TO CERVICAL SPECIMENS
Organ/tissue resected or biopsied	Results of PAP smears or biopsies
Purpose of the procedure	HPV test results
Gross appearance of the organ/tissue/lesion sampled	Hormone use
	Pregnancy
Any unusual features of the clinical presentation	Use of intrauterine device (IUD)
Any unusual features of the gross appearance	DES exposure in utero[a]
Prior surgery/biopsies—results	
Prior malignancy	
Prior treatment (radiation therapy, chemotherapy, drug use that can change the histologic appearance of tissues)	
Compromised immune system	

[a] DES was used until 1971, when it was banned by the FDA because of its association with clear cell carcinomas of the cervix and vagina. Although currently most women with clear cell carcinoma do not have a history of exposure, some exposed women may develop such carcinomas at an older age.

Cervical biopsies

Describe color, number of fragments, and size, and submit the entire specimen.

Cone biopsies

Cone biopsies are resections of the entire transition zone and the endocervical canal (Fig. 22-6). They are performed when dysplasia is present within the endocervical canal (i.e., the lesion cannot be treated adequately externally). Loop electrocautery excision procedure (LEEP) specimens are discussed below.

Processing the specimen

1. The "deep" (endocervical) and "serosal" (lateral) margins are marked with India ink.
2. Open along the cervical canal using scissors. If a suture marks the 12 o'clock position, open at this point. If not, make the cut at any site.
3. Pin the opened specimen on a corkboard, with the mucosal side up, and fix overnight. Fix the cone biopsy as soon as possible.

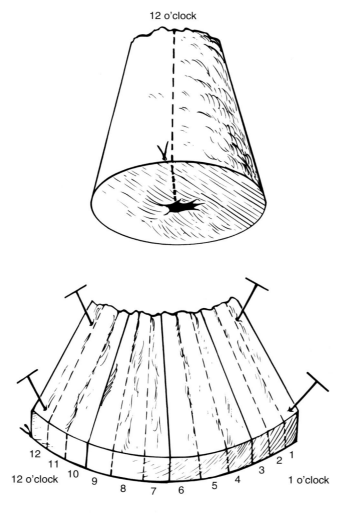

12 o'clock

12 o'clock

1 o'clock

Figure 22-6 Cervical cone biopsy.

4. Describe the length of the endocervical canal, the circumference at the external os, and the circumference at the portio. Describe any visible lesions including size, color, location, relationship to margins, and invasion. Frequently the lesions present are not evident grossly.

5. Take sections along the axis of the cervical canal in order that each section contains external os, endocervical canal, and portio. All the tissue in at least 12 sections is taken (corresponding to clock positions). If the specimen is unoriented, submit it in the same manner, starting at a random point, and state that the specimen was not oriented.

Loop electrocautery excision procedure

Most cases that would previously have been managed by cone biopsy are now dealt with by electrocautery using a thin wire loop. LEEP specimens can be distinguished grossly from cold knife cone biopsies by the presence of cauterization at the deep margin. The specimen may be submitted as a single fragment similar in appearance to a cone biopsy. More commonly, the procedure produces two or more specimens, including anterior and posterior cervix, and a deep endocervical specimen. Because of the fragmented nature of some of these specimens, it is critical that the specimen be evaluated and oriented grossly before taking sections.

Processing the specimen

1. The specimen is oriented with the mucosal side up and sectioned on the axis of the cervical canal, with portio and endocervix represented in each section, identical to the orientation of a cone biopsy.

   The mucosal side will appear either shiny and white (portio) or pink and finely granular (endocervix). The deep side will be irregular and cauterized.

2. Sections are obtained at 1 to 2 mm intervals. Inking of the specimen is not necessary, inasmuch as the cauterized margins are easily identified on histologic examination.

Special studies

There are no special studies indicated for routine examinations.

HPV testing

According to the American Society for Colposcopy and Cervical Pathology (ASCCP) guidelines, so-called "reflex" HPV DNA testing is the preferred approach for managing women with *atypical squamous cells*, qualified as "of undetermined significance" (ASC-US) if the sample was obtained using liquid-based cytology. Alternative approaches are to repeat the Papanicolaou (PAP) test or refer the patient immediately to colposcopy. The suggested indications for HPV testing may be modified in the future, but are not routinely performed on surgical specimens.

Gross differential diagnosis of cervical lesions

Squamous intraepithelial lesions (LSIL and HSIL). These appear as raised irregular plaques or papules that may be white or red. These lesions are usually removed as small biopsies and are not well appreciated grossly.

Squamous cell carcinomas appear as red papules, white plaques, or irregular ulcerated hard masses. Small carcinomas may be removed as cone biopsies.

Adenocarcinomas occur deeper in the endocervix and are usually exophytic. These carcinomas are also associated with HPV infections and can also be associated with squamous cell carcinomas.

Microscopic sections

Cervix
Entirely sectioned, with orientation from portio to endocervix.

Sample dictation

Received fresh, labeled with the patient's name and unit number and "cone," is a 1.5 cm in length by 2.3 cm in circumference intact cone biopsy with a suture marking the 12 o'clock axis. The distal 1 cm of the mucosal surface is covered by shiny white mucosa without visible lesions. The proximal 0.5 cm of the mucosal surface is finely granular and pink, consistent with endocervix. The deep, proximal, and distal margins are inked.
Cassettes #1–12: Longitudinal sections from 1 o'clock to 12 o'clock, 12 frags, ESS.

Pathologic diagnostic/prognostic features sign-out checklist for cervical carcinomas

Specimen type*
Colpectomy, hysterectomy, radical hysterectomy, pelvic exenteration.

Tumor site*
Right superior quadrant (12 to 3 o'clock), right inferior quadrant (3 to 6 o'clock), left inferior quadrant (6 to 9 o'clock), left superior quadrant (9 to 12 o'clock).

If no tumor is found (e.g., after a positive PAP smear), the adequacy of the specimen (including glandular and squamous epithelium) should be documented.

Tumor size*
Size in three dimensions.

Other organs present*
Ovary (right or left), fallopian tube (right or left), uterine corpus, vagina, urinary bladder, rectum, other.

Histologic type*
Squamous cell carcinoma (keratinizing or nonkeratinizing), adenocarcinoma (mucinous, endometrioid, clear cell), other rare types. The WHO classification is recommended.

Histologic grade*
Squamous cell carcinoma: Nonkeratinizing or keratinizing.

It is not clear that grading of squamous carcinomas provides prognostic information, and grading (well, moderately, and poorly differentiated) is optional.

Adenocarcinoma: The grade has prognostic value (Table 22-11).

Stromal invasion*
Depth: Millimeters of invasion as measured from the base of the epithelium (either surface or glandular) from which it originates. It is the distance from the epithelial–stromal junction of the adjacent most superficial epithelial papilla to the deepest point of invasion. Vascular space involvement is not included in the measurement.

Horizontal extent: Millimeters on mucosal surface or by using clock face labels (e.g., from 1 o'clock to 6 o'clock).

Extent of invasion*
No invasion = carcinoma in situ.

Depth of invasion.

Tissues invaded: cervical stroma, uterus, vagina (upper two thirds or lower third), pelvic wall, parametrium, obstruction of ureter, bladder mucosa, mucosa of rectum, beyond true pelvis.

If the carcinoma involves the uterine corpus, a determination of the most likely primary site (cervix or uterus) should be made.

Regional lymph nodes*
Absent (N0), present (N1).

Number of nodes examined, number of nodes with metastases.

Distant metastases*
Absent (M0), present (M1). Specify sites, if known.

Margins*
Endocervical, exocervical, and deep margin.

Uninvolved: Give distance of carcinoma from the margin.

Involved: Type of involvement:

invasive

intraepithelial neoplasia—give grade

focal or diffuse.

Give location if possible.

Indeterminate: For example, cautery artifact precludes diagnosis.

Venous/lymphatic (large/small vessel) invasion
Absent, present, indeterminate.

Other findings
Carcinoma in situ of cervix, glandular dysplasia or carcinoma in situ of endocervix, inflammation.

This checklist incorporates information from the ADASP (see www.panix.com/~adasp/) and the CAP Cancer Committee protocols for reporting on cancer specimens (see www.cap.org/). The asterisked elements are considered to be scientifically validated or regularly used data elements that must be present in reports of cancer-directed surgical resection specimens from ACS CoC-approved cancer programs. The specific details of reporting the elements may vary among institutions.

The AJCC/FIGO classification is given in Table 22-12.

Table 22-11 Grading of cervical adenocarcinoma

GRADE	DIFFERENTIATION	FEATURES
1	Well differentiated	Small component of solid growth and mild to moderate nuclear atypia
2	Moderately differentiated	Intermediate between 1 and 3
3	Poorly differentiated	Solid pattern with severe nuclear atypia

Undifferentiated carcinomas (those with no or minimal differentiation in only rare small foci), are classified as grade 4

Table 22-12 AJCC and FIGO (6th edition) classification of cervical carcinomas

AJCC (TNM)	FIGO	DEFINITION
Primary tumor		
TX	—	Primary tumor cannot be assessed
T0	—	No evidence of primary tumor
Tis	—	Carcinoma in situ
T1	I	Cervical carcinoma confined to uterus (extension to corpus should be disregarded)
T1a	IA	Invasive carcinoma diagnosed only by microscopy. All macroscopically visible lesions—even with superficial invasion—are T1b/IB. Stromal invasion with a maximal depth of 5.0 mm measured from the base of the epithelium and a horizontal spread of 7.0 mm or less. Vascular space involvement, venous or lymphatic, does not affect classification
T1a1	IA1	Measured stromal invasion 3.0 mm or less in depth and 7.0 mm or less in horizontal spread
T1a2	IA2	Measured stromal invasion more than 3.0 mm and not more than 5.0 mm with a horizontal spread 7.0 mm or less
T1b	IB	Clinically visible lesion confined to the cervix or microscopic lesion greater than T1a2/IA2
T1b1	IB1	Clinically visible lesion 4.0 cm or less in greatest dimension
T1b2	IB2	Clinically visible lesion more than 4.0 cm in greatest dimension
T2	II	Cervical carcinoma invades beyond uterus but not to pelvic wall or to the lower third of vagina
T2a	IIA	Tumor without parametrial invasion
T2b	IIB	Tumor with parametrial invasion
T3	III	Tumor extends to the pelvic wall and/or involves the lower third of the vagina and/or causes hydronephrosis or nonfunctioning kidney
T3a	IIIA	Tumor involves lower third of the vagina, no extension to the pelvic wall
T3b	IIIB	Tumor extends to pelvic wall and/or causes hydronephrosis or nonfunctioning kidney

Table 22-12 AJCC and FIGO (6th edition) classification of cervical carcinomas—*cont'd*

AJCC (TNM)	FIGO	DEFINITION
Primary tumor		
T4	IVA	Tumor invades mucosa of the bladder or rectum and/or extends beyond the true pelvis (bullous edema is not sufficient to classify a tumor as T4)
M1	IVB	Distant metastasis (excludes peritoneal metastasis)
Regional lymph nodes		
NX		Regional lymph nodes cannot be assessed
N0		No regional lymph node metastasis
N1		Regional lymph node metastasis
		Regional lymph nodes include paracervical, parametrial, hypogastric (obturator), common, internal, and external iliac, presacral and sacral nodes
Distant metastasis		
MX	—	Presence of distant metastasis cannot be assessed
M0	—	No distant metastasis
M1	IVB	Distant metastasis

■ VAGINA

Primary neoplasms of the vagina are very rare. Specimens from the vagina are usually biopsies or form part of a larger resection (e.g., radical hysterectomies or bladder resections).

Relevant clinical history (in addition to age)

See Table 22-13.

Vaginal biopsies

Describe the color, number of fragments, and size, and submit the entire specimen.

Vaginal resections

Vaginal resections are rare specimens. Resection is usually performed in cases of squamous cell carcinoma.

If the uterus is also removed, the specimen can be processed as a radical hysterectomy with sampling of the primary tumor and deep soft tissue paravaginal margin.

If the uterus has been removed previously, the vagina ends in a blind pouch and this portion of the specimen will not be a margin. The vagina can be opened and processed similar to a large skin excision. The distal margin and deep soft tissue margins are sampled.

Schiller's or Lugol's solution stains glycogenated epithelium brown (either normal or glycogenated tumors). These solutions do not stain areas of vaginal adenosis or immature squamous metaplasia and can be useful to identify such areas. Microscopically, dark brown-black deposits are seen on the surface of epithelium. If the solution is too concentrated, the cells can become shrunken with nuclear pyknosis and can mimic squamous dysplasia.

Table 22-13 Relevant clinical history

HISTORY RELEVANT TO ALL SPECIMENS	HISTORY RELEVANT TO VAGINAL SPECIMENS
Organ/tissue resected or biopsied	Dysplasia or cervical carcinoma
Purpose of the procedure	DES exposure in utero[a]
Gross appearance of the organ/tissue/lesion sampled	Gross features of vagina (cervical hypoplasia, pseudopolyps, coxcomb deformity, vaginal adenosis, or vaginal ridge) that are suggestive of DES exposure (present in about one third of exposed patients).
Any unusual features of the clinical presentation	
Any unusual features of the gross appearance	
Prior surgery/biopsies—results	
Prior malignancy	
Prior treatment (radiation therapy, chemotherapy, drug use that can change the histologic appearance of tissues)	
Compromised immune system	

[a] DES exposure: Clear cell adenocarcinoma of the upper vagina and cervix is related to DES exposure in utero although rare cases occur in women without such exposure. The actual risk of developing this type of carcinoma after DES exposure is estimated to be approximately 1 in 10,000. DES is no longer used in pregnant women and this type of tumor is vanishingly rare. However, some women may develop this carcinoma at a later age.

Pathologic diagnostic/prognostic features sign-out checklist for vaginal carcinomas

Specimen type*
Excisional biopsy, partial vaginectomy, radical vaginectomy.

Tumor site*
Upper third, middle third, lower third.
Circumferential, anterior, posterior, left lateral, right lateral.

Tumor size*
Greatest dimension (additional dimensions optional).

Histologic type*
Squamous cell carcinoma, adenocarcinoma, clear cell carcinoma, other rare carcinomas. The WHO classification is recommended.

Histologic grade*
Well, moderately, poorly differentiated, undifferentiated.

Extent of invasion*
Carcinoma in situ (pTis), tumor confined to vagina (pT1), tumor invades paravaginal tissues but not to pelvic wall (pT2), tumor extends to pelvic wall (pT3), tumor invades mucosa of bladder or rectum and/or extends beyond the true pelvis (pT4).
Report depth in mm. Microinvasive carcinoma is not a recognized entity in the vagina. Carcinomas that invade ≤0.3 cm and lack lymphovascular invasion are very unlikely to have lymph node metastases.

Regional lymph nodes*
Absent (N0), present (N1).
Number of nodes examined, number of nodes with metastases.

Distant metastases*

Absent (M0), present (M1), specify site if known.

Margins*

Uninvolved, involved, distance of carcinoma to closest margin.

Invasive or carcinoma in situ.

Distal vagina, paravaginal soft tissue.

Venous/lymphatic (large/small vessel) invasion

Absent, present.

Other findings

Condyloma acuminatum, endometriosis, adenosis, atypical adenosis, dysplasia.

Table 22-14 AJCC and FIGO (6th edition) classification of vaginal carcinomas		
AJCC (TNM)	FIGO	DEFINITION
Primary tumor		
TX	—	Primary tumor cannot be assessed
T0	—	No evidence of primary tumor
Tis	0	Carcinoma in situ
T1	I	Tumor confined to the vagina
T2	II	Tumor invades paravaginal tissues but not to the pelvic wall
T3	III	Tumor extends to the pelvic wall
T4	IV	Tumor invades the mucosa of the bladder or rectum and/or extends beyond the true pelvis (bullous edema is not sufficient to classify a tumor as T4). If the bladder mucosa is not involved, the tumor is classified as T3
Regional lymph nodes		
NX	—	Regional lymph nodes cannot be assessed
N0	—	No regional lymph node metastasis
N1	—	Pelvic or inguinal lymph node metastasis
Distant metastasis		
MX	—	Distant metastasis cannot be assessed
M0	—	No distant metastasis
M1	IVB	Distant metastasis

This checklist incorporates information from the ADASP (see www.panix.com/~adasp/) and the CAP Cancer Committee protocols for reporting on cancer specimens (see www.cap.org/). The asterisked elements are considered to be scientifically validated or regularly used data elements that must be present in reports of cancer-directed surgical resection specimens from ACS CoC-approved cancer programs. The specific details of reporting the elements may vary among institutions.

The AJCC classification is given in Table 22-14.

Grading of vaginal carcinomas

There is no established grading system for vaginal carcinomas. The following system is suggested. Grades 1 to 3 are used for carcinomas showing glandular or squamous differentiation. Grade 4 is used for carcinomas without such differentiation.

Grade 1 Well differentiated

Grade 2 Moderately differentiated

Grade 3 Poorly differentiated

Grade 4 Undifferentiated

■ VULVA

The vulva is subject to site-specific diseases (e.g., lichen sclerosus), infectious disease (e.g., HPV infection, syphilis), and, most commonly, squamous dysplasia and neoplasia.

Vulvar biopsies

Small biopsies or excisional biopsies are processed in the same way as skin biopsies.

Vulvectomies

Most vulvectomies are performed for the treatment of invasive squamous cell carcinoma or carcinoma in situ. Most carcinomas arise on the labia (majora more frequently than minora) or less commonly on the clitoris or posterior fourchette. A total vulvectomy includes all the perineum surrounding the vagina (Fig. 22-7). More commonly, partial vulvectomies are performed; these specimens look grossly like large skin ellipses and can be processed in a similar fashion.

Linguistic note:

Singular	**Pleural**
Labium	*Labia*
Majus	*Majora*
Minus	*Minora*

Processing the specimen

1. A total vulvectomy looks like an ellipse of skin with a central defect (corresponding to the vaginal vault). Orient the specimen using the following landmarks. If inguinal fat is present, it will be in the superior portion of the specimen and to either side. The clitoris is present superiorly and midline. The hair-bearing labia majora are present laterally. Partial vulvectomies require orientation by the surgeon.

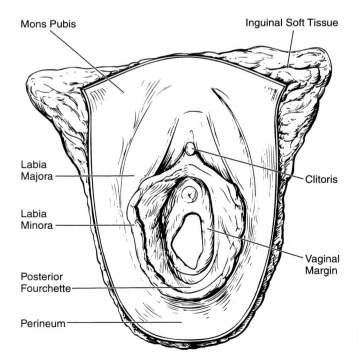

Mons Pubis

Inguinal Soft Tissue

Labia Majora

Labia Minora

Clitoris

Vaginal Margin

Posterior Fourchette

Perineum

Figure 22-7 Total vulvectomy.

Radical vulvectomies are complicated specimens with numerous resection margins including deep (soft tissue), exterior (lower abdomen, leg, groin, perineal, perianal) and central (vaginal and possibly urethral). It is prudent to study the specimen carefully to orient the probable tumor to these various resection margins. If there is any doubt as to orientation, contact the surgeon before sectioning. Before dissecting, it is usually helpful to sketch the specimen, noting any lesions and the relationship to margins.

Measure length, width, and depth. Diagrams are mandatory for complicated specimens.

Lesions may be obvious ulcerating or fungating carcinomas or may be quite subtle if the procedure was performed for vulvar intraepithelial neoplasia (VIN). VIN usually appears as a maculopapular lesion with color changes ranging from white to red to dark shades of brown. Sometimes, however, no gross lesion will be detectable. The location of prior diagnostic biopsies may be helpful to guide sectioning.

Describe each gross lesion including the distance to the nearest skin and vaginal margin.

2. Ink the exposed epithelial and soft tissue margins. It may be helpful to ink the vaginal margin with a different color.

Pin the specimen flat and fix overnight.

3. Sample all gross lesions. For invasive carcinomas, find the area of deepest invasion and sample with deep margin. Sample all close margins with perpendicular (not en face) margins.

4. If there is attached inguinal fat, search diligently for lymph nodes. Submit each node in entirety and separate right from left inguinal nodes.

Special studies

No special study is indicated for the routine evaluation of vulvar specimens.

Gross differential diagnosis of vulvar lesions

Squamous cell carcinoma

Squamous cell carcinomas are exophytic irregular masses, often with invasion into the subcutaneous tissue. Central ulceration is common.

Vulvar intraepithelial neoplasia

VIN consists of flat or papular lesions that may be white, red, gray, brown, or black. In some cases, a gross lesion may not be apparent.

Lichen sclerosus

Lichen sclerosus consists of flat white thinned plaque-like epidermis. This lesion is not usually resected but may be an incidental finding in vulvar excisions.

Microscopic sections

Tumor
Submit sections of tumor to demonstrate the deepest invasion of tumor.

Margins
Submit perpendicular sections of the margins in relationship to the tumor including the nearest skin and vaginal margins.

Other lesions
Submit sections of all other lesions (e.g., areas suspicious for VIN associated with an invasive tumor with the nearest margin).

Lymph nodes
Serially section and completely submit all lymph nodes. Separate right side and left side.

Normal
Submit sections of clitoris, fourchette, perineum, and contralateral labia majora and minora.

Sample dictation

Received fresh, labeled with the patient's name and unit number and "vulva," is an ovoid excision of white/tan skin (11 × 10 × 0.5 cm [depth]) with a centrally located circular defect (2 × 1.8 cm). The labia majora and clitoral hood are identified. There is a 1.2 × 0.9 cm white exophytic lesion located on the right labium majus which is 2.5 cm from the lateral margin and 2.1 cm from the vaginal margin. The lesion invades into the superficial soft tissue but is grossly 0.3 cm from the deep soft tissue margin. There is a depressed white fibrotic area (0.5 × 0.4 cm) located on the posterior fourchette which is 1 cm from the closest (posterior) margin. No gross invasion is seen. The remainder of the epidermal surface is unremarkable. Two lymph nodes are located in the right inguinal soft tissue, the largest measuring 0.5 cm. One lymph node is located in the left inguinal soft tissue measuring 0.6 cm. The deep and exterior epidermal margins are inked black. The vaginal epidermal margin is inked blue.

Cassettes #1–3: Exophytic lesion including deep margin, 3 frags, ESS.
Cassette #4: Closest right lateral margin, perpendicular, 1 frag, RSS.
Cassette #5: Closest vaginal margin, perpendicular, 1 frag, RSS.
Cassette #6: Flat lesion of posterior fourchette, including deep margin, 2 frags, ESS.
Cassette #7: Closest posterior margin to flat lesion, perpendicular, 1 frag, RSS.
Cassette #8: Clitoris, 1 frag, RSS.
Cassette #9: Left labium majus and minus, 2 frags, RSS.
Cassette #10: Right inguinal lymph nodes, inked green and red, 4 frags, ESS.
Cassette #11: Left inguinal lymph node, 2 frags, ESS.

Pathologic diagnostic/prognostic features sign-out checklist for vulvar carcinomas

Specimen type*
Local excision, wide excision, partial vulvectomy, total vulvectomy, radical vulvectomy.

Lymphadenectomy*
Not performed, sentinel lymph node biopsy, inguinal-femoral nodes, pelvic nodes.

Tumor site*
Right vulva (labium majus or minus), left vulva (labium majus or minus), clitoris, other.

Tumor size*
Greatest dimension (additional dimensions optional).

Histologic type*
Squamous cell carcinoma, verrucous carcinoma, Paget's disease of the vulva, adenocarcinoma, basal cell carcinoma, Bartholin's gland carcinoma, other rare malignancies. Melanomas should be reported as for skin melanomas. The WHO classification is recommended.

Histologic grade*
Well, moderately, poorly differentiated, undifferentiated.

Thickness of tumor
Squamous cell carcinoma: Report in mm, measured from the deep border of the granular cell layer or, if absent, from the surface to deepest point of invasion.

Extent of invasion*

Report in mm of invasion from the epithelial–stromal junction of the adjacent most superficial dermal papillae to the deepest extent of invasion. Squamous cell carcinomas that invade deeper than 0.1 cm may be more likely to be associated with lymph node metastasis.

Carcinoma in situ, invasion of vulva, perineum, lower urethra, vagina, anus, bladder mucosa, rectal mucosa, upper urethral mucosa, pubic bone.

Regional lymph nodes*

Absent (N0), present—unilateral (N1), present—bilateral (N2).

Number of nodes examined, number of nodes with metastases.

Absence or presence of extranodal invasion (may correlate with an increased risk of recurrence).

Distant metastasis*

Absent (M0), present (M1), specify site if known.

Tumor border

Squamous cell carcinoma: Broad pushing front (verrucous carcinoma) or infiltrating (fingerlike). The latter pattern is more likely to be associated with lymph node metastases.

Venous/lymphatic (large/small vessel) invasion

Absent, present, indeterminate.

Involvement of other structures

Tumor extending to vagina, perineum, anus.

Margins*

Uninvolved, involved, distance of carcinoma to closest margin.

Invasive or in situ carcinoma.

Cutaneous (give location as right or left, superior or inferior), perineal, vaginal, deep soft tissue.

Other vulvar findings

Lichen sclerosus, VIN3 (severe dysplasia/carcinoma in situ), condyloma acuminatum.

This checklist incorporates information from the ADASP (see www.panix.com/~adasp/) and the CAP Cancer Committee protocols for reporting on cancer specimens (see www.cap.org/). The asterisked elements are considered to be scientifically validated or regularly used data elements that must be present in reports of cancer-directed surgical resection specimens from ACS CoC-approved cancer programs. The specific details of reporting the elements may vary among institutions.

The AJCC classification is given in Table 22-15.

Report format

Reports should always be in a standardized format:

Specimen labeled "Vulvectomy"

SQUAMOUS CELL CARCINOMA, well-differentiated (keratinizing) type.

The tumor measures 5 cm in length by 4.5 cm in greatest thickness.

Capillary lymphatic space invasion is not seen.

Vulvar intraepithelial neoplasia, differentiated (simplex) type.

Lichen sclerosus.

Margins are free of intraepithelial and invasive neoplasia.

Specimen labeled "Inguinal lymph node"

Three (3) lymph nodes with no tumor identified.

Table 22-15 AJCC (6th edition) classification of vulvar carcinomas

Tumor	TX	Primary tumor cannot be assessed
	T0	No evidence of primary tumor
	Tis	Carcinoma in situ (preinvasive carcinoma)
	T1	Tumor confined to the vulva or to the vulva and perineum, 2 cm or less in greatest dimension
	T1a	Tumor confined to the vulva or vulva and perineum, 2 cm or less in greatest dimension, and with stromal invasion no greater than 1 mm
	T1b	Tumor confined to the vulva or vulva and perineum, 2 cm or less in greatest dimension, and with stromal invasion greater than 1 mm
	T2	Tumor confined to the vulva or to the vulva and perineum, more than 2 cm in greatest dimension
	T3	Tumor of any size with adjacent spread to the lower urethra and/or vagina, or anus
	T4	Tumor invades any of the following: upper urethral mucosa, bladder mucosa, rectal mucosa, or is fixed to the pubic bone
Regional lymph nodes	NX	Regional lymph nodes cannot be assessed
	N0	No regional lymph node metastasis
	N1	Unilateral regional lymph node metastasis
	N2	Bilateral regional lymph node metastasis
		Note: Regional lymph nodes are femoral and inguinal nodes.
Distant metastasis	MX	Distant metastasis cannot be assessed
	M0	No distant metastasis
	M1	Distant metastasis (pelvic lymph node metastasis is M1)

Note: This classification system is not used for malignant melanoma.

■ PLACENTA

Placentas are examined for many reasons: multiple gestation, abnormal labor, neonatal indications, unusual features of the placenta, or if there is a significant maternal medical history. Examination can often reveal significant findings relating to the health of the placenta and fetus prior to birth. The College of American Pathologists has issued a comprehensive guideline for the examination of the placenta.[2]

Relevant clinical history for placental examination

Number of gestations
History of selective termination
Any known abnormality of the gestation including:

- Low birth weight
- Low Apgar score
- Fetal demise
- Twin–twin transfusion syndrome
- Congenital malformations
- Trophoblastic disease

Unusual features of the placenta noted at delivery (e.g., small size, green discoloration, knots in the umbilical cord)
Any abnormality of labor and delivery
History of infection
Maternal history of hypertension, malignancy, or compromised immune system.

Processing the specimen

There are three major placental tissues to be examined: the umbilical cord, the membranes, and the placental parenchyma itself. Additional procedures are indicated for multiple gestation placentas (see below). The routine for processing a single gestation placenta is as follows:

1. Obtain standard measurements:

- Dimensions of disc
- Length of umbilical cord.

2. Examine the membranes and cord:

Membranes:

Color and transparency.

- Normal: shiny, translucent and thin.
- Opaque or dull: suggests chorioamnionitis.
- Green: suggests meconium staining and/or chorioamnionitis.
- Yellow or white nodules on membrane: amnion nodosum.
- Single yellow patch on membrane (possibly calcified): yolk sac.
- Fetus papyraceus: a flattened fetus may be present within the membranes in a case of selective reduction.

Point of rupture: Record distance from the point of rupture to the edge of the placenta.

Umbilical cord:

Normal: Two arteries and a vein. Examine at least 5 cm above the chorionic plate as the arteries may normally fuse near the insertion. A single umbilical cord artery is associated with fetal cardiac and renal anomalies.

Twist: Helical twisting is normal. A left-handed twist (as observed looking down the cord toward the disc) is most common.

Location of insertion of umbilical cord (central, eccentric, marginal, membranous).

In a partially membranous (velamentous) cord the cord vessels separate and run within the membrane for a distance. Measure the length of the velamentous vessels.

Furcate insertion: The cord vessels spread out over the placental disc within membranes.

True knots in umbilical cord: Note presence and tightness and differences in cord color and diameter on either side of knot. False knots appear as bulbous expansions of the cord and are formed by ectatic vessels with reduction in Wharton's jelly.

Thrombosis, congestion, thinning, or necrosis.

3. Examine the insertion of the membranes into the placental disc and estimate the percentage of each type of insertion (Fig. 22-8):

- Inserts at edge (normal situation) = *marginal*
- Inserts inside edge = *circummarginate*
- Inserts inside edge with a prominent ridge as membrane is folded back upon itself = *circumvallate*.

4. Selected sections are taken for fixation and histologic sections. The remainder of the placenta may be stored refrigerated until after final sign-out.

  Prepare one membrane roll. Cut a long strip of membrane approximately 3 cm wide from the point of rupture of the membrane inward toward the placental disc. Leave a small piece of disc at the end of the strip. Grasp the disc in a pair of flat-tipped forceps and roll the membrane tightly around it. Slip the roll off gently and drop into a formalin container.

5. Cut two sections of umbilical cord (proximal and distal) and add to the formalin container.

6. Cut off the entire umbilical cord and membranes and weigh the placenta.

  For multiple gestation placentas, record a combined weight after trimming the cords and membranes. Do not attempt to physically separate the two discs.

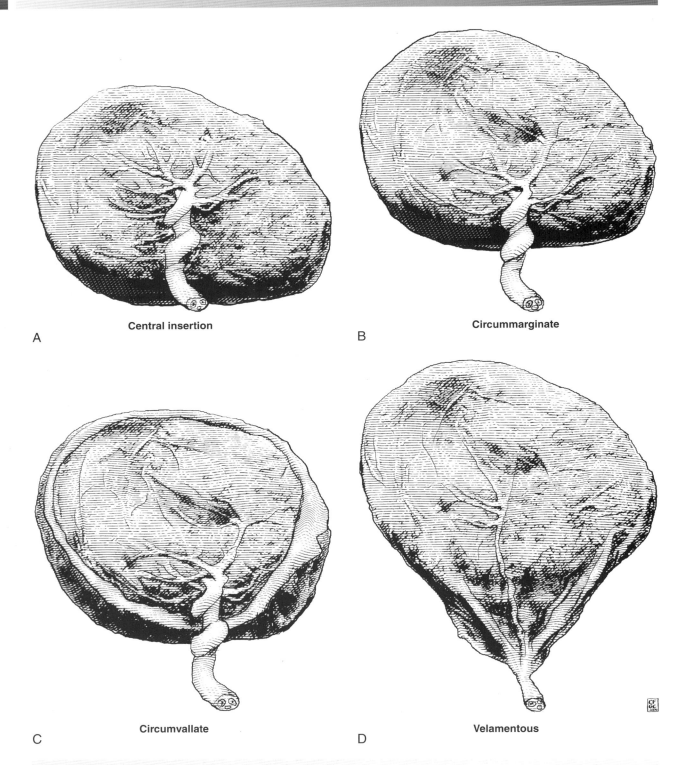

A   **Central insertion**

B   **Circummarginate**

C   **Circumvallate**

D   **Velamentous**

Figure 22-8 Insertion of membranes into the placental disc.

7. With a large sharp knife, serially section the placenta in 0.5 cm sections. Examine the parenchyma carefully for infarcts (firm white/yellow areas), intervillous thrombi, large, significant areas of hemorrhage, and any other unusual findings. Place two or three representative strips of placental parenchyma into the formalin container.

    The remainder of the placenta in routine cases is stored in the freezer until after sign-out.

8. The following day the fixed placental tissue can be sectioned. Submit two cross-sections of the umbilical cord and two cross-sections of the membrane roll. Submit sections of placental parenchyma showing both pathology (if present) and adjacent normal tissue for comparison. If the patient has a history of hypertension, diabetes, lupus erythematosus, or eclampsia, submit an additional membrane roll.

Multiple gestation placentas

At delivery, the placentas may be identified by clamping only one umbilical cord or using different numbers of clamps on the two cords. Identify the placentas using the number of clamps when present. If clamps are not present, designate the placentas arbitrarily as "A" and "B." The placentas should be identifiable after dissection. For example, the cord stump on placenta "A" may be left longer than the cord stump on placenta "B." The discs should be left attached and not physically separated.

There are four types of multiple gestation placentas (Fig. 22-9):

1. **Diamniotic/dichorionic separated twin placentas** (zygosity of the twins cannot be assessed).

    The discs are completely separate but the membranes may be adherent. The membranes are separated by pulling on them *gently*. Each placenta is described separately.

2. **Diamniotic/dichorionic fused twin placentas** (zygosity of the twins cannot be assessed). See below.

3. **Diamniotic/monochorionic fused twin placentas** (implies monozygosity); may be associated with twin–twin transfusion.

    Cases 2 and 3 consist of a single placental disc with two umbilical cords, a common outer membrane, and a twin dividing membrane separating the cords. The outer membrane may be ruptured in two separate places, or, more typically, have a single large rupture.

    In case 2, the dividing membrane consists of two complete amnions and two complete fused chorions. The dividing membrane is thick and opaque. Peel off the amnionic membranes from both sides of the membrane, leaving a part of the fused thick chorionic membrane in the middle. Grossly it appears *trilaminar* (two amnions with attached chorion and fused center of chorion).

    In case 3, the dividing membrane consists of two amnions on either side of a single chorion. The membrane is thin and almost transparent. Separate the amnions, producing two membrane leaflets. Grossly it appears *dilaminar* (two amnions with attached chorion, no thickened central chorion).

    Submit the dividing membrane for microscopic examination in addition to routine sections of each placenta.

4. **Monoamniotic/monochorionic fused twin placentas** (monozygous); associated with a high rate of complications, such as fetal death from cord entanglement.

    There are two umbilical cords, but no dividing membrane.

    Routine sections are taken from each cord, disc, and membranes.

Triplet placentas are processed similarly to twin placentas, except that there are three umbilical cords and three dividing membranes to examine.

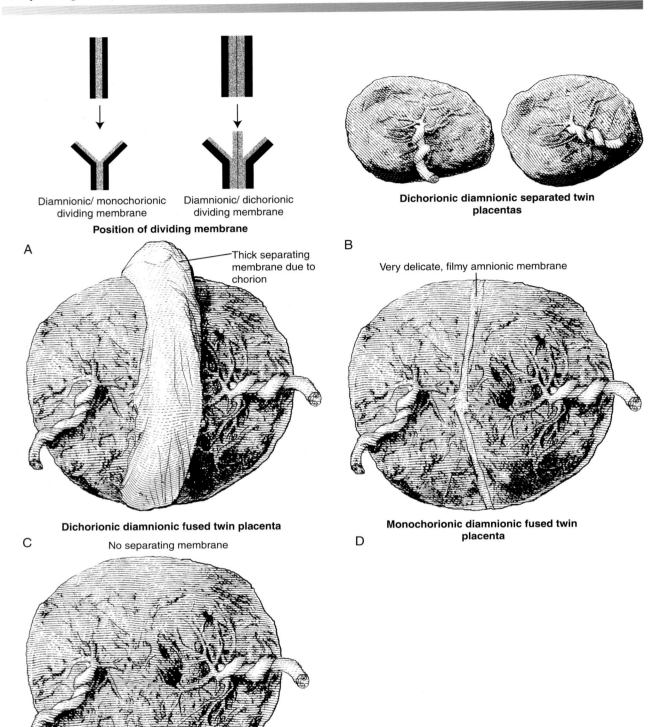

Diamnionic/ monochorionic
dividing membrane

Diamnionic/ dichorionic
dividing membrane

Position of dividing membrane

A

Thick separating
membrane due to
chorion

**Dichorionic diamnionic separated twin
placentas**

B

Very delicate, filmy amnionic membrane

Dichorionic diamnionic fused twin placenta

C

**Monochorionic diamnionic fused twin
placenta**

D

No separating membrane

**Monochorionic monoamnionic fused
twin placenta**

E

Figure 22-9 Twin placentas.

Special studies

Vascular anastomoses

Vascular anastomoses are searched for in monochorionic twin placentas. These are usually superficial artery-to-artery and vein-to-vein connections which are inconsequential, but there may be a deep artery-to-vein (AV) anastomosis which has implications for possible twin–twin transfusion syndrome. A membrane roll from between the placentas is taken first (to document the nature of the chorion). To assess the presence of anastomoses, the entire amnion is peeled away from the chorionic surface. This allows optimal visualization of the fetal vessels. Arteries and veins can then be readily traced, and artery-to-artery, vein-to-vein, and artery-to-vein anastomoses can be visualized. The arteries run *over* the veins in the chorionic plate.

Monochorionic placentas without twin–twin transfusion syndrome tend to have multiple anastomoses whereas monochorionic placentas with twin–twin transfusion syndrome almost always have a single deep anastomosis.[3]

Cytogenetics

If there is a clinical suspicion of a genetic abnormality, or multiple congenital malformations are present, or if the fetus is growth restricted or stillborn, it may be appropriate to send fresh sterile tissue taken from the midportion of the placenta for analysis. Sometimes the fetus is not available (or is very macerated) and the best tissue available is the placenta.

Infectious cases

If there is suspected chorioamnionitis, premature rupture of membranes, maternal fever, or suspected neonatal infection, it may be appropriate to take fresh tissue for culture. Cultures taken from the chorionic surface beneath the amnion may be the most representative. The most common pathogens can be detected by aerobic and anaerobic bacterial cultures. If there is a clinical suspicion of unusual infections (e.g., syphilis, tuberculosis, tularemia, listeria, toxoplasmosis, brucellosis, Q fever, or viruses), tissue can be taken and submitted for special cultures.

Potentially infectious placentas that could place pathology workers at risk (e.g., those from mothers with HIV or hepatitis) may be fixed for one week prior to processing unless there is a clinical reason for more rapid evaluation. Place the entire placenta in a large specimen container and fill it with formalin. Put paper towels underneath and over the placenta. It is very difficult to fully fix a placenta.

Metabolic diseases

In rare cases of suspected metabolic disease, 10 to 20 g of fresh tissue can be rapidly frozen.

Gross differential diagnosis of placental lesions

Chorioamnionitis. The membranes are opaque and may be yellow to green in color. Candidal infections can cause white microabscesses on the cord.

Selective reduction. In multiple gestations due to infertility treatment (i.e., when several fertilized eggs were introduced into the uterus), one or more fetuses may be terminated to reduce the total to two or three. The fetuses may be found as thickenings in the membranes and are usually markedly flattened and 1 to 2 cm in length ("fetus papyraceus").

Abnormal lobation. The placenta usually forms a single disc-shaped structure. Some placentas are comprised of two or more lobes. A smaller accessory (succenturiate) lobe may be present. These variants are associated with velamentous/intramembranous vessels and may increase the risk of fetal bleeding.

Amnion nodosum consists of multiple small (<0.1 cm) white or gray irregular nodules on the fetal surface which can easily be rubbed off. They are formed by aggregates of fetal cells (squames, vernix, hair) on the surface, associated with oligohydramnios.

Infarction. Infarcts are discrete solid lesions usually connected to the basal plate. Recent infarcts are dark red and older infarcts are orange to white. Small marginal infarcts are commonly found. Centrally located infarcts may be of clinical importance.

Intervillous thrombus. Thrombi appear as homogeneous red (recent) to white (old) aggregates of blood found within the placental disc.

Retroplacental hematoma. An aggregate of blood adheres to the basal plate. The age of the hematoma can be estimated by the degree of organization seen microscopically. The hematoma may compress the placental disc and be associated with infarctions. It may be associated with fetal hypoxia.

Subchorionic fibrin deposition. Small firm white nodules are seen below the fetal surface. Fibrin deposition can be extensive and involve the entire subchorionic area.

Chorangioma. This rare hamartoma (hemangioma) presents as a circumscribed fleshy mass that is usually subchorionic. It may resemble an infarct or an intervillous thrombus.

Microscopic sections

Umbilical cord
Two cross-sections.

Membranes
One membrane roll.
In cases of intrauterine growth retardation, pre-eclampsia (hypertension), diabetes, or lupus erythematosus, submit one additional membrane roll.

Placenta
Two full thickness sections.

Lesions
Submit additional sections of any gross lesion.

Multiple gestations
Submit separate sections as above for each placenta. In addition, submit one membrane roll of the dividing membranes.

Sample dictation

Placentas are most easily dictated using a standard template (Fig. 22-10).
Examples of gross summaries:
A 160-g singleton placenta with diffuse infarctions
A 410-g singleton placenta with a succenturiate lobe and a 3 cm area of intramembranous vessels
An 800-g diamnionic monochorionic fused twin placenta without superficial or deep vascular anastomoses
A 500-g green singleton placenta

Graphs relating umbilical cord length to gestational age and placental weight to gestational age and crown-rump length are available in Langston et al.[2] Placental weight standards are given in Table 22-16.

■ PRODUCTS OF CONCEPTION

Products of conception (POC) are not considered a routine surgical specimen by the woman, the family, or the law. These tissues represent the death of a potentially separate individual.

Placenta type

1. Singleton
2. Diamnionic, dichorionic separated twin placenta
3. Diamnionic, dichorionic fused twin placenta
4. Diamnionic, monochorionic twin placenta
5. Monoamnionic, monochorionic twin placenta
6. Triplet placenta (describe)
7. Other (describe)

If a multiple gestation placenta is examined, give each placenta a designation (e.g., one or two clamps or arbitrarily "A" and "B") and dictate each placenta separately.

Cord

Length: _____ cm.
Insertion: central/eccentric/marginal/membranous/unknown
Number of vessels: two arteries and a vein/other (describe)
Cord twist: left (most common)/right/none
Other findings:

Membranes

Insertion: _____ % marginal/ _____ % circummarginate/
_____% circumvallate

Color: normal/green/opaque/other
Point of rupture: _____ cm from edge of disc
Other findings:

Disc

Weight: _____ gm _____ (Combined weight if a multigestation placenta)

Size: _____ × _____ × _____ cm

Subchorionic fibrin: normal/patchy (1–2 nodules)/extensive (3 or more nodules)
Retroplacental hemorrhage: absent/present (describe size, old or recent, location)
Infarcts: absent/present (describe size, central or marginal, % of parenchyma infarcted)
Intervillous thrombi: absent/present (describe size, location, laminated or nonlaminated)
Other findings:

Special studies

Evaluation of vascular anastomoses
Tissue saved for cytogenetic analysis, cultures, or metabolic analysis

Gross summary

A single sentence summarizing the above findings.

Figure 22-10 Placental template for dictation.

Table 22-16 Placental weight standards

GESTATIONAL AGE	SINGLETONS PERCENTILES					TWINS (COMBINED WEIGHT) PERCENTILES				
	10	25	50	75	90	10	25	50	75	90
12			56							
14			83							
16			110							
18			137.8							
20			145			166	190	218	245	270
22	122	138	157	176	191	191	219	251	282	310
24	145	166	189	212	233	232	267	307	346	382
26	175	200	227	255	280	284	330	380	430	475
28	210	238	270	302	331	345	401	464	527	584
30	249	281	316	352	384	409	478	554	631	700
32	290	325	364	403	438	472	554	644	734	815
34	331	369	411	453	491	531	624	727	830	923
36	372	412	457	501	542	582	684	798	912	1014
38	409	452	499	547	589	619	728	850	972	1082
40	442	487	537	587	632	638	753	879	1005	1118

Clinicians should be informed about the routine procedure of specimen evaluation and disposal so that this information can be conveyed to the mother.

State law varies and must be consulted for specific requirements. In Massachusetts, fetal deaths requiring a birth certificate and death certificate include any fetus of 20 weeks' gestation or more, any fetus weighing 350 g or more, or any fetus showing signs of life at birth. If the fetal death is the result of an induced abortion, the death need not be reported. However, if the fetus shows signs of life (at any gestational age or weight), the death must be reported.

If the POC are considered to constitute a fetal death, permission must be obtained before an autopsy can be performed. It is preferable to obtain permission from both parents. The parents may wish to view the fetus. This should be done prior to the performance of the autopsy. A death certificate is required.

Types of POC and reasons for examination

Spontaneous abortion (SAB)

- First trimester "losses" (missed abortion, empty sac, blighted ovum). The most common cause is a chromosomal abnormality. Fetal tissues are often not present.
- Second trimester miscarriages. Potential causes include incompetent cervix, preterm labor, intrauterine fetal demise, structural malformations, and infections.
- Recurrent pregnancy loss (more than two losses at any gestational age).

These tissues are usually passed per vagina or removed by endometrial curettings. Examination of the tissues can document the site of the pregnancy, determine the etiology of the loss, and provide tissue for special studies.

Therapeutic abortion (TAB)

Therapeutic abortions may be performed for several reasons:

- Social (maternal request for legal termination of pregnancy)
- Maternal indications (severe diseases exacerbated by pregnancy)
- Fetal indications (structural or chromosomal anomalies).

Examination can verify the involvement of maternal disease in the gestational tissue and verify fetal anomalies.

Ectopic pregnancy

The woman presents with a first trimester pregnancy with pain and bleeding and an abnormal rise or fall in serum β-hCG levels. Endometrial curettage is performed to identify chorionic villi or placental implantation to document an in utero pregnancy (see also Chapter 6). If such a pregnancy cannot be documented, an ectopic pregnancy is likely and pelviscopy may be indicated.

Molar pregnancy

The woman presents with an abnormally enlarged uterus and elevated β-hCG for gestational age. Ultrasound reveals a cystic intrauterine mass. Examination can determine whether the mole is partial or complete.

Processing the specimen

These specimens should always be submitted fresh. This allows special studies, including karyotype analysis and microbiologic culture, to be performed. It is also much easier to identify villi in fresh tissue.

Specimens are of three types:

1. POCs without recognizable fetal parts
2. POCs with a fetus less than 12 weeks of age
3. POCs with a fetus more than 12 weeks of age.

Processing POC without recognizable fetal parts

1. Decant the tissue into a container that will allow fluid to drain. If fetal tissues are identified, follow one of the subsequent protocols according to fetal age.
2. If villous tissue is clearly identified, process one cassette of villous tissue and save the remaining tissue in formalin.

    Villi can be identified by floating the specimen in saline in a Petri dish and observing the tissue using a dissecting microscope. Blood may need to be rinsed away. Villi are usually white (but may be pink) and have acute angle branching. If gently squeezed with a forceps, villi rapidly re-expand when released. Decidualized endometrium is usually pink (but may be white) and more opaque than villi. Endometrial tissue may have glandular and vascular structures that can be mistaken for villi; however, these structures run in parallel (i.e., are not branched) and do not have the springy quality of villi.

If an *ectopic pregnancy* is suspected clinically, all tissue should be processed including the blood. These specimens are often evaluated as an OR consultation (see page Chapter 6).

If *hydropic villi* are present (any villous structure of 1 cm or more), whether or not fetal tissue is present, the specimen should be evaluated as a possible molar pregnancy. Tissue may be sent for ploidy studies (analytical cytometry; complete = diploid or tetraploid; partial = triploid) or may be cultured for karyotype analysis. Villi and fetal tissues must be sent separately for analysis. Photographs may be useful. Five to 10 cassettes of tissue should be processed.

Complete moles are recognizable by multiple tiny thin-walled fluid-filled vesicles. Look for them carefully, as they are often not suspected clinically. Fetal parts are not present (unless there is a non-molar twin). Partial moles may have fetal tissues and scattered vesicles as well, but may not be recognized until examined microscopically. If partial mole is suspected, look for syndactyly of fingers or toes, which is associated with triploidy.

Processing POC with embryonic or fetal tissue identified, less than 12 weeks

1. Obtain standard measurements (crown–rump, foot, or hand length).
2. Evaluate for developmental stage (Table 22-17).
3. Evaluate for anomalies. A complete dissection is not necessary. Gross anomalies are usually easily identified with careful visual inspection. A single incision can be performed to check for normal situs. If warranted or requested (e.g., anomalies known or suspected by prenatal ultrasound), dissection can be performed with the aid of a dissecting microscope.
4. Sterile tissue may be saved for karyotype analysis if a chromosomal abnormality is suspected (see Chapter 7).

Table 22-17 Timetable of fetal morphogenesis

GESTATIONAL AGE (WEEKS)	FOOT LENGTH	CHARACTERISTICS
6		Digital rays in hand plate, paddle limbs
7		Retinal pigment, foot plates
8		Digital rays in feet, elbow
9		Fingers
10		Toes, gut herniation (physiologic omphalocele)
11	7 mm	Eyes closing/closed
12	9 mm	Intestines in abdomen, fingernails
14	14 mm	Gender identifiable by external examination
16	20 mm	Toenails

Fetal specimen triage

Live birth with subsequent death	Autopsy
TAB <24 weeks	Surgical
Stillborn <20 weeks	Surgical
Stillborn ≥20 weeks (IUFD, liveborn)	Autopsy

5. Submit the embryonic tissue (longitudinal section or coronal sections of calvaria, thorax, abdomen, pelvis) and villous tissue.

If the procedure was a therapeutic abortion without known or suspected fetal anomalies, and the gross examination does not reveal any abnormalities, then tissue need not be examined histologically.

Processing POC with embryonic or fetal tissue identified, more than 12 weeks

Fragmented POC. A thorough examination of the tissues is required.

1. Separate the solid tissues from blood. Use a sieve or separate by hand. Do not add tap water as it will damage the tissues.
2. Examine all solid tissues.
3. Identify the major skeletal parts:

- Four extremities
- Spinal column
- Skull/base.

   Examine for number of digits, nail development, palmar creases, edema, etc. Measure foot and/or hand length (heel to great toe/wrist to middle finger).
4. Examine all organs or possible organs including placental tissues, umbilical cord (check number of vessels). Weigh organs if they are reasonably complete. Dissect the heart if possible.
5. Describe normal and abnormal findings.
6. Consider karyotypic analysis if anomalies are present or cultures if infection is suspected.
7. Submit representative sections of organs and skeleton.

Sample dictation

The specimen is received fresh, labeled with the patient's name and unit number and "POC," and consists of multiple fragments of fetal and placental tissues and blood in a stockingette (in aggregate 10 × 5 × 1 cm). All four extremities are present and include a right foot length of 12 mm and a right hand length of 10 mm. There is no syndactyly, polydactyly, or abnormal palmar crease. The nail development is normal. A portion of the vertebral column and a fragment of calvaria are intact. The right ear is present and is formed normally. Both eye globes are present. The fragmented calvaria reveals an intact hard palate. Fetal organs and tissues are present and include a relatively intact heart (1.3 g), fragments of gastrointestinal tract, two fragmented kidneys, and skin.

Dissection of the heart under a dissecting microscope reveals a small membranous ventricular septal defect and an otherwise structurally normal heart, appropriate for gestational age. The great vessels are avulsed and, therefore, the ductus arteriosus cannot be evaluated. The placental tissues include a 10 cm in length trivascular umbilical cord and fragmented villous and membranous tissues. Representative sections of fetal and placental tissues are submitted in five cassettes.

POC with an intact fetus and placenta. Intact fetuses should be examined with the placenta. The placenta is examined as described in the section on placentas.

1. Photograph the fetus with anterior, posterior, and lateral views. Photograph the face. This photograph should be appropriate to give to the family if requested.
2. Photograph any anomaly or dysmorphism.
3. Radiograph the fetus.
4. Freeze tissue (liver, skin).
5. Save tissue fresh if karyotype analysis is indicated. Usually karyotypic analysis is not indicated if the anomaly is hydrocephalus, renal agenesis/dysgenesis, or an isolated neural tube defect.

If the fetus is hydropic (ascites, pleural fluid, pericardial fluid) save fluid and tissues for bacterial and viral (HSV, parvovirus, CMV) culture.

6. Obtain the following measurements:

- Weight
- Crown–rump length (crown to ischial tuberosities, "sitting height")
- Crown–heel length (crown to heel of extended leg)
- Foot length
- Hand length
- Head circumference (above ears, as if wearing glasses)
- Chest circumference (around nipples)
- Abdominal circumference (at umbilical insertion)
- Inner canthal distance
- Outer canthal distance
- Any other potentially anomalous measurement (e.g., finger, lip, ear).

7. Make a generous Y-shaped incision.
    Examine the organs in situ. Photograph anomalies.
    Remove the thymus and gonads before evisceration. They are small and often difficult to identify after dissection.

8. Take the block from the tongue (above the larynx at a minimum) to anus. Remove and save the vertebral column. Remove the brain (see below) and spinal cord, eyes, and pituitary. CNS tissues are fixed overnight. The organ block can be dissected prior to fixation or fixed overnight if the tissues are autolyzed. Before tissues are fixed, ensure that fresh tissue is available for special studies, if needed. It is exceptional for fetuses to be embalmed. The body should be maintained in a presentable condition. Proper respect for the fetus must be maintained during the examination.

9. Remove the brain into a large vessel filled with fixative that has been weighed previously. The brain can be weighed in the container with the fixative. Dissection can be carried out once the brain is well fixed overnight. Identify each cranial nerve.

10. Submit the following tissues. More than one tissue can be placed in one cassette.

- Thymus
- Lung: portion of each lobe
- GI tract: cross-sections from each region with contents in place—do not open
- Pancreas
- Gonads
- Bivalved kidneys and adrenals (right and left)
- Cross-section of neck at thyroid with trachea and esophagus
- Skin
- Skeletal muscle
- Vertebral column (after fixation and decalcification)
- Pituitary (fixed in situ and decalcified)
- Eye: cross-section (right and left)
- Brain: include lateral ventricles, cerebellum, and brain stem.

The following sections are optional:

- Longitudinal section of long bone (if skeletal dysplasia is suspected)
- Rib or sternum
- Nuchal region (if thickened or cystic hygroma)
- Bladder
- Prostate.

Sample dictation

Received fresh and intact is a phenotypically female fetus with a fresh weight of 258 g. There is mild skin maceration with slippage over approximately 10% of the surface. The calvarial bones are not disarticulated. External examination reveals a well-developed female fetus with:

Two eyes with fused lids

Small, anteverted nose with patent nares

Intact lip and palate

Slightly recessed chin

Normally formed ears

No nuchal thickening

Two nipple buds

Sternum ends approximately half the distance from nipple line to umbilicus

No hip disarticulation

Intact vertebral column

Five digits on all extremities with no syndactyly or abnormal creases

Patent vagina and anus

No abnormal joint contractures.

Gross measurements:

Weight:

Crown–rump length:

Crown–heel length:

Foot length:

Hand length:

Head circumference:

Chest circumference:

Abdominal circumference:

Inner canthal distance:

Outer canthal distance:

Gross photographs are taken of the face, anterior, posterior, and lateral views.

A standard Y incision is made. There is approximately 3 mL of serous fluid in the abdomen. No thoracic or pericardial fluid is present. The in situ examination reveals the heart pointing to the left, the stomach and one spleen in the upper left abdomen, liver and gall bladder in right upper abdomen, and the appendix in the right side wall. The thymus is mediastinal. The diaphragms are intact.

Evisceration is performed from the tongue to anus without difficulty. The trachea and esophagus are probed to reveal no atresia or fistula. Both kidneys are present with normal fetal lobulations. Both adrenal glands are present and normally placed. The internal genitalia are female and appear grossly normal.

Dissection reveals three lobes of the right lung and two lobes of the left lung. The heart receives the pulmonary veins in the left atria and superior and inferior vena cava in the right atrium. The great vessels are normally related. Opening the heart reveals an intact atrial septum with a patent and competent valve of the foramen ovale. There is a persistence of the left superior vena cava draining into an enlarged coronary sinus. The inflow into the right ventricle is normal with a normal tricuspid valve. The right ventricular chamber is normal. The pulmonary valve is tricuspid. The left and right pulmonary arteries are patent and appear normal. The ductus arteriosis is patent into the descending aorta. The left atria, left ventricular inflow, and mitral valves are normal. There is a ventricular septal defect in the membranous septum with extension anteriorly into the conal septum. The aortic valve is tricuspid with normally placed coronary ostia. The aortic arch and branches are normal.

The esophagus empties into a stomach with scant mucous contents. The small bowel and large bowel are normal with no atresia, volvulus, or diverticulum. The large bowel contains meconium.

Both kidneys have normal fetal lobulations and their pelves are not dilated. The ureters connect to an empty bladder. The adrenal glands are normal and without hemorrhage. The liver has many subcapsular petechial hemorrhages. The spleen and pancreas are normal in appearance.

Organ weights:

Thymus:

Lungs (combined):

Heart:

Liver:

Spleen:

Adrenals (combined):

Kidneys (combined):

The vertebral column is removed. The spinal cord appears normal. The calvaria is opened. The brain in situ reveals scant subdural hemorrhage over the convexities. The corpus callosum is present. The brain and spinal cord are removed intact and fixed. The brain appears normal for gestational age. The pituitary gland is removed with the sella and is fixed and decalcified. Both orbits are removed using an interior approach.

Brain weight:

Tissue from the placenta and skeletal muscle were sent for cytogenetic analysis. A portion of the right lung was sent for microbiological culture. A portion of the skin and liver were frozen in liquid nitrogen. The fetus is fixed and returned to the specimen cabinet.

Special studies

Examination of fetuses with known or suspected anomalies

Examine the fetus for the following *external* features:
- Nuchal thickening: associated with trisomy 21 or monosomy X. Take a section through neck skin and send for chromosome analysis.
- Cleft palate/lip: associated with trisomy 13. Send for chromosome analysis.
- Skin edema, dorsal pedal edema: associated with hydrops, monosomy X. Cultures may be taken to evaluate possible infection.
- Syndactyly: associated with triploidy and partial mole. Examine the placenta carefully.
- Polydactyly: associated with trisomy 13.
- Short sternum: normally the sternum reaches halfway between the inter-nipple distance and the umbilicus. A short sternum is associated with trisomy 18.
- Ambiguous genitalia: most female fetuses have a large clitoris, which can easily be confused with a phallus. Look carefully to see if the labia/scrotum are fused, indicating a male fetus. Describe the external genitalia as being "male," "female," or "ambiguous," but do not assign a sex to the fetus without first identifying the gonads.
- Skeletal anomalies: short limbs or fractures. Be sure to obtain the history and radiographs. Submit bone sections (long bones, ribs, and vertebrae). All bony parts should be x-rayed. Arrange the bony structures on the film in their anatomic positions.
- Other features: number of hair whorls (there should be one, more than one suggests anomalies in brain genesis), dimples over the lumbosacral regions (spina bifida), abnormal hand/foot position (clenching = arthrogryposes and neural problems; short dorsiflexed great toe or thumb/little finger overlap = trisomy 18; valgus deformities of lower limbs = Potter's syndrome), protuberant tongue (Beckwith–Wiedemann syndrome).

Examine the fetus for the following *internal* features:
- Shape of liver: the gallbladder should be to the right of the umbilical vein and the slope should be up to the left.
- Spleen: polysplenia or asplenia suggests visceral heterotaxy and associated cardiac abnormalities.
- Kidneys: shape (horseshoe), bifid, cystic, absent.

- Adrenals: medullary hemorrhage (associated with infection, take cultures).
- Lobation of the lungs.
- Presence of thymus.
- Gonads and uterus.
- Diaphragm: make sure it is intact without herniations.
- Appendix: should be in the right lower quadrant.
- Tracheo-esophageal fistula; anal atresia (check for patency with a probe).
- Meckel's diverticulum.

Chromosomal analysis

Karyotype analysis may be helpful in the following cases:

- Two or more consecutive spontaneous abortions
- Developmental stage significantly discrepant from the clinical estimate of gestational age (severe intrauterine growth retardation)
- One or more malformations (isolated neural tube defects and renal agenesis/dysgenesis are possible exceptions)
- Ambiguous genitalia after 13 weeks.

Using sterile technique, remove a small sample of skin and one other tissue (e.g., lung or placenta). If the embryonic tissue is macerated, portions of placental tissue may be used.

Pathologic diagnostic features sign-out checklist for products of conception

State
Intact or fragmented, macerated or well preserved.

Gender
Male, female, intersex, or not determined.

Estimated gestational age
Crown–rump length, foot length, estimated age.

Organs examined
List all organs examined and state whether normal or abnormal for gestational age.

Congenital anomalies
Present or absent, describe.

Placenta
List relevant features (e.g., mature or immature, umbilical cord normal or abnormal, infection present or absent).

Karyotype
Indicate whether tissue was sent for analysis.

REFERENCES

1. Kurman RJ, Norris HJ. Evaluation of criteria for distinguishing atypical endometrial hyperplasia from well-differentiated carcinoma. Cancer 49:2547-2559, 1982.
2. Langston C, Kaplan C, Macpherson T, et al. Practice Guideline for examination of the placenta, developed by the Placental Pathology Practice Guideline Development task force of the College of American Pathologists. Arch Pathol Lab Med 121:449-476, 1997.
3. Bajoria R, Wigglesworth J, Fisk NM. Angioarchitecture of monochorionic placentas in relation to the twin–twin transfusion syndrome. Am J Obstet Gynecol 172:856-863, 1995.

Head and neck

23

■ SINUS CONTENTS

Functional endoscopic sinus surgery (FESS) is used as a treatment for patients with chronic sinusitis who have not responded to medical therapy. The contents of the sinuses are examined and obstructing areas and polyps are removed. A subset of these patients may have allergic sinusitis. If allergic mucin consisting predominantly of eosinophils and Charcot–Leyden crystals is seen histologically, special stains for fungi should be performed to look for the hyphae of *Aspergillus*.[1-3]

Processing the specimen

1. The specimen consists of multiple minute fragments of bone and soft tissue. Describe the color and aggregate size. If polyps are present, see the following section.
2. The specimen will generally need to be decalcified.
3. Submit a representative section of the tissue in one cassette, including mucin if present. If a portion of grossly normal nasal septum is submitted, it can be described but not examined histologically.

■ NASAL POLYPS

The most common specimen consists of inflammatory nasal polyps. These polyps are translucent, gelatinous, rounded masses ranging from 0.5 to 3 cm in diameter. The cut surface is homogeneous gray or pink. Small cystic areas may be present and areas of chronic inflammation appear as white patches. Calcification or bone may be found and, if present, must be decalcified before submission. If large, the polyps may be bisected and half of each one submitted.

Polyps consisting of firm dense white tissue may be neoplastic. Benign (but locally aggressive) papillomas or squamous cell carcinomas can occur in the nasal passages. Attempt to identify the base of firm polyps and submit as a separate section, if possible, as well as thoroughly sampling the lesion.

■ ORAL CAVITY AND TONGUE RESECTIONS

Resections of the oral cavity are often large and may include a portion of the mandible and teeth. Such resections are almost always performed for invasive squamous cell carcinomas. These specimens are often accompanied by a radical neck dissection (see below).

Processing the specimen

1. Identify structures present including bone, teeth, mucosal surfaces, palate, tongue, and muscle. Anatomically complex specimens should be reviewed with the surgeon before

processing. Record measurements for each component. Major nerves or vessels should be identified by the surgeon.

If there is any clinical or gross suspicion of bone invasion, the specimen is radiographed.

2. Describe the lesion including location, size, invasion into adjacent structures, and distance from margins.

   Squamous cell carcinomas are usually raised irregular lesions with central ulceration. If the patient has received prior irradiation, the lesion may be difficult to define and persist predominantly as a firm ulcerated area.

3. Take sections of the lesion demonstrating its relationship to mucosal and soft tissue margins and deepest extent of invasion. Margins are taken as perpendicular sections.

   Sample all margins not included in the above.

4. After all soft tissue sections have been removed, the bone can be decalcified.

   If there is possible bone invasion, take sections demonstrating the closest approach of the tumor to bone. Also take the bone margins.

   If there is no gross, radiologic, or clinical suspicion of bone invasion, the only bone submitted may be the margins.

Microscopic sections

Lesion
One to 5 sections demonstrating relationship to margins.

Margins
Mucosal and soft tissue margins not included in the lesion specimens.

Bone
Margins and any area with suspicion of invasion by tumor. Teeth are described grossly unless abnormal or thought to be involved by tumor.

Sample dictation

Received fresh, labeled with the patient's name and unit number and "Composite resection," is a resection specimen (12.5 × 10. 5 × 6.2 cm) consisting of left mandibular ramus (7 × 6 × 0.6 cm) containing three molars, base of tongue (3.9 × 3.4 × 1.9 cm), floor of mouth (5.5 × 3.5 × 0.6 cm), soft tissue on the external portion of the ramus (6.5 × 2.6 × 1.2 cm), and soft tissue posterior and lateral to the base of the tongue (3.5 × 3.8 × 1.6 cm). A raised irregular white/tan tumor mass (4.8 × 3.5 × 1.9 cm in depth) is present involving the soft tissue at the base of the tongue, extends into and through the bone, and is present in the soft tissue external to the bone. The tumor invades into the muscle of the tongue. The margins of resection are grossly free of tumor. The tumor is 0.3 cm from the lateral mucosal margin, 0.8 cm from the posterior mucosal margin, 0.8 cm from the medial mucosal margin, and 0.5 cm from the anterior mucosal margin. The tumor is 0.5 cm from the inferior soft tissue margin at the base of the tongue and 0.4 cm from the soft tissue margin in the external soft tissue to the ramus.

The specimen is radiographed and an irregular trabecular pattern is seen in the area of gross tumor involvement. The bone is fixed and decalcified prior to histologic sectioning.

Cassette #1: Anterior mucosa and tumor, perpendicular margin, 1 frag, RSS.
Cassette #2: Medial mucosa and tumor, perpendicular margin, 1 frag, RSS.
Cassette #3: Lateral mucosa and tumor, perpendicular margin, 1 frag, RSS.
Cassette #4: Posterior mucosa and tumor, perpendicular margin, 1 frag, RSS.
Cassette #5: Deepest extent of tumor at base of tongue, perpendicular margin, 1 frag, RSS.
Cassette #6: Tumor and bone, 1 frag, RSS.
Cassette #7: Tumor and soft tissue external to ramus, 1 frag, RSS.
Cassette #8: Bone, proximal margin, en face, 1 frag, ESS.
Cassette #9: Bone, distal margin, en face, 1 frag, ESS.

Pathologic prognostic/diagnostic features sign-out checklist for oral cavity and tongue tumors

Type of tumor
Squamous cell carcinoma, other rare types.

Grade
Well, moderately, or poorly differentiated.

Size
In centimeters.

Location
Oral tongue, floor of mouth, upper gingiva, etc.

Invasion
Depth of invasion (see below), invasion into adjacent structures (bone, skin, muscle).

Tumor necrosis
Present or absent, extent.

Lymphovascular invasion
Present or absent.

Perineural invasion
Present or absent.

Margins
Mucosal, soft tissue, bone.

Lymph nodes
Number and location of involved lymph nodes, size of metastatic deposits, extracapsular invasion.

Nonlesional mucosa
Carcinoma in situ, dysplasia, chronic inflammation, radiation atypia.

Depth of invasion
Endophytic tumors: Measure from the surface of the center of the tumor to the deepest area of invasion.
Exophytic tumors: Measure from the surface of the ulcer to the deepest area of invasion.
Ulcerated tumors: Measure from the ulcer base to the deepest area of invasion.

The AJCC classification is given in Table 23-1.

■ RADICAL NECK DISSECTION

Radical neck dissections are uncommon specimens; the dissection is usually performed for squamous cell carcinoma of the head and neck. Poor prognosis is associated with multiple affected nodes, bilateral as opposed to unilateral involvement, extranodal extension, and positive nodes distal from the primary site.

- The **standard** radical neck dissection includes cervical lymph nodes, sternomastoid muscle, internal jugular vein, spinal accessory nerve, and submaxillary gland; the tail of the parotid may be included.
- The **modified** radical neck dissection (functional or Bocca neck dissection) does not include the sternomastoid muscle, the spinal accessory nerve, or the internal jugular vein.
- The **extended** radical neck dissection includes retropharyngeal, paratracheal, parotid, suboccipital, and/or upper mediastinal nodes.
- The **regional** (partial or selective) neck dissection includes only the nodes of the first metastatic station.

Table 23-1 AJCC (6th edition) classification of tumors of the lip and oral cavity

Tumor	TX	Primary tumor cannot be assessed
	T0	No evidence of primary tumor
	Tis	Carcinoma in situ
	T1	Tumor 2 cm or less in greatest dimension
	T2	Tumor >2 cm but ≤4 cm in greatest dimension
	T3	Tumor more than 4 cm in greatest dimension
	T4	(Lip) Tumor invades through cortical bone, inferior alveolar nerve, floor of mouth, or skin of face (i.e., chin or nose)
	T4a	(Oral cavity) Tumor invades adjacent structures (e.g., through cortical bone, into deep (extrinsic) muscle of tongue (genioglossus, hyoglossus, palatoglossus, and styloglossus), maxillary sinus, skin of face).
	T4b	Tumor invades masticator space, pterygoid plates, or skull base and/or encases internal carotid artery
		Note: Superficial erosion alone of bone/tooth socket by gingival primary is not sufficient to classify as T4
Regional lymph nodes	NX	Regional lymph nodes cannot be assessed
	N0	No regional lymph node metastasis
	N1	Metastasis in a single ipsilateral lymph node, ≤3 cm
	N2	Metastasis in a single ipsilateral lymph node, >3 cm but not more than 6 cm in greatest dimension; or in multiple ipsilateral lymph nodes, none more than 6 cm in greatest dimension; or in bilateral or contralateral lymph nodes, none more than 6 cm in greatest dimension
	N2a	Metastasis in a single ipsilateral lymph node >3 cm but ≤6 cm
	N2b	Metastasis in multiple ipsilateral lymph nodes, none >6 cm
	N2c	Metastasis in bilateral or contralateral lymph nodes, none >6 cm
	N3	Metastasis in a lymph node >6 cm
Metastasis	MX	Distant metastasis cannot be assessed
	M0	No distant metastasis
	M1	Distant metastasis

Note: This classification does not include nonepithelial tumors.

The specific lymph node groups can only be identified in the standard and extended dissections without orientation by the surgeon.

Processing the specimen

1. Identify the type of dissection. If muscle is present, orient the specimen and divide the lymph nodes into groups (Fig. 23-1). Call the surgeon if the specimen cannot be oriented and there are any "orientable" features present (e.g., sutures, salivary gland, fragments of muscle). Record the overall dimensions.

   If not oriented by the surgeon, the specimen can be thought of as a letter Z. The upper horizontal line contains level I and can be identified by the presence of the submandibular gland; the lower horizontal line is level V; and levels II, III, and IV comprise the upper, mid, and lower thirds of the oblique line defined by the sternocleidomastoid muscle.

2. Record the dimensions and appearance of the sternocleidomastoid muscle including color and any irregular firm areas (possibly representing involvement by tumor). The jugular vein lies deep to this muscle. Record the length, diameter, and appearance (color, patency). Open the vein along its length and examine for thrombus or tumor involvement. Tumor invasion into the vein is usually found only with extensive nodal disease. The soft tissue deep to the muscle is divided into three groups—high, mid, and low jugular nodes—and placed in Bouin's in three separate labeled containers.

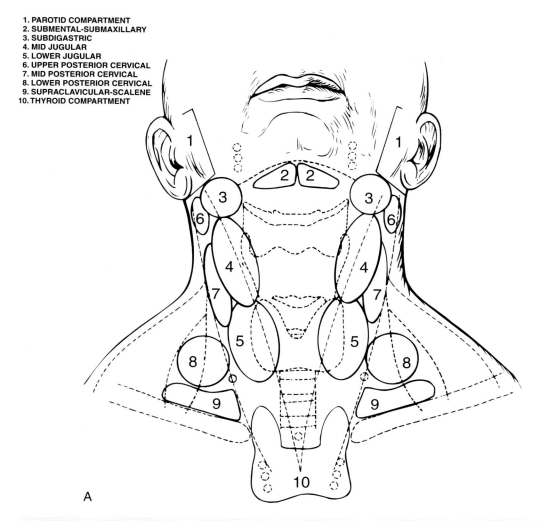

1. PAROTID COMPARTMENT
2. SUBMENTAL-SUBMAXILLARY
3. SUBDIGASTRIC
4. MID JUGULAR
5. LOWER JUGULAR
6. UPPER POSTERIOR CERVICAL
7. MID POSTERIOR CERVICAL
8. LOWER POSTERIOR CERVICAL
9. SUPRACLAVICULAR-SCALENE
10. THYROID COMPARTMENT

A

Figure 23-1 Radical neck dissection. A, Frontal view.

3. The submandibular region is the area superior to the muscle and contains the submandibular gland. Record its size, consistency, color, and lesions. Separate the soft tissue and fix in Bouin's.
4. The posterior triangle is the soft tissue inferior to the muscle. Record its dimensions and place all soft tissue in a separate container of Bouin's.
5. If gross tumor is present, evaluate the surgical margins around the tumor.

Lymph node groups should be separated and reported using standard terminology as follows:

Level I	Submental and submandibular lymph nodes
Level II	Upper jugular lymph nodes
Level III	Mid jugular lymph nodes
Level IV	Lower jugular lymph nodes
Level V	Posterior triangle lymph nodes

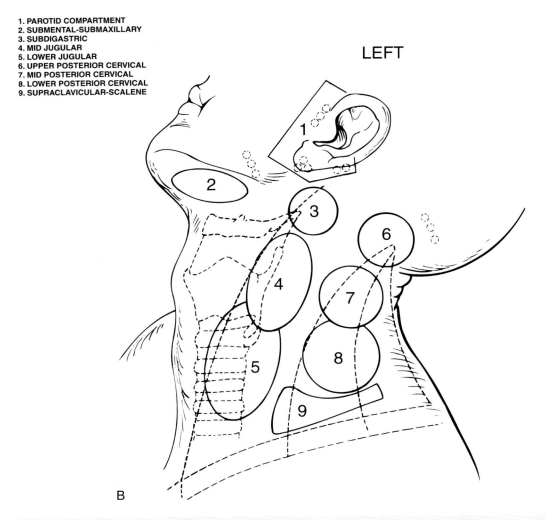

1. PAROTID COMPARTMENT
2. SUBMENTAL-SUBMAXILLARY
3. SUBDIGASTRIC
4. MID JUGULAR
5. LOWER JUGULAR
6. UPPER POSTERIOR CERVICAL
7. MID POSTERIOR CERVICAL
8. LOWER POSTERIOR CERVICAL
9. SUPRACLAVICULAR-SCALENE

LEFT

B

Figure 23-1 Radical neck dissection. B, Lateral view.

Lymph nodes
Submit representative sections of each lymph node separated into the five separate groups described above. A typical specimen contains a total of 30 to 40 lymph nodes.

Submandibular gland
One representative section.

Muscle and vein
One representative section. If these structures are grossly involved by tumor, submit one or two sections and specimen margins.

Lymph nodes
Number nodes examined, number of involved nodes, location of involved nodes, size of metastatic deposits, extracapsular invasion.

Salivary gland
Normal, involvement by tumor, inflammation.

Muscle and vein
Normal, involvement by tumor.

■ MUCOSAL BIOPSIES

Small biopsies are often obtained from the oral cavity, pharynx, or larynx to rule out carcinoma or premalignant conditions. These biopsies are usually small unorientable fragments. Diagnostic problems often include the distinction of reactive atypia from dysplasia and carcinoma in situ in tangential sections from invasive squamous cell carcinoma. Obtain three levels.

■ SALIVARY GLAND

Minor salivary gland biopsy of the lip

Patients with Sjögren's syndrome often undergo labial biopsy for diagnosis.[4] The specimen is a small fragment of tissue that is processed in its entirety. Obtain three levels.

The inflammation is scored to determine the likelihood of an autoimmune disease. A "focus" is defined as a lymphoid aggregate containing at least 50 lymphocytes, plasma cells, or macrophages. Germinal centers may be present. Foci are counted per 4-mm^2 area (close to the size of the biopsy).

Scores of more than 1 focus per 4 mm^2 are diagnostic of autoimmune sialadenitis
Scores of 1 focus per 4 mm^2 are suggestive
Scores of less than 1 focus per 4 mm^2 are nondiagnostic

Usually the lymphocytes are associated with acinar atrophy and fibrosis, and this correlates with the clinical loss of salivary gland function. Approximately 5% of patients with Sjögren's syndrome have nondiagnostic biopsies. However, re-biopsy at a later date often does reveal diagnostic changes.

Salivary gland resections

The most common specimen is a parotid gland resected for a pleomorphic adenoma (mixed tumor) or, less commonly, a Warthin's tumor. Other tumors are rare. A prior fine needle aspiration may have been performed.

Processing the specimen

1. Weigh the specimen and record the outer dimensions. Note whether any lesional tissue can be seen at the margin.
   Identify any nerves that may have been resected.
2. Ink the outer surface. Serially section through the specimen, looking for any lesions. Describe lesions including size, number (some tumors can be multifocal), color, consistency, involvement of nerve trunks, relationship to remainder of gland and capsule, and relationship to resection margin.
   Describe uninvolved parenchyma including color, fibrosis, calculi in ducts, dilated ducts, hemorrhage, and cysts. Intraparenchymal lymph nodes may be present.
3. Examine the parotid gland and surrounding soft tissue for the presence of lymph nodes.

Gross differential diagnosis

Pleomorphic adenomas (mixed tumors) are the most common type of salivary gland tumor. They are typically well circumscribed but may have small satellite nodules. They are usually white, very rubbery to firm, and translucent or cartilaginous. If diffuse infiltration or cystic degeneration is present, suspect an acinic cell or mucoepidermoid carcinoma (both can also be partially or completely circumscribed). Rarely, carcinomas arise in pleomorphic adenomas and may be recognizable grossly as areas of hemorrhage, necrosis, or frank invasion of adjacent tissue. A pleomorphic adenoma that is not well excised in the initial excision can recur as multiple nodules. Such a recurrence may be difficult to resect without also removing nerve trunks.

Warthin's tumors are circumscribed, orange/tan, and often cystic. There is usually thick brown/black fluid (like "crank case oil," but it may be clear) within the cyst spaces, which are lined by papillary nodules. Multiple tumors occur more frequently with Warthin's tumor than with any other salivary gland tumor. Approximately 12% of patients develop more than one tumor and 5% to 10% of patients have bilateral tumors.

Mucoepidermoid carcinoma may be well circumscribed if low grade. These carcinomas may have cystic areas containing mucin. Higher-grade tumors are usually infiltrative (with an appearance similar to invasive breast cancer) and solid in appearance. This is the most common malignant tumor in adults and children.

Acinic cell carcinoma is usually well circumscribed and may be grossly encapsulated. These tumors are gray/white to red/gray and lack the shiny surface of pleomorphic adenomas. Multiple cysts may be present. This is the second most common malignant tumor.

Adenoid cystic carcinoma may appear deceptively well delimited but infiltrative areas are usually present beyond the grossly apparent lesion. The tumors may show subtle effacement or blurring of normal lobular architecture. The tumors are usually solid and gray/white. Cystic areas and hemorrhage are uncommon.

Salivary duct carcinoma is rare and presents as a poorly demarcated scirrhous mass that may invade outside the gland. This carcinoma closely resembles breast carcinoma in appearance.

Lymphomas and benign lymphoepithelial lesions are very fleshy and soft to firm. These specimens should be processed like lymphomas and tissue taken for special studies. Many patients with lymphoepithelial lesions are HIV positive. These patients may develop bilateral (or, less commonly, unilateral) swelling of the parotid glands with multiple cysts.

Microscopic sections

Lesions
Up to six cassettes including relationship to uninvolved gland and capsule. Routine pleomorphic adenomas or Warthin's tumors only require three cassettes. All areas of hemorrhage, necrosis, and gross invasion of adjacent tissue should be extensively sampled.

Uninvolved gland
One or two cassettes.

Lymph nodes
All lymph nodes.

Sample dictation

Received fresh, labeled with the patient's name and unit number and "parotid," is a 6 × 5 × 3 cm parotid gland surrounded by adipose tissue measuring in thickness from 0.1 to 0.5 cm. There is a 4 × 3 × 3 cm firm tan/white homogeneous well-circumscribed lesion within the gland that is completely surrounded by salivary gland tissue but approaches to within 0.2 cm of one margin. The remainder of the gland is tan/yellow and unremarkable. No lymph nodes are identified in the surrounding soft tissue.

Cassettes 1–3: Lesion including closest margin, 4 frags, RSS.
Cassette 4: Uninvolved gland, 1 frag, RSS.

Pathologic prognostic/diagnostic features sign-out checklist for salivary gland carcinomas

Tumor site*
Resection of submandibular gland, resection of sublingual gland, superficial parotidectomy, total parotidectomy.

Laterality*
Right, left.

Tumor size*
Greatest dimension (additional dimensions optional)
≤2 cm, ≥2 cm to ≤4 cm, >4 cm but ≤6 cm, >6 cm.

Histologic type*
Adenoid cystic, mucoepidermoid, acinic cell, salivary duct carcinoma, carcinoma ex pleomorphic adenoma, adenocarcinoma, polymorphous low-grade adenocarcinoma (PLGA), other rare tumor types. The WHO classification is recommended.

Histologic grade*
See Table 23-2.
Mucoepidermoid carcinomas may be graded (see Tables 23-3 to 23-4).
Grading systems have been developed for acinic cell and adenoid cystic carcinomas but are not universally accepted. Solid areas (>30% of tumor) in adenoid cystic carcinomas are associated with a worse prognosis.

Extent of invasion*
No extraparenchymal invasion and ≤2 cm (pT1), >2 but ≤4 cm without extraparenchymal invasion (pT2), extraparenchymal invasion and/or >4 cm, without involvement of seventh nerve (pT3), invasion of skin, mandible, ear canal, or facial nerve, (pT4a), invasion of skull, pterygoid plates, or carotid artery (pT4b).

Regional lymph nodes*
Not present (pN0), present in 1 ipsilateral lymph node, ≤3 cm (pN1), present in 1 ipsilateral lymph node, >3 but ≤6 cm (pN2a), present in multiple ipsilateral lymph nodes, none >6 cm (pN2b), present in bilateral or contralateral lymph nodes, none >6 cm (pN2c), metastasis in a lymph node >6 cm (pN3). Number of lymph nodes examined, number with metastases, size of largest metastasis

Extracapsular extension of nodal metastasis
Absent, present, indeterminate.

Distant metastasis*
Absent or present.

Margins*
Uninvolved, involved (distance from closest margin), specify location if possible

Venous/lymphatic (large/small) vessel invasion
Absent, present, indeterminate.

Perineural invasion
Absent, present.

This checklist incorporates information from the ADASP (see www.panix.com/~adasp/) and the CAP Cancer Committee protocols for reporting on cancer specimens (see www.cap.org/). The asterisked elements are considered to be scientifically validated or regularly used data elements that must be present in reports of cancer-directed surgical resection specimens from ACS CoC-approved cancer programs. The specific details of reporting the elements may vary among institutions.

The AJCC classification is given in Table 23-5.

Table 23-2 Grading of salivary gland carcinomas

Low grade

Acinic cell carcinoma
Basal cell adenocarcinoma
Polymorphous low-grade adenocarcinoma

High grade

Primary squamous cell carcinoma
Undifferentiated carcinoma

Tumors of variable grade

Adenocarcinoma, NOS	Grade according to histologic features
Adenoid cystic carcinoma	Cribriform/tubular pattern versus solid (>30% of carcinoma)
Mucoepidermoid carcinoma	See Tables 23-3 to 23-4
Salivary duct carcinoma	Grade according to histologic features. Most are high grade

Table 23-3 AFIP grading system for mucoepidermoid carcinomas[5,6]

PARAMETER	POINT VALUE
Intracystic component <20%	+2
Neural invasion present	+2
Necrosis present	+3
Four or more mitoses per 10 HPF	+3
Anaplasia (nuclear pleomorphism, increased N/C ratio, large nucleoli, anisochromia, and hyperchromasia)	+4
GRADE	TOTAL POINT SCORE
Low grade	0–4
Intermediate grade	5–6
High grade	7 or more

This grading system was not predictive of outcome in submandibular tumors.

Table 23-4 Modification of AFIP grading system for mucoepidermoid carcinomas[7]

FEATURE	POINTS
Intracystic component <20%	2
Tumor front invades in small nests and islands	2
Pronounced nuclear atypia	2
Lymphatic or vascular invasion	3
Bony invasion	3
Four or more mitoses per 10 HPF	3
Perineural spread	3
Necrosis	3

GRADE	SCORE (POINTS)	CHARACTERISTIC FEATURES	DEFINING FEATURES
I	0	Prominent goblet cell component, cyst formation, intermediate cells may be prominent, circumscribed growth pattern	Lack of grade III defining features, lack of aggressive invasion pattern
II	2 to 3	Intermediate cells predominate over mucinous cells, mostly solid tumor, squamous cells may be seen	Aggressive invasion pattern, lack of grade III defining features
III	4 or more	Squamous cells predominate, intermediate and mucinous cells must also be present, mostly solid	Necrosis, perineural spread, vascular invasion, bony invasion, >4 mitoses/10 HPF, high-grade nuclear pleomorphism

Table 23-5 AJCC (6th edition) classification of tumors of major salivary glands

Tumor	TX	Primary tumor cannot be assessed
	T0	No evidence of primary tumor
	T1	Tumor ≤2 cm without extraparenchymal extension[a]
	T2	Tumor >2 cm but ≤4 cm without extraparenchymal extension[a]
	T3	Tumor more than 4 cm and/or extraparenchymal extension[a]
	T4a	Tumor invades skin, mandible, ear canal, and/or facial nerve
	T4b	Tumor invades skull base and/or pterygoid plates and/or encases carotid artery
Regional lymph nodes	NX	Regional lymph nodes cannot be assessed
	N0	No regional lymph node metastasis
	N1	Metastasis in a single ipsilateral lymph node, ≤3 cm
	N2	Metastasis in a single ipsilateral lymph node, more than 3 cm but not more than 6 cm in greatest dimension, or in multiple ipsilateral lymph nodes, none more than 6 cm in greatest dimension, or in bilateral or contralateral lymph nodes, none more than 6 cm in greatest dimension
	N2a	Metastasis in a single ipsilateral lymph node >3 cm but ≤6 cm
	N2b	Metastasis in multiple ipsilateral lymph nodes, none >6 cm
	N2c	Metastasis in bilateral or contralateral lymph nodes, none >6 cm
	N3	Metastasis in a lymph node >6 cm
Metastasis	MX	Distant metastasis cannot be assessed
	M0	No distant metastasis
	M1	Distant metastasis

[a] Extraparenchymal extension is defined as clinical or macroscopic evidence of invasion of skin, soft tissues, bone, or nerve. Microscopic extension alone is not extraparenchymal extension for classification purposes.

■ STAPES

The stapes is sometimes removed because of "otosclerosis" or "otospongiosis." The footplate of the stapes attaches to the oval window leading to the inner ear. In this disease of unknown etiology, immature bone is produced in the area, resulting in fixation of the stapes to the oval window. This process is a relatively frequent cause of conductive deafness in young persons. Surgical repair involves reimplantation of the stapes.

Early lesions show collagen disarray with increased osteoclastic and osteoblastic activity. Older lesions look like woven bone. The modern surgical procedure resects a portion of the stapes but does not remove the focus of sclerotic bone. The specimen usually consists of a minute fragment of bone, usually not identifiable as the stapes footplate. The specimen is described grossly, but usually not submitted for histologic sections.

■ TEETH

Teeth are generally removed because of caries or as part of a larger resection (e.g., mandible) and only require gross documentation.

Rarely, tumors of teeth or teeth from patients with systemic diseases involving teeth (e.g., some types of osteogenesis imperfecta) are removed. Teeth, like any other surgical specimen, need to be fixed well and not allowed to dry out if they are of diagnostic importance.

Processing the specimen (documentation)

1. Count the number of intact teeth and measure in aggregate. Measure the remaining fragments in aggregate. Note the presence of caries and dental fillings.

   Dentists and oral surgeons designate teeth by number: #1 is the left maxillary third molar, proceeding on the maxilla to #16 (the right maxillary third molar); #17 is the right mandibular third molar, proceeding to #32 (the left mandibular third molar).
2. Describe, if possible, the identity of the teeth (molars, premolars or canine, and incisors).
3. In some cases, including wisdom tooth extractions, teeth are removed with attached (pericoronal) cysts. If so, describe the location and size of attached soft tissue and submit in a separate cassette.
4. Sections of the teeth should not be submitted except in exceptional cases.

■ TONSILS AND ADENOIDS

Tonsils and/or adenoids are commonly removed for the treatment of recurrent tonsillitis, middle ear disease, or sleep apnea. Rarely, tonsils are involved by lymphomas or leukemias, infections (e.g., CMV, fungi, EBV), carcinomas, or granulomatous diseases.

In rare instances, one or both tonsils are removed from a patient with a squamous cell carcinoma metastatic to a cervical lymph node with no known primary. In such cases, the tonsil from the ipsilateral side should be examined completely microscopically to evaluate the possibility of a clinically occult primary arising in the tonsil. The presence of a basaloid morphology, p16 positivity, and HPV is highly suggestive of a tonsil primary (see Chapter 7).

Examination of "routine" specimens from patients with a routine clinical history is controversial.[8] A large study found that only 1% of such examinations resulted in a diagnosis other than benign, tonsillitis, or hyperplasia and that in none of these cases was patient care affected. However, the decision not to examine these specimens can only be made if an adequate clinical history is available and the surgeon is sufficiently experienced to recognize unusual cases. Significant pathologic findings were found in 87% of specimens if there was a significant clinical history.

Relevant clinical history (in addition to age and gender)

See Table 23-6.

Processing the specimen

1. Record the dimensions. Describe the outer surface, which is usually a convoluted squamous mucosa overlying a broad base of tan/pink soft tissue.
2. Serially section through the specimen. The convolutions can be better appreciated on cross-section. Friable yellow/green "sulfur" granules (sometimes mistaken for necrosis) are large colonies of *Actinomycetes* that colonize the crypts.
3. Submit one representative section of each tonsil.

Special studies

Basaloid carcinomas in young patients

In patients younger than 40 years, tonsillar carcinomas with nonkeratinizing basal cell morphology are usually associated with HPV16 (rarely HPV31).[9] These carcinomas are strongly positive for p16. HPV can be identified by PCR on formalin-fixed tissue.

Sample dictation

The specimen is received fresh in two parts, each labeled with the patient's name and unit number. The first part, labeled "right tonsil," consists of a 4 × 3 × 3 cm tonsil covered by tan/white convoluted squamous mucosa overlying tan/pink unremarkable soft tissue. Small focal friable yellow/green nodules are present in the tonsillar crypts.

Cassette #1: 1 frag, RSS.

The second part, labeled "left tonsil," consists of a 4.5 × 3.5 × 3 cm tonsil covered by tan/white convoluted squamous mucosa overlying tan/pink unremarkable soft tissue.

Cassette #2: 1 frag, RSS.

Table 23-6 Relevant clinical history

HISTORY RELEVANT TO ALL SPECIMENS	HISTORY RELEVANT TO TONSILLAR SPECIMENS
Organ/tissue resected or biopsied	Recurrent tonsillitis
Purpose of the procedure	Obstructive sleep apnea
Gross appearance of the organ/tissue/lesion sampled	Sleep apnea ("pickwickian syndrome" or sleep apnea due to pharyngeal obstruction): usually both palatine tonsils as well as uvula and possibly additional tissue from Waldeyer's ring are resected
Any unusual features of the clinical presentation	Infections (e.g., CMV, fungi, EBV)
Any unusual features of the gross appearance	Granulomatous disease (e.g., sarcoid)
Prior surgery/biopsies—results	
Prior malignancy	
Prior treatment (radiation therapy, chemotherapy, drug use that can change the histologic appearance of tissues)	
Compromised immune system	

REFERENCES

1. de Carpentier JP, et al. An algorithmic approach to aspergillus sinusitis. J Laryngol Otol 108:314-318, 1994.

2. Hartwick RW, Batsakis JG. Sinus aspergillosis and allergic fungal sinusitis. Ann Otol Rhinol Laryngol 100:427-430, 1991.

3. Katzenstein et al. Pathologic findings in allergic aspergillus sinusitis. A newly recognized form of sinusitis. Am J Surg Pathol 7:439-443, 1983.

4. Daniels TE. Labial salivary gland biopsy in Sjogren's syndrome: Assessment as a diagnostic criterion in 362 suspected cases. Arthritis Rheum 27:147-156, 1984.

5. Auclair PL, Goode RK, Ellis GL. Mucoepidermoid carcinomas of intraoral salivary glands. Evaluation and application of grading criteria in 143 cases. Cancer 69:2021-2030, 1992.

6. Goode RK, Auclair PL, Ellis GL. Mucoepidermoid carcinoma of the major salivary glands; clinical and histopathologic analysis of 234 cases with evaluation of grading criteria. Cancer 82:1217-1224, 1998.

7. Brandwein MS, Ivanov KI, Wallace DI, et al. Mucoepidermoid carcinoma. A clinicopathologic study of 80 patients with special reference to histological grading. Am J Surg Pathol 25:835-845, 2001.

8. Netser JC, et al. Value-based pathology; a cost–benefit analysis of the examination of routine and nonroutine tonsil and adenoid specimens. Am J Clin Pathol 108:158-165, 1997.

9. El-Mofty SK, Lu DW. Prevalence of human papillomavirus type 16 DNA in squamous cell carcinoma of the palatine tonsil, and not the oral cavity, in young patients: a distinct clinicopathologic and molecular disease entity. Am J Surg Pathol 27:1463-1470, 2004.

Hernia sac

24

Hernia sacs are common surgical specimens derived from the frequent repair of inguinal, femoral, and umbilical hernias. The sacs usually consist of a small portion of fibrous connective tissue lined by mesothelial tissue. Approximately 22% of men undergoing hernia repair also have a cord lipoma. Only 0.1% of hernia sac operations yielded an incidental liposarcoma.[1] The two patients with liposarcoma were older than the average patient with cord lipoma (56 and 64 years versus 35 years) and the tumors were larger (13 and 10 cm versus 5.5 cm). Other rare soft tissue sarcomas have been reported from this region.

Occasionally a groin mass (often an enlarged lymph node) is mistaken clinically for an inguinal hernia. If a lymph node is found, it should be processed as a lymph node biopsy as the node may be involved by metastatic tumor or infection. Not infrequently, there are other findings in hernia sac specimens that may be of clinical significance. Some of the more common are listed below.

Occasional findings in hernia sacs

- Endometriosis (may be present in a true hernia or can simulate a hernia).
- Incarcerated bowel.
- Vas deferens or epididymis (usually an inadvertent transection) is found in 0.53% of specimens from pediatric patients.[2] These structures must be distinguished from glandular inclusions, as there are medical and legal issues in such cases. A vas deferens should have a well-defined muscular coat.
- Glandular inclusions from mullerian remnants in prepubertal males.[3-5]
- Lymph nodes or metastatic tumor in inguinal nodes simulating a hernia.
- Mesothelial hyperplasia, which may closely mimic a neoplastic process.
- Tumors: a hernia may sometimes be the initial presentation of malignant mesothelioma, pseudomyxoma peritonei, or an intra-abdominal tumor (most frequently colon or ovarian carcinoma).

Processing the specimen

1. The specimen is a portion of thin tan/pink fibrous connective tissue with one shiny surface (the peritoneum) and one dull surface. Examine the specimen carefully to make sure that other structures are not present (see above).
2. Submit one cassette containing three representative cross-sections. Submit any focal lesions or additional structures.

Sample dictation

Received fresh, labeled with the patient's name and unit number and "hernia," is a 4 × 3 × 0.4 cm fragment of pink/tan connective tissue. One side has a glistening surface.
Cassette: 3 frags, RSS.

REFERENCES

1. Montgomery E, Buras R. Incidental liposarcomas identified during hernia repair operations. J Surg Oncol 71:50-53, 1999.
2. Steigman CK, Sotelo-Avila C, Weber TR. The incidence of spermatic cord structures in inguinal hernia sacs from male children. Am J Surg Pathol 23:880-885, 1999.
3. Gomez-Ramon JJ, Mayorga M, Mira C, Buelta L, Fernandez F, Val-Bernal F. Glandular inclusions in inguinal hernia sacs: a clinicopathologic study of six cases. Pediatr Pathol 14:1043-1049, 1994.
4. Popek EJ. Embryonal remnants in inguinal hernia sacs. Hum Pathol 21:339-349, 1990.
5. Walker AN, Mills SE. Glandular inclusions in inguinal hernia sacs and spermatic cords. Am J Clin Pathol 82:85-89, 1984.

Larynx

25

The reason for removal of the larynx is virtually always squamous cell carcinoma occurring near the true and false vocal cords. See Chapter 13 for biopsy specimens.

■ LARYNGECTOMY

Laryngectomies are difficult specimens because the complicated anatomy and the calcification of cartilage in older individuals necessitate decalcification of parts of the specimen. Most specimens are total laryngectomies performed to resect invasive squamous cell carcinoma (i.e., thyroid, cricoid, and arytenoid cartilages with all attached soft tissue and mucosa; hyoid bone either totally or partially excised; strap muscles; thyroid gland partially or totally excised; several tracheal rings; base of tongue not usually included). Refer to Figure 25-1 for orientation and terminology. There is often an accompanying radical neck dissection.

Laryngectomy may also be performed to control chronic aspiration in mentally retarded patients. In these cases, grossly normal specimens can be examined in three sections from the epiglottis, vocal cords, and trachea.

Processing the specimen

1. Carefully examine the outer surface of the specimen and record any evidence of tumor extension to a surgical resection margin. Although the anterior strap muscles form the anterior margin of the specimen, these muscles retract after they are cut and may not

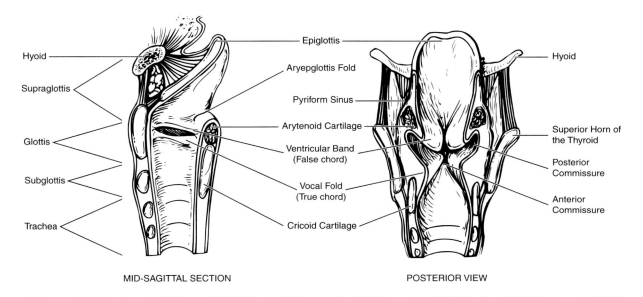

MID-SAGITTAL SECTION   POSTERIOR VIEW

Figure 25-1 Anatomy of the larynx.

completely cover this area. It may be necessary to contact the surgeon to determine the true surgical margins if areas suspicious for tumor are present at an apparent margin.

Record overall dimensions and all identifiable attached structures including the hyoid bone.

2. Ink the outer portion of the specimen, including all mucosal margins.

3. Open the specimen longitudinally along the posterior surface. The larynx can be opened to reveal the true and false vocal folds and the ventricle. Describe any lesions including color, size, quality (exophytic, flat, verrucous, ulcerated, necrotic), location, and extent of involvement of anatomic landmarks (e.g., vocal folds, ventricle, epiglottis, commissures, across midline). See Figure 25-1 for the relevant anatomical structures. Include the number of tracheal rings present.

4. Document the location of lesions by means of photography or diagrams. It is usually necessary to prop the posterior incision open (the cut ends of cotton swabs work well) or to hold the larynx open with hemostats. If the cartilage is not extensively calcified, the specimen can be cut in half and each cross-section photographed.

Often a diagram is necessary to record adequately the location of the tumor and the location of microscopic sections.

5. Fix the specimen overnight in formalin.

6. If the cartilages are calcified, submit as many soft tissue sections as possible and then decalcify the remainder of the specimen before submitting the sections with cartilage. Document the point of maximum tumor invasion through cartilage (if any). If there is soft tissue around the specimen (often there is not), identify all lymph nodes.

Microscopic sections

Tumor
Up to four cassettes of tumor including relationship to anatomical landmarks (see "Diagnostic/prognostic features" and Fig. 25-1) and deepest extent of tumor into, around, or through the surrounding cartilage.

Margins
Lowest tracheal ring, all mucosal edges, strap muscles (anterior), base of tongue, soft tissue of lateral and posterior larynx. Mucosal margins not close to the gross tumor can be taken en face.

Normal structures
True and false cords (vertical sections) bilaterally if uninvolved, anterior commissure, bilateral arytenoids and aryepiglottic folds, epiglottis.

Sample dictation

Received fresh, labeled with the patient's name and unit number and "larynx," is a total laryngectomy specimen (11 × 5 × 3.5 cm) including hyoid bone (8 × 0.3 × 0.3 cm), larynx from epiglottis to subglottis, and six tracheal rings. There is an irregular tan/white mass with central ulceration (2.5 × 1.5 × 0.9 cm) located in the glottis completely involving the left true vocal cord. The mass crosses the midline and involves the medial aspect of the right true vocal cord. The false vocal cords are not involved. The mass is 2.8 cm from the closest proximal mucosal margin (left aryepiglottic fold) and 5 cm from the distal tracheal margin. The mass invades into the lamina propria and focally appears to invade into, but not through, the thyroid cartilage. The anterior surface is covered by red/brown strap muscles, which are grossly unremarkable. 0.5 cm from the distal margin there is a 1.5 × 1 cm tracheal stoma. The cartilage is calcified and is fixed and decalcified prior to histologic sectioning.

Cassette #1: Left aryepiglottic fold, en face margin, 1 frag, ESS.
Cassette #2: Right aryepiglottic fold, en face margin, 1 frag, ESS.
Cassette #3: Epiglottis, margin, en face margin, 1 frag, ESS.

Cassette #4: Right arytenoid mucosa, en face margin, 2 frags, ESS.
Cassette #5: Left arytenoid mucosa, en face margin, 2 frags, ESS.
Cassette #6: Right anterior strap muscle, perpendicular margin, 1 frag, RSS.
Cassette #7: Left anterior strap muscle, perpendicular margin, 1 frag, RSS.
Cassette #8: Right lateral soft tissue, perpendicular margin, 1 frag, RSS.
Cassette #9: Left lateral soft tissue, perpendicular margin, 1 frag, RSS.
Cassette #10: Posterior soft tissue, perpendicular margin, 1 frag, RSS.
Cassette #11: Distal tracheal margin, en face, 1 frag, ESS.
Cassette #12: Mass including left true cord, 1 frag, RSS.
Cassette #13: Mass including right true cord, 1 frag, RSS.
Cassette #14: Mass including left false cord, 1 frag, RSS.
Cassette #15: Right false cord, 1 frag, RSS.
Cassette #16: Mass and deepest involvement of cartilage, 1 frag, RSS.
Cassette #17: Hyoid bone, 3 frags, RSS.
Cassette #18: Tracheal stoma site, 1 frag, RSS.

Pathologic prognostic/diagnostic features sign-out checklist for laryngeal carcinomas

Type of tumor
Squamous cell carcinoma, all other types rare (use the WHO modified classification).

Grade
Well, moderately, poorly differentiated, or undifferentiated.

Size
In centimeters.

Location
Supraglottis, glottis, subglottis.

Anatomic involvement
Supraglottis: ventricular bands (false cords), arytenoids, epiglottis, aryepiglottic folds; the inferior boundary is a horizontal plane through the apex of the ventricle.
Glottis: true vocal cords, anterior and posterior commissures; the lower boundary is a plane passing 1 cm below the apex of the ventricle.
Subglottis: area from the lower boundary of the glottis to the lower margin of the cricoid cartilage; thyroid and cricoid cartilages, post-cricoid area, medial wall of pyriform sinus, pre-epiglottic tissue (base of tongue).

Depth of invasion
Lamina propria, muscle, cartilage, perilaryngeal soft tissue.

Lymphovascular invasion
Present or absent.

Perineural invasion
Present or absent.

Lymph nodes
Size (≤ 3, ≤ 6, > 6 cm), ipsilateral versus contralateral, extracapsular invasion. Keratin debris may be evidence of previous tumor.

Margins
Involved or not involved, location.

Nonlesional tissue
Normal, dysplasia.

This checklist incorporates the recommendations of the ADASP (see www.panix.com/~panix/).

Table 25-1 AJCC (6th edition) classification of laryngeal tumors

Tumor	TX	Primary tumor cannot be assessed
	T0	No evidence of primary tumor
	Tis	Carcinoma in situ
Supraglottis	T1	Tumor limited to one subsite of the supraglottis with normal vocal cord mobility
	T2	Tumor invades mucosa of more than one adjacent subsite of supraglottis or glottis or region outside the supraglottis (e.g., mucosa of base of tongue, vallecula, medial wall of pyriform sinus) without fixation of the larynx
	T3	Tumor limited to larynx with vocal cord fixation and/or invades any of the following: postcricoid area, pre-epiglottic tissues, paraglottic space, and/or minor thyroid cartilage erosion (e.g., inner cortex)
	T4a	Tumor invades through the thyroid cartilage, and/or invades tissues beyond the larynx (e.g., trachea, soft tissues of neck including deep extrinsic muscle of the tongue, strap muscles, thyroid, or esophagus)
	T4b	Tumor invades prevertebral space, encases carotid artery, or invades mediastinal structures
Glottis	T1	Tumor limited to the vocal cord(s) (may involve anterior or posterior commissures) with normal mobility
	T1a	Tumor limited to one vocal cord
	T1b	Tumor involves both vocal cords
	T2	Tumor extends to supraglottis and/or subglottis, and/or with impaired vocal cord mobility
	T3	Tumor limited to the larynx with vocal cord fixation and/or invades paraglottic space, and/or minor thyroid cartilage erosion (e.g., inner cortex)
	T4a	Tumor invades through the thyroid cartilage and/or invades tissues beyond the larynx (e.g., trachea, soft tissues of neck including deep extrinsic muscle of the tongue, strap muscles, thyroid, or esophagus)
	T4b	Tumor invades prevertebral space, encases carotid artery, or invades mediastinal structures
Subglottis	T1	Tumor limited to the subglottis
	T2	Tumor extends to the vocal cord(s) with normal or impaired mobility
	T3	Tumor limited to the larynx with vocal cord fixation
	T4a	Tumor invades cricoid or thyroid cartilage and/or invades tissues beyond the larynx (e.g., trachea, soft tissues of neck including deep extrinsic muscles of the tongue, strap muscles, thyroid, esophagus)
	T4b	Tumor invades prevertebral space, encases carotid artery, or invades mediastinal structures
Regional lymph nodes	NX	Regional lymph nodes cannot be assessed
	N0	No regional lymph node metastasis
	N1	Metastasis in a single ipsilateral lymph node, ≤3 cm
	N2	Metastasis in a single ipsilateral lymph node, more than 3 cm but not more than 6 cm in greatest dimension, or in multiple ipsilateral lymph nodes, none more than 6 cm in greatest dimension, or in bilateral or contralateral lymph nodes, none more than 6 cm in greatest dimension
	N2a	Metastasis in a single ipsilateral lymph node >3 cm but ≤6 cm
	N2b	Metastasis in multiple ipsilateral lymph nodes, none >6 cm
	N2c	Metastasis in bilateral or contralateral lymph nodes, none >6 cm
	N3	Metastasis in a lymph node >6 cm
		Note: Midline metastases are classified as ipsilateral. Selective neck dissections should include at least 6 nodes. A radical or modified radical neck dissection should include at least 10 nodes
Metastasis	MX	Distant metastasis cannot be assessed
	M0	No distant metastasis
	M1	Distant metastasis

Note: This classification system does not apply to nonepithelial tumors.

Lung and pleura

26

■ LUNG

Non-neoplastic diseases of the lung are usually diagnosed by bronchoalveolar lavage, transbronchial biopsies, and open lung biopsies. In locations with lung transplant programs, chronically diseased recipient lungs are also submitted for examination and these patients are monitored by serial biopsies to exclude rejection or infection.

Lung tumors may be sampled by fine needle aspiration or endo/transbronchial biopsy, but often the patient proceeds directly to mediastinal staging, video-assisted closed chest lung biopsy, or open lung surgery.

Relevant clinical history (in addition to age and gender)

See Table 26-1.

Table 26-1 Relevant clinical history	
HISTORY RELEVANT TO ALL SPECIMENS	HISTORY RELEVANT TO LUNG SPECIMENS
Organ/tissue resected or biopsied	Organ transplantation
Purpose of the procedure	Occupational lung disease
Gross appearance of the organ/tissue/lesion sampled	Asbestos exposure
Any unusual features of the clinical presentation	Tobacco use
Any unusual features of the gross appearance	→ single mass, multiple masses, diffuse lung disease
Prior surgery/biopsies—results	Infection (known or suspected)
Prior malignancy	Systemic disease that affect the lungs (e.g., rheumatoid arthritis, sarcoidosis)
Prior treatment (radiation therapy, chemotherapy, drug use that can change the histologic appearance of tissues)	
Compromised immune system	

Endobronchial and transbronchial biopsies

Bronchial biopsies are processed as described in Chapter 13. Special stains for organisms (Gram, AFB, MSS) are ordered if the patient is immunocompromised or if infection is suspected clinically. Cytology specimens (e.g. bronchial brushings and/or bronchial lavage) are also often obtained during these procedures.

Transplant lung biopsies

Transbronchial biopsies of transplant lungs may be performed on an emergency basis for symptomatic patients or as routine follow-up biopsies after transplantation. These specimens are processed as transbronchial biopsies (8 levels, 3 H&E, MSS, Gram, 2 unstained). Other studies (e.g., immunoperoxidase, EM, immunofluorescence) are only ordered for specific clinical indications.

The revised working formulation for classification and grading of lung allograft rejection: 1995
(Tables 26-2 to 26-4.[1-3])

Table 26-2 Acute rejection[a]	
GRADE	HISTOPATHOLOGIC FINDINGS
A0 (none)	No mononuclear inflammation, hemorrhage, or necrosis
A1 (minimal)	Scattered infrequent perivascular mononuclear infiltrates not obvious at low magnification (40×)
	Blood vessels, particularly venules, are cuffed by small round, plasmacytoid, and transformed lymphocytes forming a ring 2 to 3 cells thick in the perivascular adventitia
A2 (mild)	Frequent perivascular mononuclear infiltrates surrounding venules and arterioles readily recognizable at low magnification and usually consisting of activated lymphocytes, small round lymphocytes, plasmacytoid lymphocytes, macrophages, and eosinophils
	Frequent subendothelial infiltration by the mononuclear cells with hyperplastic or regenerative changes in the endothelium (endotheliitis); although there is expansion of the perivascular interstitium by inflammatory cells, there is no obvious infiltration by mononuclear cells into the adjacent alveolar septa or airspaces
	Concurrent lymphocytic bronchiolitis is not uncommon. A solitary perivascular mononuclear infiltrate of significant intensity to be noted at low magnification still warrants a diagnosis of grade A2 (or greater) rejection
A3 (moderate)	Readily recognizable cuffing of venules and arterioles by dense perivascular mononuclear cell infiltrates, which are usually associated with endothelialitis; eosinophils and occasional neutrophils are common
	By definition, there is extension of the inflammatory cell infiltrate into perivascular and peribronchiolar alveolar septa and airspaces
	Collections of alveolar macrophages are common in the airspaces in the zones of septal infiltration
A4 (severe)	Diffuse perivascular, interstitial, and airspace infiltrates of mononuclear cells and prominent alveolar pneumocyte damage usually associated with intra-alveolar necrotic cells, macrophages, hyaline membranes, hemorrhage, and neutrophils; there may be associated parenchymal necrosis, infarction, or necrotizing vasculitis
	The obvious presence of numerous perivascular and interstitial mononuclear cells seen with grade A4 rejection permits distinction from perioperative (reperfusion/ischemic) lung injury

[a] Pathologists should mention airway inflammation and may choose to grade B lesions (see below).

Table 26-3 Chronic airway rejection (bronchiolitis obliterans)

CLASSIfiCATION	HISTOPATHOLOGIC FINDINGS
Active	In addition to the fibrosis, there are intra- and/or peribronchiolar submucosal and peribronchiolar mononuclear cell infiltrates usually associated with ongoing epithelial cell damage
Inactive	Dense fibrous scarring without cellular infiltrates; this represents old cicatricial change in the small airways with a lack of significant submucosal and peribronchiolar inflammatory infiltrates

Chronic vascular rejection

refers to the vaso-obliterative process affecting arteries and veins that affects most solid organ transplants, and reflects accelerated atherosclerosis with fibrointimal thickening of the subendothelial area by loose myxomatous connective tissue. A mononuclear cell and foamy cell infiltrate is common.

Table 26-4 Airway inflammation[a]

GRADE	HISTOPATHOLOGIC FINDINGS
B0 (none)	No airway inflammation
B1 (minimal)	Rare scattered mononuclear cells within the submucosa of the bronchi and/or bronchioles
B2 (mild)	Circumferential band of mononuclear cells and occasional eosinophils within the submucosa of bronchi and/or bronchioles unassociated with epithelial cell necrosis (apoptosis) or significant transepidermal migration by lymphocytes
B3 (moderate)	Dense band-like infiltrate of activated mononuclear cells in the lamina propria of bronchi and/or bronchioles including activated lymphocytes and eosinophils, accompanied by evidence of satellitosis of lymphocytes, epithelial cell necrosis (apoptosis) and marked lymphocyte transmigration through epithelium
B4 (severe)	Dense band-like infiltrate of activated mononuclear cells in the lamina propria of bronchi and/or bronchioles associated with dissociation of epithelium from the basement membrane, epithelial ulceration, fibrinopurulent exudates containing neutrophils, and epithelial cell necrosis
BX	Ungradeable because of sampling problems, infection, tangential cutting, etc.

[a] All cases of acute rejection should have a designation indicating whether coexistent airway inflammation is present and may choose to grade the intensity.

Open biopsies

Open lung biopsies are usually performed on critically ill patients with a wide differential diagnosis, usually for diffuse pulmonary disease. These specimens are usually processed during an OR consultation (see Chapter 6).

Wedge resection

Wedge resections are open lung or video-assisted closed chest biopsies performed to sample focal suspicious areas (e.g., pleural-based nodules) or to resect tumors if the patient cannot tolerate a more extensive procedure. Bullectomy may be performed on a patient with severe emphysema to improve pulmonary function.

Processing the specimen

1. The specimen is usually a triangular segment of lung and pleura with two intersecting staple lines at the margin. Record the dimensions of the specimen. Examine the pleura for any evidence of disease:

- **Smooth and glistening, freely mobile over an underlying mass:** normal pleura not invaded by tumor. There is no need to ink normal pleura. The absence of pleural involvement is important to document for staging lung carcinomas and can usually be determined by a good gross examination.
- **Retracted pleura over a tumor:** invasion by tumor into the pleura. The pleura will be fixed to the underlying mass. If the pleura is smooth, it will be recognizable microscopically and there is no need to ink it. If tissue (fat or muscle) is adherent this may be an indication of chest wall invasion. Use a different color of ink to distinguish this area from the lung parenchymal margin.
- **Tumor implants:** usually gray/white nodules within the pleura.
- **Lymphangitic spread of tumor:** white anastomosing lines running through the pleura.
- **Pleural lymph nodes:** small black firm nodules in the pleura.
- **Adhesions:** roughened dull areas of pleura with attached tissue—usually adipose tissue.

2. Record the length of the margin, which is usually a staple line. It is a worthless effort to try to remove all the staples as the tissue will be shredded and uninterpretable. Cut the staple line off the specimen with a pair of scissors, staying as close to the staples as possible. The cut surface of the lung now visible is the margin, which can be taken en face or, if the tumor is close, perpendicularly after inking the open surface. Blot the lung free of any fluid before inking to prevent the ink from smearing.
3. Serially section through the remainder of the specimen looking for any focal lesions. Describe all lesions including size, color, involvement of pleura, and distance from margin.
4. Describe the remainder of the lung parenchyma (emphysematous changes, consolidation, fibrosis).
5. The histologic appearance of even small specimens can be improved by inflating the fragment with a syringe filled with formalin. However, great care must be taken not to injure unprotected fingers.
6. Submit representative sections of any lesion including relationship to the pleura and uninvolved lung. Submit the closest margin. Submit one cassette of uninvolved lung parenchyma.

Pneumonectomy or lobectomy

Pneumonectomies and lobectomies are almost always performed to resect tumors. An exception is the recipient pneumonectomy performed prior to lung transplant, which is described under "Transplant pneumonectomies," below. Extrapleural pneumonectomies are used to resect mesotheliomas and are also described below.

Lung tumors

Processing the specimen

1. Weigh the specimen (Box 26-1) and record the dimensions of the bronchial margin (length and circumference). Identify the lung (right or left) or lobe/s (upper, lower, or middle)

Box 26-1 Normal lung weights

Right lung: 680 g (male); 480 g (female)

Left lung: 600 g (male); 420 g (female)

resected. Carefully examine the pleural surface for any evidence of disease (smooth and glistening = normal; dull and irregular = tumor implants or adhesions; retraction = invasion by tumor; delicate white reticular pattern on pleural surface = lymphangitic spread of tumor).

2. Inflate intact specimens through the remaining bronchus. If the bronchial resection margin has not already been removed as an OR consultation, do so before inflating. Cut an en face section and place in a labeled cassette. After the lung is inflated, clamp off the bronchus with a hemostat. *Note:* This should *not* be done if there is gross abnormality of the bronchus (e.g., invasion by tumor, dysplasia suggested by frozen section) that will be evaluated histologically. The appropriate sections are taken and a cotton swab can be used to plug the remaining bronchial stump.

   If the specimen is not intact (e.g., several sections have been cut into it), the specimen can be inflated using a syringe. Some of the formalin will leak out, but the microscopic appearance will still be much improved over no inflation at all. Many sites may need to be injected. *Great care is needed to avoid hand injuries.*

   The overall dimensions are measured after inflation.

3. Fix the specimen overnight. Previously uncut specimens are cut with a long knife in a parasagittal plane (lateral to medial). However, other methods of sectioning may be appropriate (see "Special studies," below). Photograph all lesions.

4. Describe lesions including size, color, consistency (e.g., firm = squamous or adenocarcinoma, soft = lymphoma or bronchioloalveolar carcinoma), location (bronchopulmonary segment), relationship to major bronchi (document tumor arising from a bronchus and/or obstruction of bronchi), vascular invasion, relationship to (invading through, retracting) or distance from pleura, distance from bronchial resection margin, and presence of postobstructive pneumonia.

5. Describe the remainder of the lung parenchyma including emphysematous changes (almost always centriacinar with sparing of the peripheral alveoli), fibrosis, consolidation, bullae, etc. Describe any abnormalities of the bronchi (bronchiectasis, mucous plugging).

6. Remove the soft tissue around the hilum and look for lymph nodes. Describe number, range in size, color, and consistency (anthracotic and firm or white and hard).

7. Incidental ribs removed during thoracotomies can be processed as described on page chapter 14.

   If a portion of the chest wall is attached, see "Pneumonectomies with partial chest wall resection" for processing.

Special studies

Alternative methods for sectioning lungs may best demonstrate the pathologic lesions present.

Coronal sections (anterior to posterior)

These sections are better for demonstrating hilar lesions as the bronchi and major vessels are seen in longitudinal section.

Superior to inferior (CT plane)

These sections are useful for showing the relationship of mediastinal lesions to the adjacent lung and for correlation with CT images. However, surgical specimens rarely involve such extensive resections.

Dissection of blood vessels

This type of dissection is useful for demonstrating vascular lesions (usually pulmonary emboli). Such lesions would be unusual in surgical specimens. The lung is approached from the lateral aspect within the fissure(s). A pair of scissors is used to cut towards the hilum until the pulmonary artery is entered. The major vessels can then be opened with the scissors. The vessels will not cross airways in this type of dissection.

Gross differential diagnosis (Fig. 26-1)

Squamous cell carcinomas are usually central and arise from bronchi. The tumors often obstruct the airway, leading to atelectasis of the distal lung. They are usually gray/white, firm, and commonly demonstrate necrosis or central cavitation.

Adenocarcinomas are more often peripheral and frequently involve the pleura. The tumors are gray/yellow and rarely cavitate.

Undifferentiated large cell carcinomas are more often peripheral and do not have a distinctive gross appearance.

Bronchioloalveolar carcinomas (BACs) form indistinct soft (because there is no desmoplastic response) gray nodules. Lymphomas and focal areas of inflammation can also have this gross appearance. BACs are commonly multifocal and may be associated with copious extracellular mucin.

Small cell carcinomas are rarely seen as surgical resections due to their propensity to metastasize early. These carcinomas are most commonly seen centrally.

Carcinoid tumors may be central or peripheral. Central carcinoids form polypoid endobronchial masses covered by non-ulcerated bronchial mucosa. They often extend into adjacent soft tissue to form a "dumbbell" shape. Peripheral carcinoids are seen as one or more discrete gray/yellow nodules near the pleura. Carcinoids are usually fleshy and homogeneous in appearance and have circumscribed borders.

Pulmonary chondroid hamartomas are not uncommon incidental findings on chest radiographs. The lesions are very well circumscribed, glistening white to gray, and may "pop out" of the adjacent lung parenchyma.

Microscopic sections

Tumor
Up to five cassettes including relationship to uninvolved lung, pleura, and adjacent vessels and bronchi.

Margins
Bronchial resection margin. Chest wall margins if attached chest wall is present (inferior, superior, anterior, posterior, and external). Pulmonary staple margin if the specimen is a lobectomy.

Lymph nodes
All hilar lymph nodes.

Pleura
Pleura closest to tumor if not previously submitted.

Uninvolved lung
One representative section of all lobes in the specimen.

Rib
If unattached to lung, a marrow squeeze may be performed. If attached to the lung, submit both margins and a section showing deepest point of invasion of tumor in relation to the bone.

Sample dictation

Received fresh, labeled with the patient's name and unit number and "lung," is a 150-g upper lobe of the right lung (12 × 10 × 6 cm) and bronchial remnant (1.1 cm in length × 0.6 cm in diameter). In the

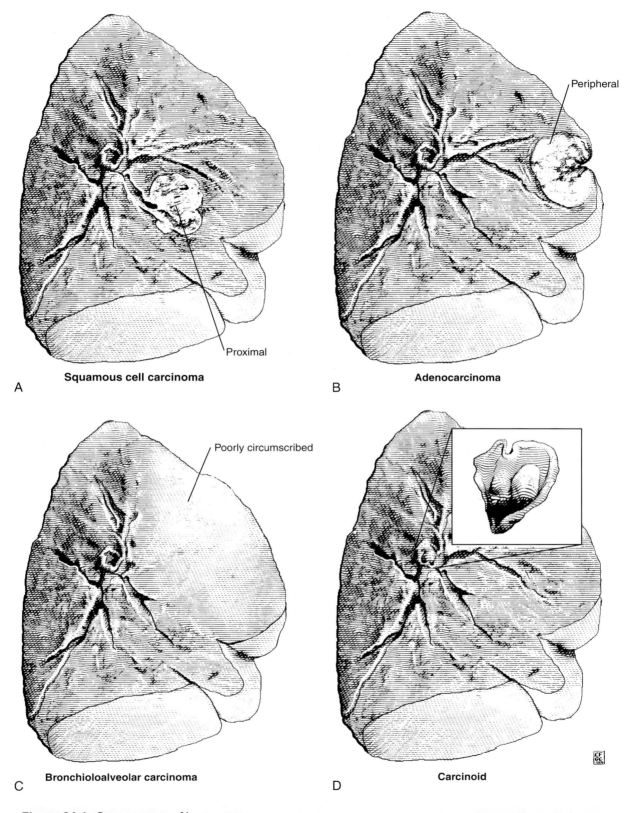

A **Squamous cell carcinoma**

Proximal

B **Adenocarcinoma**

Peripheral

C **Bronchioloalveolar carcinoma**

Poorly circumscribed

D **Carcinoid**

Figure 26-1 Gross anatomy of lung tumors.

anterior segment, there is a poorly circumscribed firm gray/white tumor (3 × 2.5 × 2.2 cm) with central necrosis, which is 5 cm from the uninvolved bronchial margin. The tumor causes retraction of the overlying pleura but does not grossly invade through the pleura, which has a smooth glistening surface. The tumor grossly invades an adjacent bronchus. There are mild emphysematous changes in the remainder of the lung parenchyma and a fibrous pleural scar (1.3 × 1.0 × 0.5 cm) at the apex of the lung. There are three anthracotic hilar lymph nodes, the largest measuring 1.4 cm in greatest dimension. The bronchial resection margin was frozen for intraoperative diagnosis. Tumor (0.5 × 0.5 × 0.5) and normal tissue (1 × 1 × 1) were given to Dr. Smith for special studies.

Cassette #1: Bronchial resection margin, en face, frozen-section remnant, 1 frag, ESS.
Cassettes #2 and 3: Tumor and pleura, 2 frags, RSS.
Cassettes #4 and 5: Tumor and adjacent lung, 2 frags, RSS.
Cassette #6: Tumor invading bronchus, 1 frag, RSS.
Cassette #7: Apical scar, 1 frag, RSS.
Cassette #8: Representative lung parenchyma, 2 frags, RSS.
Cassette #9: Three hilar lymph nodes, 3 frags, ESS.

Pathologic prognostic/diagnostic features sign-out checklist for lung carcinomas

Specimen type*
Major airway resection, wedge resection, segmentectomy, lobectomy, pneumonectomy.

Laterality*
Right, left.

Tumor site*
Upper lobe, middle lobe, lower lobe.

Tumor size*
Greatest dimension (optional: additional dimensions).

Histologic type*
Squamous cell carcinoma, adenocarcinoma, large cell carcinoma, bronchioloalveolar carcinoma, large cell neuroendocrine carcinoma, carcinoid tumor, atypical carcinoid tumor (well differentiated neuroendocrine carcinoma), small cell carcinoma (rarely resected) (Table 26-5), other rare types. The WHO classification is recommended.

Histologic grade*
Well, moderately, poorly differentiated, undifferentiated (squamous cell and adenocarcinoma) (Box 26-2).

Extent of invasion*
Lobar bronchus, main bronchus, carina.
Associated atelectasis or obstructive pneumonia of the entire lung.
Pleura: not involved, into but not through visceral pleura, through visceral pleura into parietal pleura (Fig. 26-2). Elastic stains may be used to define the elastica of the visceral pleura.[5] Invasion has been shown to have prognostic significance.[6]
Mediastinum, heart, great vessels, esophagus, trachea, vertebral body.
Separate nodules in the same lobe or a malignant pleural effusion.
If the carcinomas are of similar histology, multiple primary tumors in the same lobe are staged as T4, and those in different lobes as M1. If the carcinomas are of different histology, they are each staged separately.

Regional lymph nodes*
Absent, present (number involved, number examined). Includes nodes involved by direct extension of the primary tumor (but include description in report).

Location of lymph nodes.
Locations designated by the surgeon must be faithfully transcribed in the final report. Extracapsular invasion should be mentioned if present.

Distant metastasis*
Absent, present (includes separate tumor nodule/s in a different lobe; specify site if known).

Margins*
Uninvolved, involved (distance from closest margin).
Note whether squamous cell carcinoma is present at the bronchial margin.
Specify margin (bronchial, vascular, parenchymal, parietal pleural, chest wall, other attached tissue)

Venous (large vessel) invasion*
Absent, present.

Arterial (large vessel) invasion*
Absent, present.

Lymphatic (small vessel) invasion
Absent, present.

Nonneoplastic lung*
Pneumonia, metaplasia, granulomas, atelectasis, emphysema, fibrosis.

This checklist incorporates information from the ADASP (see www.panix.com/~adasp) and the CAP Cancer Committee protocols for reporting on cancer specimens (see www.cap.org/). The asterisked elements are considered to be scientifically validated or regularly used data elements that must be present in reports of cancer-directed surgical resection specimens from ACS CoC-approved cancer programs. The specific details of reporting the elements may vary among institutions.

The AJCC classification is given in Table 26-6.

Pneumonectomies with partial chest wall resection

Lung tumors that focally invade into the chest wall, but do not show evidence of metastatic spread, may be resected in continuity with the portions of several ribs. The patient usually will have been treated with radiation and/or chemotherapy.

The portion of chest wall should be oriented and the ribs present identified. Posterior resections may include portions of the vertebral bodies. Anterior resections may include costal cartilage. Specimens should be radiographed to identify all bones present and to evaluate possible bone destruction by tumor. The entire specimen should be fixed.

Soft tissue margins on the chest wall include the superficial soft tissue (lying beneath the subcutaneous tissue of the chest wall) as well as superior, inferior, medial, and lateral soft tissue around the ribs. Parietal pleura in these areas should also be sampled. These margins, as well as sections of the tumor and lung, are taken first. After soft tissue sections have been removed, the lung may be removed from the chest wall portion. The bones are then decalcified. Rib margins are taken from the anterior and posterior portion of each rib. Additional sections are taken demonstrating the relationship of the tumor to the adjacent ribs, including areas suspicious for bone destruction on the specimen radiograph.

Transplant pneumonectomies

The common indications for lung transplantation are idiopathic pulmonary fibrosis, emphysema, cystic fibrosis, and pulmonary hypertension. The pathologist's role is to document the underlying disease in the recipient lung and to identify any clinically unsuspected disease process. Occasionally unused donor lungs will be submitted. If the contralateral lung has been transplanted, it is important to look for unsuspected disease processes that may affect the recipient (e.g., infection, malignancies).

Both recipient and donor lungs may be processed in the same manner.

Processing the specimen

1. Weigh and measure the lung. Examine the pleura for evidence of disease (smooth and glistening, dull and irregular, adhesions). Sterile tissue is submitted for cultures (bacterial, fungal, and viral) from an unused donor lung if the contralateral lung has been transplanted.
2. Inflate the lung with formalin, either through the bronchus or by using a syringe, and fix overnight.

Table 26-5 Classification of pulmonary neuroendocrine (NE) tumors[4]

FEATURE	TYPICAL CARCINOID	ATYPICAL CARCINOID	LARGE-CELL NE CARCINOMA	SMALL-CELL LUNG CARCINOMA
Necrosis	Absent	Almost always	Almost always	Almost always
Mitoses/10 HPF	<1 (0 to 1)	3–4 (range 0 to 8)	66 (range 22–138)	46 (range 28–124)
Chromatin pattern	Finely granular	Fine to coarsely granular	Coarse or finely granular, may be vesicular	Finely granular, uniform
Nucleoli	May be present	May be present	Often present, may be prominent or faint	Absent or faint
Pleomorphism	Rare	Mild	Moderate	Absent
Cell size			Large	Small <3 lymphocytes
Nuclear molding	Absent	Absent	Uncharacteristic	Characteristic
Cytoplasm	Moderate	Moderate	Ample	Scant
Nuclear smear and basophilic staining of vessels and stroma	Absent	Absent	Rare	Frequent
Nuclear/cytoplasmic ratio			Low	High

Box 26-2 Grading system for lung carcinomas

Grade 1	Well differentiated
Grade 2	Moderately differentiated
Grade 3	Poorly differentiated
Grade 4	Undifferentiated

The least differentiated portion of the carcinoma is used for grading. Undifferentiated carcinomas do not exhibit either squamous or glandular differentiation. Small cell and large cell carcinomas are designated grade 4.

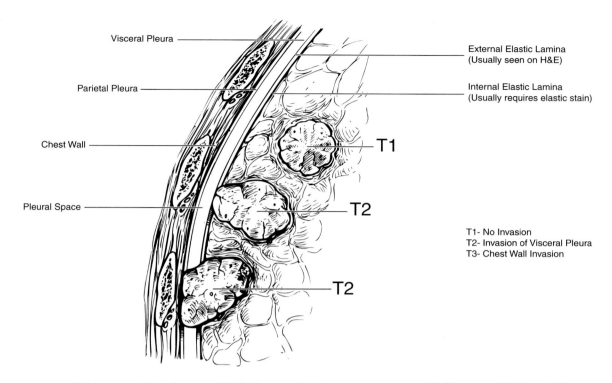

Visceral Pleura

Parietal Pleura

Chest Wall

Pleural Space

External Elastic Lamina
(Usually seen on H&E)

Internal Elastic Lamina
(Usually requires elastic stain)

T1

T2

T2

T1- No Invasion
T2- Invasion of Visceral Pleura
T3- Chest Wall Invasion

Figure 26-2 Pleural involvement by carcinomas. The inner pleural elastic lamina is best seen using special elastic stains.[5,6] Invasion has been shown to have prognostic significance.

3. Cut the lung into sagittal sections.
4. Examine the parenchyma carefully looking for focal lesions or evidence of infection, ischemia (variations in color or texture), or trauma.
5. Submit from 6 to 10 cassettes including central and peripheral lung parenchyma, bronchial resection margin, smaller airways, pulmonary vessels (both large and small), hilar lymph nodes, and any focal lesions. If infection is suspected, order AFB, Gram, and MSS stains on a representative cassette.

Special studies

Pulmonary hypertension

Angiograms may be performed on surgical specimens by filling the vessels with contrast agent using the pressures observed clinically. Although this is unlikely to be necessary for clinical management of the patient, the demonstration of markedly diminished pulmonary vasculature can provide an excellent teaching example. The tissue slices can also be radiographed.

Extrapleural pneumonectomies

Extrapleural pneumonectomy is a commando resection of malignant mesothelioma and, on rare occasions, of carcinoma of the lung that is restricted to the lung, pleura, and local lymph nodes. The lung with attached hemidiaphragm is resected together with the surrounding parietal and mediastinal pleura and a portion of the pericardium.

Extrapleural pneumonectomy is associated with a better prognosis in mesothelioma. However, whether this is because this population tends to be younger, healthier, and with more limited disease, or whether the procedure itself is beneficial, is still unclear (but under investigation).

Table 26-6 AJCC (6th edition) classification of lung tumors		
Tumor	TX	Primary tumor cannot be assessed, or tumor proven by the presence of malignant cells in sputum or bronchial washings but not visualized by imaging or bronchoscopy
	T0	No evidence of primary tumor
	Tis	Carcinoma in situ
	T1	Tumor ≤3 cm in greatest dimension and surrounded by lung or visceral pleura without bronchoscopic evidence of invasion more proximal than the lobar bronchus (i.e., not in the main bronchus). The uncommon superficial tumor of any size with its invasive component limited to the bronchial wall, which may extend proximal to the main bronchus, is also classified as T1
	T2	Tumor with any of the following features of size or extent: >3 cm in greatest dimension Involves main bronchus, 2 cm or more distal to the carina Invades the visceral pleura Associated with atelectasis or obstructive pneumonitis that extends to the hilar region but does not involve the entire lung
	T3	Tumor of any size that directly invades any of the following: chest wall (including superior sulcus tumors), diaphragm, mediastinal pleura, parietal pericardium; or tumor in the main bronchus less than 2 cm distal to the carina, but without involvement of the carina; or associated atelectasis or obstructive pneumonitis of the entire lung
	T4	Tumor of any size that invades any of the following: mediastinum, heart, great vessels, trachea, esophagus, vertebral body, or carina; or separate tumor nodules in the same lobe; or tumor with a malignant pleural effusion
Regional lymph nodes	NX	Regional lymph nodes cannot be assessed
	N0	No regional lymph node metastasis
	N1	Metastasis to ipsilateral peribronchial and/or ipsilateral hilar lymph nodes, and intrapulmonary nodes including involvement by direct extension of the primary tumor
	N2	Metastasis to ipsilateral mediastinal and/or subcarinal lymph node(s)
	N3	Metastasis to contralateral mediastinal, contralateral hilar, ipsilateral or contralateral scalene, or supraclavicular lymph node(s)
Distant metastasis	MX	Distant metastasis cannot be assessed
	M0	No distant metastasis
	M1	Distant metastasis present—includes separate tumor nodule(s) in a different lobe (ipsilateral or contralateral)

Note: This classification does not apply to noncarcinomas.

Relevant clinical history includes prior exposure to asbestos (e.g., by occupation), radiation exposure, extent of disease by radiologic studies, prior procedures and diagnoses, and prior treatment (e.g., talc poudrage).

Processing the specimen

1. Weigh the specimen and record the outer dimensions (total dimensions, dimensions of lung, dimensions of diaphragm, size of pericardium, bronchial margin).
2. Identify areas of tumor involvement in the pleura. Distinguish tumor from pleural plaque (see item 4). The bases tend to be involved more extensively than the apex.

    It may be useful to take fresh tissue for EM and cytogenetics. Match tissue taken for special studies with a formalin-fixed section at the same site to evaluate the corresponding tissue for histologic features and viability.
3. Inflate the lung through the bronchus and fix overnight.
4. Examine and describe the outer surface of the pleura (i.e., the parietal pleura).

- Rents in the parietal pleura. Location and size.
- Percentage involvement of pleura by tumor. Occasionally the full extent of parietal pleural involvement is evident only after examining the inner aspect, either via rents in the pleura or after coronal sectioning. Describe the range of size of the nodules (three dimensions), and the range in thickness of the unfused pleura (leave until after sectioning in areas fused with visceral pleura).
- Chest wall tissue. Look for areas of muscle or soft tissue adherent to the parietal pleura that may indicate invasion into the chest wall.
- Pericardium. Involvement by tumor, penetration through to pericardial surface (present or absent).

  Plaques are discrete patches of flat thickened hard white pleura, often with a shelf-like margin, and sometimes with calcification. The surface is relatively smooth with characteristic small pits. The thickness is usually about 0.3 to 0.5 cm.

  Mesothelioma is usually less dense than plaque, firm (not as hard as plaque), gray/white, frequently nodular, and occasionally myxoid in appearance.

5. Serially section the specimen at 1 cm intervals in the coronal (frontal) plane. These sections are easy to cut, easy to orient, and well demonstrate the pleural involvement.
6. Describe the tumor involvement of the diaphragm including distance from margins (anterior, posterior, medial, and lateral), depth of invasion into the diaphragm (noting any invasion of skeletal muscle), and involvement of the peritoneal surface of the diaphragm (this is rare).
7. Describe visceral pleura involvement including the percentage of visceral pleura fused to parietal pleura, the range in thickness of fused and unfused pleura, the percentage of unfused visceral pleura involved by tumor, the range of size of the nodules (unfused visceral pleura in three dimensions), and the site and size of any loculated effusion.

   Describe the lung parenchyma including any tumor involvement. Usually mesothelioma does not directly invade into lung parenchyma but pushes pleura ahead of it as it bulges into the lung. However, tumor often invades into and thickens interlobar fissures (note site and extent). Describe parenchymal fibrosis, emphysematous changes, and consolidation.

   Rarely, a second malignancy may be detected within the lung parenchyma.
8. Describe (number and size) any hilar lymph nodes (anthracotic and soft = normal; white and hard = tumor). Mesothelioma may metastasize to lymph nodes and this is an adverse prognostic feature.
9. Selectively ink (before taking sections) areas of the resection margins that demonstrate the closest extension of tumor involvement to the pleural surface (tumor involvement of margins is an adverse prognostic factor) and diaphragmatic margins. Take sections (perpendicular to the pleura, 2 to 3 per cassette if the pleura is less than 0.5 cm thick) from the apex of the lung, from the anterior, posterior, medial, and lateral pleura at one level and perpendicular sections from the anterior, lateral, medial, posterior, and deep (= inferior) margins of the diaphragm.
10. A small segment of rib is usually resected. Describe dimensions, color of bone, and color of marrow cavity. A marrow squeeze can be submitted (see chapter 14) unless gross lesions are identified or the bone is attached to the chest wall. In the latter case, the bone should be radiographed and all sections suspicious for bony involvement submitted. If a portion of chest wall is received attached to the specimen, the margins of the chest wall are submitted.

Special studies

Mesotheliomas

Usually the diagnosis has been well established prior to resection. Mesotheliomas can be distinguished from other tumors by characteristic findings by immunohistochemistry, EM, and cytogenetics (see chapter 7). It may be helpful to save tissue for these studies.

Fiber analysis

Formalin-fixed lung tissue (not tumor) for particle analysis by energy dispersive x-ray analysis (quantitative asbestos fiber counts and identification as chrysotile, amosite, tremolite, crocidolite) may be used for these studies. The periphery of the lower lobe is preferred. The counts are not performed on tumor or on pleural plaques.

Gross differential diagnosis

Mesotheliomas. Mesothelioma is usually white to gray, firm, and homogeneous. Hemorrhage or necrosis is rare.

Mesotheliomas grow in a very characteristic pattern within the pleura. Early in the development of the tumor, macules, polyps, and/or nodules form, probably first in the parietal pleura. Prior to fusion of the parietal and visceral pleura, the parietal pleura is often more extensively involved. With time, the involved areas enlarge, coalesce, and thicken the pleura; the parietal and visceral pleura fuse to form a thick rind about the lung and extend into the interlobar fissure(s). Tumor is often more extensive in basal portions of the lung than in apical areas. It would be helpful to identify cases with limited early involvement that might refute or support the limited evidence that mesotheliomas originate in the parietal pleura.

The tumor is usually sharply demarcated from the lung parenchyma. However, sampling of areas in which the tumor bulges into peripheral parenchyma may reveal microscopic areas of invasion. Separate tumor nodules within lung parenchyma are exceedingly uncommon.

Invasive areas into soft tissue of the chest wall (adipose tissue, muscle, fascia, or bone) are usually small and focal in extrapleural pneumonectomy specimens, as invasion of the chest wall is generally a contraindication to surgery. Tumor is sometimes seen in soft tissue at the site of prior surgical interventions (e.g., chest tube sites). Lymph node metastasis may occur, but involvement is not usually seen on gross examination.

Carcinoma. Extrapleural pneumonectomy is rarely performed for carcinomas with pleural involvement. The carcinoma is usually present within the lung and often has central cavitation or necrosis. The involvement of the pleura may be diffuse, closely mimicking mesothelioma, but patchy involvement with focal nodule formation and sparing of large areas of the pleura are clues suggesting carcinomatous involvement, especially when the parenchymal tumor is large. Invasion into soft tissue or bone may be present. Lymph node metastases are frequent.

Talc pleurodesis. Some patients will have undergone talc pleurodesis to control symptoms from pleural effusions. The talc will be between the parietal and the visceral pleura and will have caused them to fuse. The talc is pale yellow grossly and is associated with a fibrotic reaction that can make it difficult to distinguish from tumor. If necessary, it is possible to scrape such an area and look for polarizable material to show that it is talc, to avoid taking such tissue for special studies.

Pleural plaques. These plaques are strongly related to prior asbestos exposure (see, e.g., Bianchi et al[7]). Documenting their presence may be helpful in determining the likelihood of occupational exposure to asbestos.

Microscopic sections

Tumor and pleural margins
Take sections of resection margins (after selective inking) with underlying tumor and superficial lung parenchyma perpendicular to the pleural surface.

In the usual case with extensive fusion of parietal and visceral pleura, 9 to 10 cassettes including margins of parietal pleura chosen to demonstrate the closest approach of the tumor to the resection margin (apex, and anterior, lateral, posterior, and medial pleura), and tumor and diaphragm, tumor and lung (demonstrating any invasion into lung), small and large nodules, any areas of variable appearance.

In the unusual case with limited or no areas of fusion of parietal and visceral pleura, take sections as above and also sample the unfused visceral pleura (apex, anterior, lateral, posterior, medial, and diaphragmatic) to reflect areas of minimal (gray macules, nodules, or polyps) and maximal involvement (solitary or coalesced nodules).

Pericardium

One or two sections to demonstrate tumor, deepest penetration of pericardium by tumor, closest margin.

Diaphragmatic margins

Sections (inked, perpendicular) from anterior, lateral, posterior, and medial margins. Take sections to demonstrate the site of deepest penetration of tumor into the diaphragmatic muscle.

Lung

Representative sections from periphery of each lobe and any focal lesions.

Bronchial resection margin

One section, en face. This will usually have been taken as a frozen section.

Hilar lymph nodes

Submit each lymph node.

Separate rib

A bone marrow squeeze may be performed if the rib is not attached to the specimen and is grossly normal. If the bone is attached or grossly abnormal, the bone must be decalcified and cross-sections submitted. See Chapter 14 for instructions.

Sample dictation

Received fresh, labeled with the patient's name and unit number, are two specimens.
The first specimen is labeled "rib" and consists of a 5 × 2 × 0.8 cm segment of grossly unremarkable rib. A marrow squeeze is performed.

Cassette #1: Rib, marrow squeeze, 1 frag, RSS.

The second specimen is labeled "lung" and consists of a 750-g right extrapleural pneumonectomy specimen (26 × 20 × 15 cm) consisting of lung (24 × 18 × 14 cm), parietal pleura, pericardium (10 × 7 × 0.2 cm), and hemidiaphragm (21 × 14 × 0.3 to 1.4 cm). The parietal pleura is thickened, white, and intact except for a 6 × 0.5 cm linear rent over the lateral aspect of the mid portion of the lung. A few tags of fibrous tissue are adherent to the surface. Approximately 75% of the parietal pleura is occupied by nodules of firm gray tumor, ranging in size from 0.2 cm in diameter to 1.5 × 1.2 × 1.0 cm. Tumor is grossly present at the lateral pleural resection margin at the junction of upper and middle thirds of the lung. Apical and adjacent upper lobe pleura is relatively spared by tumor. The visceral and parietal pleura are thickened (to 1.2 cm maximum thickness, greatest basally) and are fused (75% of surface) except posteriorly and inferiorly where there is a loculated area of effusion (9 × 5 × 2 cm) filled with red cloudy fluid. Unfused visceral pleura (adjacent to the effusion) is thickened (0.2 cm) and contains scattered tumor nodules ranging from 0.2 to 0.5 cm in greatest dimension. The tumor bulges (0.5 cm) into lung parenchyma in several foci (lower lobe) and thickens (to 0.5 cm) an interlobar septum for a distance of approximately 4 cm. The diaphragmatic parietal and visceral pleura are thickened (1.2 cm) and fused. The diaphragmatic margins are grossly free of tumor with the closest approach of tumor being 0.2 cm at the lateral margin. Tumor invades to a depth of 0.3 cm into the muscle of the diaphragm, but the inferior surface is free of tumor. A flattened hard white pleural plaque (5 × 4 × 0.5 cm) is present in the lateral aspect of the parietal pleura. There are mild emphysematous changes in the peripheral lung parenchyma. The bronchial margin is free of lesions and was examined by frozen section with an en face section. There are three firm anthracotic lymph nodes in the perihilar soft tissue, the largest measuring 1.5 cm in greatest dimension. Tumor is saved for snap freezing, electron microscopy, and cytogenetics. Fixed tissue (5 × 5 × 5 cm) from the periphery of the lower lobe is given to Dr. J. Godleski for asbestos fiber analysis. Photographs are taken.

Cassette #2: Tumor, quick fix in formalin, 2 frags, area taken for special studies, RSS.

Cassette #3: Apical pleural margin, perpendicular, 1 frag, RSS.

Cassette #4: Medial pleural margin, perpendicular, 1 frag, RSS.

Cassette #5: Lateral pleural margin, site of gross extension to inked margin, perpendicular, 2 frags, RSS.

Cassette #6: Anterior pleural margin, perpendicular, 1 frag, RSS.

Cassette #7: Posterior pleural margin, perpendicular, 1 frag, RSS.

Cassette #8: Medial diaphragm margin, perpendicular, 1 frag, RSS.

Cassette #9: Lateral diaphragm margin, perpendicular, 1 frag, RSS.

Cassette #10: Anterior diaphragm margin, perpendicular, 1 frag, RSS.

Cassette #11: Posterior diaphragm margin, perpendicular, 1 frag, RSS.

Cassette #12: Tumor and diaphragm, central portion, deepest extent of tumor, 1 frag, RSS.

Cassettes #13 and 14: Tumor and interlobar fissure, 2 frags, RSS.

Cassette #15: Largest tumor nodule, parietal pleura, 2 frags, RSS

Cassette #16: Smallest and larger tumor nodules, visceral pleura, 3 frag, RSS

Cassette #17: Pleural plaque, 3 frags, RSS.

Cassette #18: Bronchial resection margin, frozen-section remnant, 1 frag, ESS.

Cassette #19: Upper lobe parenchyma, 1 frag, RSS.

Cassette #20: Middle lobe parenchyma, 1 frag, RSS.

Cassette #21: Lower lobe parenchyma, 1 frag, RSS.

Cassette #22: Perihilar lymph nodes, 3 frags, ESS.

Cassettes #23 and 24: Pericardium, closest approach of tumor, 4 frags, RSS.

Pathologic diagnostic/prognostic sign-out checklist for mesotheliomas

Specimen type*
Pleural resection, pericardial resection, extrapleural pneumonectomy.

Tumor site*
Right pleura/lung, left pleura/lung, pericardium.

Tumor configuration and size
Localized—greatest dimension.
Diffuse—maximum thickness.

Histologic type*
Mesothelioma, epithelial type (best prognosis), sarcomatoid type, mixed epithelial and sarcomatoid type, mesothelioma (usually sarcomatoid) with extensive desmoplasia (desmoplastic mesothelioma), undifferentiated, other rare types.

Extent of invasion
Parietal pleura, visceral pleura, invasion of lung parenchyma, invasion of diaphragmatic muscle, invasion of endothoracic fascia, invasion of mediastinal fat, invasion of pericardium (partial or transmural), invasion of bone (rib or spine), invasion of contralateral pleura, invasion of myocardium, invasion of brachial plexus .

Involvement of anatomic structures
Percentage of parietal and of visceral pleura involved by tumor, thickening of pleura by tumor (range/minimum and maximum), involvement of diaphragmatic muscle/pericardium/rib, involvement of adipose tissue/endothoracic fascia/skeletal muscle of chest wall, lung parenchyma or tissues in the contralateral chest.

Margins
Parietal pleura (anterior, posterior, medial, lateral), chest wall, diaphragm (anterior, posterior, medial, lateral, inferior or caudal), bronchus. A positive margin is defined as ink on tumor cells.

Pleura

Plaque (present/absent), talc pleurodesis.

Nonlesional lung

Fibrosis, pneumonia, emphysema, atelectasis, granulomas, ferruginous bodies, talc, etc.

Lymph nodes

Involved or not involved, number, location, extracapsular invasion if present.

This checklist incorporates information from the CAP Cancer Committee protocols for reporting on cancer specimens. The asterisked elements are considered to be scientifically validated or regularly used data elements that must be present in reports from ACS CoC-approved cancer programs. The specific reporting of some data elements may vary among institutions.

Three suggested staging systems are given in Tables 26-7, 26-8 and 26.9.

■ PLEURA

The pleura is usually biopsied when mesothelioma is a possible diagnosis (e.g., a typical radiologic appearance or effusion). This diagnosis may be very difficult to make on small specimens.

Biopsy

Determine from the clinician whether mesothelioma is in the clinical differential diagnosis. If there is sufficient lesional tissue, tissue is taken for special studies. In the OR consultation room, pathologists must be aggressive and timely about requesting additional tissue, especially whenever most or all of the lesional tissue has been taken for a frozen section, since freezing of the tumor may alter the immunoreactivity and prevent a definitive diagnosis. For example, calretinin may only be weakly positive in previously frozen tissue from mesotheliomas. The most important studies, after adequate tissue is made available for light microscopy, are EM followed by cytogenetics.

Pleurectomy

Pleurectomy is occasionally performed for debulking of mesothelioma if the tumor is unresectable. The specimen consists of multiple fragments of pleura with tumor implants. Pleurectomy may also be performed for diagnosis in a case of chronic fibrosing pleuritis to rule out the presence of a desmoplastic mesothelioma.

Table 26-7 Revised Sugarbaker staging system for malignant pleural mesothelioma[8]

STAGE	DESCRIPTION
I	Disease completely resected within the capsule of the parietal pleura without lymph node involvement (originally designated "adenopathy" in the published system), ipsilateral pleura, lung, pericardium, diaphragm, or chest wall disease limited to previous biopsy sites
II	All of stage I with positive resection margins and/or intrapleural lymph node involvement
III	Local extension of disease into the chest wall or mediastinum; heart, or through diaphragm, peritoneum; or with extrapleural lymph node involvement (mediastinal and peridiaphragmatic lymph nodes not located within the pleural reflection)
IV	Distant metastatic disease

Table 26-8 AJCC (6th edition) classification of pleural mesothelioma

Tumor	TX	Primary tumor cannot be assessed
	T0	No evidence of primary tumor
	T1	Tumor involves the ipsilateral parietal with or without focal involvement of visceral pleura
	T1a	Tumor involves ipsilateral parietal (mediastinal, diaphragmatic) pleura. No involvement of visceral pleura
	T1b	Tumor involves ipsilateral parietal (mediastinal, diaphragmatic) pleura, with focal involvement of the visceral pleura
	T2	Tumor involves any of the ipsilateral pleural surfaces with at least one of the following: Confluent with visceral pleural tumor (including fissure)
		Invasion of diaphragmatic muscle
		Invasion of lung parenchyma
	T3	Tumor involves any of the ipsilateral pleural surfaces, with at least one of the following: Invasion of the endothoracic fascia
		Invasion into mediastinal fat
		Solitary focus of tumor invading soft tissue of the chest wall
		Non-transmural involvement of the pericardium
		T3 describes locally advanced, but potentially resectable tumor
	T4	Tumor involves any of the ipsilateral pleural surfaces, with at least one of the following:
		Diffuse or multifocal invasion of soft tissue of the chest wall
		Any involvement of rib
		Invasion through the diaphragm to the peritoneum
		Invasion of any mediastinal organ(s)
		Direct extension to the contralateral pleura
		Invasion into the spine
		Extension to the internal surface of the pericardium
		Pericardial effusion with positive cytology
		Invasion of the myocardium
		Invasion of the brachial plexus
		T4 describes locally advanced, technically unresectable tumor
Regional lymph nodes	NX	Regional lymph nodes cannot be assessed
	N0	No regional lymph node metastasis
	N1	Metastasis to ipsilateral peribronchial and/or ipsilateral hilar lymph nodes including involvement by direct extension of the primary tumor
	N2	Metastasis to ipsilateral mediastinal, internal mammary, and/or subcarinal lymph node(s)
	N3	Metastasis to contralateral mediastinal, internal mammary, contralateral hilar, ipsilateral or contralateral scalene, or supraclavicular lymph node(s)
Distant metastasis	MX	Distant metastasis cannot be assessed
	M0	No distant metastasis
	M1	Distant metastasis present

Table 26-9 International Mesothelioma Interest Group staging system[9]

Primary tumor T	T1	
	T1a	Tumor limited to the ipsilateral parietal pleura, including mediastinal and diaphragmatic pleura. No involvement of the visceral pleura
	T1b	Tumor involving the ipsilateral parietal pleura, including mediastinal and diaphragmatic pleura. Scattered foci of tumor also involving the visceral pleura
	T2	Tumor involving each of the ipsilateral pleural surfaces (parietal, mediastinal, diaphragmatic, and visceral pleura) with at least one of the following features:
		Involvement of diaphragmatic muscle
		Confluent visceral pleural tumor (including the fissures) or extension of tumor from visceral pleura into the underlying pulmonary parenchyma
	T3	Tumor involving all of the ipsilateral pleural surfaces (parietal, mediastinal, diaphragmatic, and visceral pleura) with at least one of the following features:
		Involvement of the endothoracic fascia
		Extension into the mediastinal fat
		Solitary, completely resectable focus of tumor extending into the soft tissues of the chest wall
		Nontransmural involvement of the pericardium
	T4	Tumor involving all of the ipsilateral pleural surfaces (parietal, mediastinal, diaphragmatic, and visceral pleura) with at least one of the following features:
		Diffuse extension or multifocal masses of tumor in the chest wall with or without associated rib destruction
		Direct transdiaphragmatic extension of tumor to the peritoneum
		Direct extension to the contralateral pleura
		Direct extension of tumor to one or more mediastinal organs
		Direct extension of tumor into the spine
		Tumor extending through to the internal surface of the pericardium with or without a pericardial effusion; or tumor involving the myocardium
Regional lymph nodes	NX	Regional lymph nodes cannot be assessed
	N0	No regional lymph node metastasis
	N1	Metastasis to ipsilateral bronchopulmonary or hilar lymph nodes
	N2	Metastasis to the subcarinal or the ipsilateral mediastinal lymph nodes, including the ipsilateral internal mammary nodes
	N3	Metastasis to contralateral mediastinal, contralateral internal mammary, ipsilateral or contralateral supraclavicular lymph node(s)
Distant metastasis	MX	Distant metastasis cannot be assessed
	M0	No distant metastasis
	M1	Distant metastasis present

Processing the specimen

1. Describe each fragment of pleura separately including size and thickness. However, if three or more fragments are present, describe the number of fragments, overall dimensions, and dimensions of smallest and largest fragment. Describe any lesions including color, consistency, size, percentage of pleural involvement, any variability in appearance, and distance from margins (if received as a single fragment). Record the presence, size, and tumor involvement of any other structures (e.g., lung, skeletal muscle, adipose tissue, pericardium).

   Note the presence or absence of pleural plaques and give dimensions.

2. Take lesional tissue for EM, cytogenetics, and snap freezing.

3. Selectively ink margins that appear involved by tumor if a single fragment is received.

4. Submit approximately one cassette for every cm of greatest dimension of tumor. Document representative involved margins if a single fragment is received (ink selectively or submit en face if grossly involved).

5. If the differential diagnosis is fibrosing pleuritis versus desmoplastic mesothelioma, search carefully for all areas suspicious for tumor nodules. Extensive sampling is often necessary in such cases to confirm, or exclude, a desmoplastic mesothelioma.

REFERENCES

1. Yousem SA, Berry GJ, Cagle PT, et al. Revision of the 1990 working formulation for the classification of pulmonary allograft rejection; Lung Rejection Study Group. J Heart Lung Transplant 15:1-15, 1996.

2. Yousem S. A perspective on the Revised Working Formulation for the grading of lung allograft rejection. Transplant Proc 28:477-479, 1996.

3. http://tpis.upmc.edu/ The University of Pittsburgh Organ Transplant site.

4. Travis WD, Linnoila RI, Tsokos MG, et al. Neuroendocrine tumors of the lung with proposed criteria for large-cell neuroendocrine carcinoma. Am J Surg Pathol 15:529-553, 1991.

5. Bunker ML, Raab SS, Landreneau RJ, Silverman J. The diagnosis and significance of visceral pleural invasion in lung carcinoma: histologic predictors and the role of elastic stains. Am J Clin Pathol 112:777-783, 1999.

6. Gallagher B, Urbanski SJ. The significance of pleural elastica invasion by lung carcinomas. Hum Pathol 21:512-517, 1990.

7. Bianchi C, Brollo A, Ramani L, Zuch C. Pleural plaques as risk indicators for malignant pleural mesothelioma: a necroscopy-based study. Am J Industrial Med 32:445-449, 1997.

8. Sugarbaker DJ, Flores RM, Jaklitsch MT, et al. Resection margins, extrapleural nodal status, and cell type determine postoperative long-term survival in trimodality therapy of malignant pleural mesothelioma: results in 183 patients. J Thorac Cardiovasc Surg 117:54-65, 99.

9. Rusch VW. A proposed new international TNM staging system for malignant pleural mesothelioma from the International Mesothelioma Interest Group. Chest 108:1122-1128, 1995.

Lymph nodes, spleen, and bone marrow

27

The lymph nodes, spleen, and bone marrow are affected by a wide variety of neoplastic, infectious, and systemic diseases.

Relevant clinical history (in addition to age and gender)

See Table 27-1.

Table 27-1 Relevant clinical history	
HISTORY RELEVANT TO ALL SPECIMENS	HISTORY RELEVANT TO LYMPH NODE, SPLEEN, AND BONE MARROW SPECIMENS
Organ/tissue resected or biopsied	Lymphadenopathy
Purpose of the procedure	Organomegaly (liver or spleen)
Gross appearance of the organ/tissue/lesion sampled	Hematologic findings (e.g., pancytopenia or lymphocytosis)
Any unusual features of the clinical presentation	*Helicobacter pylori* infection
Any unusual features of the gross appearance	LDH level (a poor prognostic factor that correlates with tumor burden)
Prior surgery/biopsies—results	Constitutional symptoms (e.g., night sweats, fever)
Prior malignancy	
Prior treatment (radiation therapy, chemotherapy, drug use that can change the histologic appearance of tissues)	Congenital immune disorders
	Organ transplantation (solid organ or bone marrow)
	Serology (e.g., HTLV-1, Epstein–Barr virus)
Compromised immune system	Autoimmune disease

■ BONE MARROW

Bone marrow biopsies are performed to evaluate suspected hematologic disorders or for the staging of carcinomas and lymphomas.

Processing the specimen

1. Biopsies are optimally fixed in Zenker's, which provides excellent histologic detail as well as decalcification of the specimen.
2. Specimens should ideally remain in Zenker's for a minimum of 12 hours and for no more than 30 hours. If the specimen is easily bent, decalcification is adequate. Always check the

date on the requisition form (i.e., specimens may arrive the same day or the day after the biopsy) to make sure that specimens are not left in Zenker's for too long.

3. Describe the number of fragments, shape (tubular, irregular), and dimensions (length and diameter). Wrap in lens paper and submit the entire specimen. The cassette is rinsed in one or more water baths with stirring (use a magnetic stirrer) for 20 to 30 minutes. Mercury waste, including the initial water baths, must be disposed of into a special waste container.

4. Describe any blood smears received with the biopsy. Unstained smears should be stained with Wright Giemsa.

5. Order one H&E and two Giemsa stains for routine cases.

Special studies on bone marrow biopsies

Suspected infectious disease (e.g., in immunocompromised patients)

Special stains for organisms can be ordered on fixed sections (e.g. AFB and silver stains).

Myelodysplastic or myeloproliferative syndromes

Reticulin stains may be ordered to evaluate marrow fibrosis. Iron stains are examined to evaluate ring sideroblasts.

Sample dictation

Received in Zenker's fixative, labeled with the patient's name and unit number and "right iliac," is a 1.5 cm in length by 0.4 cm in diameter bone marrow biopsy stained yellow by the fixative. Accompanying the specimen are two unstained coverslips that are submitted for Wright Giemsa staining. The specimen is decalcified in Zenker's fixative prior to submission.

Cassette #1: 1 frag, ESS.

■ LYMPH NODES

Lymph nodes: Suspected lymphoproliferative disease

A single enlarged lymph node is often biopsied. Common diagnoses are reactive hyperplasia, lymphoma, and occasionally metastatic carcinoma. Appropriate processing of fresh tissue is necessary in order to use the special techniques available for analyzing lymphoproliferative disorders (immunoperoxidase studies on frozen sections, flow cytometry, cytogenetics, and DNA analysis). In general, if there is enough lesional tissue, some tissue is fixed in formalin as non-lymphoid antigens may not be optimally preserved in B5 (e.g., keratin) and the lacunar variants of Reed–Sternberg cells in nodular sclerosing Hodgkin's lymphoma are seen best in formalin-fixed tissue.

If infectious disease is suspected, appropriate precautions are taken (see Chapter 8) and tissue sent for culture if not already submitted by the surgeon.

Processing the specimen

1. Record the outer dimensions of the lymph node. Make very thin (2 to 3 mm) serial sections perpendicular to the long axis looking for focal lesions. Describe the node including color (uniform or irregular, pigmentation), nodularity, consistency (rubbery, hard), cystic areas, necrosis, or hemorrhage. If infectious disease is suspected, save a small amount of sterile tissue for cultures (viral and bacterial).

   A touch prep can be useful to make a preliminary diagnosis to guide the distribution of tissue.

2. Fresh tissue is submitted for special studies if indicated (see below).

3. Fix most of the tissue (after slicing thinly) in B5 for 3 to 5 hours and representative sections

in formalin. After fixation in B5, the tissue can be placed in formalin. Overfixation in B5 will make the tissue brittle.

4. All tissue is allowed to fix for at least 24 hours before it is submitted for processing. B5 fixed tissues must be washed in one or more water baths with a magnetic stirrer for 20 to 30 minutes. The water must be discarded in a mercury waste container. The tissue is then washed for an additional hour in cool running water. If there is sufficient tissue, one cassette may be processed the same day.

Special studies

Frozen tissue

Some immunohistochemical markers in hematopathology are most sensitive on frozen tissue. Frozen tissue can also be used for mRNA and DNA analysis. Frozen tissue is saved for all lymph nodes with a suspicion of a lymphoproliferative disorder or without a prior diagnosis. Save approximately 5 to 10 fragments (0.4 to 0.5 cm in greatest dimension) for snap freezing.

Flow cytometry

Flow cytometry may be useful for suspected lymphoproliferative disorders, difficult to classify processes, or typing of tissues from HIV-positive patients. Tissue is not submitted for flow cytometry in cases of Hodgkin's lymphoma or small fragmented specimens as the only diagnostic lesion might be in the fragment submitted for flow cytometry.

DNA analysis

DNA analysis may be useful for some difficult to classify lymphoproliferative disorders, processes with a suspected diagnostic rearrangement, EBV analysis, or leukemias. Fresh or frozen tissue may be used.

Cytogenetics

Cytogenetics may be useful for processes with suspected diagnostic chromosomal abnormalities. The cells must be viable for karyotype analysis. In some cases, FISH on fixed tissue may be useful.

Electron microscopy

EM may be useful for unusual tumors or metastatic tumors.

Gross differential diagnosis

Lymphoma. Lymphomas often cause diffuse expansion of the node so that it appears rounded and loses the normal bean-shaped contour. Lymphomas have a homogeneous tan/white fleshy appearance.

Hodgkin's lymphoma. The node looks very similar to non-Hodgkin lymphomas. The nodular sclerosing variant may have gross areas of nodularity with sclerotic bands and a thick capsule.

Reactive nodes. The nodes can be quite large but are usually softer than in lymphomas and are tan brown in color. Focal necrosis can be seen in cases of Kikuchi disease.

Carcinoma. The nodes are often white and hard with necrotic areas. Cystic spaces may be present (especially in papillary thyroid carcinoma or teratoma). Focal involvement of the node is common.

Tuberculosis. There are usually areas of geographic (caseating) necrosis. Tissue should be sent for culture and handled as little as possible prior to fixation. Avoid performing frozen sections as this may aerosolize infectious organisms. A presumptive diagnosis can usually be made using touch preparations, if necessary.

Sarcoidosis. Lymph nodes are diffusely firm and white.

Microscopic sections

Lymph node

Usually the entire lymph node can be submitted. If it is very large, one cassette per cm is sufficient. Order H&E on all sections and one Giemsa (on the second level) on the best B5 fixed tissue, in cases of suspected lymphoma. Six to eight unstained sections for immunohistochemistry on one block (B5 if there is a suspected lymphoid proliferation; formalin for nonlymphoid tumors) should only be ordered for special cases. Order levels if the specimen is small (e.g., in one cassette).

Pathologic diagnostic/prognostic features checklist for sign-out for lymphomas

Specimen type*

Lymphadenectomy, other.
Excisional biopsy, incisional biopsy, core needle biopsy.

Specimen site*

Involvement of specific lymph node regions, spleen, bone marrow, organs.

Histologic type*

Hodgkin's lymphoma, non-Hodgkin lymphomas (WHO classification).

Histologic grade

Follicular lymphoma and nodular sclerosing Hodgkin's lymphoma (Table 27-2, Box 27-1).

Extent of pathologically examined tumor*

Involvement of a single lymph node region; specify site.
Involvement of multiple lymph node regions; specify.
Splenic involvement.
Liver involvement.
Bone marrow involvement.
Other organ involvement; specify.

Phenotyping*

Performed, not performed.

Immunoperoxidase studies

Often used to classify lymphomas into B and T cell types and for further subclassification. The method used should be included (flow cytometry versus IHC, paraffin sections versus frozen tissue). Use CD nomenclature and specific antibody designations when relevant.

Other special studies

Information obtained from other studies (e.g., Southern blot, FISH, cytogenetics, RT-PCR, viral identification) should be incorporated into the report.

This checklist incorporates information from the ADASP (see www.panix.com/~adasp/) and the CAP Cancer Committee protocols for reporting on cancer specimens (see www.cap.org/). The asterisked elements are considered to be scientifically validated or regularly used data elements that must be present in reports of cancer-directed surgical resection specimens from ACS CoC-approved cancer programs. The specific details of reporting the elements may vary among institutions.

The AJCC classification is provided in Tables 27-3 and 27-4.

Table 27-2 Grading of follicular lymphoma

GRADE	FEATURES
1	0–5 centroblasts per HPF
2	6–15 centroblasts per HPF
3	>15 centroblasts per HPF
3a	Centrocytes are still present
3b	Centroblasts form solid sheets with no residual centrocytes

Reporting of pattern

Follicular	>75% follicular
Follicular and diffuse	25–75% follicular
Focally follicular	<25% follicular

Counts are for a 0.159 mm^2 HPF. Count 10 HPF and divide by 10. See Chapter 9, "Measuring with the microscope," for methods to determine field size.

Box 27-1 Grading of nodular sclerosing Hodgkin's lymphoma[1]

Grade I (NSI)

1. <25% of nodules show lymphocyte depletion, or
2. <25% of nodules show numerous anaplastic Hodgkin cells without depletion of lymphocytes

Grade II (NSII)

1. 25% or more of nodules show lymphocyte depletion, or
2. 25% or more of nodules show numerous anaplastic Hodgkin cells without depletion of lymphocytes

Lymph nodes for tumor staging[2-11]

Lymph nodes are the most important part of any major tumor resection. The absence of lymph node metastasis is evidence that the disease may be localized and that a surgical cure might have been achieved. The presence of lymph node metastasis usually predicts systemic dissemination and a poor outcome for the patient. Because lymph node status is so important for prognosis and therapeutic decision making, lymph nodes must always be diligently sought after and examined. For some treatment protocols, a minimum number of lymph nodes must be examined.

Retroperitoneal lymph node dissections for testicular cancer often require extra sections (see page 411).

If there is a clinical suspicion of infection or sarcoidosis, sterile tissue may be sent for cultures. Frozen sections or cytologic preparations may be helpful to guide tissue processing.

Processing the specimen

1. Often nodes are submitted surrounded by a large amount of adipose tissue.

   Fresh dissection. This method is useful for OR consultations or when there is a small amount of tissue to examine. If there is any question of a lymphoproliferative disorder, the lymph nodes *must* be examined prior to fixation in order to apportion tissue for appropriate special studies.

   Fixative does not penetrate well through an intact capsule, resulting in poor histologic preservation of the lymphocytes (but usually adequate preservation for the evaluation of metastatic tumors).

STAGE	EXTENT OF INVOLVEMENT
Table 27-3 AJCC (6th edition) classification of non-Hodgkin lymphomas	
I	Involvement of a single node region (I) or localized involvement of a single extralymphatic organ or site in the absence of any lymph node involvement (I_E) (rare in Hodgkin's lymphoma)
II	Involvement of two or more lymph node regions on the same side of the diaphragm (II), or localized involvement of a single extralymphatic organ or site in association with regional lymph node involvement with or without other lymph node regions on the same side of the diaphragm (II_E). The number of lymph node regions involved may be indicated by a subscript (e.g., II_3)
III	Involvement of lymph node regions on both sides of the diaphragm (III) which also may be accompanied by extralymphatic extension in association with adjacent lymph node involvement (III_E), by involvement of the spleen (III_S), or both ($III_{E,S}$)
IV	Diffuse or disseminated involvement of one or more extralymphatic organs with or without associated lymph node involvement, or isolated extralymphatic organ involvement in the absence of adjacent regional lymph node involvement, but in conjunction with disease in distant site(s). Any involvement of the liver or bone marrow, or nodular involvement of the lung(s). The location of stage IV disease is identified further with the following notations:

Spleen	S
Waldeyer's (tonsil naso-oropharynx)	W
Pulmonary (lung)	L
Bone marrow	M
Osseous (bone)	O
Hepatic	H
Gastrointestinal	GI
Pericardium	Pcard
Skin	D
Pleura	P
Soft tissue	Softis
Thyroid	Thy

Note: There are separate staging systems for mycosis fungoides and multiple myeloma that use clinical parameters. The St. Jude staging system is used for children with NHL (usually Burkitt's lymphoma, lymphoblastic lymphoma, or diffuse large cell lymphoma).

Lymph nodes are firmer than fat and can be found by gently "squashing" the fat with one finger. The nodes are discrete ovoid areas that cannot be completely compressed. When bisected, they are well circumscribed and more tan than the surrounding yellow fat. In some lymph nodes the central portion may be extensively replaced by fat, leaving only a thin rim of lymphoid tissue.

If no or only a few lymph nodes are found using this method, the remainder of the specimen can be fixed in Bouin's and processed as described below to look for small lymph nodes. Small nodes can sometimes be found adjacent to blood vessels.

Dissection after fixation. Bouin's is a good fixative for detecting nodes. However, this fixative may not preserve hormone receptors and is not a good choice if the primary site is unknown and immunoperoxidase studies may be needed. Other special fixatives have been used for the same purpose.[2,3]

Fix the entire specimen for several hours or overnight. Specimens fixed in formalin can be postfixed in Bouin's. Serially section through the specimen. The lymph nodes will be white and the surrounding fat yellow. When a lymph node is encountered, blunt dissect it free. This is a good method for finding very small (<0.5 cm) nodes.

Soft tissue attached to an organ (e.g., stomach, colon, kidney) can be stripped and placed in Bouin's after all the margins have been identified. Most nodes are located in the tissue close to the organ. Leave the soft tissue directly beneath the tumor in place in order to distinguish satellite nodules from nodes completely replaced by tumor.

2. Record the total dimensions of the specimen, number of lymph nodes, and size of the largest node. Describe the nodes:

STAGE	EXTENT OF INVOLVEMENT
Table 27-4 AJCC classification of Hodgkin's lymphoma	
I	Involvement of a single node region (I) or localized involvement of a single extralymphatic organ or site in the absence of any lymph node involvement (I_E) (rare in Hodgkin's lymphoma). Multifocal involvement of a single extralymphatic organ is classified as stage IE and not stage IV
II	Involvement of two or more lymph node regions on the same side of the diaphragm (II), or localized involvement of a single extralymphatic organ or site in association with regional lymph node involvement with or without involvement of other lymph node regions on the same side of the diaphragm (II_E) Note: The number of lymph node regions involved may be indicated by a subscript, e.g. II_3. For stage I to IIIA disease, involvement of 4 or more nodal regions adversely affects rates of disease-free and overall survival
III	Involvement of lymph node regions on both sides of the diaphragm (III) which also may be accompanied by extralymphatic extension in association with adjacent lymph involvement (III_E), or by involvement of the spleen (III_S), or both ($III_{E,S}$)
IV	Diffuse or disseminated involvement of one or more extralymphatic organs, with or without associated lymph node involvement, or isolated extralymphatic organ involvement in the absence of adjacent lymph node involvement, but in conjunction with disease in distant site(s); or any involvement of the liver or bone marrow, or nodular involvement of the lung(s). The location of stage IV disease is identified further by specifying the site according to the notations given above

E signifies extralymphatic disease and includes extension of disease into the lung, anterior chest wall, pericardium, bone, or thyroid. It does not include involvement of Waldeyer's ring, Peyer's patches, appendix, the thymus, or the spleen as these are not "extralymphatic" sites

Each stage can also be designated as to whether or not clinical findings were present in the six months prior to diagnosis:

A: Symptoms absent
B: Unexplained fever (>38°C)
   Unexplained weight loss (more than 10% of body weight)
   Drenching night sweats that require a change of bedclothes

Note: Pruritus, alcohol intolerance, fatigue, or a short, febrile illness associated with a suspected infection is not included under B symptoms.

- Tan, homogeneous, firm: normal nodes
- Black: anthracotic pigment in mediastinal or lung nodes, some metastatic melanomas
- White, firm to hard: metastatic carcinoma, sarcoid
- White/fleshy: lymphoma
- Cystic: metastatic teratoma, metastatic papillary thyroid carcinoma
- Necrosis: metastatic carcinoma, infection (e.g., TB).

Normal lymph nodes have a smooth outer surface. Describe the capsule: irregular or effaced. If there is extensive extracapsular extension and the nodes are matted together (corresponding to "fixed" or "matted" nodes on physical examination), estimate the number of nodes present and take a representative section of each separately identifiable involved node.

3. Each node is serially sectioned into 0.2 to 0.3 cm slices.

Metastases first enter along the midline of the node. Although the node may be sectioned through the hilum and submitted so that this portion of the node is sectioned first in order to find small metastases, in practice this is difficult to do. Slicing the node into thin sections is more important than the exact plane of section.

CAP and ADASP have recommended that all grossly negative nodes be serially sectioned and completely submitted if removed for the evaluation of metastatic disease.[4,5]

The total number of involved nodes must be determined. Small intact lymph nodes can be grouped into one cassette. Larger sectioned lymph nodes can be combined in a cassette if the nodes are inked different colors. Sections of nodes can also be combined with other tissue sections. Dictate how many nodes are in each cassette in order to count accurately the number of involved nodes.

If a gross metastasis is present, submit *one* representative section of the area most suspicious for extracapsular invasion. Record the gross size of the metastatic deposit. This method will detect all macrometastases (>0.2 cm). The clinical significance of smaller metastases (micrometastases) has not been definitely established and is under investigation. There is no practical routine method that will detect all metastases to lymph nodes and no published study has used methods that would detect every micrometastasis.

Special studies

Levels

In order to consistently find metastatic deposits smaller than 0.2 cm, additional levels need to be performed through the thickness of the tissue (Table 27-5).[6]

In order to sample the entire tissue slice, the levels need to be cut deeply into the block. Typical "levels" ordered from a histopathology laboratory are usually cut at a spacing of 10 to 20 μm. Thus three "typical" levels might examine less than 10% of the thickness of the tissue. To completely examine a 0.2 to 0.3 cm thick slice (or 2000 to 3000 μm), the levels need to be 500 to 1000 μm apart. These very deep levels need to be specifically requested from the histotechnologist. In some protocols, intervening unstained slides are saved for possible later studies.

The additional work necessary to find 0.1 cm metastases by examining three levels may be possible, if limited numbers of nodes are submitted for examination (see "Sentinel lymph nodes," below). However, it is beyond the capacity of diagnostic pathology laboratories to find smaller metastases in all cancer cases by examining numerous levels.

If multiple fragments of tissue are present in the block, levels may also ensure that all fragments are adequately sampled. Levels can also be helpful in determining the best size of a small metastasis.

Immunoperoxidase studies

Immunoperoxidase studies are used to further evaluate cells seen by H&E or to find very small metastases not seen by H&E.

IHC for the evaluation of cells seen by H&E. There are many types of benign cells present in lymph nodes that can resemble tumor cells (e.g., nevus cell nests, histiocytes, megakaryocytes).[7,8] Alternatively, tumor cells can closely resemble benign cells (e.g., lobular breast cancer cells can mimic lymphocytes or histiocytes). IHC can help identify the type of

Table 27-5 Extent of sampling necessary to find all metastases of a given size

SIZE OF METASTATIC DEPOSIT TO BE DETECTED	NUMBER OF EQUALLY SPACED LEVELS THAT NEED TO BE EXAMINED TO FIND ALL METASTASES
>0.2 cm (a macrometastasis)	1
0.1 cm	3
0.05 cm	6
0.02 cm	20
Single cell	500

cell present. Keratin is often used to identify metastatic carcinoma. However, other types of benign keratin-positive cells may need to be excluded:

- Mullerian inclusions (usually pelvic or peritoneal lymph nodes)
- Breast lobules (axillary lymph nodes; rare)
- Mesothelial cells (mediastinal lymph nodes)
- Thyroid follicles (lymph nodes of the anterior neck)
- Interstitial reticulum cells (particularly with CAM5.2)
- Plasma cells.

IHC is also used to distinguish melanoma metastases from other benign S100 cells in lymph nodes (see below).

IHC used to find small metastases not seen by H&E. Individual tumor cells or very small clusters of tumor can be detected by using IHC. The slide used for IHC is also a deeper level. Thus in some cases the new finding of metastatic tumor may be due to the level, rather than to the use of IHC.

IHC detects metastases not detected by H&E depending on how many IHC studies are performed and how deeply the tissue is leveled. In general, the number of metastases found increases with the number of IHC levels examined. No study has attempted to examine every cell in a lymph node.

False positive results can occur when benign cells are immunoreactive for the markers used (see above for keratin and the melanoma section in Chapter 18). False negative results are less common, but can occur when the tumor is not immunoreactive for the marker used.

The clinical significance of micrometastases (i.e., <0.2 cm) to lymph nodes is currently unknown but is under investigation.[9] "Isolated tumor cell clusters" measuring <0.02 cm are currently classified as N0 for breast carcinomas.

Small foci of metastatic melanoma are often more difficult to diagnose by H&E than small foci of metastatic carcinoma.[10] S100 is a sensitive marker, but it is also positive in nevus cells and dendritic cells, as well as nerves and ganglion cells. HMB45 and MART-1 can be used to identify tumor cells more specifically, but these markers are negative in 5% to 20% of metastatic melanomas.

It has been recommended by CAP and ADASP that IHC be used for the evaluation of sentinel lymph nodes in breast carcinoma only in the context of clinical protocols to determine the significance of these small metastases.[4,5]

Reverse transcriptase-polymerase chain reaction

RT-PCR can potentially detect one tumor cell among 10^6 to 10^7 cells by amplifying mRNA transcripts only produced by tumor cells. However, there are limitations to this method:

- Nontumor cells may transcribe "tumor specific" genes (e.g., nevus cells produce tyrosinase).
- Some tumors may not produce the transcript used for the assay.
- There is no histologic correlation for the RT-PCR findings (to rule out benign cells).
- The size of the metastatic deposit cannot be determined.
- The significance of very rare tumor cells undetectable by other methods is unknown.

These methods remain experimental and require clinical validation. If a portion of a node is taken for RT-PCR, metastases can be missed that would have been found by conventional methods.[11]

Sentinel lymph nodes

The sentinel lymph node is the first lymph node in the line of drainage from a tumor. If the sentinel node is free of tumor, it is highly unlikely that other nodes are involved and patients can be spared full lymph node dissections.

Methods to detect the sentinel node use either a dye (usually methylene blue) or radioactive isotopes. If a radioactive isotope is used, the radiation safety department should be contacted to determine the best method of handling the node and the potential risks to pathology personnel. The type of isotope, the dose, and the method of injection vary among institutions. The half-lives of the isotopes used are generally short, and often the passing of hours or a day will markedly decrease the amount of radioactivity remaining in the specimen. In most cases, the radioactive substances used can be handled safely by pathology personnel and do not require any special procedures or disposal.[12,13]

The best method for processing sentinel nodes has not been determined. Typically, additional levels and/or IHC are performed (see above). At a minimum, the node(s) is thinly sectioned and completely submitted in order to detect all macrometastases. Many protocols involve multiple H&E levels with intervening unstained slides. If the H&E slides are negative, the unstained slides may be used for additional studies.

Protocols for examining sentinel nodes from different sites must be developed at each institution. Additional studies beyond H&E examination are preferably performed in the context of protocols designed to determine the clinical significance of micrometastases.

The reporting of sentinel nodes should include their appearance (blue or not blue), the presence of radioactivity as provided by the surgeon (hot or not hot or specific counts), and the methods used to examine the nodes.

Processing the specimen

1. Grossly identify each node. On average, there will be two sentinel nodes for breast carcinomas.
   Describe each node:
   - Size
   - Color (may be blue if dye is used)
   - Capsule—smooth or irregular.
2. Ink each node a different color if they are to be submitted in the same cassette.
   Slice each node thinly at 0.2 to 0.3 cm intervals.
   If a frozen section is requested, freeze all the slices.
3. Submit all slices for histologic examination.

Pathologic diagnostic/prognostic features checklist for sign-out for lymph node staging for carcinomas

Number
Number of lymph nodes examined. Some protocols require that a minimum number of lymph nodes be examined for adequate staging.

Location
Location in relation to the primary tumor when appropriate, location as defined by the surgeon.

Number of metastatic deposits
Number of lymph nodes with metastatic deposits. Most staging systems require this information.

Size of metastasis
Size of the largest metastatic deposit. Macrometastases are defined as being >0.2 cm in size. For some carcinomas, the size of the largest metastatic deposit is used for staging.
Isolated tumor cell clusters ≤0.02 cm (approximately the size of a linear array of 20 tumor cells) are staged as N0 (i+) for breast cancers.

Method of detection
If a micrometastasis is only found by immunohistochemistry or RT-PCR, this should be stated as very small tumor deposits detected by these methods may not be equivalent to finding metastases by H&E.

Extracapsular invasion

Present or absent, invasion extending to other structures (e.g., adjacent lymph nodes, muscle). In some cases the extranodal invasion is so extensive that individual lymph nodes cannot be counted. The number of involved lymph nodes may need to be estimated. The clinical impression may be of "fixed" or "matted" lymph nodes.

■ EXTRANODAL LYMPHOMAS

Lymphomas are most commonly diagnosed in lymph node specimens, but occasionally lymphomas present in extranodal sites in stomach, lung, breast, colon, or other unusual sites. Tissue is taken for special studies as described under "Lymph nodes."

■ STAGING LAPAROTOMIES FOR HODGKIN'S DISEASE

Staging laparotomies should only be performed after a diagnosis of Hodgkin's disease (HD) has been made. However, if the diagnosis is uncertain, consider saving tissue (formalin, B5, snap frozen, etc.) to exclude a non-Hodgkin's lymphoma. If the diagnosis is well established, special studies are not required. If unusual lesions are encountered during the gross examination of the specimens, proceed as if the tissue were a diagnostic specimen (see sections above).

Processing the spleen

1. Weigh the spleen (normal weight is 125 to 195 g) and record the outer dimensions. Cut away the fatty tissue at the hilum and process this tissue for lymph nodes (see below). Describe the capsule including texture (smooth, irregular, nodular, plaques) and intactness.
2. Slice the spleen *very* thinly (2 to 3 mm), noting any small white lesions. These lesions may represent prominent white pulp, HD, or granulomata associated with HD. The number of lesions is important for clinical decision making. Each lesion is described including color, size, location (subcapsular, parenchymal), and consistency. Estimate the percentage of total splenic tissue occupied by the nodules. The sections are re-examined and recut into thinner sections the following day after fixation to look for additional lesions.

    Describe the uninvolved splenic tissue including color, consistency, congestion, hemorrhage, and prominence of white pulp.
3. Cut cassette-sized sections of all nodules and five additional noninvolved representative sections. Fix in small container(s) of B5. Fix the remainder of the spleen in a *large* container of formalin.
4. Wash the spleen briefly in water the following day and section further to identify any additional small nodules. Submit sections for processing. Do not submit more than one lesion per cassette in order to count accurately the total number of involved nodules. Submit all lesions up to a maximum of ten. If no lesions are encountered, submit a total of five cassettes. Order one level (H&E) on each cassette. If a lesion is very small, order two to three levels on that block.

Processing the lymph nodes

1. Thinly section each specimen and describe the number of lymph nodes, and their size and appearance. Fix in B5 for 3 to 5 hours and then transfer to formalin. Dispose all B5 into a mercury waste container as well as the formalin, which may contain mercury salts.
2. Submit sections the following day. Order two levels (H&E).

Processing the liver biopsies

1. Note the type of biopsy (needle or wedge), the size, the color, and the presence of any focal lesions. Slice wedge biopsies thinly and fix in B5 (see above).
2. Sections may be submitted after fixation for at least 3 hours or the following day. Order three levels (H&E).

■ SPLEEN: HEMATOLOGIC DISEASE

Occasionally spleens are removed for idiopathic thrombocytopenic purpura (ITP), chronic myeloproliferative disorders, lymphomas, or other cases of splenomegaly. The spleen can be processed as described above for a staging laparotomy. For all cases submit one section of formalin-fixed tissue and five sections of B5 fixed tissue (make sure B5 is disposed of properly). A PAS stain is ordered on the best B5 block.

Gross differential diagnosis

Idiopathic thrombocytopenic purpura. The spleen is usually normal in size and appearance or only mildly enlarged.

Chronic myeloid leukemia and hairy cell leukemia. The spleen may be massively enlarged (over 5000 g). Splenic infarctions may be present. The spleen of hairy cell leukemia is usually dark red in color. In both conditions the lymph nodes are also enlarged.

Chronic lymphoid leukemia. There may be mild splenic enlargement (300 to 400 g) with prominent malpighian corpuscles.

Lymphomas. Low-grade lymphomas usually show miliary (innumerable minute white nodules) or diffuse involvement of the spleen. High-grade lymphomas may form a single or multiple large nodules. The lymph nodes are often involved.

■ SPLEEN: NON-HEMATOLOGIC DISEASE

Spleens are occasionally removed after trauma or as part of a larger resection for non-hematologic malignancies (e.g., distal pancreatectomy).

Simple splenectomy

Processing the specimen

1. Weigh the spleen (normal weight 125 to 195 g) and record the outer dimensions. If the splenectomy has been performed due to trauma, photograph the specimen. Cut away the fatty tissue at the hilum and process like lymph nodes (see above). Describe the capsule including texture (smooth, irregular, nodular, plaques) and the presence of lacerations. It is generally not possible to distinguish preoperative lacerations from those occurring after removal of the spleen.
2. Slice the spleen thinly, noting any lesions. If lesions are present, the case is processed as a possible lymphoproliferative order (B5, snap freezing, possibly other studies). Each lesion is described including color, size, location (subcapsular, parenchymal), and consistency.

    Describe the uninvolved splenic tissue including color, consistency, congestion, hemorrhage, and prominence of white pulp.
3. Submit two representative sections including capsule (if no lesions are present).

REFERENCES

1. MacLennan KA, Bennett MH, Tu A, et al. Relationship of histopathologic features to survival in nodular sclerosing Hodgkin's disease. Cancer 64:1686-1693, 1989.

2. Koren R, Kyzer S, Paz A, Veltman V, Klein B, Gal R. Lymph node revealing solution: A new method for detection of minute axillary lymph nodes in breast cancer specimens. Am J Surg Pathol 21:1387-1390, 1997.

3. Koren R, Siegal A, Klein B, Halpern M, Kyzer S, Veltman V, Gal R. Lymph node-revealing solution: Simple new method for detecting minute lymph nodes in colon carcinoma. Dis Colon Rectum 40:407-410, 1997.

4. Association of Directors of Anatomic and Surgical Pathology (ADASP) recommendations for processing and reporting of lymph node specimens submitted for evaluation of metastatic disease. Mod Pathol 14:629-632, 2001.

5. Fitzgibbons PL, Page DL, Weaver D, et al. Prognostic factors in breast cancer: College of American Pathologists Consensus Statement 1999. Arch Pathol Lab Med 124:966-978, 2000.

6. Zhang PJ, Reisner RM, Nangia R, Edge SB, Brooks JJ. Effectiveness of multiple-level sectioning in detecting axillary nodal micrometastasis in breast cancer: a retrospective study with immuno-histochemical analysis. Arch Pathol Lab Med 122:687-690, 1998.

7. Xu S, Roberts SA, Pasha TL, Zhang PJ. Undesirable cytokeratin immunoreactivity of native nonepithelial cells in sentinel lymph nodes from patients with breast carcinoma. Arch Pathol Lab Med 124:1310-1313, 2000.

8. Gould VE, Bloom KJ, Franke WW, et al. Increased numbers of cytokeratin-positive interstitial reticulum cells (CIRC) in reactive, inflammatory and neoplastic lymphadenopathies: Hyperplasia or induced expression? Virchows Arch 425:617-630, 1995.

9. Weaver DL. Sentinel lymph nodes and breast carcinoma: which micrometastases are clinically significant? Am J Surg Pathol 27:842-845, 2003.

10. Roberts AA, Cochran AJ. Pathologic analysis of sentinel lymph nodes in melanoma patients: current and future trends. J Surg Oncol 85:152-161, 2004.

11. Smith PAF, Harlow SP, Krag DN, Weaver DL. Submission of lymph node tissue for ancillary studies decreases the accuracy of conventional breast cancer axillary node staging, Mod Pathol 12:781-785, 1999.

12. Miner TJ, Shriver CD, Flicek PR, Miner FC, Jaques DP, Maniscalco-Theberge ME, Krag DN. Guidelines for the safe use of radioactive materials during localization and resection of the sentinel lymph node. Ann Surg Oncol 6:75-82, 1999.

13. Morton R, Horton PW, Peet DJ, Kissin MW. Quantitative assessment of the radiation hazards and risks in sentinel node procedures. Br J Radiol 76:117-122, 2003.

Medical devices and foreign material

28

All foreign material removed from humans, whether of medical origin or not, is generally sent to pathology for documentation (with the exception of temporary medical devices such as intravenous catheters). Some of these specimens will be of legal significance (e.g., silicone implants, bullets) and others will be subject to legislation that requires the tracing of certain medical devices.

The Safe Medical Devices Act of 1990

The Federal Safe Medical Devices Act of 1990 (PL 101-629) went into effect in August of 1993. This act requires manufacturers of medical devices, healthcare personnel who use or install them, and hospitals to keep records of patients and the history of specific medical devices ("tracking"). This will allow manufacturers to remove devices from the market and/or notify patients should problems arise. The subsequent Food and Drug Administration Modernization Act (FDAMA) in 1997 eliminated automatic mandatory tracking for certain devices. Additional information can be found at www.fda.gov/medwatch.

The types of devices tracked include those with the following features:

- If the device failed it would be reasonably likely to have serious adverse health consequences.
- The device is intended to be implanted in the human body for more than one year.
- The device is intended to be life sustaining or life supporting.

The patient with a tracked device is allowed to refuse to release personal information for the purpose of tracking.

Pathologists play an important role in recognizing complications associated with medical devices. Reports of problems with medical devices can be entered on forms available at the MEDWATCH home page at www.fda.gov/medwatch. The medical device should be saved.

Devices that are currently subject to tracking by manufacturers

- Glenoid fossa prosthesis
- Mandibular condyle prosthesis
- Temporomandibular joint (TMJ) prosthesis
- Abdominal aortic aneurysm stent grafts
- Automatic implantable cardioverter/defibrillator
- Cardiovascular permanent implantable pacemaker electrode
- Implantable pacemaker pulse generator
- Replacement heart valve (mechanical only)
- Implanted cerebellar stimulator
- Implanted diaphragmatic/phrenic nerve stimulator
- Implantable infusion pumps
- Dura mater

Orthopedic hardware

All orthopedic hardware (joint prosthesis, screws, plates, etc.) is usually sent to the pathology department for documentation. The gross description includes the number, color, composition (plastic, metal), and any identifying numbers on the hardware. Obvious cracks or worn areas should be noted. There is no need to photograph these specimens unless there is a history of trauma or there is obvious damage to the hardware. Many patients request the return of their orthopedic hardware. The specimen is preferably washed clean of blood and placed in a leak-proof permanently sealed bag before return.

Foreign bodies

Foreign bodies are defined as non-medical objects within the human body. Photographs are frequently useful because there is the potential for lawsuits in some cases.

Hospitals are not required to report to the police illegal substances taken from patients (e.g., a bag of heroin extracted from a smuggler's GI tract); all information pertaining to such objects is medically confidential. The hospital lawyers may be contacted before such objects are disposed of or returned to the patient.

Bullets

The most important principle in handling bullets (or any other specimen likely to be used as evidence in a legal case) is to establish an "unbroken chain of evidence," identifying the bullet from the time it is removed by the surgeon to the time that it is released to the police. Any lapse in this procedure could be legal grounds to have the bullet removed as evidence in a trial.

Documenting the specimen

A doctor or nurse should transfer the bullet from the operating room directly to a pathologist. The names of the people delivering and receiving the bullet and the time of transfer are documented in the report.

Do *not* touch bullets or bullet fragments with metal tools (e.g., forceps) because scratches will obscure rifling marks used to identify the gun of origin. The gross description should be sufficiently detailed (including accurate measurements, color, size, and shape) to allow identification of the bullet at a future date, including numbers and letters if present. Descriptive terms (e.g., "conical silver metallic fragment") are preferred unless the prosector is a ballistics expert and can positively identify the specimen as a bullet (e.g., "bullet from a .32 automatic pistol"). The description could potentially become evidence in a trial.

Three photographs, including the surgical number and ruler, are useful for documentation. Multiple pictures may be useful if there is more information to be gained by different angles. Include any tissue submitted with the bullet. If soft tissue or bone is present, it is submitted as a surgical specimen, up to one cassette for soft tissue and one cassette for bone.

The bullet should be kept in a locked secure storage compartment until requested by the police. The name of the policeman or policewoman, his or her badge number, and the name of the person releasing the bullet should be documented as well as the day and time of transfer. Bullets should otherwise not be released. If a question about releasing a bullet arises, legal advice should be sought.

Neuropathology specimens

29

Neuropathology includes all brain and spinal cord specimens, pituitary glands, muscle and nerve biopsies, and eyes.

Relevant clinical history (in addition to age and gender)

See Table 29-1.

Table 29-1 Relevant clinical history	
HISTORY RELEVANT TO ALL SPECIMENS	HISTORY RELEVANT TO BRAIN SPECIMENS
Organ/tissue resected or biopsied	Results of previous CNS biopsies
Purpose of the procedure	Renal function tests (BUN and creatinine)
Gross appearance of the organ/tissue/lesion sampled	Duration of symptoms (e.g. rapidly progressive dementia and myoclonus is suggestive of Creutzfeldt–Jakob disease)
Any unusual features of the clinical presentation	Family history (present in 16% of patients with brain tumors): neurofibromatosis type 1 (optic system gliomas), neurofibromatosis type 2 (acoustic neuroma, multiple meningiomas, spinal cord ependymoma), tuberous sclerosis (subependymal giant cell astrocytoma), von Hippel–Lindau syndrome (hemangioblastomas of the cerebellum), Turcot syndrome (medulloblastomas and glioblastomas)
Any unusual features of the gross appearance	
Prior surgery/biopsies—results	
Prior malignancy	
Prior treatment (radiation therapy, chemotherapy, drug use that can change the histologic appearance of tissues)	
Compromised immune system	Imaging features

■ BRAIN BIOPSIES

Biopsies and resections are often small. Most will be evaluated intraoperatively to ensure that diagnostic tissue is present and to provide a specific diagnosis. Cytologic smear preparations in addition to frozen sections are often needed for rapid diagnosis (see Chapter 6, "Neuropathology: Stereotactic brain biopsies"). Biopsies may be performed for focal lesions (primary tumors, metastases, infectious disease) or to evaluate nonsurgical diseases (e.g., dementia).

Processing the specimen

The specimen often consists of small fragments of tissue or a stereotactic core needle biopsy measuring approximately 1 × 0.2 × 0.2 cm. It is sometimes possible to distinguish gray and white matter. If tissue is to be taken for intraoperative diagnosis or for special studies, a careful gross examination is necessary to select the areas most likely to be diagnostic (see below). A magnifying lens or dissecting microscope may be helpful.

All small fragments of brain for permanent sections are wrapped in saline-moistened lens paper and submitted in entirety. The fragments must be handled gently as there is little supporting tissue and specimens are easily distorted. If possible, fix the tissue before processing it.

Do not use sponges or toothed forceps with brain biopsies as artifacts are introduced when the soft tissue is pressed into the interstices of the sponge or the forceps teeth.

Special studies

Pituitary tumors

Lesions of the pituitary are almost always adenomas; Rathke's cleft cysts, lymphocytic hypophysitis, abscesses, and metastatic carcinomas are rare cases. Immunoperoxidase studies on formalin-fixed tissue can be used to detect cell products (FSH, LH, TSH, PL, GH, ACTH).

Vascular malformations

Elastic and trichrome stains are useful to evaluate the types of vessels present.

Meningioma

Immunoperoxidase studies for EMA are often positive; GFAP can be helpful to evaluate invasion into brain tissue. MIB-1 (Ki-67) is used to assess the proliferation index in atypical lesions. Immunoperoxidase studies on fixed tissue and a PAS stain may be helpful in the diagnosis of the secretory type of meningioma (CEA-positive, keratin-positive, with PAS-positive globules in glandular lumina).

Gliomas (oligodendrogliomas)

A portion of tissue should be submitted for FISH to evaluate 1p/19q deletions. If tumor tissue is limited, air-dried touch preps can also be used for FISH.

Medulloblastoma

DNA ploidy studies are useful for prognosis. This determination can be made using touch preps and image analysis or by flow cytometric analysis on fresh (preferred) or fixed tissue.

Metastatic tumors

The most common source is lung if the primary site is unknown. Metastases may also arise from breast, melanoma, renal cell carcinoma, and colon carcinoma. If the primary site is unknown, immunohistochemistry on formalin-fixed tissue may be useful to determine the most likely site of origin.

Pineal region tumors

It may be helpful to take tissue for EM to classify neoplasms in this region. Germ cell tumors can be subclassified using immunoperoxidase studies (PLAP, β-hCG, AFP).

Creutzfeldt–Jakob disease

Creutzfeldt–Jakob disease must be suspected in any patient with a rapidly progressive dementia. Most patients die within 10 months. Immunoperoxidase studies and Western blotting for protease K-resistant PrP^{SC} are useful for diagnosis.

In the US, specimens may be sent to the National Prion Disease Pathology Surveillance Center (www.cjdsurveillance.com) for confirmation of the diagnosis:

Dr. Pierluigi Gambetti, Director
National Prion Disease Pathology Surveillance Center
Institute of Pathology
Case Western Reserve University
2085 Adelbert Road, Room 418
Cleveland, OH 44106
Telephone: 216-368-0587 or 216-368-0822
Fax: 216-368-4090
e-mail: cjdsurv@cwru.edu

The Center can be contacted for questions related to shipping specimens.

Prion proteins are highly resistant to normal decontamination procedures and every effort must be made to prevent exposure of pathology personnel.[1,2] *Fixed and stained tissue on glass slides can transfer the disease.*

All tissue (neural and non-neural) for histology must be fixed in formalin for 24 hours. The tissue is then placed in formic acid for 1 hour and then placed again in formalin. The specimen must be clearly labeled as coming from a patient with *known or suspected Creutzfeldt–Jakob disease*. The fixation is followed by a 1-hour treatment with formic acid followed by an additional 24-hour fixation in formalin.

If the biopsy is of adequate size, it is useful to freeze a sample at −80°C for potential Western blotting.

Everything that touches the tissue (both disposable and non-disposable) must be soaked in bleach for 1 hour prior to discarding or washing.

Lymphoma

Frozen tissue is useful for typing by immunoperoxidase studies. However, many antibodies are now available for use on tissues fixed in formalin or B5.

Infections

Immunoperoxidase studies for viral antigens (e.g., Herpes) or *Toxoplasma* may be performed on formalin-fixed tissue. In a case of suspected encephalitis it may be helpful to save tissue for EM to look for viral particles. Parasites are usually evident by light microscopy. Progressive multifocal leukoencephalopathy (JC virus) is usually diagnosable from light microscopy although antibodies are available to detect the virus in tissues. There should be coordination with the surgeon at the time of OR consultation in order that microbiologic cultures can be performed as appropriate.

Metabolic diseases/storage disorders

Brain biopsies for metabolic diseases are more often performed in children but may be performed in adults as well. It is important to sample gray and white matter (ideally separately) for standard histology, frozen sections, EM, and biochemical studies.

Gross differential diagnosis

Normal tissue. Gray matter and white matter can often be identified, even in small core biopsies. The tissue is slightly firm and maintains its shape. Inflammatory lesions may have a similar appearance, but may be congested or softened.

Tumors. The color is usually abnormally yellow/gray and necrosis may be grossly apparent. The tissue is soft and gelatinous and does not maintain the shape of the biopsy.

Meningiomas are usually firmer than normal tissue but can be soft or gelatinous or whorled. Calcifications are commonly present. If attached dura and brain tissue can be identified, take sections to demonstrate the relationship of the meningioma to these structures. If the specimen is large, submit at least one section per cm of tumor.

Metastatic tumors. The tissue is often gray in color and necrosis may be present. The boundary with the normal brain, if present, is usually sharp.

Vascular malformations. These lesions in general are not biopsied but removed in one piece and are, therefore, usually larger than other lesional biopsies. The tissue usually appears hemorrhagic and small vascular structures may be apparent.

Acoustic neuromas. The tissue is usually firm and fibrotic.

Sample dictation

Received fresh, labeled with the patient's name and unit number and "parietal," are five fragments of gelatinous soft yellow/gray tissue, each measuring 0.5 × 0.3 × 0.2 cm. Normal gray and white matter is not apparent. One fragment was used for cytologic preparations for intraoperative consultation and a second fragment was used for frozen section.

Cassette #1: frozen-section remnant, 1 frag, ESS.
Cassette #2: remainder of specimen, 3 frags, ESS.

Pathologic diagnostic/prognostic features checklist for sign-out for brain tumors

Type of specimen*
Core needle biopsy, open biopsy, subtotal/partial resection, total resection.

Specimen size*
Greatest dimension.

Tumor site*
Meninges, cerebrum (the lobe may be specified), basal ganglia, thalamus, hypothalamus, suprasellar, pineal, cerebellum, cerebellopontine angle, ventricle, brain stem, spinal cord, nerve root.

Histologic type*
Astrocytomas, oligodendrogliomas, medulloblastomas, ependymal and choroid plexus tumors, etc. (use WHO classification).

Tumor size*
Greatest dimension.

Grade*
Specify the grading system used (see Tables 29-2 to 29-5).
Astrocytomas, oligodendrogliomas, ependymomas, and meningiomas are graded.

Margins*
Involved, uninvolved, cannot be assessed, not applicable.
Margins are often not applicable except for completely resected gliomas of the temporal or frontal tip. Meningeal or dural margin assessment may be important for meningiomas. Cranial or spinal nerve sheath tumor resection margins should be evaluated.
Invasion into the brain is prognostically important for meningiomas.

Change over time
If the tumor is a recurrence, compare to previous biopsies to determine whether there has been a change in grade.

Treatment effects
Evaluate treatment effects (usually radiation) on tumor and adjacent brain (extent of necrosis, viability).

This checklist incorporates information from the ADASP (see www.panix.com/~adasp) and the CAP Cancer Committee protocols for reporting on cancer specimens (see www.cap.org/). The asterisked elements are considered to be scientifically validated or regularly used data elements that must be present in reports of cancer-directed surgical resection specimens from ACS CoC-approved cancer programs. The specific details of reporting the elements may vary among institutions.

A formal AJCC classification and staging system is not available for tumors of the brain and spinal cord. For more information on the WHO classification and grading systems, see Kleihues and Cavenee.[3]

Table 29-2 WHO grading of astrocytomas

GRADE	DESCRIPTION
I	Pilocytic astrocytomas
II	Astrocytomas: well-differentiated neoplasms composed primarily of astrocytes without mitoses (fibrillary, protoplasmic, gemistocytic, combinations of these)
III	Anaplastic astrocytoma: focal or diffuse anaplasia, e.g., increased cellularity, pleomorphism, nuclear atypia, and mitotic activity. Vascular proliferation and necrosis are absent
IV	Glioblastoma: an anaplastic, often cellular tumor, composed of poorly differentiated, fusiform, round or pleomorphic cells and occasional multinucleated giant cells. Essential for histologic diagnosis is the presence of prominent vascular proliferation and/or necrosis

Note: Although this grading scheme appears to represent a continuum, pilocytic astrocytoma is a distinct entity that only becomes high grade in extremely rare circumstances. In contrast, grade II/IV fibrillary astrocytomas typically do progress in grade over time, with recurrences eventually showing higher-grade histologic features (grade III/IV or IV/IV).

Table 29-3 WHO grading of oligodendrogliomas

GRADE	DESCRIPTION
II	Oligodendroglioma: moderately cellular with infrequent mitoses. Endothelial hyperplasia is absent or mild
III	Anaplastic (malignant) oligodendroglioma: focal or diffuse anaplasia (e.g., high cellularity, nuclear polymorphism, and brisk mitotic activity). Occasional multinucleated giant cells, vascular proliferation, mitotic activity, and foci of necrosis may also be seen
IV	Some tumors with areas showing oligodendroglial features may have other areas that may be morphologically indistinguishable from glioblastoma

Note: Cytogenetic changes may also aid in classification and predict response to treatment (see "Cytogenetic Changes in Solid Tumors" Table 7-33).

Table 29-4 WHO grading of ependymomas

GRADE	DESCRIPTION
I	Myxopapillary ependymoma: a variant that occurs almost exclusively in the region of the cauda equina and originates from the filum terminale. This lesion is distinct from other forms of ependymoma
II	Ependymoma: moderately cellular with low mitotic activity. Occasional mitoses, nuclear atypia, and foci of necrosis may be present
III	Anaplastic (malignant) ependymoma: anaplasia (e.g., high cellularity, variable nuclear atypia, marked mitotic activity, and often prominent vascular proliferation). Necrosis may be widespread

Table 29-5 WHO grading of meningiomas

GRADE	DESCRIPTION
I	Meningioma
II	Clear cell meningioma
	Chordoid meningioma
	Atypical meningioma—several of the following features are evident: frequent mitoses (>4/10 HPF), increased cellularity, small cells with high nuclear–cytoplasmic ratios and/or prominent nucleoli, uninterrupted patternless or sheet-like growth and foci of "spontaneous" or geographic necrosis. Nuclear atypia alone or simply invasion of dura or bone does not qualify a tumor for the designation "atypical"
III	Papillary meningioma—an aggressive highly cellular variant
	Rhabdoid meningioma
	Anaplastic (malignant) meningioma—has obviously malignant cytology, a high mitotic index, and conspicuous necrosis. Brain invasion is a separate predictor of recurrence, independent of other histologic features

■ BIOPSIES OF THE DURA

Dural biopsies are rarely performed for the evaluation of pachymeningitis or vasculitis. The specimen is small and can be entirely submitted and examined in fixed permanent sections.

■ CAVITRON ULTRASONIC SURGICAL ASPIRATOR SPECIMENS

The Cavitron Ultrasonic Surgical Aspirator (CUSA) causes localized ultrasonic fragmentation of tissue that can then be removed by irrigation and suction. This technique minimizes the effects of surgery on adjacent normal tissues. It is used to remove some intracranial tumors. The procedure may be performed without a prior histologic diagnosis.

The specimen consists of small fragments of tissue in a volume of fluid. The fragments can be collected by straining the fluid through gauze pads. The tissue is gently placed in mesh bags or wrapped in paper. Tissue sufficient to fill two or three cassettes is usually adequate for diagnosis. If the tissue fragments are quite small, cytologic smears and cell blocks prepared from the fluid are often diagnostic and can be used for immunohistochemical studies, if necessary.

■ SUBDURAL AND SUBARACHNOID HEMATOMA EVACUATIONS

Blood removed for therapeutic reasons after intracranial bleeding may be submitted for histologic examination. Any tissue fragments within the blood are identified grossly and submitted for histologic examination.

Occasionally, congophilic (amyloid) angiopathy is diagnosed in such specimens. Amyloid can be detected in meningeal or cortical vessel walls using a Congo red stain or immunoperoxidase studies on fixed tissue for beta-amyloid.

Metastatic carcinoma can also be the cause of a hematoma and must be excluded by careful sampling and microscopic analysis.

■ BRAIN RESECTIONS

Large areas of the brain are resected sometimes to remove an epileptic focus and rarely for other lesions. Failure to find an abnormality may correlate with recurrence of seizures after surgery.

Processing the specimen

1. Determine the location of the resection and orient the specimen. A photograph of the intact specimen is helpful. Describe each component.

   Meninges: Describe any areas of fibrosis or hemorrhage.

   Brain surface: Describe the gyral pattern including normal, distorted, tubers (tuberous sclerosis), or polymicrogyria.

   Identify white matter and gray matter. Measure the width of the gray matter and the range of widths. Describe the gray–white junction (distinct or blurred).

   Describe any other abnormalities present (e.g., alteration in color or consistency, focal masses).

   In general, it is not necessary to ink margins. However, colored inks are sometimes useful to indicate orientation.

2. The specimen is sliced (perpendicular to the pial surface) at thicker intervals than the final sections to be submitted for processing (about 1.0 to 1.5 cm). Examine the gray and white matter for abnormal appearance or consistency. Samples of gray and white matter should be frozen for histology (in embedding medium), taken for EM, and snap frozen in liquid nitrogen.

   After sectioning, the slices should be photographed as a composite in an oriented manner. Individual slices containing lesions should be photographed separately as well.

   Prior to placing the slices in formalin (in a manner that will preserve orientation), small pieces of paper towel are placed against each face of the slice to minimize retraction.

3. Fix the slices in 20× volume of formalin overnight.

4. Serially submit sections from the slices but maintain orientation. The photograph will help document the areas used for histologic examination. One section per 1 to 1.5 cm of greatest dimension is submitted for the initial evaluation.

   The orientation of the specimen can be maintained by separating each piece of tissue in a specimen container with a paper towel and stacking in order. If diagnostic abnormalities are found in one of the initial sections, it is possible to find the same area and submit more sections at a later time.

■ EYES

An eye may be removed because of a primary tumor (most commonly melanoma), because it is nonfunctioning and painful, or as part of a large face resection for deeply invasive tumors.

Processing the specimen (Fig. 29-1)

1. If part of a larger face resection, the eye is removed by cutting around the extraocular muscles.

   The eye is fixed intact for at least 24 hours. Slicing the unfixed globe or injecting fixative into the vitreous will disrupt the intraocular structures.

   Wash in tap water for at least 1 hour.

2. Orient the globe by observing the posterior surface. The posterior ciliary vessels are on the medial aspect of the optic nerve. The superior and inferior oblique muscles are lateral to the optic nerve.

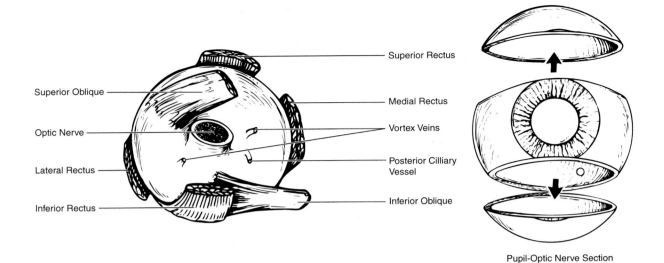

Figure 29-1 Eye anatomy and dissection.

Take the following measurements:

Globe:
- Anterior/posterior
- Horizontal
- Vertical.

Optic nerve:
- Length.

Cornea:
- Vertical (normal 11 mm) and horizontal (normal 11.5 mm).

Describe corneal clarity or opacities, size and shape of pupil, iris color and abnormalities (e.g., arcus senilis), scars of the superior limbus (present after surgery for glaucoma or cataracts), or a silicone band or sponge (present after surgery for retinal detachment).

Tumors: If melanoma is present, examine the outer surface for tumor including the vortex veins. If retinoblastoma is present, examine the optic nerve for involvement (this is an important margin).

3. Transilluminate the globe in a darkened room using a bright light source. Increased light transmission can be seen in defects of the iris. Decreased light transmission may be due to hemorrhage or tumor. Mark any abnormal shadows on the sclera with a marking pencil. The cornea and sclera are best examined under a dissecting microscope. Radiography is indicated if an intraocular foreign body or retinoblastoma is suspected.

4. Cut off the distal segment of the optic nerve and submit en face.

5. The globe is sectioned to demonstrate best any lesions present. A razor blade is adequate for sectioning.

If no lesion is apparent, section the globe in a plane to include the optic nerve, macula, and pupil. Make a horizontal section 0.5 cm superior to the optic nerve and 0.5 cm central to the superior limbus. After this section is removed, examine the eye contents (lens, iris, ciliary body, vitreous, choroid, retina, and optic nerve) under a dissecting microscope. Note the size and location of any lesions. If a lesion is present, note its location with respect to the ora serrata, optic disc, and macula. Finish sectioning the eye by making a parallel section just below, through the inferior limbus.

If a focal lesion is present, the globe is sectioned vertically or obliquely to include the lesion in the plane with the optic nerve and pupil.

6. Usually only the tissue in the central section is submitted for histologic examination. Portions of the other sections can be submitted if additional lesions are present. Include sections of optic nerve (transverse), retina, choroid, ciliary body, pupil, lens, and cornea. A PAS stain should be obtained.

Gross differential diagnosis

Malignant melanoma. Lobulated pigmented masses arise in the choroid or ciliary body. Choroid tumors may extend into the subretinal space and form a mushroom-shaped tumor. The size, presence at ciliary body, and location over the optic nerve are poor prognostic factors. Some melanomas may extend beyond the sclera into scleral canals with vortex veins or into the subconjunctival space.

Retinoblastoma. The majority of retinoblastomas present before the age of 3 years and approximately one third are due to a germline mutation. These latter tumors are more likely to be multifocal or bilateral. The tumors are chalky white and arise from the retina. The tumor may grow into the vitreous, the subretinal space, or both.

AJCC (6th edition) classification of tumors of the eye

There are separate classification systems for carcinoma of the eyelid, carcinoma of the conjunctiva, malignant melanoma of the conjunctiva, malignant melanoma of the uvea, retinoblastoma, carcinoma of the lacrimal gland, and sarcoma of the orbit. The Sixth Edition of the AJCC Cancer Staging Manual should be consulted for the specifics of these systems.

■ LENS

Lenses are removed when they are involved by cataracts.

Describe the specimen grossly including diameter, thickness, shape (lentiform, ovoid), color, and the presence of opacities (central or peripheral).

These specimens are usually not examined histologically but may be examined if requested. A PAS stain should be obtained.

■ CORNEA

The central portion of the cornea may be removed during transplantation and can be involved by endothelial decompensation, postinflammatory scarring and traumatic changes, or keratoconus. The specimen may be a failed graft. The specimen is embedded and cut on edge, perpendicular to the epithelial surfaces. A PAS stain should be obtained.

■ NERVE BIOPSIES

Peripheral nerve biopsies are usually performed to evaluate peripheral neuropathy. The final diagnosis should be correlated with clinical and neurophysiologic data (e.g., a history of an inherited metabolic disease or toxic insult, biopsy of other tissues).

Processing the specimen

Nerve biopsies are processed routinely for light microscopy and EM, and a small portion is saved frozen.

Electron microscopy. Submit a 5- to 6-mm length of nerve—preferably from the center of a larger segment so that crush artifact from the ends can be avoided. Semithin sections can be examined to determine whether EM is necessary.

Light microscopy. After specimens have been taken for special studies, the remainder of the specimen is kept intact. Wrap the specimen in lens paper. Longitudinal and cross-sections may be prepared by the histology laboratory. Routine stains are H&E (two levels) and a trichrome stain.

Frozen tissue. A small cross-section should be frozen in embedding medium.

Special studies

Vasculitis or history of collagen vascular disease

Immunofluorescence studies may be indicated. Either fresh or frozen tissue can be used.

Demyelinating disease

Evaluation of demyelinating diseases requires an extra portion of nerve for "teasing." A 5-mm length of nerve is saved in formalin. The nerve must be flat, but not stretched, during fixation. Individual nerve fibers are gently separated under a dissecting microscope. The fibers can then be embedded and sectioned longitudinally and stained with osmium to look for segmental loss of myelin or the "onion balls" seen in remyelination.

■ MUSCLE BIOPSY

Muscle biopsy is performed to evaluate myopathies or neurogenic atrophy. Specimens are often processed for electron microscopy and saved as frozen sections for enzyme studies.

Processing the specimen

1. Two unfixed specimens wrapped in saline-moistened gauze may be submitted. #1 is submitted on a clamp and #2 is unclamped.
2. Specimen #1 (clamped):
   - **EM:** Submit a specimen large enough to be oriented for cross-sections. Place in glutaraldehyde.
   - **Histochemistry:** A cross-section is frozen in isopentane (see Box 29-1).
3. Specimen #2 (unclamped):
   - **Paraffin sections:** Submit both a cross-section and longitudinal section.

An additional section is frozen for special studies if needed.

Box 29-1 Freezing muscle biopsies

1. Label a scintillation vial with the surgical pathology number and place in the cryostat to cool. A second vial will be needed if biochemistry studies are required.

2. Pour liquid nitrogen into a large Dewar flask kept cold in a freezer.

3. Pour cold isopentane into a pre-cooled small metal cup, but only enough to cover the specimen, and immerse the base of the clamp in liquid nitrogen.

4. The isopentane bath is ready to use when white drops form on the bottom of the cup.

5. Cut one section from the middle of the specimen, approximately 5 to 7 mm in length.

6. Lightly powder the muscle with baby powder to prevent the outer fibers from detaching. This step is optional.

7. Take a small piece of stiff paper (e.g., a piece of index card small enough to fit in a vial) and write the surgical number on one end. Fold the other end to form an L shape. The bottom of the L is where the tissue will be placed for freezing.

8. Place a drop of OCT on the short arm of the paper. Orient the muscle cross-section and place on this end. *Do not* cover the muscle with OCT as this interferes with the freezing process.

9. Immerse the paper and specimen in the isopentane for about 10 seconds. Place the frozen specimen on the paper in the pre-cooled vial and store in the −70°C freezer.

10. Tissue for biochemical studies can be frozen en bloc in liquid nitrogen and placed in another pre-cooled vial.

REFERENCES

1. Brown P, Wolff A, Gafdusk DC. A simple and effective method for inactivating virus infectivity in formalin-fixed tissue samples from patients with Creutzfeldt-Jakob disease. Neurology, 40:887-890, 1990.

2. Budka H, Aguzzi A, Brown P, et al. Tissue handling in suspected Creutzfeldt-Jakob disease (CJD) and other human spongiform encephalopathies (prion diseases). Brain Pathol 5:319-322, 1995.

3. Kleihues P, Cavenee WK. Pathology and Genetics: Tumors of the Nervous System. WHO Classification of Tumours. IARC Press, Lyon, 2000.

Paraganglioma

The adrenal medullary paraganglioma, pheochromocytoma, is discussed in Chapter 11. The extra-adrenal paragangliomas are classified according to their location and site of origin, which corresponds to the paravertebral sympathetic chain:

Abdominal extra-adrenal paragangliomas

- Organ of Zuckerkandl
- Urinary bladder

Paragangliomas of the head and neck
Carotid body paraganglioma
Jugulotympanic paraganglioma
Vagal paraganglioma
Laryngeal paraganglioma
Aortic pulmonary paraganglioma.

Relevant clinical history (in addition to age and gender)

See Table 30-1.

Processing the specimen

1. Examine the specimen to identify any attached structures. Usually the tumor is surrounded by a small amount of soft tissue. Record the overall specimen dimensions. Ink the outer surface.

Table 30-1 Relevant clinical history

HISTORY RELEVANT TO ALL SPECIMENS	HISTORY RELEVANT TO PARAGANGLIOMA SPECIMENS
Organ/tissue resected or biopsied	Signs and symptoms due to excess catecholamine production.
Purpose of the procedure	Family history (see "Hereditary Cancer Syndromes") Table 7-36
Gross appearance of the organ/tissue/lesion sampled	
Any unusual features of the clinical presentation	
Any unusual features of the gross appearance	
Prior surgery/biopsies—results	
Prior malignancy	
Prior treatment (radiation therapy, chemotherapy, drug use that can change the histologic appearance of tissues)	
Compromised immune system	

2. Serially section through the specimen. Describe the tumor including size, color, consistency, borders (well-circumscribed, infiltrating, multinodular), capsule, necrosis or hemorrhage.
3. Carefully examine the surrounding soft tissue for adjacent lymph nodes.
4. Submit one cassette per 1 cm of greatest dimension of tumor. Submit sections of all lymph nodes present.

Microscopic sections

Paraganglioma
One section per 1 cm of greatest dimension.

Lymph nodes
Submit any lymph nodes present.

Special studies

Paraganglioma

The gross and microscopic appearance is similar to a pheochromocytoma. These tumors are usually well circumscribed with a thin capsule and have a homogeneous fleshy yellow surface. They often adhere to the carotid artery (if present) but this is not a sign of malignancy. Special studies are not required for the diagnosis of paragangliomas and should only be considered if the diagnosis is uncertain or the gross appearance is atypical. The diagnosis can be confirmed on formalin-fixed tissue by immunoperoxidase staining ("zellballen" are positive for chromogranin and the surrounding sustentacular cells are positive for S100).

Pathologic prognostic/diagnostic features sign-out checklist for paragangliomas

Tumor size
Greatest dimension.

Tumor configuration
Single or multiple nodules.

Invasion
Encapsulated or with invasion into surrounding tissue.

Necrosis
Present or absent.

Criteria for malignancy in paragangliomas[1,2]

Approximately 10% of paragangliomas are malignant based on either extensive local invasion or metastasis. Histologic features may be suggestive of, but cannot accurately predict, malignant behavior. The likelihood of such behavior can be determined using the four features listed. Of malignant paragangliomas, 71% have two or three of these features, whereas 89% of benign tumors have none or one of the features.

- Extra-adrenal location
- Coarse nodularity or multiple nodules on gross examination
- Confluent tumor necrosis
- Absence of hyaline globules

REFERENCES

1. Linnoila RI, Keiser HR, Steinberg SM, Lack EE. Histopathology of benign vs malignant sympathoadrenal paragangliomas, clinicopathologic study of 120 cases including unusual features. Hum Pathol 21:1168-1180, 1990.
2. Solcia E, Kloppel G, Sobin LH. World Health Organization—Histological Typing of Endocrine Tumors. 2000, IARC, Lyon pp. 38-44.

Penis

31

Amputations of the penis are almost always performed for the resection of invasive squamous cell carcinoma. Foreskin evaluation is discussed in Chapter 18.

Processing the specimen (Fig. 31-1)

1. Record the dimensions of the total specimen (length, circumference) and foreskin (length, width, thickness).

   Tumors usually affect the glans and coronal sulcus. Describe the lesion including size, color, growth pattern (fungating, papillary, verrucous, ulcerated), consistency (friable, soft, rubbery, hard), contour (well-defined, infiltrating, pushing margins), location, and distance from the proximal resection margin.

2. Open the urethra along the ventral aspect where it is closest to the surface. Extend this cut deeper to bisect the penis. Record the depth of invasion and involvement of foreskin, frenulum, glans, meatus, corpora cavernosa, urethra, and corpus spongiosum.

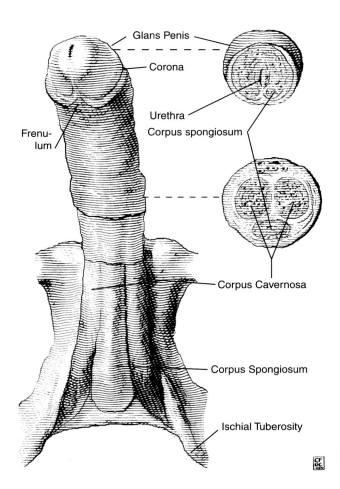

Figure 31-1 Penis anatomy.

3. Fix the specimen overnight in formalin.

4. Microscopic sections may be taken the following day. Additional cuts can be taken at right angles to further evaluate the tumor.

Microscopic sections

Tumor
Up to four cassettes demonstrating deepest extent of invasion and relationship to adjacent structures.

Margin
Up to two cassettes of proximal resection margin, including skin, corpora, and urethra. Submit more if there is grossly suspicious involvement.

Other structures
Any structure not included above.

Pathologic diagnostic/prognostic features sign-out checklist for tumors of the penis

Type of procedure
Penectomy, partial penectomy.

Type of tumor*
Squamous cell carcinoma (and subtypes), others rare.

Grade
Well, moderately, or poorly differentiated.

Size*
In centimeters.

Extent*
In situ, subepithelial connective tissue (depth in cm), corpus spongiosum (depth in cm), cavernosum (depth in cm), urethra, prostate, other adjacent structures.

Lymphovascular invasion
Present or absent.

Blood vessel invasion
Present or absent.

Perineural invasion
Present or absent.

Nodal status
Regional lymph nodes are inguinal. Single vs. multiple, unilateral vs. bilateral.

Margins*
Involved or not involved: urethral, corpus spongiosum, corpus cavernosum, cutaneous.

Associated lesions
Squamous hyperplasia, balanitis xerotica obliterans, condyloma acuminatum, bowenoid papulosis, Paget's disease, basal cell carcinoma.

This checklist includes recommendations from the ADASP (see www.panix.com/~adasp/). Asterisked elements and AJCC classification are considered to be required elements.

AJCC classification is produced in Table 31-1.

Table 31-1 AJCC (6th edition) classification of tumors of the penis

Tumor	TX	Primary tumor cannot be assessed
	T0	No evidence of primary tumor
	Tis	Carcinoma in situ
	Ta	Noninvasive verrucous carcinoma
	T1	Tumor invades subepithelial connective tissue
	T2	Tumor invades corpus spongiosum or cavernosum
	T3	Tumor invades urethra or prostate
	T4	Tumor invades other adjacent structures
Regional lymph nodes	NX	Regional lymph nodes cannot be assessed
	N0	No regional lymph node metastasis
	N1	Metastasis in a single, superficial, inguinal lymph node
	N2	Metastasis in multiple or bilateral superficial inguinal lymph nodes
	N3	Metastasis in deep inguinal or pelvic lymph node(s) unilateral or bilateral

Note: Regional lymph nodes include superficial inguinal (femoral), deep inguinal (Rosenmüller's or Cloquet's node), external iliac, internal iliac (hypogastric), and pelvic nodes

Distant metastases	MX	Distant metastasis cannot be assessed
	M0	No distant metastases
	M1	Distant metastases

Soft tissue tumors (sarcomas)

32

Soft tissue tumors are among the most difficult neoplasms to diagnose. Special studies (immunoperoxidase studies, EM, cytogenetics) often are required for the appropriate classification of these tumors and for reliable distinction from carcinomas, melanomas, and lymphomas.

Relevant clinical history (in addition to age and gender)

See Table 32-1.

Table 32-1 Relevant clinical history	
HISTORY RELEVANT TO ALL SPECIMENS	HISTORY RELEVANT TO SARCOMA SPECIMENS
Organ/tissue resected or biopsied	Location of mass
Purpose of the procedure	Involvement of soft tissue or bone
Gross appearance of the organ/tissue/lesion sampled	Rate of growth
Any unusual features of the clinical presentation	
Any unusual features of the gross appearance	
Prior surgery/biopsies—results	
Prior malignancy	
Prior treatment (radiation therapy, chemotherapy, drug use that can change the histologic appearance of tissues)	
Compromised immune system	

■ BIOPSIES

Biopsies are usually performed before definitive surgery because resections often must be large in order to obtain adequate margins and preoperative adjunctive therapy may be indicated. Either incisional or needle biopsies are used. It may not be possible to provide a specific diagnosis or grade based on very small specimens.

Processing the specimen

1. Relevant clinical history should be provided or obtained to establish a preoperative differential diagnosis (i.e., patient gender, age, location of mass, involvement of soft tissue and/or bone, prior history of malignancies). The likely diagnosis will aid in deciding how to apportion limited amounts of lesional tissue.

2. Describe the specimen including type (needle, incisional), size, color, necrosis or hemorrhage. Indicate what proportion of the specimen appears to be lesional and nonlesional (fibrous, fatty, etc.).

3. Very small or very heterogeneous (i.e., little tissue is available and viable tumor may be difficult to identify grossly) specimens are fixed in formalin and submitted in entirety.

Larger specimens should be apportioned for special studies if lesional tissue can be identified, see also Chapters 6 and 7.

In selected cases, a frozen section or cytologic preparation may be helpful to narrow the differential diagnosis to guide apportionment of limited tissue.

Special studies

Formalin

Formalin-fixed tissue remains the cornerstone of diagnosis. Make sure there are sufficient representative samples in formalin before submitting tissue for the special studies listed in order of importance below.

Electron microscopy

EM requires a small amount of tissue that can be also examined by light microscopy. If the tumor is heterogeneous, submit multiple specimens paired with formalin sections. EM is useful for distinguishing carcinoma from sarcoma (intercellular junctions), melanoma (premelanosomes), and subtyping round cell sarcomas (e.g., rhabdomyosarcoma) and some spindle cell sarcomas (e.g., malignant peripheral nerve sheath tumors). See Chapter 7, "Electron microscopy".

Frozen tissue

One or more fragments of 1 cm^3 are required. The tissue can be used for molecular analysis (DNA, RNA, FISH, Southern blotting, PCR, RT-PCR).

Cytogenetics

It is helpful to save tissue for cytogenetics if sarcoma is suspected clinically and there is a sufficient sample. Cytogenetics is a very useful technique for classifying some tumors (see Chapter 7, "Cytogenetics") but may require a large volume of tissue that cannot be examined histologically. An amount equivalent to two needle biopsies may be sufficient for highly cellular tumors, but 1 to 2 cm^3 of tumor is preferred.

■ LIPOMAS

Lipomas are common benign soft tissue tumors that are often removed for cosmetic reasons. However, malignancy must always be excluded. The likelihood of malignancy is increased if any of the following are present:

- Large size (over 5 cm)
- Infiltration into surrounding tissues
- Location in deep tissues
- Recurrence
- Unusual gross appearance: any appearance other than apparently normal fat (e.g., white or cream colored, homogeneous, firm, fibrotic areas, attached tissues).

Approximately 22% of patients undergoing hernia repair will also have a cord lipoma.[1] In this study, only 0.1% of hernia sac operations yielded an incidental liposarcoma. The two patients with liposarcoma were older than the average patient with cord lipoma (56 and 64 years versus 35 years) and the tumors were larger (13 and 10 cm versus 5.5 cm). Palpable cord tumors are more likely to be malignant.

Lipomas are usually enucleated without removal of the adjacent tissue. Thus, the lesion is often fragmented. There is no reason to ink these specimens as the lesion is present at the margin and margins are irrelevant for the vast majority of benign lesions.

Processing the specimen

1. Record overall or aggregate measurements if the specimen is fragmented. Thinly section through the specimen. Evaluate the specimen for tissues present (usually adipose tissue, occasionally muscle, all else rare).
2. Sample the lesion with one section per cm of greatest dimension, including all areas of varying appearance. Two fragments can be placed in one cassette.
3. It is helpful to send tissue for cytogenetics if any of the following pertain:

   - Subcutaneous lipomas larger than 5 cm
   - Subfascial lipomas
   - Lipomas in deep-seated locations (e.g., intra-abdominal)
   - Unusual gross appearance
   - Requested by surgeon.

■ RESECTIONS

Resections are often large and may include organs and limbs. It is usually advisable to discuss and orient large complicated resections with the surgeon at the time of resection and to identify all anatomic landmarks.

Margins are extremely important. Complete resection of the tumor with adequate margins (1 to 2 cm for sarcomas) is an important determinant of long-term outcome. Distance from the margin may determine the need for further surgery or postoperative radiation therapy.

Processing the specimen

1. Evaluate the outer surface of the specimen for structures present (muscle, bone, nerve, vessels, organs) and gross tumor involvement. Record measurements (outer dimensions, structures present). For very large retroperitoneal lesions, the weight may be requested by clinicians.
2. Selectively ink the outer margins if they appear closer than 2 cm, excluding skin if present. Avoid inking any non-marginal tissue (e.g., soft tissue exposed by overlying retracted muscle). In general, margins more than 2 cm from the tumor need not be inked and those more than 5 cm from the tumor need not be sampled.
3. Serially section, leaving the sections attached at one side. Describe the lesion including size in three dimensions (very important!), color, borders (infiltrating, pushing, satellite nodules), necrosis (percentage of tumor involved) or hemorrhage, variation in gross appearance, involvement of adjacent structures (arising from a structure such as nerve, vessel, or muscularis propria), and location (skin, subcutaneous tissue, fascia, muscle, visceral).

   The closest gross distance from all margins and the type of tissue at each margin (e.g., fascial plane, periosteum, muscle, strands of soft tissue) are documented. Most specimens should have at least six margins evaluated (visualize the specimen as if it were a box with six sides).

   Complicated specimens will require a diagram documenting the location of the tumor and adjacent structures and the site of microscopic sections.

If bone is included in the specimen, a specimen radiograph is performed to document the location of the bone(s) and areas of possible tumor involvement. See also Chapter 12.

Lymph nodes are not usually resected along with soft tissue sarcomas and are rarely involved. However, any lymph nodes present in a resection specimen should be submitted.

4. Pin the oriented specimen on wax and fix in an adequate volume of formalin for at least 10 to 12 hours to facilitate taking sections from the margins and the interface between normal and tumor tissue.

5. Submit tumor for special studies as indicated above. It is helpful to take tissue from all areas that have a different gross appearance (e.g., different consistencies or colors) and to match adjacent sections submitted for light microscopy and special studies. *Avoid necrotic areas when taking tissue for special studies.* If the specimen is a re-excision and gross tumor is not apparent, do not submit tissue for special studies.

As a general rule, at least one section per cm of the tumor's greatest dimension should be examined, including all areas of different gross appearance.

Take sections to document the extent of necrosis. Margins are taken perpendicular to the margin to assess the distance of the tumor from the margin. If the margin is more than 5 cm from the tumor, it need not be sampled except in cases of epithelioid sarcoma and angiosarcoma. Margin involvement by these two types of sarcoma may be difficult to evaluate grossly. En face blocks of margins are not recommended.

Special studies

Tissue may be taken for special studies as described under "Biopsies," above.

Gross differential diagnosis

Sarcomas. In general, sarcomas grow as circumscribed white tan fleshy masses, often with a pseudocapsule. The invasion into adjacent tissues may be subtle and not appreciated grossly. Some sarcomas have distinctive appearances.

Lipomas. These tumors are well circumscribed or lobulated and have a thin delicate capsule. The tumor usually resembles normal adipose tissue. Lipomas are often enucleated and, thus, are often fragmented and the capsule cannot be appreciated.

Liposarcomas. Low-grade lipoma-like liposarcomas may be soft and resemble normal fat. However, these tumors are usually paler and have a more coarsely lobulated appearance. Higher-grade liposarcomas are more likely to have firm solid areas as well as areas of necrosis.

Schwannoma is a circumscribed encapsulated mass consisting of tan/white to yellow firm tissue. It may be possible to identify an associated nerve.

Neurofibroma is a circumscribed mass with a thin capsule consisting of soft tan/white tissue. The nerve is incorporated into the lesion and may not be separately identified. In patients with neurofibromatosis, the lesions may be plexiform (multiple lesions along a nerve—"bag of worms").

Malignant peripheral nerve sheath tumor is often infiltrative and hemorrhage and necrosis may be present. These tumors sometimes arise from a nerve that may be identifiable as it enters one side of the tumor. Tumors arising in patients with neurofibromatosis may be plexiform, taking the form of multiple finger-like projections of tumor in the surrounding tissue: the "bag of worms" appearance.

Leiomyosarcomas. These tumors are often found in association with the smooth muscle from which they arise (e.g., a large vein or the myometrium). They often have a whorled appearance.

Angiosarcoma. The tumor may subtly infiltrate the tissue, producing a grossly indistinct mass. Extensively involved areas are often very hemorrhagic.

Microscopic sections

Tumor

The general rule of thumb is one cassette per cm of greatest dimension. Document all areas with a different appearance, edges (e.g., capsule, infiltration), and involvement of any adjacent structures or organs.

Margins

Document all close margins with at least one cassette. If the tumor is very close to a margin (i.e., within 2 cm), multiple sections may be submitted. Take only perpendicular margins. If a margin is more than 5 cm from the tumor, and the tumor is not an angiosarcoma or an epithelioid sarcoma, the margin need not be submitted.

Margins should be 1 to 2 cm or a fascial plane for sarcomas.

Other structures

Document any other anatomic structures present. Document any prior biopsy scars/sites.

Pathologic diagnostic/prognostic features sign-out checklist for soft tissue tumors

Type of specimen

Needle core biopsy, incisional biopsy, excisional biopsy, wide excision, compartmentectomy, radical excision, amputation.

Histologic type*

Liposarcoma, rhabdomyosarcoma, leiomyosarcoma, malignant peripheral nerve sheath tumor, numerous other types. If the tumor type is unknown, the term "unclassified sarcoma" with a qualifier such as pleomorphic, spindle cell, myxoid, or round cell, is useful. The WHO classification system is suggested.

Histologic grade*

Some tumors are by definition high grade or low grade and some cannot be graded. Other types can be divided into grades and this provides prognostic information (see Table 32-3). This system is increasingly preferred by most professional groups.

Mitoses

Documented as number of mitoses per 10 HPF (40×) in the most mitotically active area of the tumor. Count at least 50 HPF. If specific grading systems are used (see Table 32-3), the mitotic count should be adjusted for the size of the HPF.

Necrosis

Present or absent and extent.

Tumor size*

Measure size in three dimensions; 5 cm is used for AJCC classification and staging.

Tumor margin characteristics

Circumscribed, focally infiltrative, diffusely infiltrative.

Site and depth*

Anatomic location and involvement of anatomic structures.

Superficial (tumor does not involve the superficial fascia).

Deep (all intraperitoneal visceral lesions, retroperitoneal lesions, intrathoracic lesions). The majority of head and neck lesions are considered deep.

Tumor is deep to, or involves, the superficial fascia.

Specify location of the tumor.

Nodal status*

Rarely involved. Most common in alveolar rhabdomyosarcomas, angiosarcomas, epithelioid sarcomas, and synovial sarcomas.

Vascular invasion
Optional—may be prognostic.

Invasion
Invasion of adjacent nerve, blood vessels, lymphatics, or bone.

Margins*
The distance to each margin should be specified. Margins less than 2 cm should be specified as to location and distance. In re-excision specimens, the distance of scarring or granulation tissue from margins should also be measured. Margins bounded by a fascial plane or periosteum should be specified as a smaller distance may be adequate.

Preexisting lesion*
If the tumor is a nerve sheath neoplasm, state whether there is evidence of a preexisting benign lesion

Special studies*
Immunohistochemistry, EM, cytogenetics, etc., when appropriate.

Inflammatory response
Optional (no known relevance)—present or absent, extent, type.

Response to therapy
If patient has received prior treatment: extent of tumor necrosis, presence of viable tumor.

Note: This list incorporates recommendations from the ADASP (see www.panix.com/~adasp/). Asterisked elements are considered to be required.

The AJCC classification system is provided in Table 32-2.

Pathologic diagnostic/prognostic features sign-out checklist for pediatric rhabdomyosarcoma and related neoplasms

Specimen type*
Excision (local, wide, or radical), compartmentectomy, amputation (type, neural, vascular, soft tissue margins), other (e.g., piecemeal, needle core biopsy, incisional biopsy).
Give distance in cm to the closest margin.

Tumor depth*
Dermal, subcutaneous, subfascial, intramuscular, intra-abdominal, retroperitoneal.

Tumor size*
Greatest dimension (additional dimensions optional).

Laterality*
Right, left.

Tumor site*
Bladder/prostate, cranial, extremity, genitourinary, head and neck (excluding parameningeal), orbit, parameningeal, other.

Histologic type*
Embryonal (botryoid, spindle cell, or not otherwise specified), alveolar (solid or not otherwise specified), mixed (give percentage of each type), undifferentiated.

Anaplasia*
Absent, focal, diffuse, indeterminate.
May be associated with any histologic type.
Defined as large, lobate hyperchromatic nuclei (at least three times the size of neighboring nuclei) and atypical (obvious, multipolar) mitotic figures.

Focal anaplasia (group I): A single or a few cells scattered amongst non-anaplastic cells.
Diffuse anaplasia (group II): Clusters or sheets of anaplastic cells present.

Mitotic rate
Give number of mitoses per 10 HPF using a 40× objective in the most proliferative area.

Necrosis
Absent, present (extent in %).

Regional lymph nodes*
Cannot be assessed, negative, metastases present (specify number of nodes examined and number with metastases).

Distant metastases*
Cannot be assessed, present (specify sites, if known).

Margins*
Cannot be assessed, uninvolved, distance from closest margin, involved margin (specify).

Venous/lymphatic (large/small) vessel invasion
Absent, present.

This checklist incorporates information from the CAP Cancer Committee protocols for reporting on cancer specimens (see www.cap.org/). The asterisked elements are considered to be scientifically validated or regularly used data elements that must be present in reports of cancer-directed surgical resection specimens from ACS CoC-approved cancer programs. The specific details of reporting the elements may vary among institutions.

The Intergroup Rhabdomyosarcoma Study Post-Surgical Clinical Group System is given in Box 32-1.

Table 32-2 AJCC (6th edition) classification of soft tissue sarcomas

Tumor	TX	Primary tumor cannot be assessed
	T0	No evidence of primary tumor
	T1	Tumor ≤5 cm in greatest dimension
	T1a	Superficial tumor
	T1b	Deep tumor
	T2	Tumor >5 cm in greatest dimension
	T2a	Superficial tumor
	T2b	Deep tumor
	Superficial: lack of any involvement of the superficial investing muscular fascia in extremity or trunk lesions	
	Deep: the tumor is located exclusively beneath the superficial fascia, or superficial to the fascia with invasion of or through the fascia, or superficial yet beneath the fascia	
	Intraperitoneal visceral tumors, pelvic tumors, retroperitoneal tumors, intrathoracic (mediastinal) tumors, and the majority of head and neck tumors are classified as deep	
Regional lymph nodes	NX	Regional lymph nodes cannot be assessed
	N0	No regional lymph node metastasis
	N1	Regional lymph node metastasis
	Note: Patients whose nodal status is not determined to be positive for tumor, either clinically or pathologically, should be designated as N0	
Metastases	MX	Distant metastasis cannot be assessed
	M0	No distant metastasis
	M1	Distant metastasis

Note: This classification system does not apply to angiosarcoma, Kaposi's sarcoma, dermatofibrosarcoma protuberans, inflammatory myofibroblastic tumor, fibromatosis (desmoid tumor), mesothelioma, or sarcomas arising in tissues apart from soft tissue (e.g., parenchymal organs, dura mater, brain, or hollow viscera). It does include gastrointestinal stromal tumor and Ewing's sarcoma/primitive neuroectodermal tumor.
There is an alternative staging system for rhabdomyosarcoma of children and young adults.[2]

Box 32-1   The Intergroup Rhabdomyosarcoma Study (IRS) post-surgical clinical grouping system

If applicable, the appropriate stage group may be assigned by the pathologist.

Group I

A Localized tumor, confined to site of origin, completely resected

B Localized tumor, infiltrating beyond site of origin, completely resected

Group II

A Localized tumor, gross total resection, but with microscopic residual disease

B Locally extensive tumor (spread to regional lymph nodes), completely resected

C Locally extensive tumor (spread to regional lymph nodes), gross total resection, but with microscopic residual disease

Group III

A Localized or locally extensive tumor, gross residual disease after biopsy only

B Localized or locally extensive tumor, gross residual disease after major resection (>50% debulking)

Group IV

Any size primary tumor, with or without regional lymph node involvement, with distant metastases, without respect to surgical approach to primary tumor

Grading of soft tissue sarcomas

The Federation Nationale des Centres de Lutte Contre le Cancer (FNCLCC) grading system

See Tables 32-3 to 32-5. The three scores from Table 32-3 are added together to determine the histologic grade as shown in Table 32-4.

See also Weiss and Goldblum.[6]

The following tumors should not be graded:

- Treated tumors
- Benign lesions
- Bone sarcomas
- Visceral sarcomas (uterine and gastrointestinal sarcomas—grading is currently under investigation)
- Pediatric sarcomas
- Dermatofibrosarcoma protuberans, atypical fibroxanthoma
- Fine needle or core biopsies (sampling error is likely to be high).

However, recurrent tumors should be graded.

Grading of breast angiosarcoma

Breast angiosarcomas in younger women are usually primary (and high grade); in older women they are usually related to prior treatment for breast carcinoma (radiation therapy or, less often, therapy related edema). See Table 32-6.

Table 32-3 The Federation Nationale des Centres de Lutte Contre le Cancer (FNCLCC) grading system for soft-tissue sarcomas of adults (updated version)

Tumor differentiation[a]

Score 1	Sarcomas closely resembling normal, adult, mesenchymal tissue (e.g., well-differentiated liposarcoma)
Score 2	Sarcomas for which the histologic typing is certain (e.g., alveolar soft part sarcoma)
Score 3	Sarcomas of uncertain histologic type, including embryonal and undifferentiated sarcomas, synovial sarcomas, extraskeletal osteosarcomas, Ewing's/PNET, rhabdoid tumors, undifferentiated sarcomas

Mitotic count[b]

Score 1	0–9 mitoses per 10 HPF
Score 2	10–19 mitoses per 10 HPF
Score 3	20 or more mitoses per 10 HPF

Tumor necrosis[c]

Score 0	No tumor necrosis on any examined slides
Score 1	≤50% tumor necrosis over all the examined tumor surface
Score 2	>50% tumor necrosis over all the examined tumor surface

[a] See Table 32-5.
[b] *Mitotic count:* The count is made in the most mitotic areas in 10 successive fields (a high-power field ×400 measured 0.174 mm^2). This count is taken to establish the score. Ulcerated, necrotic, and hypocellular areas should not be counted. Only definitive mitotic figures (not pyknosis or apoptotic cells) should be counted.
[c] *Tumor necrosis:* The necrosis should appear spontaneous and not related to prior surgery or ulceration. Areas of hyalinization or hemorrhage are not scored.

Table 32-4 Histologic grade—FNLCC system

SCORE	GRADE
Total score = 2 or 3	I
Total score = 4 or 5	II
Total score = 6, 7, or 8	III

■ ABDOMINAL FAT PAD BIOPSY FOR THE DIAGNOSIS OF AMYLOIDOSIS

There are several methods of sampling tissues to establish the diagnosis of systemic amyloidosis. Rectal biopsies are reported to be the most sensitive (97%), followed by fine needle aspiration of the abdominal fat pad (75%), oral biopsy (64%), and biopsy of the abdominal fat pad (50%). These latter biopsies can be either excisional or core biopsies.

The tissue can be fixed in formalin and stained with Congo red. Both false positive and false negative results have been reported. If there is sufficient tissue, some can be saved for EM, which may be helpful in confirming a diagnosis. Immunohistochemical studies can be used to identify subtypes of amyloid.

The abdominal fat pad biopsy technique is not helpful in the evaluation of dialysis patients with β$_2$-microglobulin amyloidosis as this type of amyloid is preferentially found near joints.

Table 32-5 Tumor differentiation score—FNCLCC system[3-5]

HISTOLOGIC TYPE	SCORE
Liposarcoma	
Well differentiated	1 (always grade I)
Myxoid	2
Round cell	3
Pleomorphic	3 (always grade III)
Dedifferentiated	3
Fibrosarcoma	
Well differentiated	1
Conventional	2
Poorly differentiated	3
Malignant peripheral nerve sheath tumor	
Well differentiated	1
Conventional	2
Poorly differentiated	3
Epithelioid	3
Malignant triton tumor	3
Leiomyosarcoma	
Well differentiated	1
Conventional	2
Poorly differentiated/pleomorphic/epithelioid	3
Embryonal/alveolar/pleomorphic rhabdomyosarcoma	3 (always grade III except spindle cell and botryoid)
Chondrosarcoma	
Well differentiated	1
Myxoid	2
Mesenchymal	3 (always grade III)
Extraskeletal osteosarcoma	3 (always grade III)
Angiosarcoma	(always grade III, except for breast)
Conventional	2
Poorly differentiated/epithelioid	3
Hemangiopericytoma	
Well differentiated malignant	2
Conventional malignant	3
Malignant fibrous histiocytoma	
Myxoid	2
Typical storiform/pleomorphic	2
Giant-cell and inflammatory	3
Ewing's sarcoma/PNET	3 (always grade III)
Alveolar soft part sarcoma	3
Epithelioid sarcoma	3
Malignant rhabdoid tumor	3
Clear cell sarcoma	3
Synovial sarcoma, biphasic or monophasic	3
Undifferentiated sarcoma	3

Table 32-6 Breast angiosarcoma—grade

	LOW	INTERMEDIATE	HIGH
Histologic features			
Endothelial tufting	Minimal	Present	Prominent
Papillary formations	Absent	Focal	Present
Solid and spindle cell foci	Absent	Absent or minimal	Present
Mitoses	Rare or absent	Present in papillary areas	Numerous, even in low-grade areas
Blood lakes	Absent	Absent	Present
Necrosis	Absent	Absent	Present
Clinical features			
Percentage of patients	40%	19%	41%
Median age	43	34	29
5- and 10-year survival	76%	70%	15%
Median DFS	15 years	12 years	15 months

Modified from reference 7

REFERENCES

1. Montgomery E, Buras R. Incidental liposarcomas identified during hernia repair operations. J Surg Oncol 71:50-53, 1999.
2. Qualman SJ, et al. Protocol for the examination of specimens from patients (children and young adults) with rhabdomyosarcoma. Arch Pathol Lab Med 127:1290-1297, 2003.
3. Trojani M, Contesso G, Coindre J-M, et al. Soft-tissue sarcomas of adults: study of pathological prognostic variables and definition of a histopathological grading system. Int J Cancer 33:37-42, 1984.
4. Guillou L, Coindre JM, Bonichon F, et al. A comparative study of the NCI and FNCLCC grading systems in a population of 410 adult patients with soft tissue sarcoma. J Clin Oncol 15:350-362, 1997.
5. Guillou L, Coindre J-M. How should we grade soft tissue sarcomas and what are the limitations? Pathology Case Reviews 3:105-110, 1998.
6. Weiss SW, Goldblum JR. In: Enzinger and Weiss's Soft Tissue Tumors, 4th edn Mosby, Philadelphia. Chapter 1.
7. Rosen PP. Rosen's Breast Pathology, 2nd edn Lippincott Williams, New York.

Thymus

33

The thymus may be removed because of disease (both benign and malignant tumors), for the treatment of myasthenia gravis, or rarely incidentally during thoracic surgery (e.g., open heart surgery). If the specimen is of an anterior mediastinal mass, one must consider lymphoma and teratoma as well as thymoma.

Relevant clinical history (in addition to age and gender)

See Table 33-1.

Table 33-1 Relevant clinical history	
HISTORY RELEVANT TO ALL SPECIMENS	HISTORY RELEVANT TO THYMUS SPECIMENS
Organ/tissue resected or biopsied	Myasthenia gravis
Purpose of the procedure	Findings at surgery (infiltration of adjacent structures)
Gross appearance of the organ/tissue/lesion sampled	
Any unusual features of the clinical presentation	
Any unusual features of the gross appearance	
Prior surgery/biopsies—results	
Prior malignancy	
Prior treatment (radiation therapy, chemotherapy, drug use that can change the histologic appearance of tissues)	
Compromised immune system	

Processing the specimen

1. Record outer dimensions and weight of the specimen (normal weight 15 to 30 g).

   Examine the outer portion of the specimen looking for adherent structures such as pleura or pericardium. Capsular and soft tissue invasion is one of the criteria distinguishing benign from malignant neoplasms: these areas should be well sampled.

   Ink the outer surface if the specimen is intact.

2. Serially section the specimen. Describe any lesions including size, color, external appearance (lobulated or smooth), relationship to capsule and surrounding structures, edges (encapsulated, infiltrating), fibrous bands, calcification, necrosis or hemorrhage, and relationship to uninvolved thymus.

   Describe uninvolved thymus including color, consistency (cystic, nodular, gritty, uniform), and relative proportions of fat and thymic parenchyma.

3. Carefully look for lymph nodes in any attached soft tissue.
4. If a lymphoma is suspected, tissue is saved in B5 and submitted for snap freezing and possibly flow cytometry. The remainder of the specimen can be fixed in formalin.

Special studies

Suspected lymphoma

Save tissue for hematopathologic work-up (see above).

Thymic carcinomas versus carcinomas originating from other sites

The epithelial cells of most thymic carcinomas (but not thymomas or invasive thymomas) are immunoreactive for CD5, whereas carcinomas from other sites are CD5 negative.

Thymomas and invasive thymomas versus other tumors

Thymomas and invasive thymomas (but not thymic carcinomas or non-thymic neoplasms) retain a complement of immature cortical thymocytes. These cells can be detected by immunohistochemistry for CD99 (=HBA-17 or O13 or MIC-2), TdT, or CD19.

Gross differential diagnosis

Normal thymus. The thymus is usually atrophic in adults. Tan lobules of thymic parenchyma are separated by fibrous septa and abundant adipose tissue. Hassall's corpuscles may be prominent and must be distinguished from metastatic squamous cell carcinoma in a lymph node.

Myasthenia gravis. Thymectomy is performed as a treatment for myasthenia gravis. The thymus may be normal in size or slightly enlarged but has a grossly normal appearance.

Thymomas are solid, yellow/gray, and divided into lobules by fibrous septa. Most are surrounded by a distinct capsule. Invasion into adjacent soft tissue is an important prognostic factor. Cystic degeneration is common.

Thymic carcinomas may be hard and white with areas of necrosis and hemorrhage. The broad fibrous septa characteristic of thymomas are absent. Invasion into adjacent soft tissue is usually grossly evident.

Germ cell tumors. Any type of germ cell tumor can occur in the anterior mediastinum. The gross appearance is similar to that seen in tumors arising in the testes.

Lymphomas. Hodgkin's and non-Hodgkin's lymphomas can occur at this site. They usually present as lobulated fleshy masses.

Microscopic sections

Lesions
Four to six cassettes (depending on the size of the specimen) including relationship to capsule, remainder of thymus.

Margins
If the specimen is intact and there is a focal lesion, submit sections of the margin.

Thymus
Submit two cassettes of uninvolved thymic parenchyma.

Other structures
Submit representative sections of lymph nodes, pleura, and pericardium if present.

Sample dictation

Received fresh, labeled with the patient's name and unit number and "mediastinal mass," is a 7.5 × 4 × 4 cm fragment of tissue composed of a mass with a smoothly lobulated surface on one side and a 5 × 3 cm portion of glistening smooth pericardium on the opposite side. The mass has two major lobes separated by a fibrous septum. The mass is pink and gelatinous with fine trabeculae throughout. There are small cystic areas filled with pink fluid (largest 0.4 cm). There are small areas of necrosis. The mass is encapsulated except for a 1 × 1 cm area where it appears to invade into the pericardium and is present at the inked margin. Tissue is taken for snap freezing, cytogenetics, and EM. The majority of the lesion is fixed in B5 and quick fixed in formalin.

Cassettes #1 and 2: B5-fixed tumor with adjacent pericardium, 2 frags, RSS.
Cassettes #3 and 4: B5-fixed tumor with areas of necrosis and cysts, 3 frags, RSS.
Cassettes #5 and 6: Formalin-fixed tumor and capsule, 2 frags, RSS.

Pathologic diagnostic/prognostic features sign-out checklist for thymic lesions

Specimen type*
Cervical thymectomy, thoracotomy, video-assisted thoracotomy.

Specimen size
Greatest dimension (additional dimensions).

Tumor site*
Thymus, anterior mediastinum, middle mediastinum, posterior mediastinum.

Tumor size*
Greatest dimension (optional: additional dimensions).
Tumors over 15 cm have a worse prognosis.

Histologic type*
Thymoma, thymic carcinoma (several classification schemes are used)

Extent of invasion*
Grossly and microscopically encapsulated.
Microscopic capsular invasion.
Macroscopic capsular invasion.
Macroscopic invasion into adjacent adipose tissue and/or pleura.
Macroscopic invasion into adjacent structures of mediastinum including pericardium, great vessels and lung.
Hematogenous or lymphatic dissemination.

Regional lymph node metastasis*
Absent, present (number of nodes involved, number of nodes examined).

Distant metastasis*
Absent, present (specify site if known).

Margins*
Uninvolved, distance from closest margin, involved-specify margin(s).

Invasion of pulmonary parenchyma*
Absent, present.

Pleural invasion*
Absent, present.

Vascular (small/large vessel) invasion
Absent, present.

This checklist incorporates information from the CAP Cancer Committee protocols for reporting on cancer specimens (see www.cap.org/). The asterisked elements are considered to be scientifically validated or regularly used data elements that must be present in reports of cancer-directed surgical resection specimens from ACS CoC-approved cancer programs. The specific details of reporting the elements may vary among institutions.

Staging systems are provided in Tables 32-2, 32-3 and 32-4.

Table 33-2 Masaoka's clinical stage as modified by Koga et al[1,2]

STAGE	EXTENT
I	Grossly and microscopically completely encapsulated (including microscopic invasion into the capsule)
IIa	Microscopic transcapsular invasion
IIb	Macroscopic capsular invasion into thymic or surrounding fat, or grossly adherent but not breaking through mediastinal pleura or pericardium
III	Macroscopic invasion into neighboring organs (e.g., pericardium, great vessels, or lung)
IVa	Pleural or pericardial dissemination
IVb	Lymphogenous or hematogenous metastasis

Table 33-3 Yamakawa–Masaoka TNM classification and staging[3]

T	T1	Macroscopically completely encapsulated and microscopically no capsular invasion
	T2	Macroscopically adhesion or invasion into surrounding fatty tissue or mediastinal pleura, or microscopic invasion into capsule
	T3	Invasion into neighboring organs, such as pericardium, great vessels, and lung
	T4	Pleural or pericardial dissemination
N	N0	No lymph node metastasis
	N1	Metastasis to anterior mediastinal lymph nodes
	N2	Metastasis to intrathoracic lymph nodes except anterior mediastinal lymph nodes
	N3	Metastasis to extrathoracic lymph nodes
M	M0	No hematogenous metastasis
	M1	Hematogenous metastasis

Table 33-4 Proposed pathologic TNM and staging of thymic epithelial tumor (thymomas and thymic carcinomas)[4]

pT	pT1	Completely encapsulated tumor
	pT2	Tumor breaking through capsule, invading thymus or fatty tissue (may be adherent to mediastinal pleura but not invading adjacent organs)
	pT3	Tumor breaking through the mediastinal pleura or pericardium, or invading neighboring organs, such as great vessels or lung
	pT4	Tumor with pleural or pericardial implantation
pN	pN0	No lymph node metastasis
	pN1	Metastasis in anterior mediastinal lymph nodes
	pN2	Metastasis in intrathoracic lymph nodes excluding anterior mediastinal lymph nodes
	pN3	Metastasis in extrathoracic lymph nodes
pM	M0	No distant organ metastasis
	M1	With distant organ metastasis

REFERENCES

1. Masaoka A, Monden Y, Nakahara K, Tanioka T. Follow-up study of thymomas with special reference to their clinical stages. Cancer 48:2485-2495, 1981.
2. Koga K, Matsuno Y, Noguchi M, et al. A review of 79 thymomas: modification of staging system and reappraisal of conventional division into invasive and non-invasive thymoma. Pathol Int 44:359-367, 1994.
3. Yamakawa Y, Masaoka A, Hashimoto T, et al. A tentative tumor-node-metastasis classification of thymoma. Cancer 68:1984-1987, 1991.
4. Tsuchiya R, Koga K, Matsuno Y, Mukai K, Shimosato Y. Thymic carcinoma: proposal for pathological TNM and staging. Pathol Int 44:505-512, 1994.

Thyroid and parathyroid glands

34

■ THYROID

Thyroidectomies are usually performed to remove solitary nodules, either benign or malignant, or multinodular goiters, and rarely for the treatment of Graves' disease. Most thyroidectomies are total but some may be unilateral. Many nodules will have been evaluated prior to excision by fine needle aspiration.

Relevant clinical history (in addition to age and gender)

See Table 34-1.

Table 34-1 Relevant clinical history	
HISTORY RELEVANT TO ALL SPECIMENS	HISTORY RELEVANT TO THYROID SPECIMENS
Organ/tissue resected or biopsied	Thyroid function test results
Purpose of the procedure	Autoantibodies
Gross appearance of the organ/tissue/lesion sampled	History of radiation exposure
Any unusual features of the clinical presentation	Results of prior FNA
Any unusual features of the gross appearance	Single or multiple nodules
Prior surgery/biopsies—results	Family history of thyroid disease or MEN syndromes
Prior malignancy	
Prior treatment (radiation therapy, chemotherapy, drug use that can change the histologic appearance of tissues)	Drug use (amiodarone or minocycline)
Compromised immune system	

Processing the specimen

1. Weigh and record the dimensions of the right and left lobes and isthmus. Glands can usually be easily oriented because the posterior surface is concave, the lobes taper superiorly, and the isthmus is inferior. The posterior surface should be examined carefully for parathyroid glands (brown or yellow/brown ovoid bodies, 2 to 3 mm in size). Save these in a separate cassette if found.
2. Ink the entire outer surface. Serially section through the entire gland. Describe each lesion including size, color, consistency (papillary, rubbery, firm, gelatinous, or friable), cysts, necrosis or hemorrhage, location (upper, lower, right, left), encapsulation or infiltration, and relationship to capsule (intact or with invasion of capsule).

- **Normal**: beefy red/brown.
- **Pale**: lymphocytic thyroiditis or Hashimoto's thyroiditis.
- **Amber colored with a plastic-like consistency**: amiodarone thyroid disease.
- **Black**: side effect of minocycline therapy.

Whenever possible, nodules that have been previously sampled by FNA should be identified and specifically designated in the cassette code to facilitate correlation between the cytologic and histologic findings.

3. Describe the remainder of the parenchyma including color (dark red/brown), consistency (fibrotic, hard, friable, soft), contour (lobulated, multinodular, uniform), and calcifications.

Evaluate any adjacent soft tissue for composition (adipose tissue, skeletal muscle, nerves, parathyroid glands), presence of lymph nodes, or extension of tumor into soft tissue.

Gross differential diagnosis (Fig. 34-1)

Adenoma. This is the most common thyroid neoplasm. An adenoma is usually a solitary, completely encapsulated, pale tan to gray, soft gelatinous or fleshy mass, rarely larger than 3 cm. There may be areas of hemorrhage, fibrosis, or calcification. The capsule is usually thin.

Papillary carcinoma. This is the most common type of thyroid malignancy. The tumor is usually white/tan and may have a granular or finely nodular texture due to the papillae. Tumors are often firm because of fibrosis but may be soft. Calcification is common. The tumor may have a poorly developed capsule but rarely has a complete capsule, which may be thick or thin. The tumor may grossly invade the capsule. Cysts may be present. The size ranges from microscopic to huge (average 2 to 3 cm), and 20% to 60% are multicentric. An occult papillary carcinoma may appear as a tiny pale gray depressed scar.

Follicular carcinomas are less common than papillary carcinomas or adenomas: fewer than 20% of follicular lesions are carcinomas. The tumor may be a small encapsulated mass that can only be distinguished from adenoma by histologic examination (i.e., microscopic evidence of capsular or vascular invasion). Larger tumors may have areas of hemorrhage and necrosis and have infiltrative borders. The capsule may be thick. These tumors are usually solitary.

Medullary carcinoma. These tumors are less common than papillary and follicular carcinomas. The tumors are often multicentric and non-encapsulated but are well circumscribed, with a soft and fleshy or firm and gritty consistency. The color ranges from gray/white to yellow/brown. Areas of necrosis and hemorrhage may be present. The size ranges from less than 1 cm to replacement of the entire thyroid. Small carcinomas may be located at the junction of the middle and upper third of the lobe, in the area where the most C cells are seen. Approximately 25% are associated with germline mutations. An intraoperative diagnosis may be important so that the gland can be evaluated for multiple tumors and the parathyroid glands can be evaluated.

Patients at risk for familial medullary carcinoma may undergo a prophylactic thyroidectomy. Serial sections of each lobe from superior to inferior with separate sections of the isthmus should be taken. C cells are located within the middle and upper thirds of the lateral lobes. Immunoperoxidase studies for calcitonin and CEA may be helpful to evaluate C-cell hyperplasia.

Anaplastic carcinoma. This is a very rare tumor. It is often pale gray and firm to hard in consistency. Necrosis and hemorrhage are often present. Its tendency to invade locally and widely means that a recognizable thyroid may not be present. Skeletal muscle may be resected with infiltrating tumor.

Nodular hyperplasia (multinodular goiter). The gland is enlarged and distorted (one lobe is usually larger than the other). There is a diffuse heterogeneous nodularity and some of the nodules may appear to be encapsulated. There may be random irregular scarring, hemorrhage, calcifications, and cysts. It is often difficult to distinguish a dominant nodule in hyperplasia

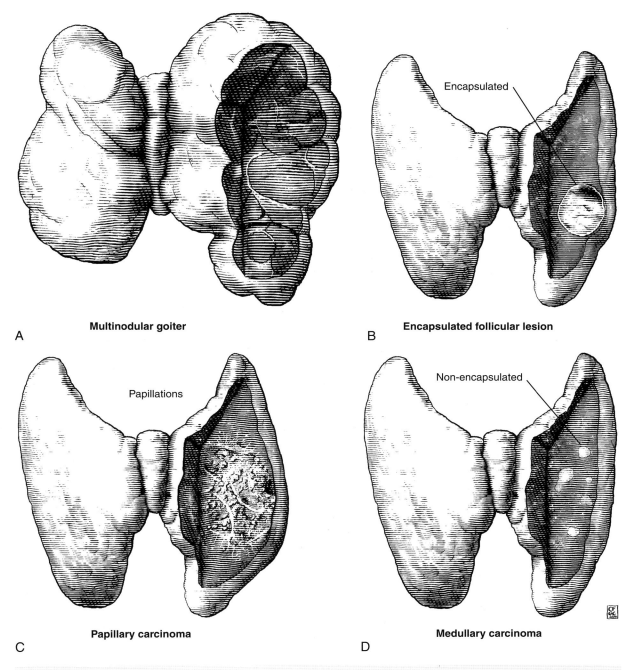

A   **Multinodular goiter**

B   **Encapsulated follicular lesion**

Encapsulated

C   **Papillary carcinoma**

Papillations

D   **Medullary carcinoma**

Non-encapsulated

Figure 34-1 Thyroid lesions.

from an adenoma. Therefore, the surrounding parenchyma must be carefully evaluated grossly (for multiple nodules) and microscopically.

Graves' disease. The gland is diffusely enlarged but with a very homogeneous texture without nodularity. It is usually a beefy red color.

Lesions

Follicular lesions:
It is very important to submit the entire tumor capsule, as invasion of the capsule distinguishes carcinomas from adenomas.

Papillary carcinoma:
At least one section per 1 cm including relationship to any perithyroidal tissue.

Nodular hyperplasia:
Submit one representative section of each nodule, up to five nodules.

Thyroid

Two representative uninvolved sections from each lobe. Submit all areas that show discoloration or increased consistency.

Lymph node/parathyroid

Submit representative sections.

Sample dictation

Received fresh, labeled with the patient's name, unit number, and "thyroid," is a 75-g total thyroidectomy specimen consisting of right lobe (6 × 3.5 × 3 cm), left lobe (8 × 5 × 4 cm), and isthmus (2 × 2 × 1 cm). A 4 × 3 × 3 cm ovoid white/tan firm tumor mass with a finely granular appearance is present in the left lobe. The central portion is densely white and firm and depressed. The tumor is poorly circumscribed and grossly invades into the adjacent capsule but is 0.1 cm from the inked resection margin. The remainder of the parenchyma is red/brown and homogeneous without other lesions noted. There is a small (0.5 × 0.5 × 0.3 cm) soft tan/brown ovoid nodule adherent to the capsule of the right lobe.

Cassettes #1 and 2: Tumor and capsular margin, 2 frags, ESS.
Cassettes #3–7: Remainder of tumor, 7 frags, ESS.
Cassettes #8 and 9: Left lobe, away from tumor, 2 frags, RSS.
Cassette #10: Isthmus, 1 frag, RSS.
Cassettes #11 and 12: Representative section of right lobe, 2 frags, RSS.
Cassette #13: Small brown nodule, 2 frags, ESS.

Pathologic diagnostic/prognostic features sign-out checklist for thyroid tumors

Specimen type*
Nodulectomy, lobectomy, subtotal thyroidectomy (right or left lobe), total thyroidectomy.

Tumor site*
Right lobe, left lobe, isthmus.

Tumor focality*
Unifocal, multifocal.

Tumor size*
Largest nodule: greatest dimension (additional dimensions optional).

Histologic type*
Papillary carcinoma: classical, follicular variant, solid variant, macrofollicular variant, microcarcinoma (1 cm or less), encapsulated variant, diffuse sclerosing, tall cell variant, others.
Follicular and Hürthle cell carcinoma: minimally invasive, widely invasive, medullary.
Anaplastic (undifferentiated) carcinoma: presence or absence of residual well-differentiated component, poorly differentiated carcinoma: insular, trabecular, solid, NOS, other rare types.
The WHO classification is recommended.

Extent of invasion*
Tumors except for anaplastic carcinoma:
Tumor size ≤2 cm, limited to thyroid (T1), tumor >2 cm but ≤4 cm, limited to the thyroid (T2), tumor >4 cm, limited to the thyroid, or with minimal extrathyroidal extension (e.g., extension to sternothyroid muscle or perithyroid soft tissues) (T3), extension beyond the thyroid capsule to invade subcutaneous soft tissues, larynx, trachea, esophagus, or recurrent laryngeal nerve (T4a), invasion of perivertebral fascia or encases carotid artery or mediastinal vessels.
Anaplastic carcinoma:
Tumor within the thyroid and surgically resectable (T4a), tumor outside of the thyroid and not resectable (T4b).

Regional lymph nodes*
Absent (N0), nodal metastases to level IV (N1a), nodal metastases to cervical or superior mediastinal lymph nodes (ipsilateral or contralateral) (N1b).
Number of nodes examined, number with metastases, size of largest metastasis.
Extranodal invasion: present or absent.

Distant metastasis*
Absent (M0), present (M1), specify site, if known.

Margins*
Uninvolved (distance of carcinoma from nearest margin optional), involved, site of involvement.

Venous/lymphatic (large/small vessel) invasion
Absent, present, indeterminate.
Extent (focal versus multiple foci).

Grade
Not universally used but thought by some to be useful.[1] The following is a grouping of carcinomas according to their clinical behavior:
Low-grade group:
Most papillary carcinomas, minimally invasive follicular carcinoma.
Intermediate-grade group:
Widely invasive follicular carcinoma, tall cell, columnar cell, and diffuse sclerosing papillary carcinoma variants, poorly differentiated carcinoma, medullary carcinoma.
High-grade group:
Anaplastic carcinoma.

Capsular invasion
Invasion of the tumor capsule: absent, minimally present, extensively present (most important for follicular and Hürthle cell carcinomas) (see Box 34-2 and Fig. 34-2).

Blood vessel invasion
Present or absent. Blood vessels should be the size of veins and located outside the tumor but within or immediately outside the capsule. Tumor cells are attached to the vessel wall and protrude into the lumen and are usually covered by endothelial cells (see Box 34-1).

Extrathyroidal extension
Invasion into adipose tissue or skeletal muscle outside the limits of the thyroid: absent, grossly present, microscopically present ("extrathyroidal extension" is preferred over "invasion through thyroid capsule" to avoid confusion with invasion through the tumor capsule).

Multicentricity
Single versus multiple tumors, approximate number, same or differing morphologies, location, some estimation of bulk (e.g., "each measuring 0.1 cm").

Uninvolved thyroid
Hashimoto's or lymphocytic thyroiditis, nodular hyperplasia.

C-cell hyperplasia (associated with familial cases of medullary carcinoma):
Diffuse: involves both lobes with ≥50 C cells per low-power field
Nodular: extensive, bilateral, multifocal.

Parathyroid glands

Number, location (if possible, indicate intra- versus extrathyroidal, right versus left, upper versus lower), normal versus abnormal (specify).

This checklist incorporates information from the CAP Cancer Committee protocols for reporting on cancer specimens. The asterisked elements are considered to be scientifically validated or regularly used data elements that must be present in reports from ACS CoC-approved cancer programs (although the details of reporting each element may vary). This list also incorporates recommendations from the ADASP (see www.panix.com/~adasp/).

Table 34-2 AJCC (6th edition) classification of thyroid tumors

Tumor	TX	Primary tumor cannot be assessed
	T0	No evidence of primary tumor
	T1	Tumor ≤2 cm limited to the thyroid
	T2	Tumor >2 cm but ≤4 cm, limited to the thyroid
	T3	Tumor >4 cm limited to the thyroid or any tumor with minimal extrathyroidal extension (e.g., extension to sternothyroid muscle or perithyroid soft tissue)
	T4a	Tumor of any size extending beyond the thyroid capsule to invade subcutaneous soft tissues, larynx, trachea, esophagus, or recurrent laryngeal nerve
	T4b	Tumor invades prevertebral fascia or encases carotid artery or mediastinal vessels
	All anaplastic carcinomas are classified as T4	
	T4a	Intrathyroidal anaplastic carcinoma—surgically resectable
	T4b	Extrathyroidal anaplastic carcinoma—surgically unresectable
Regional lymph nodes	NX	Regional lymph nodes cannot be assessed
	N0	No regional lymph node metastasis
	N1	Regional lymph node metastasis
	N1a	Metastasis to level VI (pretracheal, paratracheal, and prelaryngeal/Delphian lymph nodes)
	N1b	Metastasis to unilateral, bilateral, midline, or contralateral cervical or superior mediastinal lymph node(s)
	Note: Regional lymph nodes are central compartment, lateral cervical and upper mediastinal lymph nodes. Paralaryngeal, paratracheal, prelaryngeal (Delphian) nodes adjacent to the thyroid are now included in staging	
Distant metastasis	MX	Distant metastasis cannot be assessed
	M0	No distant metastasis
	M1	Distant metastasis

Box 34-1 Blood vessel invasion

The involved blood vessels must be located within or outside the fibrous capsule (i.e., not within the tumor). The vessels should be of large caliber with an identifiable wall and there should be lining endothelial cells. The intravascular polypoid tumor growth must be covered by endothelium or it must be attached to the wall of the vessel and associated with a thrombus. Clusters of epithelial cells floating in a vascular lumen, unattached to the wall, may be an artifact and should not be considered vascular invasion.

Box 34-2 Criteria for capsular invasion (Fig. 34-2)

A. A tumor bud has invaded beyond the contour of the capsule, but is still covered by a thin new fibrous capsule.

B. A tumor bud has extended through the outer capsular surface.

C. The classic mushroom-shaped bud has completely transgressed the fibrous capsule and grown out into the surrounding thyroid.

D. A satellite nodule with cytoarchitectural and cellular features identical to the tumor cells is present outside of the capsule. The point of capsular rupture is not seen in the sections.

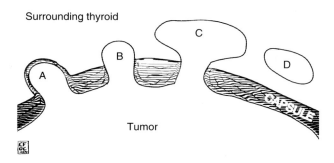

Figure 34-2 Thyroid capsular invasion.

■ PROPHYLACTIC THYROIDECTOMY

Prophylactic thyroidectomy may be performed for patients with a history of familial medullary carcinoma (familial MTC, MEN2, or variants) if a germline mutation in the *RET* proto-oncogene has been detected.

The thyroid should be examined to document the extent of C-cell hyperplasia and to determine whether a small medullary carcinoma is present. Multiple sections from each lobe should be submitted from superior to inferior and should include any gross lesions. The isthmus should be sampled separately. Normal C cells are restricted to a zone within the middle to upper third of the lateral lobes and are normally absent from the extreme upper and lower poles of each lobe and the isthmus.

■ PARATHYROID GLAND

Parathyroidectomy is performed for hyperparathyroidism caused either by adenoma or by hyperplasia (most commonly secondary to chronic renal failure). Malignancies are vanishingly rare. The specimens are usually evaluated intraoperatively (Chapter 6). However, intraoperative PTH assays may replace frozen-section evaluation.

Relevant clinical history (in addition to age and gender)

See Table 34-3.

Processing the specimen

1. Record the dimensions of each specimen and the weights of large intact glands. Describe, including color (brown to brown/yellow) and any lesions (an adenoma may compress normal adjacent parenchyma). It should be evident from the description whether the specimen is the entire gland (smoothly contoured surface) or a biopsy (small irregular fragment of tissue).

Table 34-3 Relevant clinical history

HISTORY RELEVANT TO ALL SPECIMENS	HISTORY RELEVANT TO PARATHYROID SPECIMENS
Organ/tissue resected or biopsied	Primary hyperparathyroidism (elevated serum calcium)—usually due to one adenoma, rarely due to multiple adenomas or primary hyperplasia
Purpose of the procedure	
Gross appearance of the organ/tissue/lesion sampled	
Any unusual features of the clinical presentation	Secondary hyperparathyroidism (decreased serum calcium)—usually due to chronic renal failure: all four glands enlarged
Any unusual features of the gross appearance	
Prior surgery/biopsies—results	Intraoperative PTH assays—if PTH did not decrease, the adenoma may not have been removed
Prior malignancy	
Prior treatment (radiation therapy, chemotherapy, drug use that can change the histologic appearance of tissues)	Personal or family history of MEN syndrome
	Gross appearance of gland at surgery—adherence to adjacent tissue could suggest carcinoma
Compromised immune system	

Average normal weight:
- 30 ± 3.5 mg for men (any gland >50 mg is enlarged)
- 35 ± 5.2 mg for women.
  Normal size:
- 2–7 mm × 2–4 mm × 0.5–2 mm.
2. Submit small specimens in entirety. Larger glands have representative sections submitted in a single cassette.

Gross differential diagnosis

Adenomas (85% of surgical cases). These are almost always solitary lesions (96%) and usually weigh from 300 mg to several grams (size 1 to 3 cm). There is loss of stromal fat and the adjacent normal gland may be compressed. Rarely, a parathyroid gland may be located completely within the thyroid gland.

Hyperplasia (15% of surgical cases, almost all secondary). Hyperplasia usually involves multiple glands but each gland may not be involved to the same degree. Fat may be decreased or absent.

Secondary:

Usually due to renal disease. All four glands are markedly increased in size but may vary in size. Three may be removed and the fourth biopsied.

Primary:

All four glands may be increased in size. However, only one or two glands may be enlarged or all glands may be minimally enlarged. Twenty per cent of patients will have an MEN syndrome (usually MEN 1 or 2A). Primary hyperplasia is very rare.

Carcinoma (rare, 2% of cases). Carcinoma is more common in older adults (fourth to sixth decade). The carcinoma is usually a firm lobulated tan/gray mass that is often adherent to adjacent soft tissue. The tumors are often large (2 to 6 cm; over 40 g). Histologically there may be capsular or vascular invasion, mitoses, and necrosis.

Microscopic sections

Enlarged glands

Representative sections (one cassette). If there is attached soft tissue and a possibility of carcinoma (i.e., potential invasion into soft tissue), more sections should be taken.

Small glands or biopsies

Entire specimen (one cassette).

Sample dictation

The specimen is received fresh, labeled with the patient's name and unit number, in three parts. The first part, labeled "right upper adenoma," consists of a 100-mg ovoid smoothly surfaced gland (2 × 2 × 1 cm) with a homogeneous tan brown parenchyma. A representative portion was used for a frozen section A.

Cassette #1: FSR A, 1 frag, ESS.
Cassette #2: Representative sections, 2 frags, RSS.

The second part, labeled "right lower," consists of an irregular fragment of tan brown soft tissue measuring 0.5 × 0.5 × 0.4 cm which was entirely frozen for FSB.

Cassette #3: FSR B, 1 frag, ESS.

The third part, labeled "left upper," consists of an irregular fragment of tan brown soft tissue measuring 0.6 × 0.3 × 0.2 cm which was entirely frozen for FSC.

Cassette #4: FSR C, 1 frag, ESS.

Pathologic diagnostic/prognostic features sign-out checklist for parathyroid glands

Type of lesion

Adenoma, atypical adenoma, carcinoma, hyperplasia, cysts, parathyromatosis, normal gland, or secondary tumors.

Size and weight

Specify for glands completely excised.

Prognostic factors

For carcinomas, some histologic features may be associated with malignant behavior (see below).

Percentage adipose tissue

Usually 15% to 20% in normal glands; reduced in young individuals, adenomas, and hyperplasia.

Parathyroid adenoma versus atypical adenoma versus carcinoma

Parathyroid carcinomas are very rare, accounting for less than 5% of cases of primary hyperparathyroidism. In the absence of metastasis, a definitive diagnosis of malignancy is difficult to make. Some cases differ minimally from chief cell adenomas, while others are obviously anaplastic. The histologic features in Table 34-4 can be used to help predict malignant behavior.

Table 34-4 Features predicting malignancy in parathyroid adenoma

HISTOLOGIC FEATURE	ADENOMA	ATYPICAL ADENOMA	CARCINOMA
Relationship to surrounding tissue	Confined within capsule	Adherence of tumor to adjacent structures	Invasion through the capsule into adjacent soft tissues or thyroid in approximately one half
Thick fibrous bands	Usually absent	Usually present	Usually present
Mitotic activity	May be present	Present (<5 per 50 HPF or Ki-67 <3%)	Present (>5 per 50 HPF or Ki-67 >6% is more common in carcinomas)
Perineural invasion	Absent	Absent	May be present
Vascular invasion	Absent	Absent	May be present
Necrosis	May be present	May be present	Present in approximately one third
Nuclear atypia	Scattered cells with markedly atypical nuclei may be present	Scattered cells with markedly atypical nuclei may be present	Marked nuclear pleomorphism with macronuclei may be present in approximately half of tumors

REFERENCE

1. Gilliland FD, Owen C, Gilland SS, Key CR. Prognostic factors for thyroid carcinoma. Cancer 79:564-573, 1997.

Index